Ultrasound

Ultrasound

Edited by

Leslie M. Scoutt, MD, FACR, FAIUM, FSRU

Professor of Diagnostic Radiology and Vascular Surgery
Vice Chair of Education
Chief, Ultrasound Section
Medical Director, Non-Invasive Vascular Laboratory
Associate Program Director
Department of Radiology and Biomedical Imaging
Yale University School of Medicine
New Haven, Connecticut

Ulrike M. Hamper, MD, MBA, FACR, FAIUM, FSRU

Professor of Radiology, Urology, and Pathology
Russell H. Morgan Department of Radiology and Radiological Science
Johns Hopkins University School of Medicine
Baltimore, Maryland

Teresita L. Angtuaco, MD, FACR, FAIUM, FSRU

Professor of Radiology, Obstetrics, and Gynecology
Director, Division of Body Imaging
Chief of Ultrasound
Department of Radiology
University of Arkansas for Medical Sciences
Little Rock, Arkansas

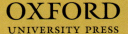

OXFORD
UNIVERSITY PRESS

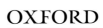

OXFORD
UNIVERSITY PRESS

Oxford University Press is a department of the University of Oxford. It furthers
the University's objective of excellence in research, scholarship, and education
by publishing worldwide. Oxford is a registered trade mark of Oxford University
Press in the UK and certain other countries.

Published in the United States of America by Oxford University Press
198 Madison Avenue, New York, NY 10016, United States of America.

Library of Congress Cataloging-in-Publication Data
Names: Scoutt, Leslie M., editor. | Hamper, Ulrike M., editor. | Angtuaco,
Teresita L., 1949– , editor.
Title: Ultrasound / edited by Leslie M. Scoutt, Ulrike M. Hamper, Teresita L. Angtuaco.
Other titles: Ultrasound (Scoutt)
Description: Oxford ; New York : Oxford University Press, [2017] | Includes
bibliographical references and index.
Identifiers: LCCN 2015042572 | ISBN 9780199988105 (hard cover : alk. paper)
Subjects: | MESH: Ultrasonography—methods—Handbooks.
Classification: LCC RC78.7.U4 | NLM WN 39 | DDC 616.07/543—dc23
LC record available at http://lccn.loc.gov/2015042572

This material is not intended to be, and should not be considered, a substitute for medical or other professional advice. Treatment for the
conditions described in this material is highly dependent on the individual circumstances. And, while this material is designed to offer
accurate information with respect to the subject matter covered and to be current as of the time it was written, research and knowledge
about medical and health issues is constantly evolving and dose schedules for medications are being revised continually, with new side
effects recognized and accounted for regularly. Readers must therefore always check the product information and clinical procedures
with the most up-to-date published product information and data sheets provided by the manufacturers and the most recent codes of
conduct and safety regulation. The publisher and the authors make no representations or warranties to readers, express or implied, as
to the accuracy or completeness of this material. Without limiting the foregoing, the publisher and the authors make no representations
or warranties as to the accuracy or efficacy of the drug dosages mentioned in the material. The authors and the publisher do not accept,
and expressly disclaim, any responsibility for any liability, loss or risk that may be claimed or incurred as a consequence of the use and/or
application of any of the contents of this material.

9 8 7 6 5 4 3 2 1

Printed by Sheridan Books, Inc., United States of America

To our families for their unwavering support and encouragement, to our residents and fellows who inspire us to be better teachers, to all the contributing authors for their hard work and dedication to this project, to our sonographers for their expertise and commitment to patient care, and to our colleagues both at our home institutions and in the medical community who constantly stimulate us through their passion for and commitment to the field of ultrasound.

Leslie M. Scoutt

Ulrike M. Hamper

Teresita L. Angtuaco

Preface

One of the most rewarding aspects of the medical profession is the opportunity, even necessity, for continuing education, and ultrasound is no exception. Ultrasound has been an integral part of the diagnostic workup algorithm for patients over many years and is often used to evaluate the acutely ill patient, to follow chronic illness or response to therapy, and for screening purposes. Readily accessible, without harmful bioeffects and relatively inexpensive, ultrasound has a wide range of clinical applications, ranging from gynecology, obstetrics, urology, and endocrinology to evaluation of vascular, abdominal, and musculoskeletal pathology. As such, ultrasound can be effectively used for diagnosis and screening, to guide recommendations for further imaging, and to direct interventional procedures. Currently, the field of ultrasound is undergoing a renaissance due to rapid evolution and advances in technology such as three-dimensional imaging, elastography, and intravenous ultrasound contrast agents. In addition, the use of ultrasound by clinical subspecialists has also served to stimulate new applications of ultrasound not previously explored by most radiologists, such as imaging of the lung, critical care, and rheumatologic disease.

This case series covers a wide spectrum of clinical applications of ultrasound. A total of 187 cases have been grouped into six sections: Gynecology; First Trimester (Obstetrics); Second and Third Trimester (Obstetrics); Abdomen (gastrointestinal, urology, and retroperitoneal pathology); Small Parts (thyroid, scrotal, and musculoskeletal pathology); and Vascular. Although the book focuses on diagnoses that are commonly addressed by ultrasound and content that should be mastered during residency, more unusual pathology is also included. The cases also vary in terms of difficulty. Cases are presented as unknowns with a short clinical history, and on subsequent pages explanation of the imaging features, differential diagnosis, salient teaching points, and a brief discussion of clinical management are provided. Information is presented in a concise bullet-point format, and correlation with other imaging modalities—including plain films, computed tomography, magnetic resonance, positron emission tomography/computed tomography, and angiography—is provided as appropriate. Although often considered the first line or screening imaging modality of choice, ultrasound should not be practiced in an isolated imaging vacuum. Hence, these correlative images have been included not only to emphasize and clarify the ultrasound findings but also to help the reader understand when additional imaging is helpful. In addition, correlative cases have also been provided in numerous instances to demonstrate normal anatomy for comparison, additional imaging features to illustrate the spectrum of ultrasound findings for the entity under discussion, or related pathology. It is hoped that these additional cases will help the reader to better analyze the important discriminatory imaging and/or clinical features of the entities included in the differential diagnosis. Lastly, pertinent key references are provided at the end of each case for the reader who wishes to learn more about the index case pathology.

As educators, we believe that case review and self-assessment are extremely important in developing the breadth and depth of knowledge required to become a skilled sonologist. We believe this format will be useful to readers at all levels of training and in multiple specialties. The beginner will find the material presented in a concise format that highlights the most important teaching points and can use this book to complement a more detailed reference textbook. The more advanced learner will be able to use the book as a self-assessment module by approaching the cases as unknowns and using the detailed explanations and differential diagnosis provided on the following pages to gauge image interpretation, knowledge base, and critical thinking. More experienced sonologists may find the book helpful as a handbook demonstrating the classic ultrasound features of both common and unusual pathology.

Finally, we thank Andrea Knobloch, who proposed this project to us several years ago and has waited patiently and graciously throughout the many iterations of the case material. She unfailingly and generously provided us with the guidance and resources that we needed to complete this volume. This book would never have happened without the support, encouragement, and unfailing good humor of Andrea and her fantastic team at Oxford University Press.

Leslie M. Scoutt
Ulrike M. Hamper
Teresita L. Angtuaco

Contents

Section V.   Small Parts

Section VI. Vascular

Assistant Editor: Gowthaman Gunabushanam

Contributors

Sindhura Alapati, MD
Resident
Department of Radiology
University of Arkansas for Medical Sciences
Little Rock, Arkansas
Cases 38, 45, 51, 54, and 58

Michael J. Angtuaco, MD
Assistant Professor
Department of Pediatrics
Division of Pediatric Cardiology
University of Arkansas for Medical Sciences
Little Rock, Arkansas
Cases 49 and 50

Melanie Atkins, MD
Attending Radiologist
Fairfax Radiological Consultants, PC
Fairfax, Virginia
Former Instructor of Radiology
Russell H. Morgan Department of Radiology and
    Radiologic Science
Johns Hopkins University, School of Medicine
Baltimore, Maryland
Cases 1, 11, 12, 13, and 15

Claire B. Beaumont, MD
Resident
Department of Radiology
University of Arkansas for Medical Sciences
Little Rock, Arkansas
Cases 24, 26, 44, 59, and 63

Marcus M. Brown, MD
Resident
Department of Radiology
University of Arkansas for Medical Sciences
Little Rock, Arkansas
Cases 25, 37, 57, 62 and 64

Linda C. Chu, MD
Assistant Professor
Russell H. Morgan Department of Radiology and
    Radiologic Science
Johns Hopkins University, School of Medicine
Baltimore, Maryland
Cases 68, 69, 83, 84, 85, and 86

Stephanie Coquia, MD
Assistant Professor
Russell H. Morgan Department of Radiology and
    Radiological Science
Johns Hopkins University, School of Medicine
Baltimore, Maryland
Cases 4, 10, 71, 78, and 86

Nafisa K. Dajani, MD
Associate Professor
Department of Obstetrics and Gynecology
Division of Maternal Fetal Medicine
University of Arkansas for Medical Sciences
Little Rock, Arkansas
Cases 39 and 40

Swati Deshmukh, MD
Resident
Russell H. Morgan Department of Radiology and
    Radiological Science
Johns Hopkins University, School of Medicine
Baltimore, Maryland
Cases 73, 96, 97, 98, and 99

Melissa Durand, MD, MS
Assistant Professor
Department of Radiology and Biomedical Imaging
Yale University School of Medicine
New Haven, Connecticut
Cases 2, 5, 8, 14, and 22

Gowthaman Gunabushanam, MD
Assistant Professor
Department of Radiology and Biomedical Imaging
Yale University School of Medicine
New Haven, Connecticut
Cases 87, 102, 107, 126, 139, 146, 159, 161, 163, 166, 167,
173, 176, and 184

Brian M. Haas, MD
Resident
Department of Diagnostic Radiology
Yale University School of Medicine
New Haven, Connecticut
Cases 32, 80, 107, 116, 118, 128, 145, 162, 167, 174, 177, and 179

Steffen Huber, MD
Assistant Professor
Department of Radiology and Biomedical Imaging
Yale University School of Medicine
New Haven, Connecticut
Cases 148, 157, 165, 170, and 175

Christopher Jones, MD
Assistant Professor
Russell H. Morgan Department of Radiology and Radiological
    Science
Johns Hopkins University, School of Medicine
Baltimore, Maryland
Cases 76, 81, 114, and 135

Jonathan D. Kirsch, MD
Assistant Professor
Department of Radiology and Biomedical Imaging
Yale University School of Medicine
New Haven, Connecticut
Cases 86, 92, 133, 134, 136, 168, 172, and 177

Amanda Lackey, MD
Resident
Department of Radiology
University of Arkansas for Medical Sciences
Little Rock, Arkansas
Cases 28, 29, 41, and 67

Igor Latich, MD
Assistant Professor
Department of Radiology and Biomedical Imaging
Yale University School of Medicine
New Haven, Connecticut
Cases 149, 150, 153, 155, 169, and 185

Mahan Mathur, MD
Assistant Professor
Department of Radiology and Biomedical Imaging
Yale University School of Medicine
New Haven, Connecticut
Cases 72, 95, 111, 118, 123, and 186

Vijayanadh Ojili, MD
Associate Professor
Department of Radiology
University of Texas Health Center at San Antonio
San Antonio, Texas
Cases 112, 125, 141, 152, 158, 180, and 181

Jay K. Pahade, MD
Assistant Professor
Department of Radiology and Biomedical Imaging
Yale University School of Medicine
New Haven, Connecticut
Cases 21, 77, 90, 93, and 113

Kristin Porter, MD, PhD
Assistant Professor
Russell H. Morgan Department of Radiology and Radiological Science
Johns Hopkins University, School of Medicine
Baltimore, Maryland
Cases 18, 74, 75, 114, and 120

Madhavi Raghu, MD
Assistant Professor
Department of Radiology and Biomedical Imaging
Yale University School of Medicine
New Haven, Connecticut
Cases 132, 151, 154, 156, and 187

Siva P. Raman, MD
Assistant Professor
Russell H. Morgan Department of Radiology and
    Radiological Science
Johns Hopkins University, School of Medicine
Baltimore, Maryland
Cases 117, 131, 178, 182, and 183

Balaji Rao, MD
Assistant Professor
Department of Radiology and Biomedical Imaging
Yale University School of Medicine
New Haven, Connecticut
Cases 87, 101, 129, and 171

Ananth K. Ravi, MD
Resident
Department of Radiology
University of Arkansas for Medical Sciences
Little Rock, Arkansas
Cases 47, 60, and 65

Margarita V. Revzin, MD, MS
Assistant Professor
Department of Radiology and Biomedical Imaging
Yale University School of Medicine
New Haven, Connecticut
Cases 6, 9, 20, 23, 79, 88, 91, 94, 95, 103, 104, 105, 106, 108, 109, 110,
115, and 121

William M. Reyenga, MD
Resident
Department of Radiology
University of Arkansas for Medical Sciences
Little Rock, Arkansas
Cases 30, 33, 42, and 46

Charles D. Sessions, MD
Resident
Department of Radiology
University of Arkansas for Medical Sciences
Little Rock, Arkansas
Cases 34, 48, 52, and 53

Sheila Sheth, MD
Associate Professor
Russell H. Morgan Department of Radiology
    and Radiological Science
Johns Hopkins University, School of Medicine
Baltimore, Maryland
Cases 7, 16, 19, 70, 82, 122, and 124

Artur Velcani, MD
Assistant Professor
Department of Radiology and Biomedical Imaging
Yale University School of Medicine
New Haven, Connecticut
Cases 142, 143, 144, and 160

Susanna Catherina Sucari Vlok, MD
Resident
Department of Radiology
Tygerberg Hospital
Cape Town, South Africa
Cases 66 and 87

Andrew West, MD
Resident
Department of Radiology
University of Arkansas for Medical Sciences
Little Rock, Arkansas
Cases 36, 43, 55, and 56

Section I

Gynecology

History

► 20-Year-old pregnant female with left-sided pelvic pain (Figs. 1.1–1.3)

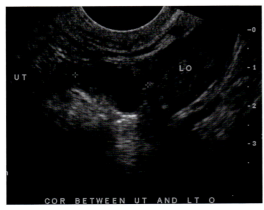

Fig. 1.1

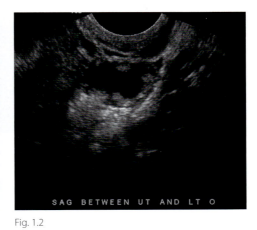

Fig. 1.2

Fig. 1.3

Case 1 Hydrosalpinx

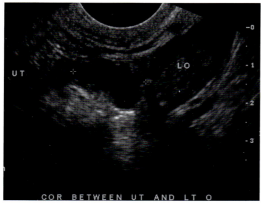

Fig. 1.4

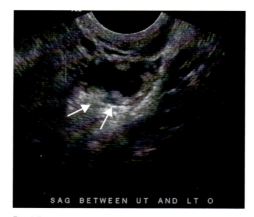

Fig. 1.5

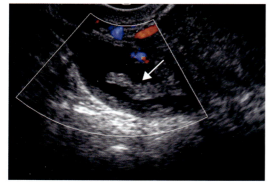

Fig. 1.6

Imaging Findings

▶ Dilated avascular tubular anechoic structure between the uterus (UT) and left ovary (LO) (Fig. 1.4) containing short round projections and a "beads on a string" or "cogwheel" appearance (arrows in Fig. 1.5) representing thickened endosalpingeal folds and incomplete septation due to the tube folding on itself (arrows in Fig. 1.5 and Fig. 1.6)

Differential Diagnosis

▶ Pyosalpinx
▶ Hematosalpinx
▶ Fallopian tube torsion
▶ Fallopian tube carcinoma
▶ Peritoneal inclusion cyst

Teaching Points

▶ Obstruction of the fallopian tube most commonly from adhesions secondary to prior episodes of pelvic inflammatory disease. Other causes: adhesions from endometriosis, prior surgery, or hysterectomy
▶ Normal fallopian tube: 1–4 mm in diameter, frequently not visualized
▶ Dilated tubular cystic structure between ovary and uterus with "S," "V," or "U" shape
▶ May see thickened endosalpingeal folds with "beads on a string" or "cogwheel" appearance in cross section at junction of fimbriated and ampullary portion of tube and incomplete septation or "waist sign" (indentation on opposite sides). Separate from ipsilateral ovary
▶ Three-dimensional US with inversion mode imaging or cine clips are useful for diagnosis in equivocal findings on two-dimensional US
▶ Pyosalpinx/hematosalpinx: low-level echoes and/or fluid–fluid levels in the dilated tube, representing pus, often-hyperemic walls on color Doppler US
▶ Fallopian tube torsion: more common in prepubertal girls due to excessive mobility of the adnexa and results from rotation of the tube on its pedicle

- Fallopian tube carcinoma: most often in postmenopausal women with a US appearance similar to ovarian carcinoma
- Peritoneal inclusion cysts: after prior pelvic surgery, pelvic inflammatory disease, or endometriosis. US features: cystic mass, following the contour of adjacent pelvic structures with the ovary located at the edge of the mass or suspended within it

Management

- Asymptomatic hydrosalpinx: no additional treatment—patients may be at increased risk for ectopic pregnancy
- In the setting of infertility: tubal recanalization
- Nonclassic US appearance: further imaging with MRI or follow-up US

Further Reading
1. Rezvani M. Fallopian tube disease in the nonpregnant patient. *RadioGraphics*. March 2011; 31: 527–548.
2. Levine D, Brown DL, Andreotti RF, et al. Management of asymptomatic ovarian and adnexal cysts imaged at US: Society of Radiologists in Ultrasound consensus conference statement. *Ultrasound Q*. 2010; 26(3): 121–131.

Case 2

History

► 23-Year-old female admitted with fever, leukocytosis, and pelvic pain (Figs. 2.1–2.4)

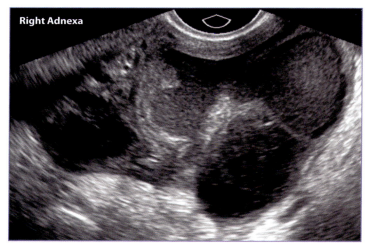

Fig. 2.1

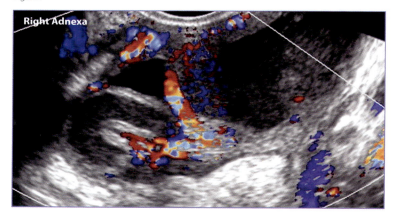

Fig. 2.2

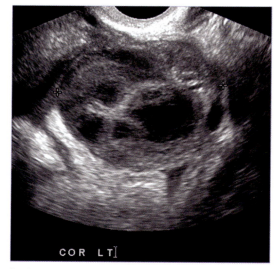

Fig. 2.3

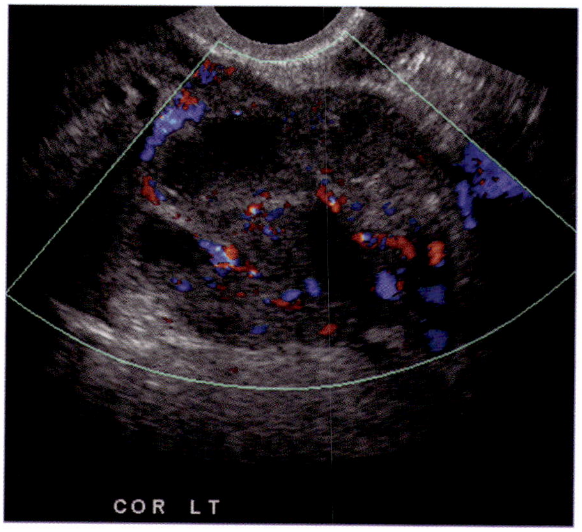

Fig. 2.4

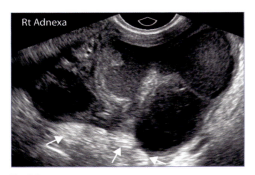

Fig. 2.5

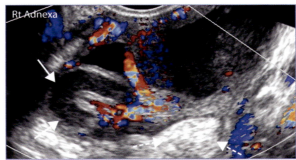

Fig. 2.6

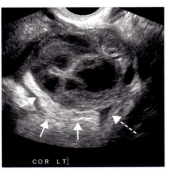

Fig. 2.7

Imaging Findings

▶ Complex, multilocular cystic bilateral adnexal masses with internal echoes (Fig. 2.5 and calipers in Fig. 2.7) and no distinguishable ovary
▶ Color flow imaging demonstrates increased vascularity, right adnexa shown (Fig. 2.6)
▶ Adjacent dilated tubular structure (solid arrows in Fig. 2.6) consistent with hydrosalpinx
▶ Increased echogenicity of the adjacent pelvic fat (arrows in Fig. 2.5, dotted arrows in Fig. 2.6, and solid arrows in Fig. 2.7)
▶ Complex intraperitoneal free fluid (dotted arrow in Fig. 2.7)

Differential Diagnosis

▶ Perforated appendix
▶ Crohn's colitis
▶ Endometriomas
▶ Complex ovarian mass

Teaching Points

▶ Pelvic inflammatory disease: Ascending infection of the female reproductive tract begins with cervicitis progressing to endometritis, salpingitis, and tubo-ovarian abscess (TOA)
▶ Due to sexually transmitted infection from *Neisseria gonorrhoeae, Chlamydia trachomatis*, or polymicrobial infection involving vaginal flora
▶ Clinical presentation: dull, aching, or acute pelvic pain; fever; leukocytosis; foul-smelling vaginal discharge; cervical motion tenderness
▶ US findings
   ▪ Cervicitis: usually normal
   ▪ Endometritis: indistinct endometrium; fluid, pus, ± air in endometrial canal; increased vascularity and diastolic flow (low resistive index)
   ▪ Salpingitis: thickened, vascular fallopian tube
   ▪ Hydrosalpinx: distended tubular "S"- or "V"-shaped adnexal structure with indentations or "waist sign" and/or "incomplete septations" due to folding of tube on itself
   ▪ Pyosalpinx: internal echoes ± fluid/debris levels, mural vascularity
   ▪ Uterine serositis: hypoechoic rim around uterine serosal surface
   ▪ Tubo-ovarian complex: ovary engulfed by infection but still recognizable
   ▪ TOA: ovary no longer distinct, multilocular cystic adnexal collections with thick walls and debris, vascular
   ▪ Increased echogenicity and vascularity of adjacent pelvic fat secondary to inflammation and/or infection

- Complex free fluid due to pus ± hemorrhage and debris
- Often bilateral and tender
▶ Pelvic abscess from perforated appendix, Crohn's disease, or other bowel pathology can mimic findings but would be more likely unilateral
▶ Endometriomas or cystic epithelial neoplasms can cause bilateral complex adnexal masses but would not present with symptoms suggesting infection

Management

▶ Antibiotics with drainage if TOA does not resolve
▶ Increases risk of infertility, ectopic pregnancy, chronic pelvic pain

Further Reading

1. Horrow MM. Ultrasound of pelvic inflammatory disease. *Ultrasound Q.* 2004; 20(4): 171–179.
2. Brown DL, Dudiak KM, Laing FC. Adnexal masses: US characterization and reporting. *Radiology.* 2010; 254: 342–354.

History

► 72-Year-old female with history of septated left adnexal mass seen on outside sonogram (Figs. 3.1–3.3)

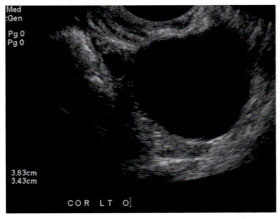

Fig. 3.1

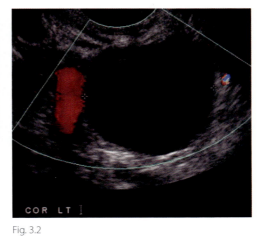

Fig. 3.2

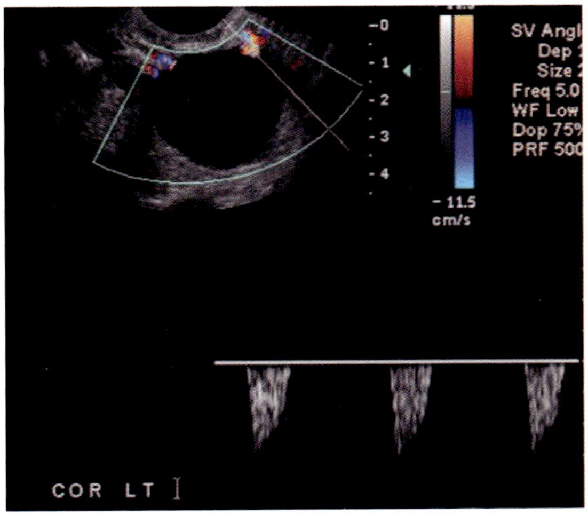

Fig. 3.3

Case 3 Simple Postmenopausal Ovarian Cyst

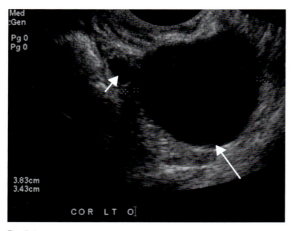

Fig. 3.4

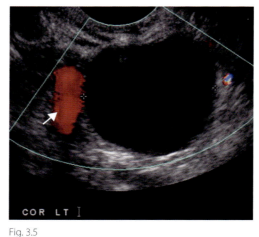

Fig. 3.5

Fig. 3.6

Imaging Findings

▶ Simple 3.5 × 3.5 × 3.4-cm left ovarian cyst (long arrow in Fig. 3.4)
▶ Adjacent iliac vessel (short arrow in Fig. 3.4) mistaken on outside US for a septation shows flow on color Doppler US (short arrow in Fig. 3.5)
▶ High resistance flow on spectral Doppler US at the periphery of the cyst (Fig. 3.6) supporting benign etiology

Differential Diagnosis

▶ Serious epithelial ovarian neoplasm
▶ Hydrosalpinx
▶ Paraovarian cyst

Teaching Points

▶ Postmenopausal simple ovarian cysts
  ▪ Seen in up to 15% of postmenopausal women
  ▪ Unrelated to postmenopausal state or hormone use
  ▪ If simple: regardless of age, almost always benign
  ▪ Can be followed with serial transvaginal US based on recommendations from the Society of Radiologists in Ultrasound (SRU) consensus conference (see Management section)
▶ Clinical symptoms: often asymptomatic; however, may present with lower abdominal and pelvic pain and/or palpated during pelvic exam
▶ US findings
  ▪ Round or oval in shape
  ▪ No internal echoes

- Thin, smooth walls
- No solid internal or mural components
- No internal vascularity
- High resistance flow in wall or adjacent ovarian tissue
► Cystic epithelial ovarian neoplasm: suspect if cyst contains internal echoes, mural nodularity, or thick septations (> 3 mm) with vascularity
► Hydrosalpinx: dilated tubular cystic structure between ovary and uterus with "S," "V," or "U" shape; may have thickened endosalpingeal folds giving a "beads on a string" or "cogwheel" appearance in cross section at junction of fimbriated and ampullary portion of tube; incomplete septation(s) or waist sign (indentation on opposite sides), both of which are pathognomonic for hydrosalpinx; separate from ipsilateral ovary
► Paraovarian cyst: simple cystic lesion seen separate from the ovary; usually do not resolve; generally inconsequential in asymptomatic women

Management

► Recommendations based on the SRU 2010 consensus conference
- > 1 cm and < 7 cm: yearly transvaginal US follow-up. Individual practice may opt to increase lower size threshold for yearly follow-up to 3 cm
- > 7 cm: MRI or surgical removal

Further Reading

1. Levine D, Brown DL, Andreotti RF, et al. Management of asymptomatic ovarian and adnexal cysts imaged at US: Society of Radiologists in Ultrasound consensus conference statement. *Ultrasound Q.* 2010; 26(3): 121–131.
2. Brown DL, Doubilet PM, Miller FH, et al. Benign and malignant ovarian masses: Selection of the most discriminating grayscale and Doppler sonographic features. *Radiology.* 1998; 208(1): 103–110.
3. Jeong Y-Y, Outwater EK, Kang HK. Imaging evaluation of ovarian masses. *RadioGraphics.* 2000; 20(5): 1445–1147.

Case 4

History

▶ 37-Year-old female with enlarging right ovarian cyst. Figures 4.1 and 4.2 are from two different exams, performed 5 months apart. Figure 4.2 is from the later exam, which was performed because of increasing pelvic pain.

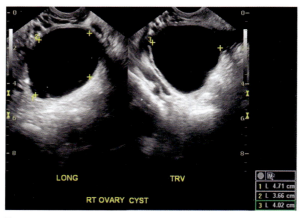

Fig. 4.1

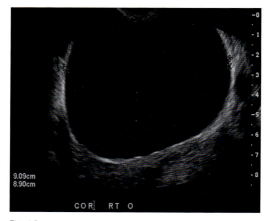

Fig. 4.2

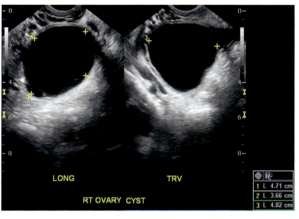

Fig. 4.3

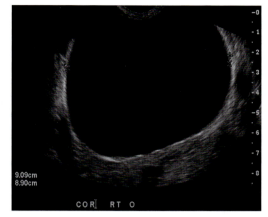

Fig. 4.4

Imaging Findings

► Approximately 9-cm simple cyst within the right ovary (between calipers Fig. 4.4); 5 months earlier, it measured 4.7 cm
► No solid components, septations, debris, or internal vascularity on Doppler US (not shown)

Differential Diagnosis

► Simple ovarian cyst
► Paraovarian cyst
► Serous cystadenoma

Teaching Points

► Simple adnexal cysts less than 10 cm are most likely benign, with a less than 1% chance of malignancy
► US criteria for the diagnosis of a simple cyst include an anechoic structure with a thin, imperceptible wall; no internal echoes, septations, or internal vascularity; and increased through-transmission or posterior wall enhancement
► However, there is overlap in the US appearance of simple ovarian cysts and cystic epithelial neoplasms as this case demonstrates. Follow-up was performed for increasing pelvic pain
► Cystic epithelial neoplasms account for 60% of all ovarian neoplasms but comprise 85% of all malignant neoplasms
► The most common cystic epithelial neoplasms are serous and mucinous tumors; of these, serous tumors are more common
► It is difficult to differentiate the type of epithelial neoplasm on imaging, but mucinous tumors tend to be multiloculated with septations, whereas serous tumors tend to have solid mural components
► Features that suggest benign pathology include unilocularity, thin walls; few, thin septations; and the absence of soft tissue nodularity or papillary projections
► Paraovarian cysts are typically simple, almost always benign, and can be differentiated from ovarian cysts by identification of a fat plane between the ovary and the cyst

Management

► The Society of Radiologists in Ultrasound guidelines for the management of asymptomatic ovarian cysts published in 2010 recommend further workup with either MRI or surgical consultation for simple cysts measuring > 7 cm in maximum diameter in premenopausal and postmenopausal women due to the possibility of sampling error on US that might miss small mural solid nodules in a large structure
► The patient underwent MRI, which showed no solid components, and then cystectomy. Pathology showed a mucinous cystadenoma

Further Reading

1. Levine D, Brown DL, Andreotti RF, et al. Management of asymptomatic and ovarian and other adnexal cysts imaged at US: Society of Radiologists in Ultrasound consensus conference statement. *Radiology*. 2010; 256: 943–954.
2. Jeong Y-Y, Outwater EK, Kang HK. Imaging evaluation of ovarian masses. *RadioGraphics*. 2000; 20(5): 1445–1147.

Case 5

History

▶ 47-Year-old female with left lower quadrant pain and fullness (Figs. 5.1–5.3)

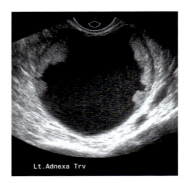

Fig. 5.1

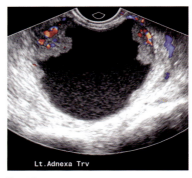

Fig. 5.2

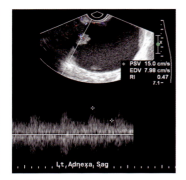

Fig. 5.3

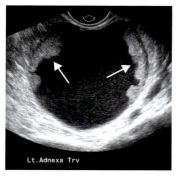

Fig. 5.4

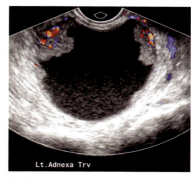

Fig. 5.5

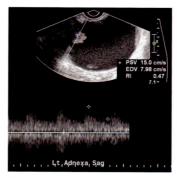

Fig. 5.6

Imaging Findings

► Complex cystic left ovarian mass with multiple mural nodules (arrows in Fig. 5.4) that are vascular on color Doppler imaging (Fig. 5.5). Note low level echoes within the central fluid
► Spectral Doppler image demonstrates a low-resistance arterial waveform pattern within the mural nodules (Fig. 5.6)

Differential Diagnosis

► Benign cystic epithelial ovarian neoplasm (serous cystadenoma)
► Cystadenofibroma
► Tubo-ovarian abscess (TOA)
► Endometrioma

Teaching Points

► Ovarian cancer is the second most common gynecologic malignancy in the United States
   ▪ 90% are serous or mucinous cystadenocarcinomas
   ▪ Five-year survival is poor
   ▪ Often "silent": no symptoms until late stage, when patients present with abdominal distension, bloating, anorexia, pelvic pain, and/or weight loss
► Risk factors: older age, high socioeconomic class, nulliparity, positive family history, obesity, hereditary syndromes
► Cystic epithelial neoplasms may be benign (cystadenomas) or malignant (cystadenocarcinomas), either borderline or invasive
   ▪ Serous (more common): solid mural nodules
   ▪ Mucinous: thick, irregular septations. Different locules may have different levels of echogenicity
► US features most concerning for malignancy
   ▪ Solid, vascular components (highest positive predictive value)
   ▪ Thick (> 3 mm) or vascular septations
   ▪ Large size
   ▪ Ascites
   ▪ Peritoneal implants
► However, significant overlap in US appearance of benign and malignant lesions
► Cystadenofibromas and Brenner's tumors
   ▪ Similar US findings
   ▪ Complex predominately cystic ovarian masses with mural nodules
   ▪ Cystadenofibromas may present as multi-septated masses without mural nodules
► TOAs or endometriomas
   ▪ Complex adnexal masses with thick vascular walls and internal echoes
   ▪ TOAs may have septations and locules
   ▪ Solid, vascular mural nodules should not be identified, unless malignant degeneration of an endometrioma (usually a clear cell or endometroid carcinoma) has occurred

Management

► Initial evaluation of a suspected adnexal mass should be with transvaginal US
  ▪ Transabdominal US helpful for large masses and to search for ascites or peritoneal implants
► Staging: CT/MRI
► Treatment: surgical debridement and chemotherapy

Further Reading

1. Brown DL, Dudiak KM, Laing FC. Adnexal masses: US characterization and reporting. *Radiology*. 2010; 254: 342–354.
2. Levine D, Brown DL, Andreotti RF, et al. Management of asymptomatic and ovarian and other adnexal cysts imaged at US: Society of Radiologists in Ultrasound consensus conference statement. *Radiology*. 2010; 256: 943–954.

History

▶ 48-Year-old female with history of gastric adenocarcinoma presents with abdominal bloating (Figs. 6.1–6.3)

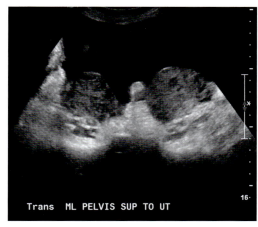

Fig. 6.1

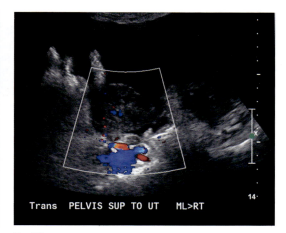

Fig. 6.2

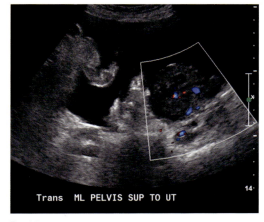

Fig. 6.3

Case 6   Bilateral Krukenberg Tumors

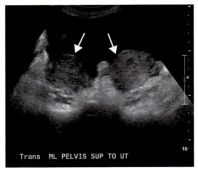

Fig. 6.4

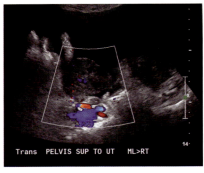

Fig. 6.5

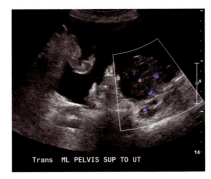

Fig. 6.6

Imaging Findings

- ► Both ovaries are enlarged and heterogeneous (arrows in Fig. 6.4) in an infiltrative pattern with loss of the normal sonographic ovarian architecture without a discrete mass
- ► Color Doppler imaging demonstrates central vascularity (Figs. 6.5 and 6.6)
- ► There is a moderate amount of free pelvic fluid

Differential Diagnosis

- ► Benign solid ovarian neoplasms (fibrothecoma/thecoma)
- ► Primary malignant solid ovarian neoplasms (dysgerminoma, granulosa cell tumor, clear cell carcinoma)
- ► Lymphoma

Teaching Points

- ► Ovarian metastases account for ~1–2% of ovarian tumors and typically occur in the setting of widespread metastatic disease
  - ▪ Most common primaries: gastric, breast, gastrointestinal tract, endometrial
  - ▪ Krukenberg tumors are drop metastases to the ovaries from gastric or colon cancer that specifically contain mucin-secreting "signet-ring" cells
- ► Clinical presentation: asymptomatic, abdominal/pelvic pain, distension, bloating, nonspecific gastrointestinal symptoms
- ► US findings
  - ▪ Bilateral ovarian enlargement—infiltrative, heterogeneous with loss of the normal sonographic architecture (nonvisualization of follicles and central, more echogenic stroma)
  - ▪ Bilateral solid ovarian masses
  - ▪ Cystic or necrotic ovarian metastases are less common and often from colon cancer. They may mimic cystic epithelial ovarian neoplasms
  - ▪ Ascites ± peritoneal carcinomatosis
- ► Other solid benign (thecomas, fibrothecomas) or malignant (dysgerminomas, endometroid tumors, granulosa cell tumors) ovarian masses may have a similar US appearance but are less likely to be bilateral
  - ▪ Fibromas are typically extremely hypoechoic with dense posterior shadowing
  - ▪ Clinical history and evidence of primary tumor or metastatic disease elsewhere may aid in the differential diagnosis
- ► Lymphomatous involvement of the ovaries also may result in bilateral solid hypoechoic ovarian masses or diffuse ovarian enlargement due to infiltrative disease
  - ▪ Associated pelvic or retroperitoneal lymphadenopathy, which may encase the pelvic vessels, suggests lymphoma

Management

- ► Patients with bilateral solid ovarian masses should be evaluated for underlying primary malignancy or lymphoma
- ► Treatment is based on the primary tumor
- ► Prognosis is poor because ovarian metastases usually occur in the setting of advanced, widely metastatic disease

Further Reading

1. Al-agha OM, Nicastri AD. An in-depth look at Krukenberg tumor: An overview. *Arch Pathol Lab Med.* 2006; 130: 1725–1730.
2. Ha HK, Baek SY, Kim SH, et al. Krukenberg's tumor of the ovary: MR imaging features. *Am J Roentgenol.* 1995; 164: 1435–1439.

History

► 45-Year-old woman with vague pelvic pain (Figs. 7.1 and 7.2)

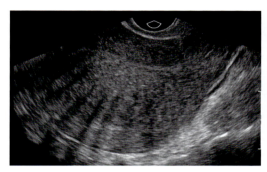

Fig. 7.1

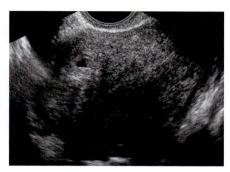

Fig. 7.2

Case 7 Adenomyosis of the Uterus

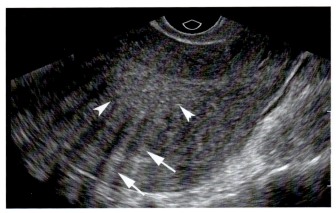

Fig. 7.3

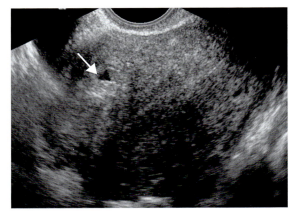

Fig. 7.4

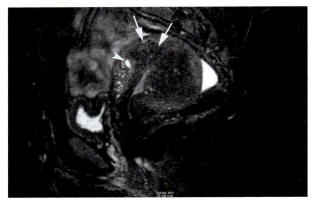

Fig. 7.5

Imaging Findings

► Enlarged globular uterus; focal tenderness elicited by vaginal transducer (Figs. 7.3 and 7.4)
► Asymmetric thickening of the posterior myometrium with heterogeneous echotexture
► Ill-defined boundaries between endometrium and myometrium (arrowheads in Fig. 7.3)
► Echogenic stripes radiating from the endometrium into the myometrium (arrows in Fig. 7.3)
► A small cyst in the anterior myometrium (arrow in Fig. 7.4)
► T2-weighted sagittal MR shows widening of the junctional zone (arrows in Fig. 7.5), cysts in the anterior myometrium (arrowhead in Fig. 7.5), and diffuse low-intensity signal in the posterior myometrium

Differential Diagnosis

► Leiomyomas, which frequently coexist with adenomyosis
► Focal adenomyoma

Teaching Points

► Adenomyosis of the uterus is characterized by the presence of ectopic endometrial glands within the uterine myometrium. Some of these ectopic glands may undergo cystic dilatation and appear as small myometrial cysts on ultrasound
► There is associated hyperplastic reaction in the smooth muscle of the surrounding myometrium
► It is a common condition usually affecting multiparous women in late reproductive age
► Clinical symptoms are nonspecific and include dysmenorrhea, dyspareunia, chronic pelvic pain, and menorrhagia. Many women are asymptomatic
► Endovaginal US is a sensitive and specific imaging modality for establishing the diagnosis in experienced hands
► Findings on US can be subtle and best appreciated on real-time evaluation or review of cine clips and include the following:
  ▪ Diffuse uterine enlargement with asymmetric thickening and diffuse heterogeneity of the myometrium

- Poor definition of the myometrial–endometrial border
- Subendometrial cysts
- Subendometrial echogenic nodules and linear striations
► Leiomyomas appear as focal hypoechoic or heterogeneous masses often with shadowing or edge refraction. The margins are classically well defined because of the presence of a pseudocapsule
► Focal adenomyomas appear as focal myometrial masses with indistinct borders and are often difficult to differentiate from leiomyomas. May be cystic in nature

Management

► MR is highly accurate and helpful in confirming the diagnosis: Findings are best displayed on sagittal T2-weighted images
► The goal of therapy is to alleviate pain and treat the menorrhagia
► Medical treatment includes estrogen suppression and oral contraceptives as well as nonsteroidal anti-inflammatory agents and gonadotropin-releasing hormone analogues. Endometrial ablation or laparoscopic myometrial electrocoagulation can be effective in superficial cases, whereas hysterectomy is reserved for more advanced intractable cases

Further Reading

1. Andreotti RF, Fleischer AC. The sonographic diagnosis of adenomyosis. *Ultrasound Q.* 2005; 21: 167–170.
2. Sakhel K, Abuhamad A. Sonography of adenomyosis. *J Ultrasound Med.* 2012; 31: 805–808.

Case 8

History

▶ 65-Year-old female with pelvic pain (Figs. 8.1–8.3)

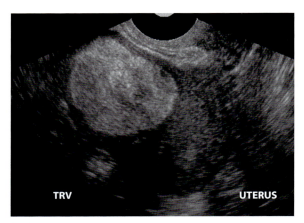

Fig. 8.1

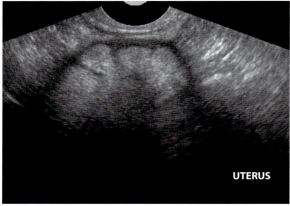

Fig. 8.2

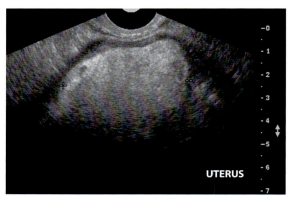

Fig. 8.3

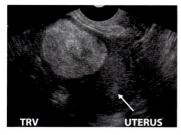

Fig. 8.4

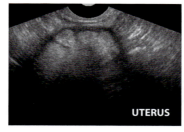

Fig. 8.5

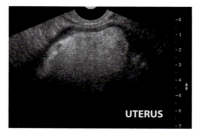

Fig. 8.6

Imaging Findings

▶ Homogeneous echogenic slightly lobular intramural myometrial mass with posterior attenuation (Figs. 8.4–8.6)
▶ Myometrium extends around the mass well seen in Fig. 8.4, confirming intramural uterine location
▶ The echogenic endometrium (arrow in Fig. 8.4) is separate

Differential Diagnosis

▶ Leiomyoma
▶ Hemorrhagic/cellular leiomyoma
▶ Leiomyosarcoma
▶ Ovarian dermoid

Teaching Points

▶ Rare benign subtype of uterine leiomyoma containing fat (lipo) and smooth muscle (leiomyoma)
  ▪ Incidence: 0.03–0.2%
  ▪ More common in postmenopausal women
▶ Thought to represent adipocyte differentiation rather than degenerative change of leiomyoma
▶ Presentation: asymptomatic, pain, bleeding
▶ US findings
  ▪ Homogeneous echogenic well-marginated myometrial mass
  ▪ Posterior attenuation suggests the presence of fat
  ▪ Usually intramural and fundal
▶ Leiomyoma: usually hypoechoic (although echogenicity is variable), round, well-marginated, homogeneous or heterogeneous, ± shadowing, focal calcification, edge refraction
▶ Hemorrhagic or cellular leiomyoma: may be echogenic (hemorrhagic often heterogeneous; cellular more likely homogeneous), may shadow or demonstrate edge refraction, but posterior attenuation unlikely
▶ Leiomyosarcoma: imaging features nonspecific
  ▪ More likely to be large, vascular, and heterogeneous with central necrosis and ill-defined, lobular or infiltrative margins
  ▪ Rapid growth
▶ Leiomyosarcoma arising from a lipoleiomyoma is very rare
▶ Ovarian dermoids: often homogeneously echogenic with posterior attenuation ("tip of the iceberg sign"), but arise from the ovary rather than the uterus

Management

▶ Consider sonographic follow-up to establish stability
▶ If there is a rapid increase in size, consider leiomyosarcoma
▶ MRI or CT can definitively demonstrate fat within these lesions and confirm uterine origin if US is indeterminate
▶ Treatment depends on size and symptoms, but most can be left alone
▶ If necessary, treatment is uterine artery embolization or surgical excision

Further Reading

1. Wang X, Kumar D, Seidman JD. Uterine lipoleiomyomas: A clinicopathologic study of 50 cases. *Int J Gynecol Pathol*. 2006; 25: 239–242.
2. Avritscher R, Iyer RB, Ro J, et al. Lipoleiomyoma of the uterus. *Am J Roentgenol*. October 2001; 177(4): 856.
3. Preito A, Crespo C, Pardo A, et al. Uterine lipoleiomyomas: US and CT findings. *Abdominal Imaging*. 2000; 25(6): 655–657.

Case 9

History

▶ 61-Year-old woman presents with vaginal bleeding (Figs. 9.1–9.3)

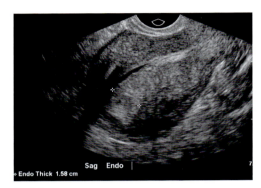

Fig. 9.1

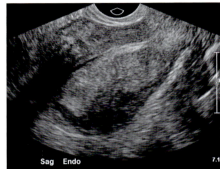

Fig. 9.2

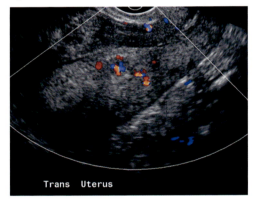

Fig. 9.3

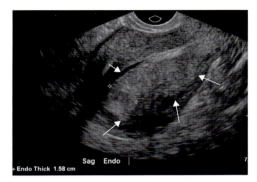

Fig. 9.4

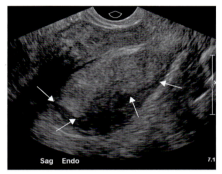

Fig. 9.5

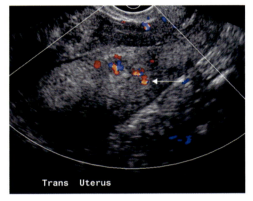

Fig. 9.6

Imaging Findings

▶ Heterogeneous asymmetric thickening (1.58 cm) of posterior endometrial layer (calipers in Fig. 9.4)
▶ Fluid in endometrial cavity (short arrow in Fig. 9.4) separates the normal, thin echogenic anterior endometrium from the posterior echogenic endometrial mass that invades the myometrium (long arrows in Fig. 9.4 and arrows in Fig. 9.5) extending close to the serosal surface, indicating > 50% myometrial invasion (stage IB)
▶ Note increased vascularity near the area of maximal myometrial invasion (arrow in Fig. 9.6)

Differential Diagnosis

▶ Endometrial hyperplasia
▶ Endometrial polyp
▶ Endometrial atrophy

Teaching Points

▶ Endometrial cancer: most common invasive gynecologic malignancy
  ▪ Risk factors: older age, increased estrogen exposure, obesity, nulliparity, diabetes, high socioeconomic class, polycystic ovarian disease
  ▪ 90% present with abnormal vaginal bleeding, although only 4–10% of women with postmenopausal bleeding (PMB) have endometrial cancer
  ▪ 70% present with stage 1 disease
  ▪ Most important prognostic factors are histologic grade, depth of myometrial invasion, stage, and lymph node involvement
▶ US findings
  ▪ Diffuse or focal heterogeneous thickening of endometrium
  ▪ Endometrial mass
  ▪ Most specific finding: irregularity of the endometrial/myometrial (E/M) interface or invasion of endometrial mass into myometrium
  ▪ Increased vascularity, low-resistance arterial waveforms, irregular distribution of blood vessels
▶ Endometrial hyperplasia: diffuse homogeneous endometrial thickening with sharp E/M interface, ± small cystic areas, ± mildly increased vascularity in regular pattern

- ► Endometrial polyp: echogenic focal endometrial mass with single feeding vessel, sharp E/M interface, ± cysts
- ► Endometrial atrophy: thin, homogeneous echogenic endometrium ≤ 5 mm, sharp E/M interface, no abnormal blood flow

Management

- ► Transvaginal US is the most appropriate initial imaging study for women presenting with PMB
  - ▪ Endometrial thickness (ET) ≤ 5 mm: Endometrial atrophy is the most likely diagnosis and endometrial sampling not indicated for most patients
  - ▪ ET > 5 mm: Tissue sampling is recommended
- ► Sonohysterography or 3D US may improve visualization of the E/M interface, and are also useful to differentiate between focal and diffuse disease
- ► MR is recommended for local staging of endometrial cancer; CT and MR equivalent for assessing pelvic and para-aortic lymph nodes

Further Reading

1. Sohaib SA, Verma H, Attygalle AD, et al. Imaging of uterine malignancies. *Semin Ultrasound CT MR.* 2010; 31: 377–387.
2. Olaya FJ, Dualde D, García E, et al. Transvaginal sonography in endometrial carcinoma: Preoperative assessment of the depth of myometrial invasion in 50 cases. *Eur J Radiol.* 1998; 26: 274–279.

History

▶ 33-Year-old female with persistent vaginal bleeding, status post-suction dilatation and curettage (D&C) 4 weeks previously, presents to the emergency department with vaginal bleeding and a drop in hematocrit (Figs. 10.1 and 10.2).

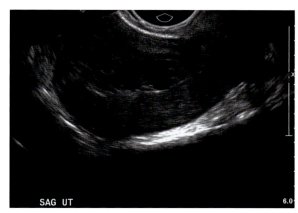

Fig. 10.1

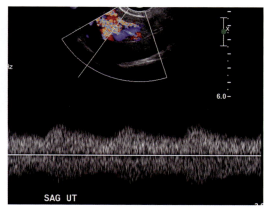

Fig. 10.2

Case 10 Myometrial Arteriovenous Fistula

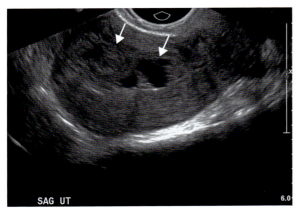

Fig. 10.3

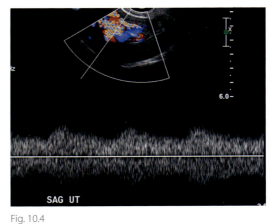

Fig. 10.4

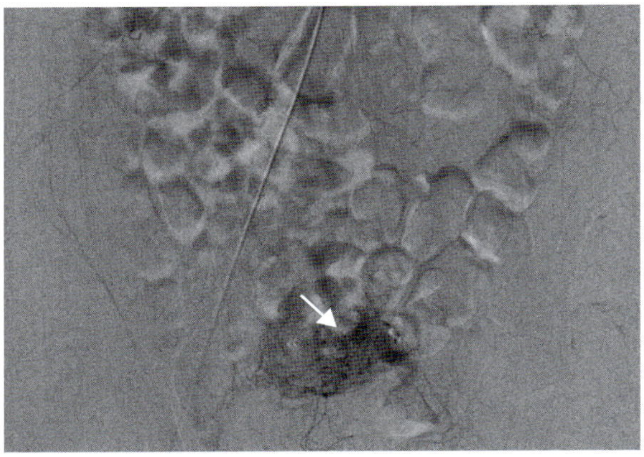

Fig. 10.5

Imaging Findings

- ▶ Complex cystic and solid myometrial lesion on grayscale US (arrows in Fig. 10.3)
- ▶ Color Doppler US: highly vascular lesion with a low-resistance spectral Doppler waveform (Fig. 10.4)
- ▶ Left uterine artery angiogram: hypertrophied left uterine artery with arteriovenous shunting on delayed images, compatible with arteriovenous fistula (arrow in Fig. 10.5)

Differential Diagnosis

- ▶ Retained products of conception
- ▶ Myometrial pseudoaneurysm

Teaching Points

- ▶ Causes of persistent vaginal bleeding post D&C include myometrial AVF, myometrial pseudoaneurysm (PSA), and retained products of conception (RPOC)
- ▶ A focal tangle of vessels with a low-resistance spectral Doppler arterial waveform is typical of AVFs
- ▶ Although RPOC can be associated with increased myometrial vascularity, RPOC are primarily located within the endometrium, whereas myometrial AVFs and PSAs are located within the myometrium
- ▶ PSAs appear as cystic structures in the myometrium on grayscale that fill in on color Doppler imaging with a "ying-yang" appearance. A "to-and-fro" appearance will be noted in the spectral waveform obtained from the neck of the PSA

Management

▸ Transcatheter arterial embolization, which does not affect future fertility

▸ It is important to distinguish this abnormality from RPOC, which are typically treated with repeat D&C. This could result in further damage to the myometrium and cause massive hemorrhage in a patient with an AVF

Further Reading

1. Kwon JH, Kim GS. Obstetric iatrogenic arterial injuries of the uterus: Diagnosis with US and treatment with transcatheter arterial embolization. *RadioGraphics*. 2002; 22: 35–46.

Case 11

History

► 23-Year-old female with right-sided pelvic pain (Figs. 11.1 and 11.2)

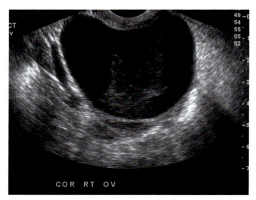

Fig. 11.1

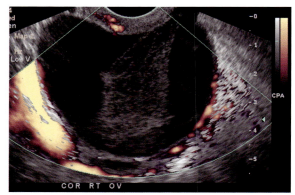

Fig. 11.2

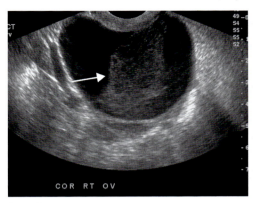

Fig. 11.3

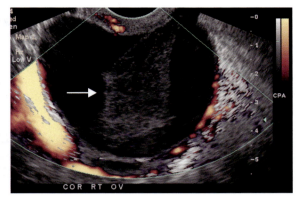

Fig. 11.4

Imaging Findings

▶ Cystic right ovarian mass demonstrating central retractile clot with straight to slightly scalloped borders (arrow in Figs. 11.3 and 11.4)
▶ No internal vascularity, although small amount of mural vascularity is present (Fig. 11.4)

Differential Diagnosis

▶ Endometrioma
▶ Tubo-ovarian abscess (TOA)
▶ Cystic ovarian neoplasm

Teaching Points

▶ Common in premenopausal patients; size variable
▶ Internal hemorrhage may occur into follicular and corpus luteal cysts
▶ Patients may present with acute pain
▶ Variable US appearance based on the amount of hemorrhage and time course
  ▪ Echogenic to diffuse low-level echoes in the acute phase may mimic appearances of solid mass, although they will demonstrate posterior acoustic enhancement (arrows in Figs. 11.5) and no internal blood flow (Fig. 11.6)

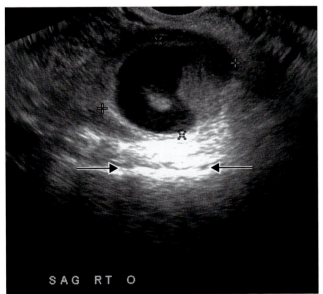

Fig. 11.5

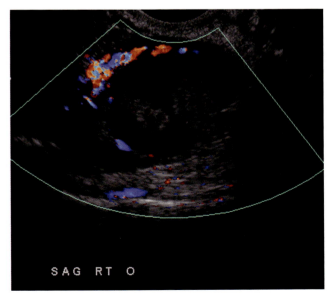

Fig. 11.6

- Lacelike or reticular pattern of internal echoes with no internal vascularity (Figs. 11.7 and 11.8)

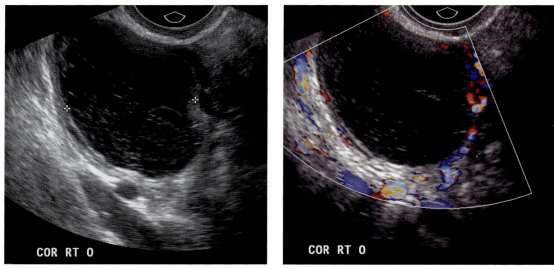

Fig. 11.7   Fig. 11.8

- Clot may appear echogenic, irregular, or lentiform and adherent to the wall
- No internal vascularity, no matter the pattern of internal echoes
- Adjacent echogenic fluid, fluid in the cul-de-sac, and a crenated appearance may occur following rupture of a hemorrhagic cyst. May occasionally result in massive hemoperitoneum
- Change in size and US appearance over time and eventual resolution
▶ Endometrioma
  - Homogeneous low-level internal echoes
  - Ground glass appearance
  - No solid components
  - May contain tiny echogenic foci in the wall
  - Little change in size and US appearance over time
▶ Tuboovarian Abscess (TOA)
  - Multiseptated complex mass with septations, scattered internal echoes, and irregular margins
  - Increased vascularity on color Doppler US
▶ Cystic ovarian neoplasm
  - Often contains true septations, thick or thin, extending from one wall to the next, ± vascularity
  - Mural nodules or solid vascular components

Management

▶ Premenopausal patient with classic appearance of hemorrhagic cyst < 5 cm: no additional follow-up
▶ Premenopausal patient with hemorrhagic cyst > 5 cm: initial follow-up 6–12 weeks to document resolution
▶ Early postmenopausal patient any size: short interval follow-up to resolution
▶ Late postmenopausal patient any size: consider surgical intervention

Further Reading

1. Levine D, Brown DL, Andreotti RF, et al. Management of asymptomatic ovarian and adnexal cysts imaged at US: Society of Radiologists in Ultrasound consensus conference statement. *Ultrasound Q.* 2010; 26(3): 121–131.

History

▶ 54-Year-old female with ovarian mass seen at an outside hospital (Figs. 12.1–12.3)

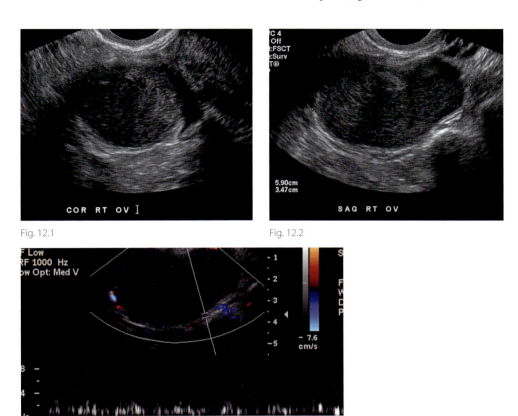

Fig. 12.1

Fig. 12.2

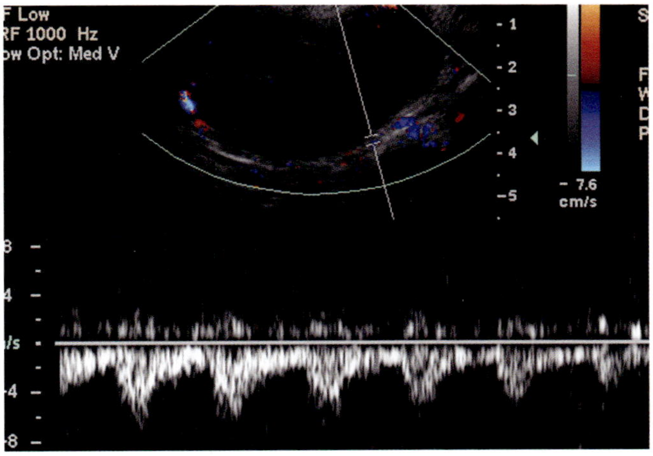

Fig. 12.3

Case 12 Endometrioma

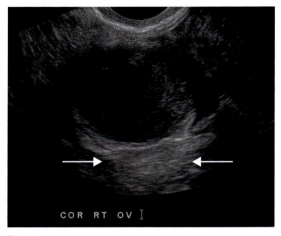

Fig. 12.4

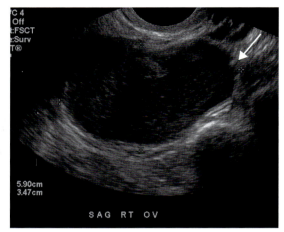

Fig. 12.5

Fig. 12.6

Imaging Findings

▶ Largely homogeneous hypoechoic mass adjacent to the right ovary with posterior acoustic enhancement (arrows in Fig. 12.4)
▶ Small echogenic foci within the wall of the endometrioma (arrow in Fig. 12.5)
▶ No internal vascularity on color Doppler US (Fig. 12.6)

Differential Diagnosis

▶ Hemorrhagic ovarian cyst
▶ Cystic ovarian neoplasm
▶ Tubo-ovarian abscess

Teaching Points

▶ Localized form of endometriosis, also called chocolate cyst, presents with a discrete mass
▶ Patients may be asymptomatic or present with cyclic pelvic pain
▶ Often associated with a history of infertility
▶ US appearance
  ▪ Homogeneous unilocular cystic mass with low-level internal echoes, and sometimes ground glass appearance
  ▪ Often multiple with angular margins due to fibrosis and retraction
  ▪ Small echogenic foci in the cyst wall likely due to small cholesterol deposits or hemosiderin
  ▪ No internal vascularity, although wall may be vascular
  ▪ Often little change between initial and follow-up examinations
▶ MRI appearance
▶ T1 hyperintense and T2 hypointense on MRI (arrows in Figs. 12.7 and 12.8)

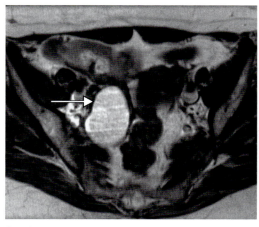

Fig. 12.7

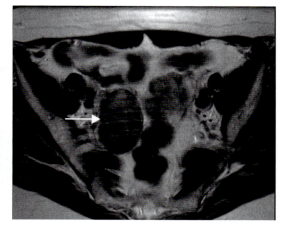

Fig. 12.8

- ▶ Hemorrhagic ovarian cyst
  - ▪ Usually present with acute pelvic pain
  - ▪ Appearance varies with time and can range from homogeneous low-level echoes to lacelike reticular pattern and retractile clot
  - ▪ Often associated with cul-de-sac fluid
  - ▪ Usually decreases in size and resolves over time
- ▶ Cystic ovarian neoplasm
  - ▪ Septated mass with internal echoes, mural nodularity, and solid components with internal vascularity
- ▶ Tubo-ovarian abscess
  - ▪ Complex multilocular cystic mass with internal echoes and/or septations and increased vascularity
  - ▪ Tender, bilateral, often associated with hydro- or pyosalpinx

Management

- ▶ At any age: initial follow-up recommended at 6–12 weeks
- ▶ Continued follow-up yearly unless surgically removed
- ▶ If equivocal or unusual US appearance, obtain MRI to also determine extent of disease

Further Reading

1. Levine D, Brown DL, Andreotti RF, et al. Management of asymptomatic ovarian and adnexal cysts imaged at US: Society of Radiologists in Ultrasound consensus conference statement. *Ultrasound Q.* 2010; 26(3): 121–131.
2. Brown DL, Doubilet, PM, Miller FH, et al. Benign and malignant ovarian masses: Selection of the most discriminating grayscale and Doppler sonographic features. *Radiology.* 1998; 208(3): 102–110.

Case 13

► 28-Year-old female with left-sided pelvic pain (Figs. 13.1 and 13.2)

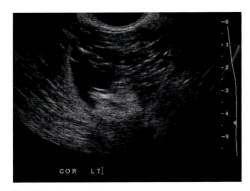

Fig. 13.1

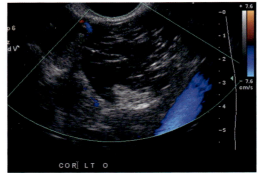

Fig. 13.2

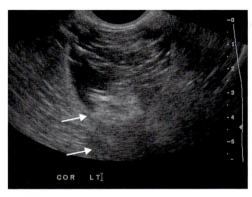

Fig. 13.3

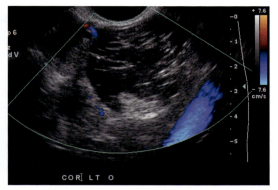

Fig. 13.4

Imaging Findings

► Heterogeneous, partially cystic, and echogenic left ovarian mass with a classic dot–dash pattern of internal echoes
► Echogenic mural focus (Rokitansky nodule) posteriorly with posterior attenuation (arrows in Fig. 13.3)
► No internal vascularity on color Doppler US (CDUS) (Fig. 13.4)

Differential Diagnosis

► Hemorrhagic cyst
► Endometrioma
► Cystic epithelial neoplasm

Teaching Points

► Account for 15–20% of ovarian neoplasms, 95% benign
► Bilateral: 10–15%
► Malignant transformation rare, approximately 1% and usually in older patients
► Variable sonographic appearance
 ▪ Homogeneously echogenic mass. May simulate "tip of the iceberg sign" (Fig. 13.5). Avascular on CDUS (Fig. 13.6)

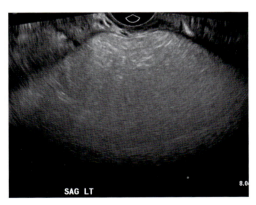

Fig. 13.5

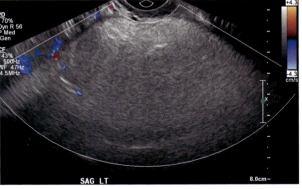

Fig. 13.6

 ▪ Cystic mass with a calcified echogenic dermoid plug or Rokitansky nodule/protuberance (arrow in Fig. 13.7). Avascular on CDUS (Fig. 13.8)

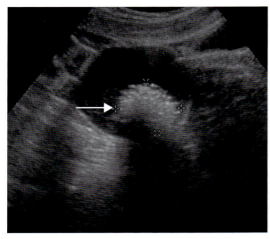

Fig. 13.7

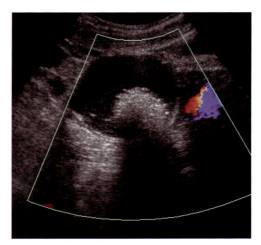

Fig. 13.8

- Shadowing calcification corresponding to bone or teeth (arrow in Fig. 13.9). CT scan shows dense calcification (arrow in Fig. 13.10)

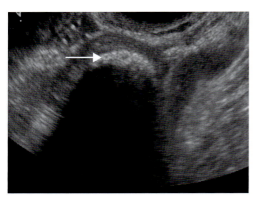

Fig. 13.9

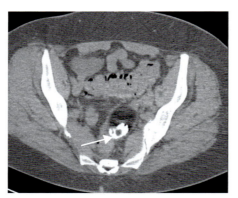

Fig. 13.10

- Dot–dash appearance or dermoid mesh corresponding to strands of hair
- Hair–fluid or fat–fluid levels
- Multiple floating mobile spherical echogenic masses
- Usually avascular on CDUS
► Complications include torsion, malignant transformation, or, rarely, rupture causing chemical peritonitis
► Homogeneously echogenic dermoid may mimic bowel gas on US exam and result in false-negative examination
► Hemorrhagic ovarian cyst or endometrioma
   - May be diffusely echogenic in the acute phase of hemorrhage
   - Demonstrates posterior acoustic enhancement rather than attenuation
   - Hemorrhagic cysts decrease in size and resolve over time, whereas a dermoid will remain stable
► Cystic epithelial neoplasm
   - Mural nodules will not be echogenic or attenuate sound and will be vascular
   - Septations go from wall to wall without demonstrating dot–dash sign and may demonstrate vascularity

Management

► If classic US appearance and < 6 cm, may not be surgically removed but yearly US follow-up recommended to ensure stability
► Growth or development of vascular solid components may herald malignant transformation
► If equivocal US appearance, further evaluation with CT or MRI
► Surgical removal for large (> 6 cm) or symptomatic lesions

Further Reading

1. Levine D, Brown DL, Andreotti RF, et al. Management of asymptomatic ovarian and adnexal cysts imaged at US: Society of Radiologists in Ultrasound consensus conference statement. *Ultrasound Q.* 2010; 26(3): 121–131.
2. Outwater E, Siegelman E, Hunt J. Ovarian teratomas: Tumor types and imaging characteristics. *RadioGraphics*. March 2001; 21: 475–490.

History

▶ 25-Year-old female with history of laparoscopic removal of "chocolate cysts" presents with chronic pelvic pain (Figs. 14.1–14.3)

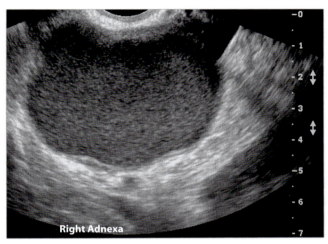

Fig. 14.1

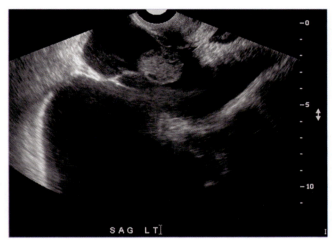

Fig. 14.2

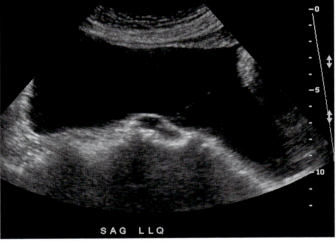

Fig. 14.3

Case 14 Peritoneal Inclusion Cyst

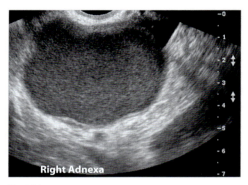

Fig. 14.4

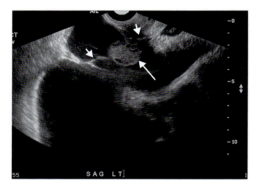

Fig. 14.5

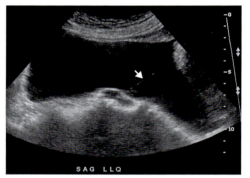

Fig. 14.6

Imaging Findings

► Homogeneous hypoechoic right adnexal cystic mass demonstrating increased through-transmission, "ground glass" appearance, and "shading" consistent with the diagnosis of endometrioma (Fig. 14.4). There was no internal vascularity on color Doppler imaging (not shown)
► Left lower quadrant anechoic, cystic mass with lobular contour, and thin septations (short arrows in Figs. 14.5 and 14.6)
► A morphologically normal-appearing ovary (long arrow in Fig. 14.5) is suspended by thin septations in the center of the cystic mass

Differential Diagnosis

► Paraovarian cyst
► Hydro/pyosalpinx
► Cystic epithelial ovarian neoplasm

Teaching Points

► Peritoneal inclusion cysts are reactive mesothelial-lined cystic structures that develop when ovarian exudate is trapped by peritoneal adhesions
► Occur most commonly secondary to adhesions from abdominal or pelvic surgery, endometriosis, pelvic inflammatory disease, inflammatory bowel disease, or trauma
► No malignant potential
► Clinical presentation: premenopausal women with above clinical history and chronic pelvic pain, bloating, or pelvic mass; may be an incidental finding
► US findings
  ▪ Anechoic, cystic mass with angular, lobular, or irregular configuration conforming to the shape of surrounding pelvic structures
  ▪ Septations
  ▪ Normal ovary found suspended centrally or at edge of the collection

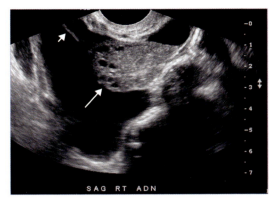 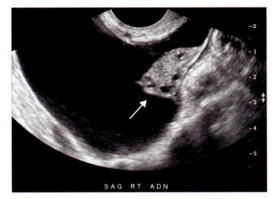

Fig. 14.7　　　　　　　　　　　　　　　　　Fig. 14.8

Second patient with a peritoneal inclusion cyst. Note lobular cystic right adnexal mass with thin septation (short arrow in Fig. 14.7) and normal ovary at periphery (long arrow in Fig. 14.7 and arrow in Fig. 14.8).

▶ Paraovarian cysts: round or oval, completely anechoic adnexal cyst, no septations, clearly separate from the ovary (echogenic fat plane often seen between paraovarian cyst and ovary)

▶ Hydro/pyosalpinx: tubular, serpiginous "S"- or "V"-shaped adnexal structure, may have "waist sign" (indentations of the wall on opposite sides of the dilated tube usually between the ampulla and body), "incomplete septation" sign due to mucosal folds or folding of the tube on itself, separate from the ovary
   ▪ Internal echoes, which may layer, indicate debris, pyosalpinx, or hematosalpinx
   ▪ Mural vascularity suggests acute infection

▶ Cystic epithelial ovarian neoplasm: arises from the ovary, may have mural nodules, septations, internal echoes; wall, mural nodules and/or septations may be vascular; will not have such an irregular/lobular shape; the normal ovary will not be identified separately within the mass engulfed by fluid

Management

▶ If imaging is classic for peritoneal inclusion cyst: no follow-up is necessary

▶ If diagnosis suspected but US appearance is not definitive (e.g., thick septations, normal ovary not clearly seen, no history consistent with formation of pelvic adhesions, postmenopausal patient): consider MRI

▶ Conservative treatment: leave alone versus oral contraceptives to suppress ovulation (decrease formation of exudative fluid)

▶ If symptomatic, can be aspirated or surgically removed: however, recurrence rate is high following surgery (30–50%)

Further Reading

1. Brown DL, Dudiak KM, Laing FC. Adnexal masses: US characterization and reporting. *Radiology*. 2010; 254: 342–354.
2. Moyle PL, Kataoka MY, Nakai A, et al. Nonovarian cystic lesions of the pelvis. *RadioGraphics*. 2010; 30: 921–938.
3. Levine D, Brown DL, Andreotti RF, et al. Management of asymptomatic and ovarian and other adnexal cysts imaged at US: Society of Radiologists in Ultrasound consensus conference statement. *Radiology*. 2010; 256: 943–954.

Case 15

History

▶52-Year-old female with intermittent pelvic pain (Figs. 15.1 and 15.2)

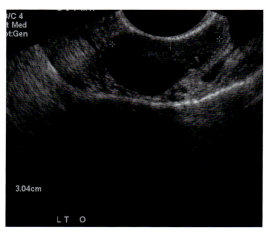

Fig. 15.1

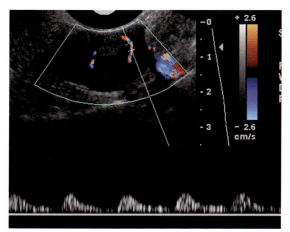

Fig. 15.2

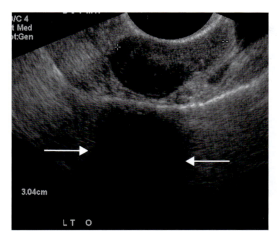

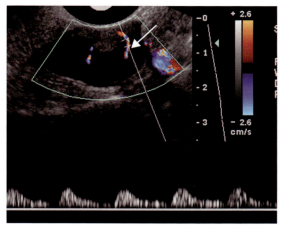

Fig. 15.3   Fig. 15.4

Imaging Findings

▶ Well-circumscribed, markedly hypoechoic solid left ovarian mass with posterior shadowing (arrows in Fig. 15.3)
▶ Arterial internal vascularity on color Doppler US (CDUS) (arrow in Fig. 15.4)

Differential Diagnosis

▶ Subserosal or broad ligament fibroid
▶ Granulosa cell tumor
▶ Dysgerminoma

Teaching Points

▶ Ovarian fibromas and fibrothecomas are benign ovarian tumors arising from the ovarian stroma accounting for 1–4% of all ovarian neoplasms
▶ 70% occur in perimenopausal or postmenopausal females
▶ Most commonly, they present as an incidental finding in asymptomatic patients
▶ Difficult to distinguish from each other on imaging or pathology
▶ Histologic differentiation is based on the percentage and density of thecal cells
▶ Can present with ascites and pleural effusion in the setting of Meig's syndrome
▶ Characteristic US appearance
   ▪ Markedly hypoechoic mass with posterior shadowing due to dense fibrous tissue arising from the ovary (arrows in Fig. 15.3, 15.5, and 15.6)

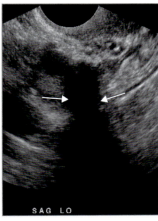

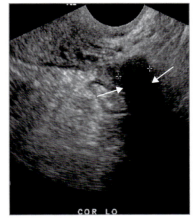

Fig. 15.5   Fig. 15.6

- May contain internal vascularity (arrow in Fig. 15.4)
- However, variable appearance and larger lesions may be more heterogeneous, and not all will have dense acoustic shadowing
► MRI appearance
  - Hypointense on both T1-weighted images (arrow in Fig. 15.7) and T2-weighted images (arrow in Fig. 15.8). MR images as well as with minimal post-contrast enhancement (arrow in Fig. 15.9)

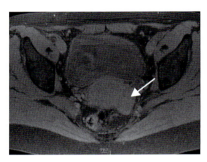 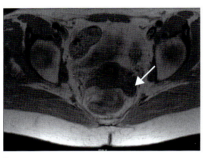 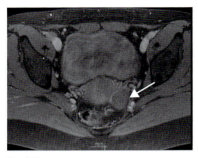

Fig. 15.7   Fig. 15.8   Fig. 15.9

► Subserosal or broad ligament fibroids may present as solid adnexal masses mimicking ovarian fibroma/fibrothecoma; however, they are connected to the uterus and on CDUS show blood supply arising from the uterus through a connecting vessel. The ovary will be seen separately
► Granulosa cell tumors have varied sonographic appearance from small solid ovarian masses to multilocular cystic lesions, sometimes with hemorrhage and fibrosis. Clinical signs of estrogen production. Low malignant potential
► Dysgerminomas are malignant germ cell tumors composed of undifferentiated germ cells. Occur predominantly in women < 30 years old. On US, solid ovarian mass with fibrous septations and increased vascularity

Management

► Imaging with MRI may confirm diagnosis
► Surgical consultation and most often surgically removed because one cannot always differentiate from other possibly malignant solid ovarian masses
► Definitive diagnosis by histologic appearance

Further Reading

1. Jeong Y-Y, Outwater EK, Kang HK. Imaging evaluation of ovarian masses. *RadioGraphics*. 2000; 20(5): 1445–1147.
2. Brown DL, Doubilet PM, Miller FH, et al. Benign and malignant ovarian masses: Selection of the most discriminating grayscale and Doppler sonographic features. *Radiology*. 1998; 208(1): 103–110.
3. Leung SW, Yuen PM. Ovarian fibroma: A review on the clinical characteristics, diagnostic difficulties, and management options of 23 cases. *Gynecol Obstet Invest*. 2006; 62: 1–6.

Case 16

History

- 22-Year-old woman, 6 weeks pregnant, presents with sudden onset of severe left lower quadrant pain (Figs. 16.1–16.4)

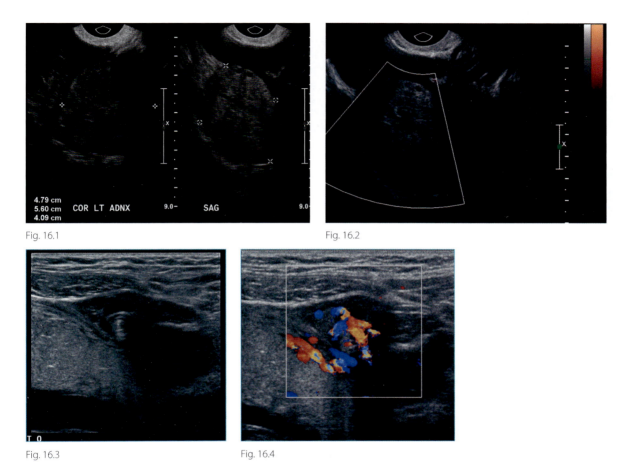

Fig. 16.1

Fig. 16.2

Fig. 16.3

Fig. 16.4

Case 16 Ovarian Torsion

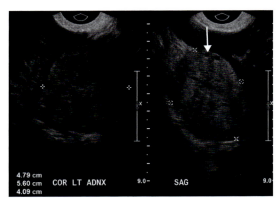

Fig. 16.5

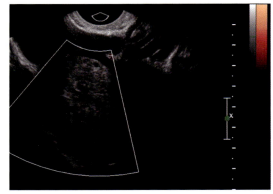

Fig. 16.6

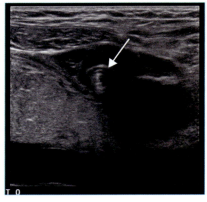

Fig. 16.7

Imaging Findings

▶ Enlarged left ovary with prominent heterogeneous central stroma and peripherally displaced tiny follicles (arrow in Fig. 16.5)
▶ Absent flow within the left ovary on power Doppler US (Fig. 16.6)
▶ Target sign of twisted pedicle on grayscale US (arrow in Fig. 16.7)

Differential Diagnosis

▶ Massive edema of the ovary
▶ Unilateral polycystic ovarian syndrome (PCOS)

Teaching Points

▶ Ovarian torsion: consequence of twisting of the adnexal vascular pedicle. In the majority of cases, the fallopian tube is involved as well. Initially, blockage of venous and lymphatic outflow from the ovary results in edematous enlargement of the affected ovary. Arterial supply is subsequently compromised, leading to ischemia and hemorrhage within the ovary and ultimately necrosis
▶ Classical clinical presentation: acute onset of severe lower abdominal pain, nausea, and vomiting. However, pain may be mild or intermittent in up to 50% of cases
▶ Women of reproductive age are most commonly affected. An underlying ovarian mass, usually a large cyst or a cystic teratoma, often is present, acting like a fulcrum and predisposing the ovary to torsion. Ovarian torsion is more common in young girls, in whom mobility of the adnexal ligament predisposes to torsion. Ovarian torsion is rare following menopause and usually related to an underlying ovarian mass. There is increased risk of ovarian torsion in pregnancy
▶ Additional findings on US include abnormal midline location of the torsed ovary as well as visualization of the twisted pedicle with coiled adnexal vessels appearing as a round or tubular mass adjacent to the enlarged ovary giving the appearance of a "target" or "whirlpool" sign (arrows in Figs. 16.8 and 16.9)

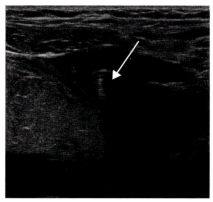

Fig. 16.8

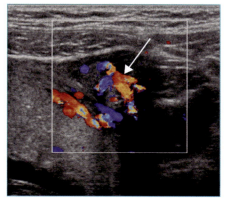

Fig. 16.9

▶ Absent or decreased vascularity within the ovary on CDUS. The presence of Doppler flow within the ovary does *not* exclude the diagnosis of ovarian torsion

▶ Massive edema of the ovary: results from venous and lymphatic blockage of the ovary and appears sonographically similar to ovarian torsion

▶ Unilateral PCOS: rare, usually a bilateral process with enlarged or normal-sized ovaries containing multiple (> 12) peripherally placed small follicles (< 10 mm)

Management

▶ Emergent surgical intervention

Further Reading

1. Albayram F, Hamper UM. Ovarian and adnexal torsion: Spectrum of sonographic findings with pathologic correlation. *J Ultrasound Med.* 2001; 20: 1083–1089.
2. Chang HC, Bhatt S, Dogra VS. Pearls and pitfalls in diagnosis of ovarian torsion. *RadioGraphics*: 2008; 28: 1355–1368.
3. Sibal M. Follicular ring sign: A simple sonographic sign for early diagnosis of ovarian torsion. *J Ultrasound Med.* 2012; 31: 1803–1809.

Case 17

History

▶28-Year-old female with history of nonviable early pregnancy, treated with misoprostol, presents to the emergency department with fever, chills, and heavy vaginal bleeding (Figs. 17.1–17.4)

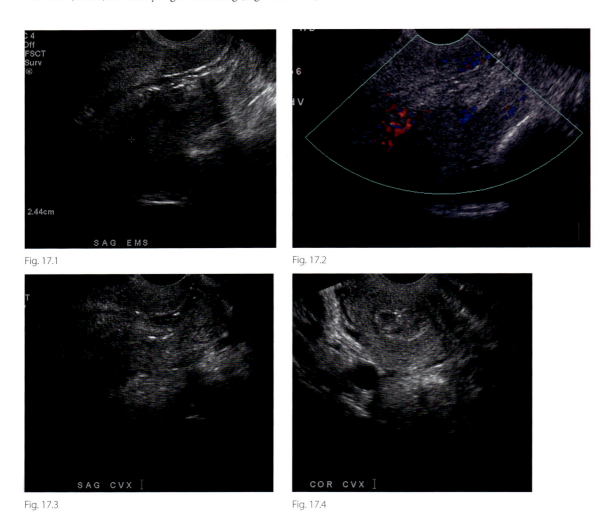

Fig. 17.1

Fig. 17.2

Fig. 17.3

Fig. 17.4

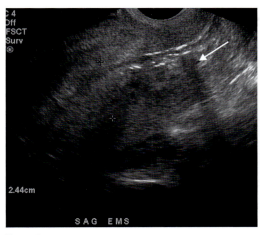

Fig. 17.5

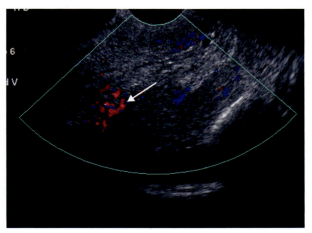

Fig. 17.6

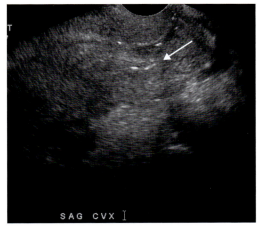

Fig. 17.7

Imaging Findings

► Thickened endometrium (up to 2.4 cm between cursors) with tiny linear echogenic foci with "dirty" posterior acoustic shadowing (arrow in Fig. 17.5)
► Increased focal vascularity on CDUS (arrow in Fig. 17.6)
► Thickened echogenic material in cervix with punctate echogenic foci without posterior shadowing (arrow in Fig. 17.7)

Differential Diagnosis

► Normal postpartum/post-abortion findings
► Bland hemorrhage

Teaching Points

► Endometritis
   ▪ Caused by infections such as chlamydia, gonorrhea, tuberculosis, or mixed normal vaginal bacteria
   ▪ Increased risk after medical procedures such as dilatation and curettage(D&C), hysteroscopy, and placement of an intrauterine contraceptive device
   ▪ Commonly found in association with pelvic inflammatory disease or postpartum
► Clinical symptoms: fever, abnormal vaginal bleeding and purulent discharge, lower abdominal and pelvic pain
► US findings

- Thickened heterogeneous endometrium
- Fluid (simple or complex) within endometrial cavity (arrow in Fig. 17.8)
- Gas—echogenic often linear or punctate foci with or without dirty distal acoustic shadowing (arrow in Fig. 17.9)
- Variable vascularity, usually increased with increased diastolic flow

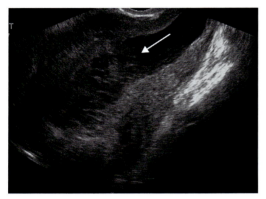 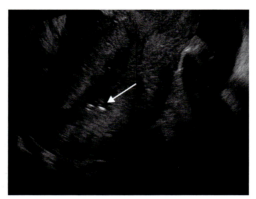

Fig. 17.8   Fig. 17.9

▶ Normal postpartum/post-abortion: important to recognize because gas can be seen in approximately 20% of normal women in the first 2–4 weeks after uncomplicated vaginal delivery
▶ Bland hemorrhage: echogenic, avascular material within the endometrial canal without focal echogenic foci or posterior shadowing

Management

▶ Clinical correlation is most important when endometrial echogenic foci suggestive of gas are seen in a postpartum or post-abortion patient
▶ Antibiotics if just endometritis
▶ D&C for definitive pathologic diagnosis if suspected associated retained products of conception

Further Reading

1. Wachsberg RH, Kurtz AB. Gas within the endometrial cavity at postpartum ultrasound: A normal finding after spontaneous vaginal delivery. *Radiology*. 1996; 199: 757–759.
2. Savelli S, Pilu G, Valeri B, et al. Transvaginal sonographic appearance of anaerobic endometritis. *Ultrasound Obstet Gynecol*. 2003; 21: 623–624.

History

▶34-Year-old female presenting with abdominal cramping, vaginal spotting, and a missing intrauterine device (IUD) string (Figs. 18.1–18.3)

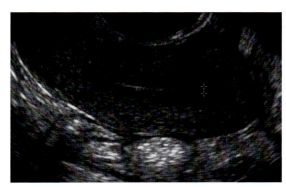

Fig. 18.1

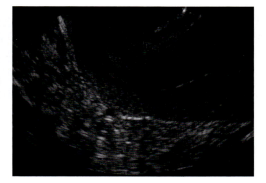

Fig. 18.2

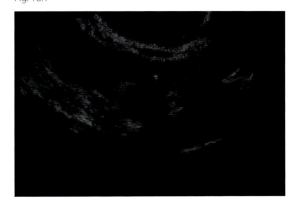

Fig. 18.3

Case 18   Misplaced Intrauterine Device

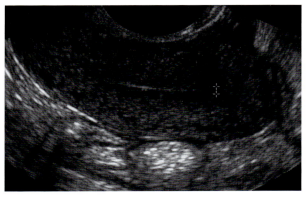

Fig. 18.4

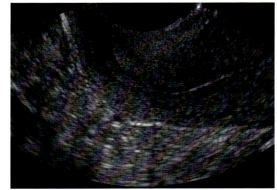

Fig. 18.5

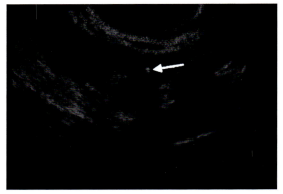

Fig. 18.6

Imaging Findings

► Empty endometrial cavity and endocervical canal (Figs. 18.4 and 18.5)
► Cross arm of the IUD presents as tiny echogenic focus adjacent to a normal-appearing right ovary in the right adnexa (arrow in Fig. 18.6)

Differential Diagnosis

► IUD expulsion
► IUD embedment
► Uterine/visceral perforation

Teaching Points

► IUD's contraceptive efficacy is related to appropriate intrauterine location
► Intra-abdominal migration may lead to more serious complications (e.g., adhesions, fistula, bowel perforation, infection, or abscess) and will not prevent pregnancy
► Radiographs in this patient demonstrate the IUD in the right side of the pelvis rotated 180° from its normal orientation, which is concerning for complete uterine perforation and migration (arrows in Fig. 18.7 and 18.8)

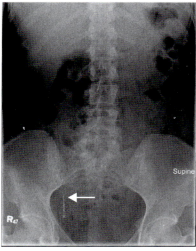
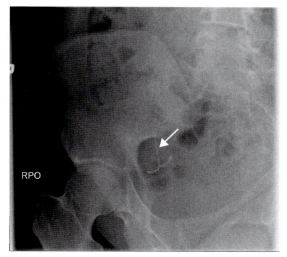

Fig. 18.7

Fig. 18.8

▶ Properly placed IUD
   ▪ Three-dimensional (3D) US is the state-of-the-art method for confirming proper IUD placement
   ▪ Stem is straight and entirely within the endometrial cavity on 2D imaging (arrow in Fig. 18.9); however, proper or improper location of the side arms is only appreciated on 3D US (Fig. 18.10)
   ▪ In proper location, side arms extend laterally in the uterine fundus (arrows in Fig. 18.10)
   ▪ In improper location, side arm displacement burrows into the adjacent myometrium (arrow in Fig. 18.11)

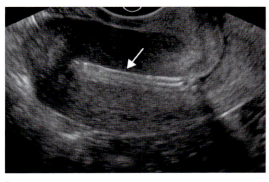
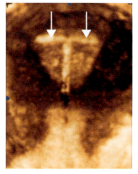

Fig. 18.9

Fig. 18.10

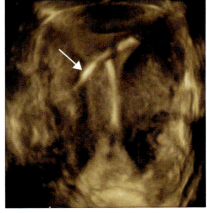

Fig. 18.11

- Intrauterine misplacement in the cervix is seen on 2D US (arrow in Fig. 18.12); however, 3D US demonstrates arms of the IUD embedded into the adjacent musculature of the cervix (arrows in Fig. 18.13)

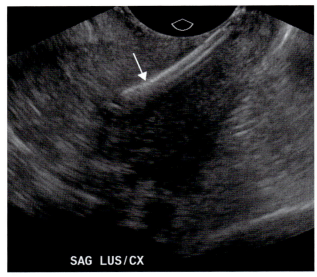

Fig. 18.12

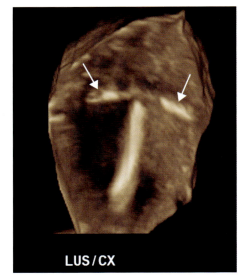

Fig. 18.13

- ▶ A missing IUD string is a common indication for US evaluation
  - 3D US can demonstrate normal position of the IUD (short arrow in Fig. 18.11), with the missing string retracted into the uterine cavity (long arrows in Fig. 18.11 and Fig. 18.12)

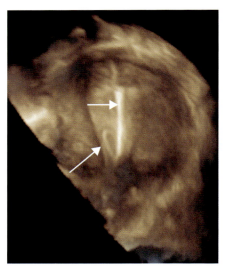

Fig. 18.14

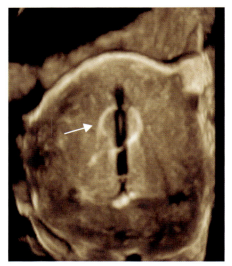

Fig. 18.15

- ▶ CT or MR or plain film X-ray may be necessary to
  - Differentiate perforation from displacement (Figs. 18.7 and 18.8)
  - Evaluate complications associated with intra-abdominal IUDs, such as visceral perforation, abscess formation, and bowel obstruction
- ▶ Visualized IUD in an inappropriate location, not embedded in the myometrium, militates against an expelled or embedded IUD
- ▶ Suspected expulsion must be conveyed in radiology report with exclusion of intraperitoneal location by abdomino-pelvic radiography
- ▶ Perforation may be partial with embedment in myometrium or complete transuterine perforation with migration into the peritoneal cavity

Management

▶ Empiric antibiotics for embedment or perforation

▶ Removal of displaced IUD recommended because it is less effective for contraception and more likely to be expelled

▶ Asymptomatic perforated IUD should be laparoscopically removed as soon as possible after diagnosis to reduce adhesion formation

▶ Urgent surgical intervention in symptomatic or complicated cases

▶ In displaced IUD and synchronous pregnancy, removal depends on location and gestational age, with risks weighed against benefits

Further Reading

1. Boortz HE, Margolis DJA, Ragavendra N, et al. Migration of intrauterine devices: Radiologic findings and implications for patient care. *RadioGraphics* April 2012; 32(2): 335–352.

2. Betlem G, Hereter L, Pascual MA, et al. Normal and abnormal images of intrauterine devices: Role of three-dimensional sonography. *J Clin Ultrasound* 2012; 40(7): 433–438.

Case 19

► 42-Year-old female with history of intermenstrual bleeding and menorrhagia (Figs. 19.1 and 19.2)

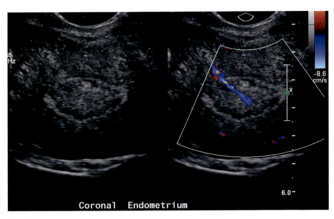

Fig. 19.1

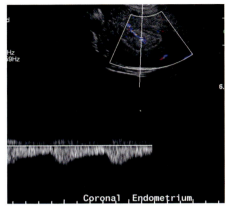

Fig. 19.2

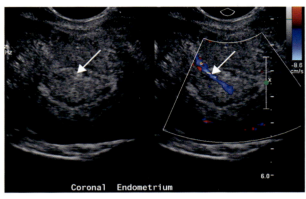
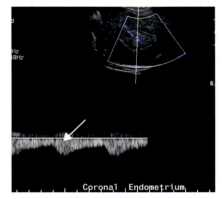

Fig. 19.3

Fig. 19.4

Imaging Findings

▶ Focal echogenic endometrial mass (arrows in Fig. 19.3)
▶ CDUS shows central feeding vessel with arterial flow (arrows in Figs. 19.3 and 19.4)

Differential Diagnosis

▶ Endometrial hyperplasia
▶ Tamoxifen changes
▶ Endometrial cancer
▶ Submucosal leiomyoma

Teaching Points

▶ Endometrial polyps
  ▪ Overgrowth of endometrial tissue covered by an epithelial layer with either broad-based or pedunculated attachment
  ▪ Solitary or multiple
  ▪ May manifest with intermenstrual bleeding, menorrhagia, or postmenopausal bleeding; however, many patients are asymptomatic
  ▪ On endovaginal US, endometrial polyps appear as a focal mass. The mass may be echogenic or contain small cystic spaces. On CDUS, a central vessel within the stalk may be seen
  ▪ Saline infusion sonohysterography (SIS) more clearly outlines the polypoid endometrial mass (arrows in Fig. 19.5)

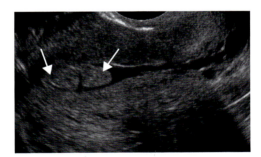

Fig. 19.5

- 3D US has proven to be an effective alternative to SIS for the diagnosis of endometrial polyps (arrow in Fig. 19.6)

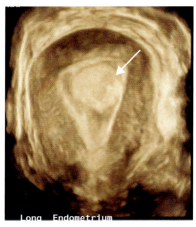

Fig. 19.6

► Endometrial hyperplasia
  - Diffuse endometrial thickening and often cystic spaces on endovaginal US
  - May have minimal vascularity; however, not central and stalk-like
► Tamoxifen changes
  - Patients on tamoxifen for treatment or prevention of breast cancer are at increased risk of endometrial hyperplasia, polyps, and possibly a slight increased risk of endometrial cancer because of the estrogen agonist effect of the drug on the estrogen receptors in the endometrium
  - Risk is related to cumulative dose
► Endometrial cancer
  - Associated with marked endometrial thickening, heterogeneous endometrial echotexture, irregular poorly defined endometrial borders, and irregular vascularity
► Submucosal leiomyomas
  - Broad-based hypoechoic masses covered by an echogenic endometrium. On CDUS, diffuse vascularity may be seen

Management

► In patients with endometrial thickening, 3D US or sonohysterography are helpful in differentiating endometrial hyperplasia, polyps, and submucosal leiomyoma
► In patients with postmenopausal bleeding and endometrial thickness > 4 or 5 mm, histologic sampling with endometrial biopsy or curettage is recommended to exclude endometrial cancer
► If a polyp is suspected or confirmed on 3D US or sonohysterography, sampling and removal under hysteroscopic guidance is performed if the polyp is large and symptomatic
► If the polyp is small and in asymptomatic patients, it may be followed sonographically

Further Reading

1. Davidson KG, Dubinsky TJ. Ultrasonographic evaluation of the endometrium in postmenopausal vaginal bleeding. *Radiol Clin North Am.* 2003; 41: 769–780.
2. Kalampokas T, Sofoudis C, Anastasopoulos C, et al. Effect of tamoxifen on postmenopausal endometrium. *Eur J Gynaecol Oncol.* 2013; 34(4): 325–328.

History

▶ 47-Year-old female with irregular vaginal bleeding (Figs. 20.1–20.3)

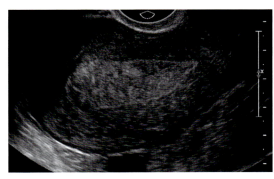

Fig. 20.1

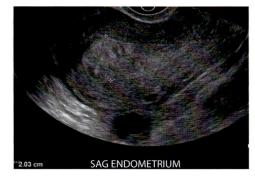

Fig. 20.2

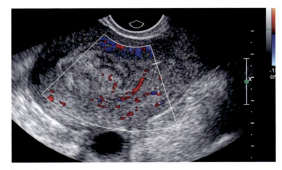

Fig. 20.3

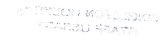

Case 20 Endometrial Hyperplasia

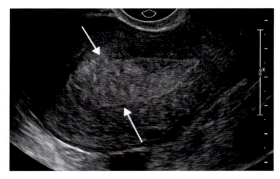

Fig. 20.4

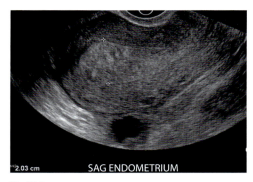

Fig. 20.5

Fig. 20.6

Imaging Findings

▶ Diffusely thickened, slightly heterogeneous endometrium (arrows in Fig. 20.4 and calipers in Fig. 20.5), measuring 20 mm
▶ Sparse vascularity on color Doppler US (CDUS) (Fig. 20.6)
▶ Sharp, regular endometrial/myometrial interface

Differential Diagnosis

▶ Normal secretory endometrium
▶ Endometrial cancer (CA)
▶ Endometrial polyp
▶ Tamoxifen effect on endometrium

Teaching Points

▶ Pathology: extensive proliferation of endometrial glands with increased ratio of glands to stroma
  ▪ Cystic dilatation of glands results in cystic endometrial hyperplasia (EH)
▶ Two categories: EH without cellular atypia and EH with cellular atypia
  ▪ EH without atypia < 2% risk of progression to endometrial CA
  ▪ 25% of patients with atypical EH will develop endometrial CA
▶ Presentation: asymptomatic, or menorrhagia, metrorrhagia, vaginal spotting
▶ Risk factors: anything that increases estrogen exposure, such as chronic anovulatory states, polycystic ovarian syndrome, unopposed exogenous estrogen, tamoxifen therapy, obesity, estrogen-secreting ovarian tumors (granulosa cell CA)
▶ Decreased risk: long-term oral contraceptives
▶ US findings
  ▪ Diffusely thickened homogeneous, echogenic endometrium, may be heterogeneous
  ▪ Endometrial thickness > 16–18 mm in premenopausal women during secretory phase, > 8 mm during proliferative phase, or > 5 mm in postmenopausal women considered abnormal
  ▪ ± Small cystic areas
  ▪ ± Increased vascularity on CDUS, may see multiple feeding vessels
  ▪ Endometrial/myometrial interface or subendometrial halo sharp and well-defined without irregularity

- ▶ Secretory endometrium: homogeneously echogenic endometrium that is indistinguishable from EH, but endometrial thickness will measure < 15–18 mm
- ▶ Endometrial CA: may mimic US findings of EH (homogeneously echogenic endometrial thickening)
  - ▪ However, endometrium more likely to demonstrate irregular thickening, heterogeneity, cystic spaces, focal mass (especially if heterogeneous and lobular), increased vascularity with an irregular pattern or distribution
  - ▪ Disruption or irregularity of endometrial/myometrial interface or subendometrial halo and direct invasion of an endometrial mass into the subjacent myometrium or cervix are the most specific findings for endometrial CA
  - ▪ May coexist with EH
  - ▪ Probability of endometrial cancer increases with age and endometrial thickness
- ▶ Polyp: echogenic endometrial mass, single feeding vessel, ± cystic spaces

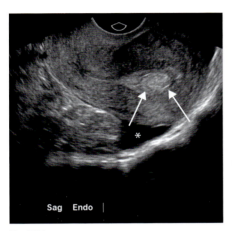

Fig. 20.7

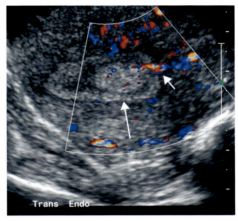

Fig. 20.8

Note focal echogenic endometrial mass (arrows in Fig. 20.7 and long arrow in Fig. 20.8) with a single feeding vessel on the color Doppler image (short arrow in Fig. 20.8) in a patient presenting with intermenstrual bleeding consistent with an endometrial polyp. The uterus is retroverted, and there is a small amount of free fluid in the cul-de-sac (asterisk in Fig. 20.7).

- ▶ Tamoxifen or selective estrogen receptor modulators: Adjuvant or prophylactic therapy for breast cancer, but have agonistic effect on endometrial receptors causing increased incidence of EH, polyps, and endometrial CA. US findings nonspecific but often see anechoic cystic areas within thickened endometrium (1.52 cm) (calipers in Fig. 20.9), as in Fig. 20.9 of a postmenopausal woman with breast cancer being treated with tamoxifen. Cysts in the subjacent myometrium may also be seen, possibly secondary to adenomyosis, which has also been associated with tamoxifen therapy

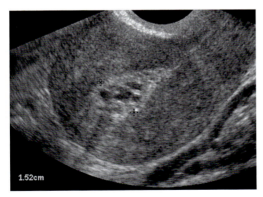

Fig. 20.9

Management

► 3D transvaginal US: best imaging modality for evaluation of a thick endometrium
► Saline infusion sonohysterography can be used to differentiate diffuse from focal pathology. Hysteroscopic sampling is generally recommended for focal disease rather than dilatation and curettage or pipelle sampling of the endometrium, which is adequate for diffuse endometrial pathology
► Conservative or hormonal therapy if no atypia
► Curettage for atypia; simple hysterectomy occasionally performed

Further Reading

1. Nalaboff KM, Pellerito JS, Ben-Levi E. Imaging the endometrium: Disease and normal variants. *RadioGraphics*. 2001; 21: 1409–1424.
2. Montgomery BE, Daum GS, Dunton CJ. Endometrial hyperplasia: A review. *Obstet Gynecol Surv*. 2004; 59: 368–378.
3. Armstrong AJ, Hurd WW, Elguero S, et al. Diagnosis and management of endometrial hyperplasia. *J Minim Invasive Gynecol*. 2012; 19: 562–571.

History

▶ 43-Year-old female presents with lower abdominal pain and palpable right adnexal mass (Figs. 21.1–21.3)

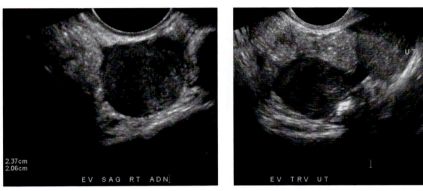

Fig. 21.1

Fig. 21.2

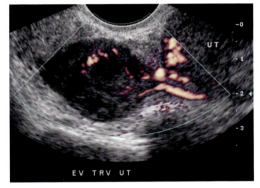

Fig. 21.3

Case 21 Pedunculated Subserosal Leiomyoma

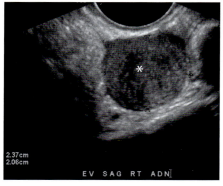

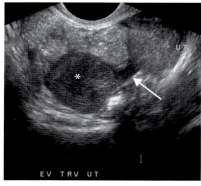

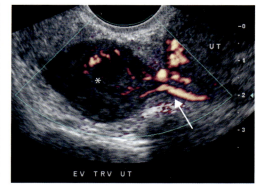

Fig. 21.4

Fig. 21.5

Fig. 21.6

Imaging Findings

▶ Solid right adnexal mass (asterisks in Figs. 21.4–21.6) with similar echotexture to myometrium (UT, uterus; Figs. 21.5 and 21.6)
▶ Note soft tissue pedicle (arrow in Fig. 21.5) connecting the mass (asterisk) to the serosal surface of the uterus (UT). The mass is similar in echotexture to the myometrium
▶ Power Doppler image (Fig. 21.6) demonstrating vascularity in mass (asterisk), pedicle (arrow), and adjacent myometrium

Differential Diagnosis

▶ Ovarian fibroma
▶ Thecoma/fibrothecoma
▶ Dysgerminoma
▶ Gastrointestinal stromal tumor (GIST)

Teaching Points

▶ Leiomyoma: benign smooth muscle uterine neoplasm found in up to 25–50% of women
  ▪ Higher incidence in African American women
▶ Presentation: asymptomatic, menometrorrhagia, anemia, infertility, or symptoms related to mass effect such as constipation, frequent urination, pelvic pain/pressure
▶ Described based on location of epicenter as submucosal, intramural, or subserosal
▶ US findings of subserosal leiomyoma
  ▪ Solid adnexal mass
  ▪ Echotexture similar to myometrium
  ▪ Broad-based or pedunculated (narrow bridge of soft tissue) attachment to serosal surface of the uterus
  ▪ Color or power Doppler imaging may demonstrate vascularity within leiomyoma (peripheral more common than central as with all leiomyomata) as well as blood vessels extending from the myometrium into the leiomyoma; especially helpful in identifying the stalk of a pedunculated leiomyoma
  ▪ Identification of ovary separate from the mass as well as direct connection of the mass to the uterus allows confident diagnosis
▶ Provocative maneuvers such as applying pressure to the anterior abdominal wall or gentle direct pressure on an adnexal mass with the transvaginal probe may help determine if the mass is connected to versus separate from the uterus or visualize the bridge of soft tissue connecting the leiomyoma to the uterus
▶ A pedunculated leiomyoma may mimic a solid ovarian mass or other solid adnexal pathology. Hence, identification of the connection to the uterus and separation of the mass from the ovary are critical US findings
▶ Ovarian fibroma: benign ovarian mass of sex cord–stromal (mesenchymal) origin, composed largely of spindle cells or fibroblasts with densely packed collagen, most common in middle-aged women
  ▪ US findings: solid ovarian mass, often extremely hypoechoic with dense posterior acoustic shadowing
  ▪ US appearance may be very similar to a leiomyoma
  ▪ Partial rim of surrounding ovarian parenchyma ("claw sign") helps confirm that the mass arises from the ovary
  ▪ 1% associated with ascites and pleural effusions (Meig's syndrome)
▶ Thecoma: also a sex cord–stromal ovarian tumor, composed of theca cells, estrogen secreting, most common in postmenopausal women of whom 60% present with postmenopausal bleeding, 20% will have endometrial cancer, also associated with endometrial hyperplasia

- US findings: solid ovarian mass of variable echogenicity, thick endometrium ± endometrial mass
▶ Fibrothecoma: combines histologic elements of fibroma and thecoma
  - US findings: solid ovarian mass, round to oval, occasionally lobular, echogenicity and degree of posterior shadowing depend on relative amount of collagen/fibrous tissue, often heterogeneous
▶ Dysgerminoma: uncommon ovarian malignancy
  - US findings: solid ovarian mass, lobular contour, no posterior shadowing, vascular, areas of cystic degeneration common (especially if large), associated with endometrial hyperplasia and thickened endometrium
▶ GIST: solid, homogeneous hypoechoic mass arising from bowel wall without posterior shadowing, large tumors may have necrotic areas, ovaries separate

Management

▶ If US findings are not diagnostic, MR is the optimal imaging modality to determine the origin of a solid adnexal mass
▶ MR appearance of pedunculated leiomyoma
  - Low signal intensity on T1- and T2-weighted images
  - Gadolinium enhancement
  - Demonstration of pedicle connecting leiomyoma to uterus
  - Visualization of the ovary separate from the mass

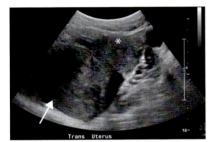 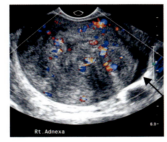 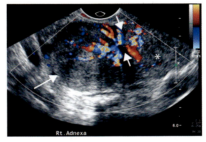

Fig. 21.7   Fig. 21.8   Fig. 21.9

Pelvic US performed in a 45-year-old female presenting with a palpable adnexal mass and bloating demonstrates a large solid, vascular right adnexal mass (arrow in Fig. 21.7 and long arrow in Fig. 21.9) adjacent to uterus (asterisks in Figs. 21.7 and 21.9). There are blood vessels (short arrow in Fig. 21.9) that appear to connect the mass to the uterus, but a direct attachment could not be convincingly visualized, and the right ovary was not identified. Note the small amount of adjacent free fluid (black arrow in Fig. 21.8) as well as substantial internal vascularity on color Doppler, increasing concern for malignancy.

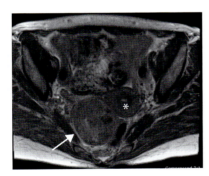 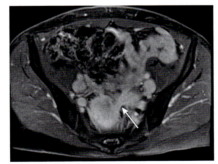

Fig. 21.10   Fig. 21.11

Follow-up pelvic MRI demonstrating a low signal intensity right adnexal mass on T2-weighted axial image (arrow in Fig. 21.10) adjacent to the uterus (asterisk in Fig. 21.10). On a more cephalad T1-weighted fat sat post contrast axial image, an enhancing pedicle (arrow in Fig. 21.11) is clearly visualized connecting the leiomyoma to the uterus.
▶ Medical management with hormonal therapy: oral contraceptives or gonadotropin-releasing hormone analogue therapy
▶ Hysteroscopic (for submucosal leiomyomata) or laparoscopic myomectomy

▸ Uterine fibroid embolization (UFE): minimally invasive treatment for leiomyomata with reported outcomes similar to standard surgical approaches
  ▪ A pedunculated subserosal leiomyoma with a thin stalk, as in this case, is a relative (although not absolute) contraindication for UFE because the infarcted tumor can be expelled into the peritoneal space and serve as a nidus for infection

Further Reading

1. Bulman JC, Ascher SM, Spies JB. Current concepts in uterine fibroid embolization. *RadioGraphics*. 2012; 32(6): 1735–1750.
2. Ghai S, Rajan DK, Benjamin MS, et al. Uterine artery embolization for leiomyomas: Pre- and postprocedural evaluation with US. *RadioGraphics*. 2005; 25(5): 1159–1172.

Case 22

History

- 27-Year-old female with history of frequent miscarriages (Figs. 22.1–22.4)

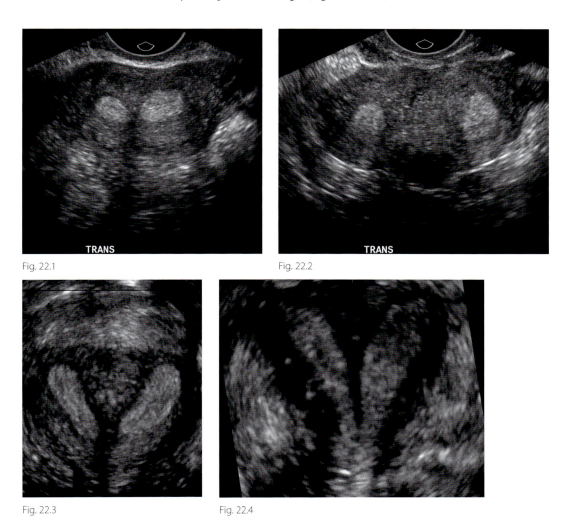

Fig. 22.1

Fig. 22.2

Fig. 22.3

Fig. 22.4

Case 22 Septate Uterus

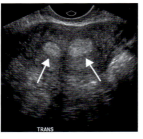

Fig. 22.5

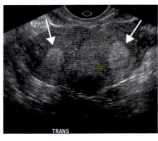

Fig. 22.6

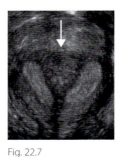

Fig. 22.7

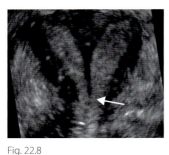

Fig. 22.8

Imaging Findings

► The two echogenic endometrial canals are close together in the lower uterine segment (arrows in Fig. 22.5) but become divergent in the uterine fundus (arrows in Fig. 22.6)
► The fundal contour (arrow in Fig. 22.7) is flat on reconstructed multiplanar 3D image, and the hypoechoic septum extends to the level of the internal os (arrow in Fig. 22.8)

Differential Diagnosis

► Arcuate uterus
► Bicornuate uterus
► Didelphys uterus

Teaching Points

► Septate uterus (American Society for Reproductive Medicine class V) is the most common Müllerian duct anomaly (MDA)
  ▪ Results from partial or complete failure of septal resorption following fusion of the Müllerian ducts
  ▪ Associated with the worst reproductive/obstetric outcomes of all MDAs, with increased risk of first-trimester pregnancy loss (65%), premature birth (20%), and intrauterine growth retardation
► Key differential feature between a septate and bicornuate uterus is the configuration of the fundal contour
  ▪ 3D ultrasound or MRI best means of depicting the fundal contour
  ▪ Hysterosalpingogram outlines endometrial cavities but not fundal contour
► US findings of septate uterus
  ▪ Convex, flat, or minimally indented (< 1 cm) fundal contour between the two uterine horns
  ▪ Endometrial cavities most commonly parallel and symmetric, but they can be divergent in fundus
  ▪ The septum usually is composed of myometrial tissue in the fundus but fibrous tissue inferiorly, appearing hypoechoic
  ▪ The septum can extend to the external cervical os (complete), end above the internal os (partial), or end in the fundus (subseptate)

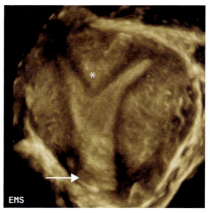

Fig. 22.9

Figure 22.9 shows 3D surface-rendered image from a patient with a subseptate uterus. The septum (asterisk) extends only partially into the endometrial canal and does not reach the level of the internal os (arrow) and cervix.

- ▶ Arcuate uterus
  - ▪ Class VI
  - ▪ Occurs secondary to nearly complete resorption of uterovaginal septum
  - ▪ Good reproductive outcome
  - ▪ Found in approximately 12% of women with repeated second-trimester pregnancy loss
  - ▪ US findings
    - • Convex external fundal contour
    - • Broad, shallow, rounded indentation of the fundal myometrium into the endometrial cavity creating a "heart-shaped" appearance of the echogenic endometrium
    - • Criteria for differentiating an arcuate from a subseptate uterus are not standardized

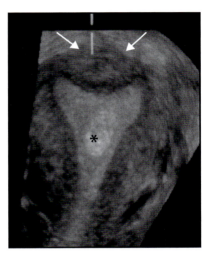 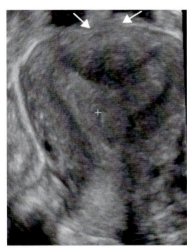

Fig. 22.10   Fig. 22.11

Figures 22.10 and 22.11 show an arcuate uterus in two different patients. 3D reconstructed multiplanar images demonstrate a convex fundal contour (arrows in Fig. 22.10) in the first patient, whereas the second patient has a flat fundal contour (arrows in Fig. 22.11). In both patients, the fundal myometrium minimally protrudes into the endometrial cavity, giving the echogenic endometrium a "heart-shaped" configuration. Note that the myometrial indentation is slightly deeper in the second patient (Fig. 22.11). There is a spectrum of appearances from the arcuate to the subseptate to the partial septate uterus, and there is no consensus on exact differential diagnostic criteria. Myometrial indentation more than 1 cm from the dome of the endometrial cavity is suggestive of a subseptate uterus. However, not all agree with this criterion. Note the echogenic endometrial polyp in the first patient (asterisk in Fig. 22.10).

- ▶ Bicornuate uterus
  - ▪ Class IV
  - ▪ Approximately 10% of Müllerian duct anomalies
  - ▪ Occurs secondary to incomplete fusion of the Müllerian ducts in the uterine fundus
  - ▪ The two horns fuse caudally, and the two endometrial cavities communicate at the isthmus above the level of the internal os
  - ▪ The cervix may be single or divided by a fibrous septum
  - ▪ 25% will have a vaginal septum
  - ▪ Often found incidentally
  - ▪ Infrequently associated with obstetrical complications
  - ▪ Increased incidence of cervical incompetence
  - ▪ US findings
    - • Deep cleft (> 1 cm) in external fundal contour between the two horns
    - • Widely divergent endometrial cavities (nonspecific finding)

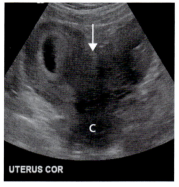

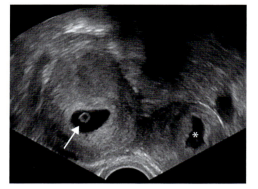

Fig. 22.12   Fig. 22.13

Transabdominal US images of a patient with a bicornuate uterus revealing a deep cleft between the two uterine horns (arrow in Fig. 22.12). Note intrauterine gestational sac in the right horn. There is a single cervix (C). On transvaginal US image, the two horns are widely splayed. Note intrauterine gestational sac with a yolk sac (arrow in Fig. 22.13) in the right horn and anechoic fluid distending the endometrial cavity of the left horn (asterisk in Fig. 22.13).

- ▶ Didelphys uterus
  - ▪ Class III
  - ▪ < 5% of Müllerian duct anomalies
  - ▪ Complete lack of fusion of the Müllerian ducts: two separate uterine horns and cervices; the two endometrial cavities do not communicate
  - ▪ 75% have a vaginal septum that may obstruct one horn
  - ▪ Non-obstructive variety usually asymptomatic and found incidentally
  - ▪ Patients with an obstructed horn may present with a pelvic or vaginal mass, dysmenorrhea, vaginal discharge, or pelvic pain
  - ▪ Increased risk of endometriosis, spontaneous abortion (21%), and preterm labor (24%)
  - ▪ US findings
    - • Two completely separate uterine horns
    - • Two cervices
    - • One horn may be obstructed

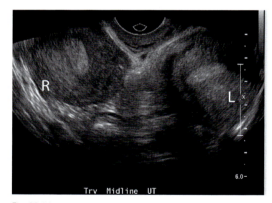

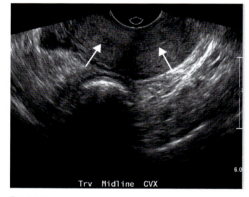

Fig. 22.14   Fig. 22.15

Figures 22.14 and 22.15 show two completely separate uterine horns (R and L in Fig. 22.14) and two separate cervices with separate endocervical canals (arrows in Fig. 22.15) in a patient with a didelphys uterus.

Management

- ▶ MDAs often associated with renal anomalies; hence, always assess both kidneys
- ▶ Septate uterus: hysteroscopic metroplasty will significantly improve reproductive outcomes and decrease spontaneous abortion rate
- ▶ Bicornuate uterus: may not require surgical intervention unless one horn is obstructed. If treatment is necessary, however, transabdominal metroplasty usually performed
- ▶ Arcuate uterus: no intervention required
- ▶ Didelphys uterus: no intervention unless obstructed

Acknowledgments

Figures 22.1–22.8 courtesy Dr. Marcela Bohm-Velez, Weinstein Imaging Associates, Pittsburgh, Pennsylvania. Figures 22.14 and 22.15 courtesy Dr. Lynwood Hammers, Hammers Healthcare, New Haven, Connecticut.

Further Reading

1. Bermejo C, Martinez Ten P, Cantarero R, et al. Three-dimensional ultrasound in the diagnosis of Müllerian duct anomalies and concordance with magnetic resonance imaging. *Ultrasound Obstet Gynecol*. 2010; 35: 593–601.
2. Steinkeler J, Woodfield C, Lazarus E, et al. Female infertility: A systematic approach to radiologic imaging and diagnosis. *RadioGraphics*. 2009; 29: 1353–1370.
3. Troiano R, McCarthy S. Mullerian duct anomalies: Imaging and clinical issues. *Radiology*. 2004; 233, 19–34.

Case 23

History

▶ 41-Year-old female presents with vaginal bleeding and inability to tolerate pelvic examination (Figs. 23.1–23.3)

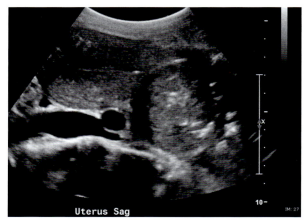

Fig. 23.1

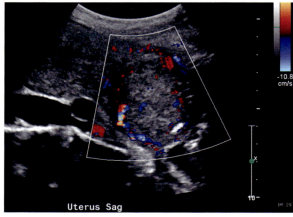

Fig. 23.2

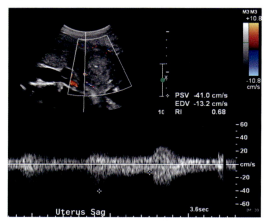

Fig. 23.3

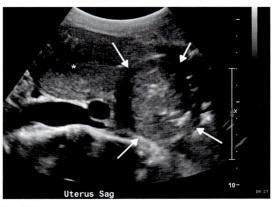

Fig. 23.4

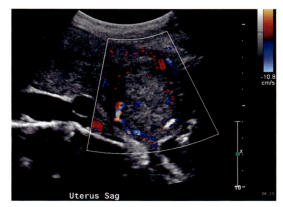

Fig. 23.5

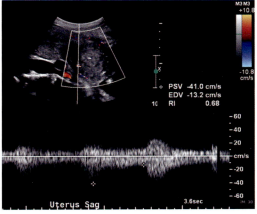

Fig. 23.6

Imaging Findings

▶ Heterogeneous well-marginated solid mass (arrows in Fig. 23.4) arising from the uterine cervix and extending into the parametrium posteriorly. The mass is primarily isoechoic relative to the myometrial echotexture

▶ The endometrium is normal (asterisk in Fig. 23.4)

▶ Note peripheral as well as internal vascularity on color Doppler image (Fig. 23.5) with low-resistance arterial waveform on spectral Doppler image (Fig. 23.6)

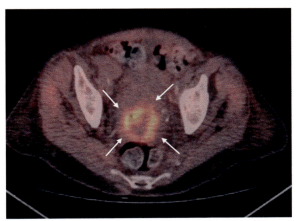

Fig. 23.7

► Follow-up positron emission tomography/CT reveals a fluorodeoxyglucose avid mass (arrows in Fig. 23.7) with central necrosis arising from the cervix, confirming the diagnosis of cervical cancer (CA)

Differential Diagnosis

► Cervical leiomyoma
► Endocervical polyp
► Cervical lymphoma
► Endometrial cancer invading the cervix

Teaching Points

► Third most common gynecologic malignancy
  ▪ Highest incidence in young women of low socioeconomic status
► Risk factors: almost all cervical cancers caused by human papilloma virus (HPV) infection, usually sexually transmitted
  ▪ Early age at first sexual intercourse, multiple sex partners, multiparity (three or more children), history of sexually transmitted diseases, use of birth control pills for more than 5 years
  ▪ HIV
  ▪ Low socioeconomic status
  ▪ Smoking
► Prevention: HPV vaccine
  ▪ Studies have definitively shown that the incidence of cervical cancer is substantially decreased in HPV-vaccinated populations
  ▪ The Centers for Disease Control and Prevention currently recommends HPV vaccine for girls and boys aged 11 or 12 years and in nonvaccinated females aged 13–26 years and nonvaccinated males aged 13–21 years
► Histology
  ▪ Squamous cell carcinoma most common (80–90% of cases)
  ▪ Adenocarcinoma second most common (10%); carries a worse prognosis
► Prognostic factors: histologic grade, tumor volume (> 4 cm diameter = worse prognosis), depth of stromal invasion, invasion of adjacent organs, lymph node metastases
  ▪ More aggressive in Hispanic, Asian, and African American women
► Clinical presentation
  ▪ Abnormal vaginal bleeding, vaginal discharge, pelvic pain, urinary symptoms
  ▪ Carcinoma in situ is usually asymptomatic, found on screening Pap smear
  ▪ Screening with Pap smears has significantly reduced the incidence of invasive cervical cancer, resulting in earlier detection and increased survival
► US findings
  ▪ Cervical mass involving cervical stroma, may extend into parametrium
    • Note large echogenic cervical mass invading the lower uterine segment (LUS) (white arrows in Fig. 23.8) and parametrium (black arrows in Fig. 23.8) in a second patient with cervical CA.

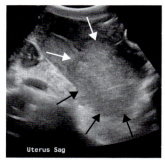
Fig. 23.8

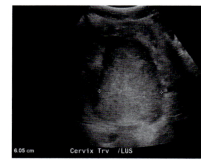
Fig. 23.9

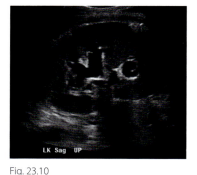
Fig. 23.10

    • The large mass (> 6 cm) (calipers Fig. 23.9) completely infiltrates the cervix and no normal cervical tissue is seen on the transverse image (Fig. 23.9)
    • Left hydronephrosis (Fig. 23.10) confirms parametrial invasion, which has obstructed the left ureter, indicating at least FIGO stage IIIB disease
  ▪ Fluid distending endometrial canal secondary to obstruction
  ▪ Local spread to endometrium relatively common

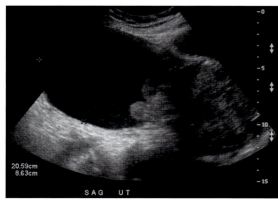

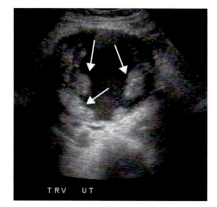

Fig. 23.11   Fig. 23.12

- Note large polypoid cervical mass infiltrating the entire cervix and extending into the LUS in a third patient with cervical cancer. The endometrial cavity (X's in Fig. 23.11) is distended and filled with fluid. The myometrium is markedly thinned
- Transverse image through the LUS demonstrating circumferential nodular invasion of the endometrium (arrows in Fig. 23.12)
► Significant overlap in US appearance with other solid cervical masses
  ▪ Leiomyoma: mass may demonstrate posterior acoustic shadowing, edge refraction, calcifications, minimal or peripheral vascularity; separate from endocervical canal which is often normal as a cervical leiomyoma arises in the wall of the cervix
  ▪ Lymphoma: mass generally hypoechoic and more homogeneous, often infiltrative without discrete mass, pelvic lymphadenopathy
  ▪ Polyp: echogenic mass located within the endocervical canal, vascular pedicle, will not invade cervical stroma or extend into parametria
  ▪ Invasion of cervix from endometrial cancer (i.e., extension of endometrial cancer into the cervix) would be contiguous with endometrial mass

Management

► Transvaginal US: limited role, usually an incidental finding, can assess local disease and measure diameter of tumor, but inadequate for staging
► MR: method of choice for local extension and parametrial invasion
► CT: used primarily to assess for abdominopelvic lymphadenopathy, distant metastasis and radiation treatment planning
► FIGO staging system
  ▪ Stage 0: carcinoma in situ
  ▪ Stage I: cervical invasion
  ▪ Stage II: invades beyond cervix, but not to pelvic sidewall or lower one-third of vagina
    • A: upper two-thirds of vagina
    • B: parametrial spread
  ▪ Stage III: spread to lower one-third of vagina or pelvic sidewall
  ▪ Stage IV: invasion of bladder or rectum or distant metastases
► Once parametrial invasion has occurred, FIGO stage IIB, the patient is no longer an operative candidate

Further Reading

1. Epstein E, Di legge A, Måsbäck A, et al. Sonographic characteristics of squamous cell cancer and adenocarcinoma of the uterine cervix. *Ultrasound Obstet Gynecol*. 2010; 36: 512–516.
2. Kaur H, Silverman PM, Iyer RB, et al. Diagnosis, staging, and surveillance of cervical carcinoma. *Am J Roentgenol*. 2003; 180: 1621–1631.

Section II

First Trimester

History

► 24-Year-old primigravida with unknown last menstrual period presents with left lower quadrant pain; serum human chorionic gonadotrophin β-subunit (hCG) level of 5600 mIU/ml (Fig. 24.1)

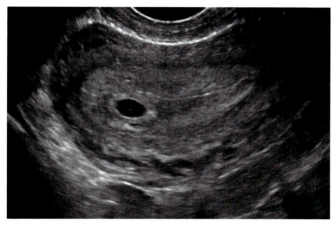

Fig. 24.1

Case 24 Normal Intrauterine Pregnancy

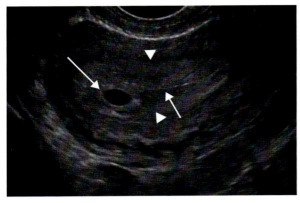

Fig. 24.2

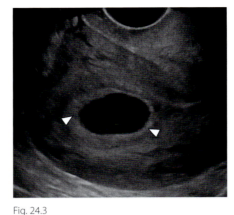

Fig. 24.3

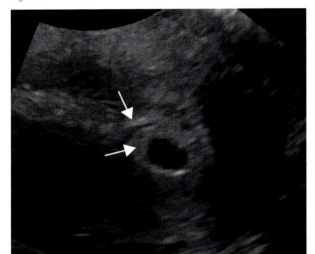

Fig. 24.4

Imaging Findings

- Normal thick decidua (arrowheads in Fig. 24.2) is seen within the uterus
- Pencil-thin endometrial cavity (short arrow in Fig. 24.2) is clearly delineated as a thin echogenic line within the decidua
- Early gestational sac (long arrow in Fig. 24.2) is seen eccentric to the endometrial canal, below the echogenic line implanted in the posterior endometrium
- Used as a criterion to decide if the fluid collection is an intrauterine pregnancy (IUP) before definite visualization of a yolk sac or embryo; yolk sac is faintly delineated within the gestational sac but seen in only one view, causing uncertainty in diagnosis; demonstration of intradecidual sign increases confidence in making the correct diagnosis
- Magnified view of an early IUP in another patient demonstrates the echogenic chorionic ring (arrowheads in Fig. 24.3) surrounding the gestational sac eccentrically located also within the posterior layer of the endometrium
- Another patient with an example of the double decidual sign (Fig. 24.4) (see Teaching Points)

Differential Diagnosis

- Anembryonic gestation
- Pseudogestational sac of ectopic pregnancy

Teaching Points

- Intradecidual sign refers to eccentric location of gestational sac (GS) subjacent to the echogenic interface between two decidual layers in early pregnancy (5 or 6 menstrual weeks); may be absent in 35% of normal gestational sacs
- Essential to clearly establish location of endometrial canal relative to the GS; normal GS implants within the endometrium (decidua) and therefore the endometrial line does not pass through the sac

- Different from "double decidual" sign also seen in early IUP; composed of hyperechoic decidua parietalis (lines the uterine cavity) and hyperechoic decidua capsularis (lines the GS), resulting in two echogenic rings separated by hypoechoic fluid within the uterine cavity (arrows in Fig. 24.4)
- The presence of yolk sac confirms an IUP but does not confirm viability until a live embryo is detected within 3 or 4 days after appearance of yolk sac
- Anembryonic gestation—diagnosed when the mean sac diameter of the GS measures ≥ 25 mm on endovaginal exam and no embryo is detected
- Pseudogestational sac of ectopic pregnancy is centrally located within the endometrial cavity and lacks an echogenic chorionic ring

Management

- Conservative follow-up with continued US and hCG levels until viability or diagnosis of failed pregnancy is established

Further Reading

1. Gupta N, Angtuaco T. Embryosonology in the first trimester of pregnancy. *Ultrasound Clin.* 2007; 2: 175–185.
2. Doubilet PM, Benson CB, Bourne T, et al. Diagnostic criteria for nonviable pregnancy early in the first trimester. *N Engl J Med.* 2013; 369: 1443–1451.

Case 25

▶ 15-Year-old primigravida 10 weeks pregnant presents with cramping and vaginal bleeding (Fig. 25.1)

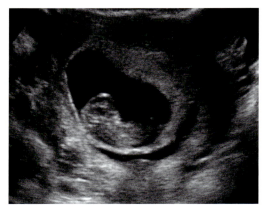

Fig. 25.1

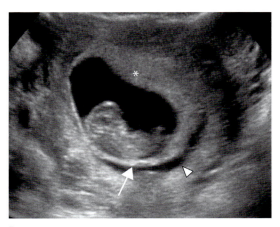

Fig. 25.2

Imaging Findings

► Perigestational hemorrhage (PGH) (arrowhead in Fig. 25.2) in intrauterine cavity separates echogenic combination of decidua capsularis and chorion laeve (arrow in Fig. 25.2) from its attachment to the decidua parietalis

► Placental site (asterisk in Fig. 25.2) is designated by combination of chorion frondosum and decidua basalis resulting in focal thickening of the chorionic ring

► Images from other first-trimester cases (Figs. 25.3–25.5) prior to detection of the yolk sac or embryo showing similar appearance that constitutes the "double decidual sign" (double arrows), namely a combination of chorion laeve and decidua capsularis separated by PGH from the decidua parietalis

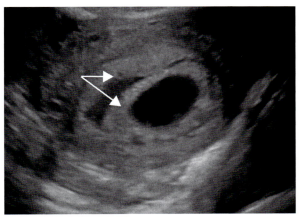

Fig. 25.3

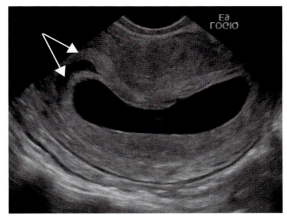

Fig. 25.4

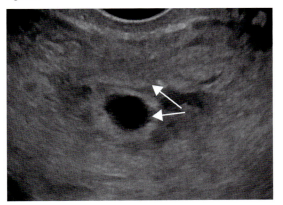

Fig. 25.5

Differential Diagnosis

► Chorioamniotic separation
► Twin gestation with demise of one twin
► Pseudogestational sac of ectopic pregnancy

Teaching Points

► PGH is synonymous with subchorionic hemorrhage and is the most common cause of first-trimester bleeding occurring in 18% of pregnancies
► Fluid collection representing hemorrhage in uterine cavity that separates the chorion laeve–decidua capsularis complex from the decidua parietalis
  ▪ Acute hemorrhage is echogenic, subacute is hypoechoic, chronic hemorrhage is sonolucent
  ▪ Large hemorrhage greater than two-thirds chorionic sac diameter, moderate 50% chorionic sac diameter, small less than one-third chorionic sac diameter
► Vast majority with good outcome: > 90% survival if PGH is small
► Overall spontaneous abortion rate 9.3%
  ▪ 18.8% for large PGH
  ▪ 9.2% for moderate PGH
  ▪ 7.7% for small PGH
► Spontaneous abortion rate for fetuses less than 8 weeks is 13.3% versus 5.9% for fetuses older than 8 weeks
► Should not be called "abruption" in first trimester
► May be associated with morbidity in second and third trimester: intrauterine growth restriction, preeclampsia, preterm delivery, pregnancy-induced hypertension, premature delivery and abruption
► Differentiated from chorioamniotic separation, which may be seen as a normal developmental variation up to 17 or 18 weeks of gestational age, after which fusion of membranes occur
► Pseudogestational sac of ectopic pregnancy (EP) of concern prior to detection of yolk sac
  ▪ Endometrial fluid collections associated with EP often have "pointy" margins
  ▪ Would not contain echogenic ring of a gestational sac
  ▪ Look for intradecidual sign
► Difficult to differentiate from demise of a twin unless prior ultrasound exam documented yolk sac/embryo in fluid collection

Management

► Follow up in 1 or 2 weeks to determine progression or evolving resolution of hemorrhage
► Fetal monitoring in the second trimester to evaluate for complications mentioned previously

Further Reading

1. Bennett GL, Bromley B, Lieberman E, et al. Subchorionic hemorrhage in first trimester pregnancies: Prediction of pregnancy outcome with sonography. *Radiology*. 1996; 200: 803–806.
2. Dighe M, Cuevas C, Moshiri M, et al. Sonography in first trimester bleeding. *J Clin Ultrasound*. 2008; 36(6): 352–366.
3. Sauerbrei EE, Pham DH. Placental abruption and subchorionic hemorrhage in the first half of pregnancy: US appearance and clinical outcome. *Radiology*. 1986; 160: 109–112.

History

▶ 28-Year-old primigravida with 9 weeks of amenorrhea, presenting with vaginal spotting and pelvic pain (Figs. 26.1–26.3)

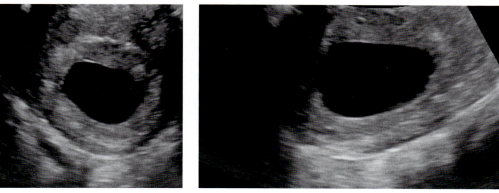

Fig. 26.1   Fig. 26.2

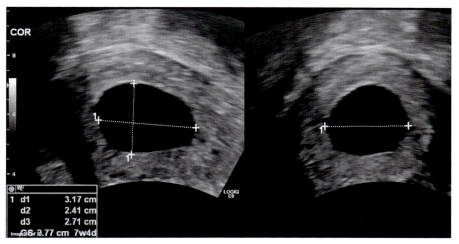

Fig. 26.3

Case 26 Anembryonic Gestation

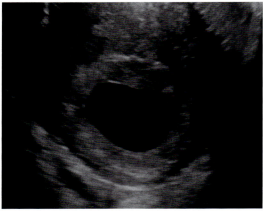

Fig. 26.4

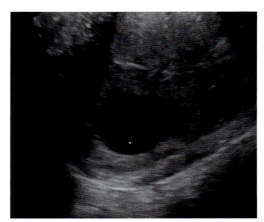

Fig. 26.5

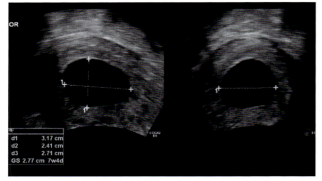

Fig. 26.6

Imaging Findings

▶ Sagittal (Fig. 26.4) and coronal (Fig. 26.5) transvaginal images of the uterus show no evidence of embryonic pole or yolk sac within the intrauterine gestational sac
▶ Measurements of the three dimensions of the sac (Fig. 26.6) result in a mean sac diameter (MSD) of 27.7 mm. An embryonic pole should be observed on transvaginal ultrasound once the MSD is > 25 mm

Differential Diagnosis

▶ Early normal intrauterine pregnancy
▶ Pseudogestational sac in ectopic pregnancy
▶ Retained products of conception
▶ Abortion in progress

Teaching Points

▶ An anembryonic gestation refers to a pregnancy in which embryonic development arrested at a very early stage or failed altogether, resulting in a gestational sac with no yolk sac or embryonic pole
  ▪ Also referred to as the "empty amnion sign" or failed intrauterine pregnancy (IUP)
▶ Newly revised criteria for evaluation of early pregnancy state that a normal intrauterine gestational sac with an MSD ≥ 25 mm should have an embryo
  ▪ Hence, an intrauterine gestational sac with an MSD ≥ 25 mm without an embryo is diagnostic of an anembryonic gestation (failed IUP)
  ▪ Older criteria used an MSD ≥ 8–10 mm without a yolk sac as diagnostic of an anembryonic gestation. However, in today's practice, such pregnancies, although considered at risk, should not be diagnosed as anembryonic gestations or failed IUPs but, rather, should be carefully monitored
▶ Early normal gestations with an MSD measuring < 25 mm may not be distinguishable from an anembryonic gestation, so it is important to do short-term follow-up US to monitor for the development of an embryo

- Pseudogestational sac of an ectopic pregnancy: usually a fluid collection that is central in location within the endometrial cavity
  - Intradecidual or double decidual signs indicative of a normal early gestation will not be present
- An abortion in progress: low position of the gestational sac close to or within the cervix
- Correlation with patient's presenting history is important in distinguishing between incomplete abortion and anembryonic gestation
  - Passage of large clots or tissue would be more consistent with incomplete abortion
  - Typically patients with an anembryonic gestation present with minimal spotting or are otherwise asymptomatic
- Follow-up ultrasound studies will show decreasing size of the sac or failure to grow at the predicted rate of 1 mm/day for normal pregnancies
- The term "blighted ovum" is no longer in use and has been replaced by "anembryonic gestation"; recent literature suggests the term "failed pregnancy" to include all those instances in which the criteria for viability have not been met

Management

- "Wait and see"—most cases of failed pregnancy will spontaneously abort
- Pelvic ultrasound should be repeated in 1 or 2 weeks to document lack of development over time, such as
  - Absence of an embryo with a heartbeat ≥ 2 weeks after initial pelvic ultrasound that showed gestational sac without a yolk sac
  - Absence of an embryo with a heartbeat ≥ 11 days after initial pelvic ultrasound showed a gestational sac with a yolk sac
- Vaginal misoprostol
- Dilatation and curettage sometimes required with persistent bleeding

Further Reading

1. Doubilet PM, Benson CB, Bourne T, et al. Diagnostic criteria for nonviable pregnancy early in the first trimester. *N Engl J Med.* 2013; 369: 1443–1451.
2. Sohaey R, Woodward P, Zwiebel WJ. First-trimester ultrasound: The essentials. *Semin Ultrasound CT MR.* 1996; 17(1): 2–14.

Case 27

History

▶ 30-Year-old gravida 2 para 1 presenting with severe nausea (Fig. 27.1)

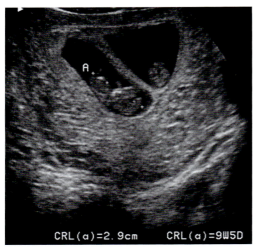

Fig. 27.1

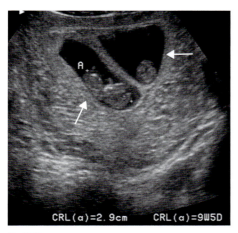

Fig. 27.2

Imaging Findings

► Transabdominal image shows two chorionic sacs each containing an embryo (arrows in Fig. 27.2) before 10 weeks gestational age, confirming dichorionic diamniotic gestation.

Teaching Points

► Chorionicity is best determined in the first trimester before 10 weeks
► Timing of egg division determines placentation in monozygotic twins
  ▪ Dichorionic, diamniotic (DC/DA) placentation occurs with division within three days post fertilization
    • All dizygotic and one-third of monozygotic twins are DC/DA
    • For DC gestations, 80–90% dizygotic and 10–20% monozygotic
    • Two separate placentas (arrows in Fig. 27.3) may be seen in second or third trimester
    • May also present with a "lambda sign" (arrow in Fig. 27.4), which refers to a triangular projection of chorionic tissue from fused dichorionic placentas, extending between layers of the intertwin membrane

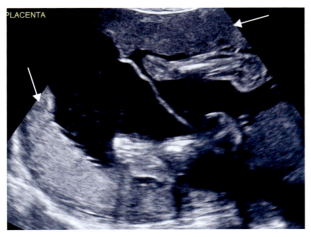

Fig. 27.3

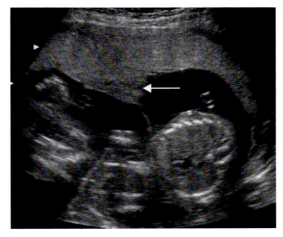

Fig. 27.4

► Monochorionic diamniotic (MC/DA) placentation occurs with division between days 4 and 8 post fertilization
  ▪ All MC twins are monozygotic and two-thirds of monozygotic twins are MC
  ▪ One gestational sac is seen before 10 weeks with two amniotic sacs (arrows in Fig. 27.5)
  ▪ In the second and third trimesters, the "T sign" may be seen, which refers to the appearance of an intertwin membrane taking off from placenta at a 90° angle (arrow in Fig. 27.6)

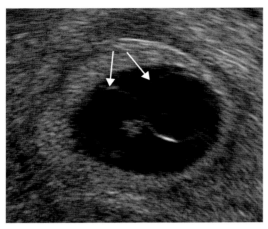

Fig. 27.5

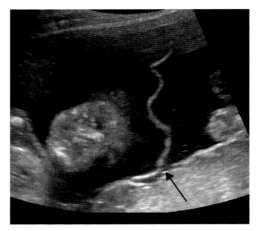

Fig. 27.6

▶ Monochorionic monoamniotic (MC/MA) placentation occurs with division between days 8 and 12 post fertilization
  ▪ One gestational sac, no separating amniotic membrane, and one yolk sac (arrow in Fig. 27.7) are diagnostic criteria

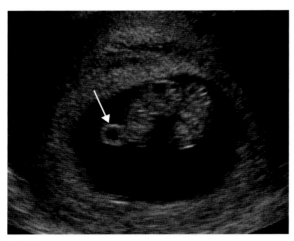

Fig. 27.7

▶ Division at or after day 13 results in conjoined twins in which certain anatomical parts such as the pelvis (arrow in Fig. 27.8) are fused

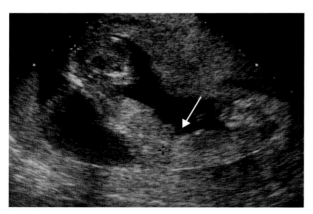

Fig. 27.8

▶ Accurate diagnosis of chorionicity is more important than zygosity
▶ MC twins are at most risk for complications, including twin transfusion syndrome, twin reversed arterial perfusion, intrauterine growth restriction, and twin demise

Management

▶ Dichorionic twins: US examination every 4–6 weeks after 20 weeks of gestation; fetal growth deceleration/discordance optimally detected between 20 and 28 weeks of gestation

▶ Monitoring of mochorionic twins includes assessment of amniotic fluid volume and fetal bladder in both twins for early detection of twin transfusion syndrome

▶ Monoamniotic twins have especially high risk of fetal death; managed with more intensive fetal surveillance, earlier delivery, and cesarean birth

Further Reading

1. Wood SL, St Onge R, Connors G, et al. Evaluation of the twin peak or lambda sign in determining chorionicity in multiple pregnancy. *Obstet Gynecol*. 1996; 88: 6–12.
2. Shetty A, Smith AP. The sonographic diagnosis of chorionicity. *Prenat Diagn*. 2005; 25: 735–740.
3. Lee YM, Cleary-Goldman J, Thaker HM, et al. Antenatal sonographic prediction of twin chorionicity. *Am J Obstet Gynecol*. 2006; 195: 863–868.

Case 28

History

► 37-Year-old primigravida with suspected embryonic anomaly on first routine checkup following in vitro fertilization (Figs. 28.1 and 28.2)

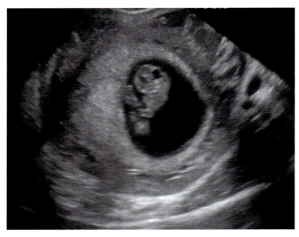

Fig. 28.1

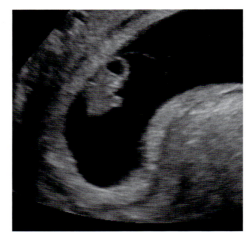

Fig. 28.2

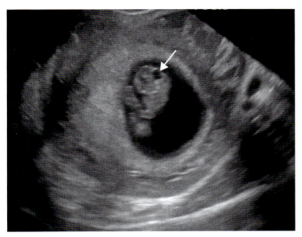

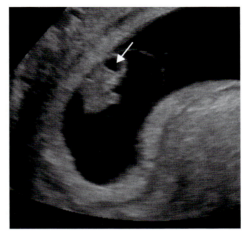

Fig. 28.3

Fig. 28.4

Imaging Findings

▶ Small cystic structure (3 or 4 mm) in the posterior aspect of the cranium corresponds to the open rhombencephalon, rhomboid fossa, or hindbrain (arrows in Figs. 28.3 and 28.4)

Differential Diagnosis

▶ Posterior fossa cyst or cephalocele
▶ Hydranencephaly
▶ Alobar holoprosencephaly

Teaching Points

▶ Open rhombencephalon is a normal first-trimester US finding, usually seen at 8–10 menstrual weeks; should not be mistaken for a congenital defect
▶ Develops into the normally proportioned fourth ventricle after the 11th menstrual week when the vermis and cerebellar hemispheres form the posterior roof to the fourth ventricle. Until then, the rhombencephalon will remain open. When imaged in the midsagittal view (Fig. 28.5), no other abnormality should be suspected

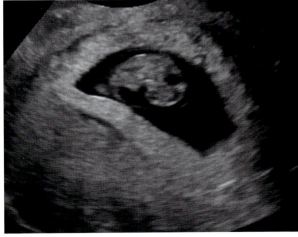

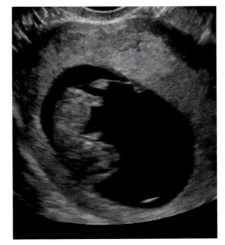

Fig. 28.5

Fig. 28.6

▶ Disappears later in the first trimester (Fig. 28.6)
▶ Can be mistaken for other cystic brain anomalies as follows
  ▪ Hydranencephaly: congenital brain defect in which fluid-filled cavities replace the cerebral hemispheres

- Result of either massive brain infarction from bilateral carotid artery occlusion or primary agenesis of the neural wall
- Usually diagnosed later in pregnancy when absence of the cerebral cortex surrounding a large intracranial fluid collection can be determined with certainty
- The falx, midbrain, and posterior fossa structures are usually normal
  - Alobar holoprosencephaly: lethal congenital anomaly characterized by complete failure of cleavage of the prosencephalon
    - Cerebral hemispheres are fused and there is a monoventricle
    - Can be diagnosed at the 10th menstrual week
    - Associated with multiple chromosomal anomalies
  - Posterior fossa cyst or cephalocele are other considerations due to the location of the cystic structure relative to the neck of the embryo/fetus
    - Usually diagnosed later in pregnancy

Management

▶ No follow-up necessary, but confirmatory study later in the first trimester often performed, especially if a perfect midsagittal view cannot be obtained

Further Reading

1. Cyr DR, Mack LA, Nyberg DA, et al. Fetal rhombencephalon: Normal US findings. *Radiology*. 1988; 166: 691–692.
2. Monteagudo A, Timor-Tritsch IE. First trimester anatomy scan—Pushing the limits. What can we see now? *Curr Opin Obstet Gynecol*. April 2003; 15(2): 131–141.
3. Bronshtein M, Zimmer EZ, Blazer S. Isolated large fourth ventricle in early pregnancy—A possible benign transient phenomenon. *Prenat Diagn*. October 1998; 18(10): 997–1000.

History

▶ 28-Year-old gravida 2 para 1 diabetic female, asymptomatic, referred for dating (Figs. 29.1 and 29.2)

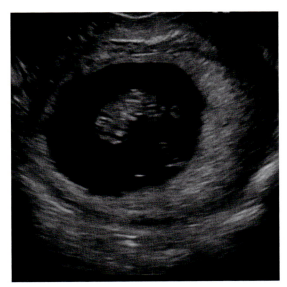

Fig. 29.1

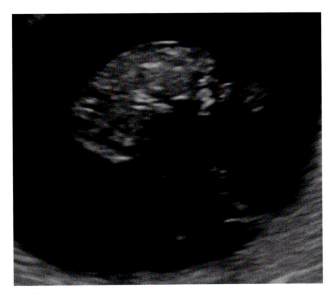

Fig. 29.2

Case 29 Physiologic Gut Herniation

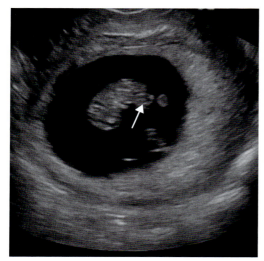 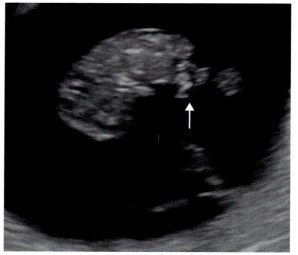

Fig. 29.3

Fig. 29.4

Imaging Findings

▶ Echogenic "mass" is seen at the base of the umbilical cord, adjacent to the anterior abdominal wall of the fetus (arrows in Figs. 29.3 and 29.4)

Differential Diagnosis

▶ Gastroschisis
▶ Omphalocele

Teaching Points

▶ During the period of rapid growth of the midgut, herniation of bowel into the proximal portion of the umbilical cord normally occurs
   ▪ While the bowel is within the umbilical cord, the midgut rotates 90° counterclockwise, and this appears on US as an echogenic mass in which the umbilical cord attaches to the anterior abdominal wall of the fetus (arrow in Fig. 29.3) measuring < 7 mm across the base
   ▪ Usually seen at 6–8 menstrual weeks; sometimes up to 11 weeks in utero
   ▪ Should not extend more than 1 cm into base of the cord
   ▪ Best seen on magnified views (arrow in Fig. 29.4)
▶ At approximately 10 or 11 weeks the abdomen enlarges, allowing the intestines to return inside the abdominal cavity, which is confirmed by observation of a normal cord insertion site in the first trimester (arrow in Fig. 29.5) or in the second trimester of pregnancy (arrow in Fig. 29.6)

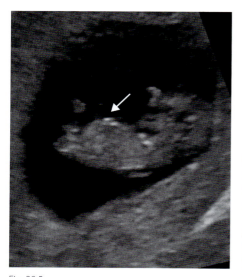 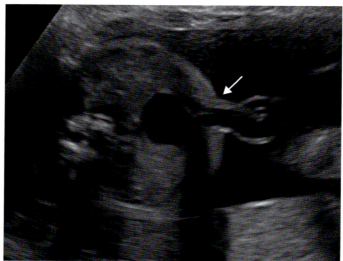

Fig. 29.5

Fig. 29.6

- The midgut then rotates an additional 180° counterclockwise and fixes to the posterior retroperitoneum
- The jejunum, ileum, and large portion of the colon are derived from midgut
- In the second trimester, a mass arising from the anterior abdominal wall is always abnormal and usually due to gastroschisis or omphalocele
- In gastroschisis, the bowel herniates through a right paramedian abdominal wall defect
  - Cord insertion is normal
  - No covering membrane is visualized
  - Does not contain liver or other solid organs
  - No known association with chromosomal abnormalities
- With omphalocele, the abdominal wall defect is midline in location with herniation of abdominal contents into base of cord
  - Covering membrane is demonstrated
  - Often contains small bowel and liver
  - Well-known association with other structural and chromosomal abnormalities (trisomy 18, Beckwith–Wiedemann syndrome)

Management

- Normal developmental phenomenon
- Further investigation necessary if seen later than 12 weeks or if contains liver or other solid organs

Further Reading

1. Achiron R, Soriano D, Lipitz S, et al. Fetal midgut herniation into the umbilical cord: Improved definition of ventral abdominal anomaly with the use of transvaginal sonography. *Ultrasound Obstet Gynecol.* 1995; 6: 256–260.
2. Cyr DR, Mack LA, Schoenecker SA, et al. Bowel migration in the normal fetus: US detection. *Radiology.* 1986; 161(1): 119.

Case 30

History

▶ 27-Year-old gravida 3 para 2 presented for dating. Initial ultrasound (not shown) did not show an intrauterine pregnancy; hCG value was 2700 mIU/ml. The patient returned 5 days later with vaginal bleeding and abdominal pain; repeat hCG level was 7200 mIU/ml (Figs. 30.1–30.4).

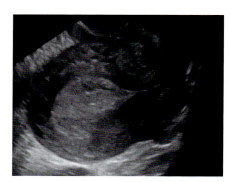

Fig. 30.1

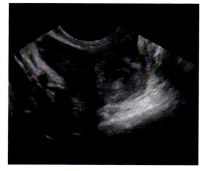

Fig. 30.2

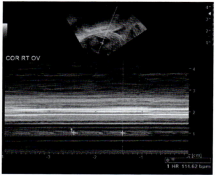

Fig. 30.3

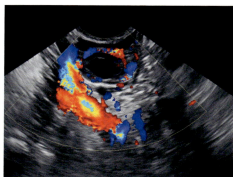

Fig. 30.4

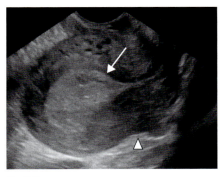

Fig. 30.5

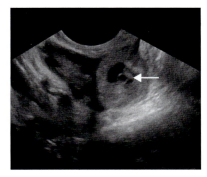

Fig. 30.6

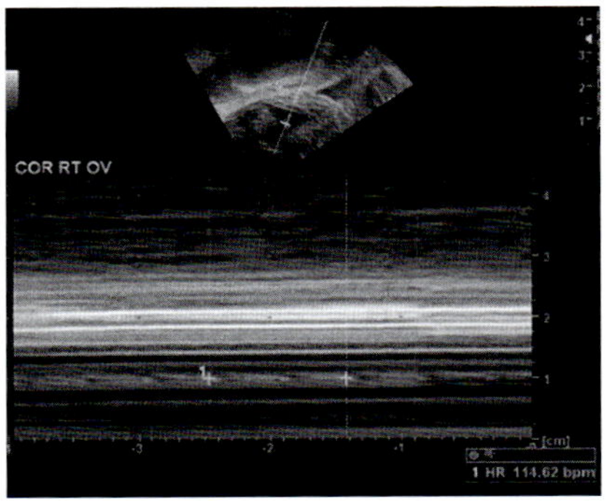

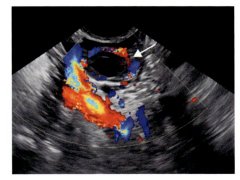

Fig. 30.7

Fig. 30.8

Imaging Findings

▶ No gestational sac seen in endometrial cavity. Note thickened endometrium (arrow in Fig. 30.5)

▶ No fluid in cul-de-sac behind cervix (arrowhead in Fig. 30.5)

▶ An intact ectopic gestational sac containing a yolk sac and embryo (arrow in Fig. 30.6) with cardiac motion (Fig. 30.7) is seen medial to the normal right ovary, suggesting tubal location

▶ Vascular flow around sac suggests an intact chorionic ring (arrow in Fig. 30.8)

▶ In another patient presenting with pain in the first trimester, note central fluid collection in the endometrial cavity with debris (arrow in Fig. 30.9) corresponding to a pseudogestational sac of ectopic pregnancy. There is no evidence of an intrauterine gestational sac

▶ There is echogenic free fluid in the cul-de-sac (arrow in Fig. 30.10) and around the uterus and adnexa (short arrow in Fig. 30.11), indicating hemoperitoneum likely due to a ruptured ectopic pregnancy

▶ Note complex adnexal mass indicative of hematoma from a ruptured tubal ectopic pregnancy (long arrow in Fig. 30.11), although the ectopic gestation sac is not directly visualized

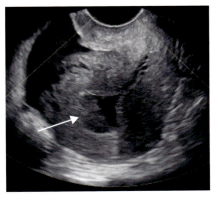

Fig. 30.9

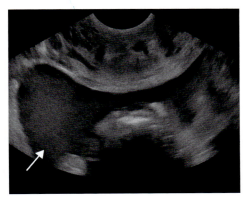

Fig. 30.10

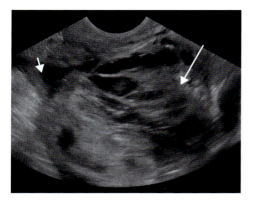

Fig. 30.11

Differential Diagnosis

▶ Very early normal pregnancy
▶ Abortion in progress or a failed intrauterine gestation
▶ Corpus luteum with "ring of fire" in adnexa
▶ Tubo-ovarian abscess with purulent fluid in cul-de-sac

Teaching Points

▶ Ectopic pregnancy (EP) is defined as the implantation of a pregnancy outside the endometrial cavity
  ▪ Most occur in the fallopian tube (90%), predominately in the ampulla or isthmus
▶ Account for approximately 2% of all pregnancies in the United States
▶ Leading cause of maternal death in the first trimester
▶ Risk factors include
  ▪ History of prior ectopic pregnancy
  ▪ Pelvic inflammatory disease
  ▪ Tubal surgery
  ▪ Assisted reproductive techniques
  ▪ Advanced maternal age
  ▪ Endometriosis
  ▪ Prior cesarean section
▶ Risk factors are additive
▶ However, 50% of patients with EPs have no known risk factors
▶ Classic symptoms of ectopic pregnancy include
  ▪ Amenorrhea
  ▪ Pelvic pain
  ▪ Vaginal bleeding
▶ Patients usually present 6–8 weeks after last menstrual period (may occur later in non-tubal ectopic pregnancies)
▶ US technique: must scan transabdominally and transvaginally to include findings in abdomen or high in the pelvis that may be beyond transvaginal range
▶ Ultrasound findings
  ▪ Definitive: extrauterine gestational sac containing a yolk sac, embryo, ± cardiac activity
  ▪ Highly suspicious findings: echogenic tubal ring, adnexa mass (hematoma) in the absence of intrauterine pregnancy (Fig. 30.11)
  ▪ Hemoperitoneum (Fig. 30.10)
  ▪ < 20% will have a pseudogestational sac (Fig. 30.9)
▶ Suspect when serum hCG is > 3000 mIU/ml with no evidence of an intrauterine gestation (IUP)
  ▪ Discriminatory hCG level for visualization of an IUP on transvaginal US previously considered to be 1500–2000 mIU/ml
  ▪ Current recommendation is that no single serum hCG level should be used to differentiate an early IUP versus failed IUP or EP
▶ May mimic an early intrauterine gestation, but the pseudogestational sac seen in some patients with EP is a central fluid collection within the endometrial cavity, whereas a true intrauterine gestational sac is eccentrically located relative to the endometrial canal

- In an incomplete abortion, the debris and hemorrhage in the uterine cavity may be difficult to differentiate from the pseudosac of an EP and correlation with patient's history or prior imaging is needed when available. Short-term follow-up ultrasound can be helpful
- "Ring of fire" indicates chorionic vascularity on color Doppler but is also seen around the corpus luteum (CL)
  - More commonly completely circumferential around the CL
  - Neither color nor spectral Doppler findings can be used to confidently differentiate between an EP and CL
- Tubo-ovarian abscess: uncommon in pregnancy
  - Complex multilocular vascular adnexal mass without yolk sac or embryo
  - Associated hemato-pyosalpinx
  - Purulent free fluid could mimic hemoperitoneum and could appear similar to the second case

Management

- If findings are inconclusive and the patient is stable: follow-up hCG and US; hCG typically rises more slowly for an ectopic than intrauterine pregnancy
- Methotrexate for patients with EPs who are hemodynamically stable, willing and able to comply with post-treatment follow-up, have an hCG level ≤ 5000 mIU/mL, no fetal cardiac activity, and ectopic mass size less than 3 or 4 cm
  - hCG level and size criteria may vary from institution to institution
- Laparoscopy/laparotomy indicated in patients who are hemodynamically unstable

Further Reading

1. Doubilet PM, Benson CB, Bourne T, et al. Diagnostic Criteria for Nonviable Pregnancy Early in the First Trimester. *N Engl J Med*. 2013; 369: 1443–1451.
2. Levine D. Ectopic pregnancy. *Radiology*. 2007; 245(2): 385–397.
3. Lin EP, Bhatt S, Dogra VS. Diagnostic clues to ectopic pregnancy. *RadioGraphics*. 2008; 28: 1661–1671.

Case 31

History

- 21-Year-old gravida 2 para 1 presents with left lower quadrant pain. She was given methotrexate at another institution several days prior to this admission due to concern for an ectopic pregnancy (Figs. 31.1–31.4).

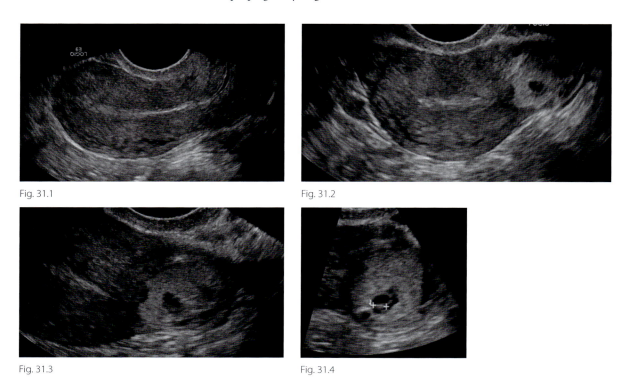

Fig. 31.1

Fig. 31.2

Fig. 31.3

Fig. 31.4

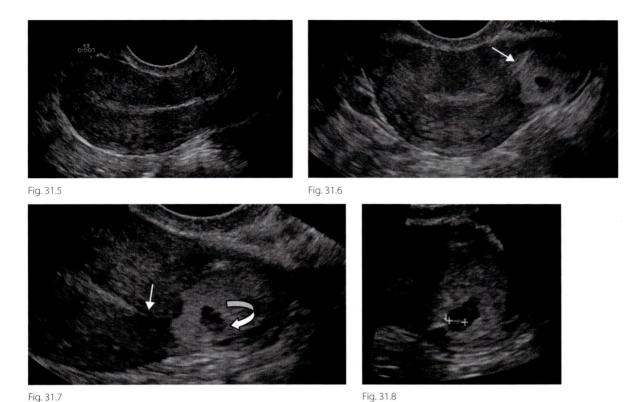

Fig. 31.5

Fig. 31.6

Fig. 31.7

Fig. 31.8

Imaging Findings

► Sagittal image of uterus shows empty endometrial canal (Fig. 31.5)
► Transverse midline image of uterine fundus shows intact gestational sac (arrow in Fig. 31.6) within myometrium but separate from endometrium
► Note yolk sac within the gestational sac (curved arrow in Fig. 31.7) and thin echogenic line (straight arrow in Fig. 31.7) extending from the endometrial canal through the myometrium to the edge of the gestational sac (interstitial line sign)
► There is an embryonic pole within the gestational sac (calipers in Fig. 31.8) with a crown–rump length of 0.52 cm corresponding to 5 weeks 6 days of gestation (Fig. 31.8). No cardiac activity was demonstrated

Differential Diagnosis

► Intrauterine pregnancy
► Isthmic tubal pregnancy
► Angular pregnancy

Teaching Points

► An interstitial pregnancy is diagnosed when a gestational sac implants in the interstitial portion of the fallopian tube (i.e., the proximal tubal segment that travels through the muscular wall of the uterus in the fundus)
► If undiagnosed, rupture may occur resulting in the protrusion of the gestational sac beyond the serosal surface of the uterine fundus on transverse (arrow on Fig. 31.9) and longitudinal (arrow on Fig. 31.10) images

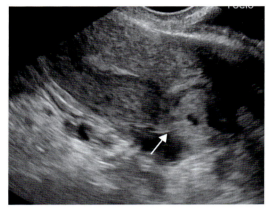
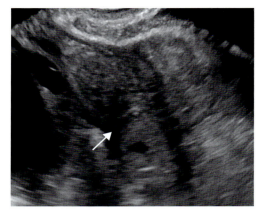

Fig. 31.9   Fig. 31.10

► US findings
  ▪ Eccentric location of the gestational sac, surrounded by a thin rim of myometrium
  ▪ Myometrial tissue will separate the medial edge of the eccentric gestational sac from the endometrium
  ▪ "Interstitial line sign"—echogenic line extending from most superior and lateral aspect of endometrium to midportion of interstitial mass or sac; likely represents interstitial portion of fallopian tube
  ▪ Can be mimicked by an intrauterine gestation displaced by a myoma or myometrial contraction; however, an intrauterine gestational sac should be located within the endometrial cavity and therefore either be surrounded by the echogenic endometrium or have a broad-based interface with the endometrium and no intervening myometrium
► The term interstitial pregnancy is often used interchangeably with "cornual pregnancy," which specifically refers to a pregnancy in the horn of bicornuate or septate uterus or in a rudimentary horn attached to a unicornuate uterus
► Isthmic tubal pregnancy: occurs in the isthmic portion of the fallopian tube outside of the uterus
  ▪ Along with the ampullary portion of tube, it is the most common site of ectopic pregnancy
  ▪ Not embedded within myometrium
► Angular pregnancy: an intrauterine pregnancy in the lateral "angle" of the endometrial cavity medial to the uterotubal junction and round ligament
  ▪ Distinction is important because angular pregnancies, unlike interstitial pregnancies, are more likely to miscarry than rupture
  ▪ Distinction may be difficult on US alone, and MRI may be helpful

Management

► Advances in early diagnosis in the 1980s facilitated use of methotrexate (MTX) as treatment of choice for tubal and interstitial ectopic pregnancy over surgery, with an overall success rate of nearly 90% in properly selected women
► Optimal candidates for MTX treatment are hemodynamically stable, willing and able to comply with post-treatment follow-up, have an hCG concentration ≤ 5000 mIU/ml, no fetal cardiac activity, and no significant hemoperitoneum
► Those who are not appropriate candidates for medical therapy should be managed surgically, including women who are hemodynamically unstable or have signs of impending or ongoing ectopic mass rupture (i.e., severe or persistent abdominal pain or > 300 ml of free peritoneal fluid outside the pelvic cavity), or contraindications such as hypersensitivity to MTX, bone marrow suppression, or abnormal liver function tests

Further Reading

1. Lau S, Tulandi T. Conservative medical and surgical management of interstitial ectopic pregnancy. *Fertil Steril*. 1999; 72: 207.
2. Ackerman TE, Levi CS, Dashefsky SM, et al. Interstitial line: Sonographic finding in interstitial (cornual) ectopic pregnancy. *Radiology*. 1993; 189: 83.
3. Auslender R, Arodi J, Pascal B, et al. Interstitial pregnancy: Early diagnosis by ultrasonography. *Am J Obstet Gynecol*. 1983; 146: 717.

History

▶ 32-Year-old pregnant female status post assisted reproduction presents with right-sided pelvic pain (Figs. 32.1–32.6)

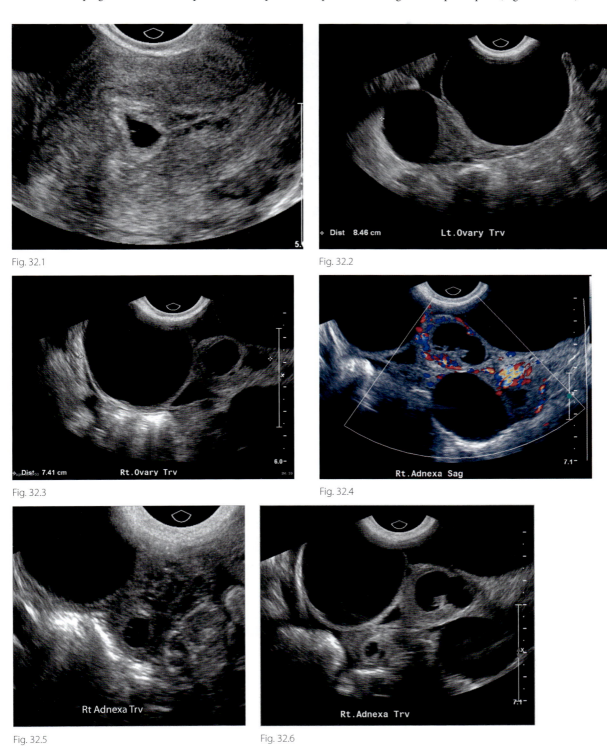

Fig. 32.1

Fig. 32.2

Fig. 32.3

Fig. 32.4

Fig. 32.5

Fig. 32.6

Case 32 Ovarian Hyperstimulation Syndrome With Heterotopic Pregnancies

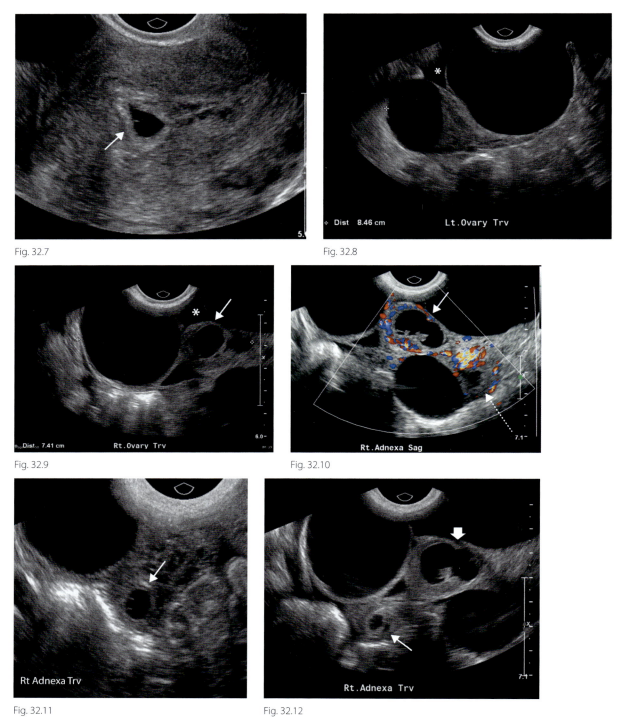

Fig. 32.7

Fig. 32.8

Fig. 32.9

Fig. 32.10

Fig. 32.11

Fig. 32.12

Imaging Findings

▶ Intrauterine gestational sac (arrow in Fig. 32.7) containing a yolk sac

▶ The left (Fig. 32.8) and right (Fig. 32.9) ovaries are massively enlarged with numerous simple cysts of varying size distorting the ovarian parenchyma. Note adjacent free fluid (star)

▶ Right corpus luteum (arrow in Figs. 32.9 and 32.10; thick arrow in Fig. 32.12) with thick vascular wall and internal echoes consistent with hemorrhage

▶ Note additional echogenic thick-walled, vascular ring-like cystic structure containing a yolk sac inferior to the right ovary (arrows in Figs. 32.11 and 32.12; dotted arrow in Fig. 32.10) consistent with an ectopic pregnancy

Differential Diagnosis

▶ Polycystic ovarian syndrome (PCOS)
▶ Ovarian torsion
▶ Theca lutein cysts from a molar pregnancy

Teaching Points

▶ Heterotopic pregnancies, namely an intrauterine pregnancy (IUP) plus an ectopic pregnancy (EP), are extremely rare in the general population, occurring in approximately 1/30,000 pregnancies
▶ However, the incidence of heterotopic pregnancies is estimated to be as high as 1/100 to 1/300 pregnancies in women undergoing assisted reproduction techniques, including ovulation induction
▶ US findings of heterotopic pregnancies
  ▪ The demonstration of yolk sacs within the intrauterine cavity (arrow in Fig. 32.13) and in the adnexa (arrow in Fig. 32.14) is confirmatory of heterotopic pregnancy in a second patient with a heterotopic pregnancy. Note, however, that the gestational sacs are different in size, reflecting different growth rates likely due to less blood supply in the adnexa

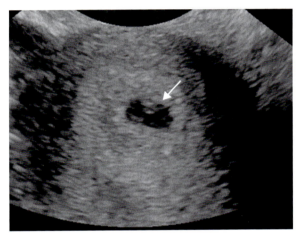

Fig. 32.13

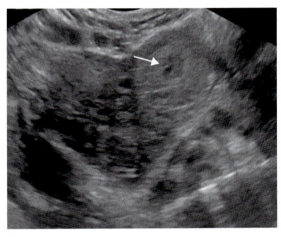

Fig. 32.14

  ▪ In a third patient with heterotopic pregnancy (Fig. 32.15 and 32.16), embryos are noted in the intrauterine (Fig. 32.15) and extrauterine (Fig. 32.16) gestational sacs. When a live embryo is demonstrated in the uterine cavity (arrow in Fig. 32.15), the coexisting embryo in the adnexa (arrow in Fig. 32.16) may be smaller, especially in a case of embryonic demise

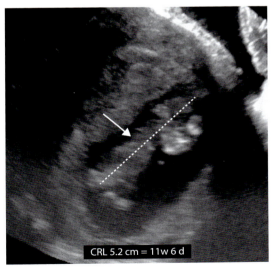

CRL 5.2 cm = 11w 6 d

Fig. 32.15

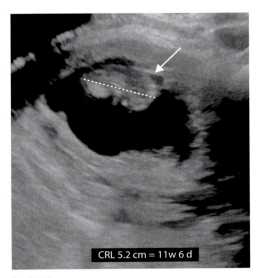

CRL 5.2 cm = 11w 6 d

Fig. 32.16

- In patients undergoing ovulation induction, enlargement of the ovaries with multiple cysts of varying sizes (theca lutein cysts) typically occurs secondary to increased hCG levels
- The term ovarian hyperstimulation syndrome (OHSS) implies that a fluid shift has also occurred
  - Mild: ovaries < 5 cm, no weight gain
  - Moderate: ovaries 5–12 cm, 5–10 lb. weight gain
  - Severe: ovaries > 12 cm, > 10 lb. weight gain
- Severe OHSS can result in life-threatening fluid shifts: hypovolemia, ascites, pleural effusion, hypotension, electrolyte imbalance, and oliguria
- Pelvic pain is common and can be multifactorial
  - Stretching of the ovarian capsule as the ovary enlarges
  - Hemorrhage or rupture of an ovarian cyst
  - Ovarian torsion
  - EP
- US findings in OHSS include the following
  - Bilateral symmetric ovarian enlargement with numerous ovarian cysts of varying size with compression and distortion of ovarian parenchyma
  - Ascites
  - ± Pleural effusions
  - Patients with pain should be evaluated for hemorrhagic cysts, cyst rupture, ovarian torsion, and EP
- PCOS
  - Bilateral moderate ovarian enlargement with numerous small (< 1 cm) peripheral follicles (string of pearls sign)
  - Preserved central ovarian architecture
  - No ascites
- Ovarian torsion
  - Unilateral ovarian enlargement
  - Unilateral pain
  - Small number of peripherally displaced small follicles
  - An ovarian mass, including a large simple cyst; mass may act as lead point
  - Decreased or absent blood flow
  - Small amount of adjacent free fluid
- Theca lutein cysts associated with gestational trophoblastic disease
  - Similar US appearance of the ovaries to this case with multiple bilateral large ovarian cysts of varying size
  - Occurs in approximately 50% of molar pregnancies
  - Endometrial mass, often with numerous cysts ("cluster of grapes" appearance) and highly vascular with low-resistance waveform pattern
  - Markedly elevated serum hCG levels
  - No increased incidence of EP

Management

- Surgical resection or direct injection of EP with either potassium chloride or methotrexate allows preservation of IUP
- Treatment of OHSS: cessation of hormonal therapy and supportive therapy

Further Reading

1. Luo X, Lim CED, Huang C, et al. Heterotopic pregnancy following in vitro fertilization and embryo transfer: 12 case reports. *Arch Gynecol Obstet.* 2009; 280(2): 325–329.
2. Baron KT, Babagbemi KT, Arleo EK, et al. Emergent complications of assisted reproduction: Expecting the unexpected. *RadioGraphics.* 2013; 33(1): 229–244.

History

▶ 30-Year-old gravida 4 para 3 presenting to the emergency room with severe vaginal bleeding; past history is positive for prior cesarean section (C-section) 3 years ago due to placenta previa (Figs. 33.1–33.4)

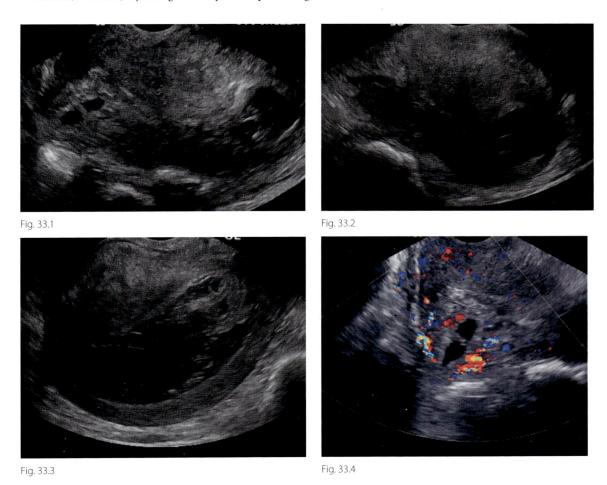

Fig. 33.1

Fig. 33.2

Fig. 33.3

Fig. 33.4

Case 33 Pregnancy in C-Section Scar

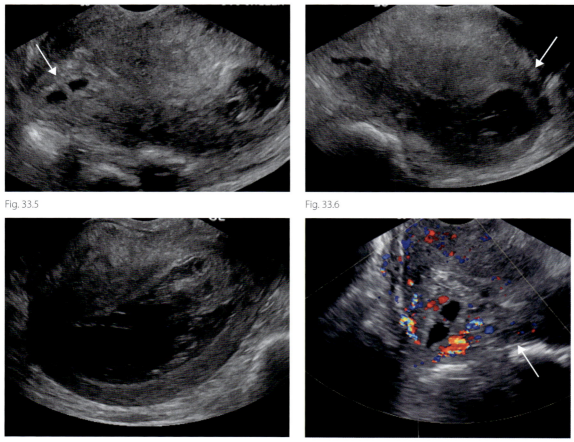

Fig. 33.5

Fig. 33.6

Fig. 33.7

Fig. 33.8

Imaging Findings

▶ Figures 33.5 and 33.6 are longitudinal transvaginal images of the retroflexed uterus; the gestational sac (arrow in Fig. 33.5) is implanted in the anterior myometrium close to the cervix in the lower uterine segment; the uterine fundus (arrow in Fig. 33.6) is located more superiorly

▶ Figure 33.7 focuses on the large heterogeneous hematoma filling the uterine cavity located superiorly and separate from the gestational sac

▶ Figure 33.8 shows intact gestational sac with color Doppler flow in surrounding trophoblast; cardiac activity was demonstrated within the embryo on real-time observation; outline of the lower anterior uterine wall (arrow in Fig. 33.8) is interrupted by the bulging gestational sac that protrudes beyond the serosal surface of the uterus

▶ Negative "sliding organs sign" was elicited. With application of gentle pressure with the transvaginal probe on the lower uterine body, the gestational sac could not be moved from its position and separated from the uterus because it was embedded in the anterior uterine wall

Differential Diagnosis

▶ Abortion in progress
▶ Cervical ectopic pregnancy
▶ Tubal ectopic pregnancy

Teaching Points

▶ C-section is the most common major abdominal operation in women in the United States, accounting for 33% of all surgeries
▶ Reported prevalence of 0.15% of women with prior C-section; prevalence of complications related to healed scar is unknown
▶ The incidence of ectopic pregnancy (EP) in C-section scars is increasing as the rate of C-sections is increasing
▶ The greatest risk of an EP in a C-section scar is uterine rupture and hemorrhage, which may require hysterectomy and occasionally may result in maternal death
▶ Transvaginal examination is the method of choice to delineate the location of the gestational sac relative to the uterine cavity with 86.4% sensitivity

- ▶ Clinical presentation
  - ▪ Painless vaginal bleeding
  - ▪ Mild to moderate pelvic pain
- ▶ Cervical ectopic pregnancy: gestational sac within the cervical wall with empty endocervical canal seen adjacent
- ▶ Abortion in progress: usually no trophoblastic flow adjacent to or in wall of gestational sac; gestational sac located within the endometrial or endocervical canal
- ▶ If endocervical and endometrial canal cannot be definitely demonstrated, the gestational sac may be mistakenly localized outside the uterus; this emphasizes the importance of meticulous demonstration of the continuity between endocervical and endometrial canals and the wall of the cervix with the myometrium

Management

- ▶ Termination of the pregnancy surgically or by methotrexate injection within the sac in cases in which the diagnosis is made prior to uterine rupture
- ▶ Once uterine rupture is documented, surgical intervention may be required to control hemorrhage
- ▶ Revision of C-section scar may be performed to minimize the possibility of recurrence

Further Reading

1. Rodgers SK, Kirby CL, Smith RJ, et al. Imaging after cesarean delivery: Acute and chronic complications. *RadioGraphics*. 2012; 32: 1693–1712.
2. Jurkovic D, Hillaby K, Woelfer B, et al. First-trimester diagnosis and management of pregnancies implanted into the lower uterine segment cesarean section scar. *Ultrasound Obstet Gynecol*. 2003; 21: 220–227.

Case 34

▶ 16-Year-old primigravida with unknown last menstrual period presents with severe vaginal bleeding, cramping, and abdominal pain; hCG = 3144 mIU/ml (Figs. 34.1–34.3)

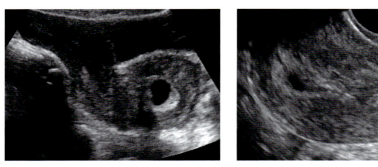

Fig. 34.1   Fig. 34.2

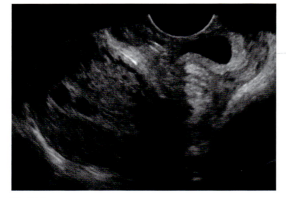

Fig. 34.3

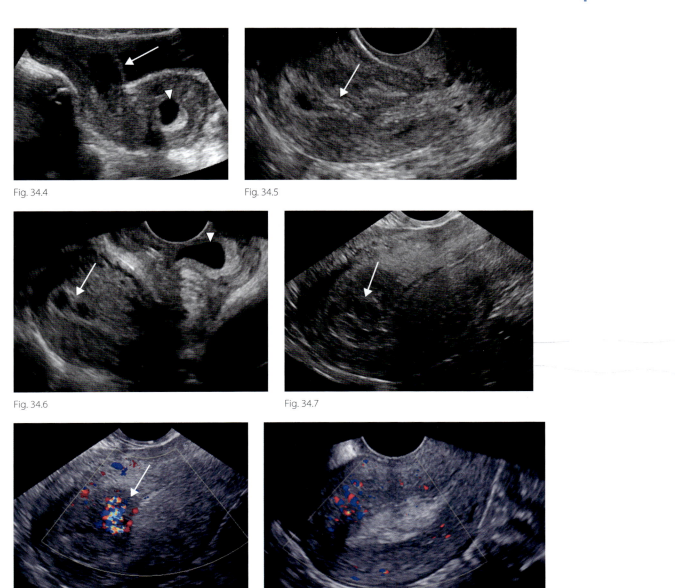

Fig. 34.4

Fig. 34.5

Fig. 34.6

Fig. 34.7

Fig. 34.8

Fig. 34.9

Imaging Findings

► Ill-defined uterine cavity (arrow in Fig. 34.4) and the recently passed gestational sac (arrowhead in Fig. 34.4) in upper vagina on transabdominal image

► Ill-defined endometrial cavity filled with debris (arrow in Fig. 34.5) on transvaginal image, probably a combination of blood and retained products of conception (RPOC)

► Progression of the gestational sac (arrowhead in Fig. Fig. 34.6) into the lower vagina; RPOC seen in the uterus (arrow in Fig. 34.6) on transvaginal US obtained minutes later

► Images from another patient show a more solid-appearing RPOC (arrow in Fig. 34.7) representing retained placenta with increased flow (arrow in Fig. 34.8), which was evacuated on dilatation and curettage

► Contrasting image of RPOC in another patient with no Doppler flow (Fig. 34.9), suggesting the absence of viable tissue; combination of blood and necrotic placenta passed in this patient status post elective abortion 2 weeks earlier

Differential Diagnosis

► Physiologic implantation hemorrhage in uterus
► Pseudosac of ectopic pregnancy
► Gestational trophoblastic disease

Teaching Points

► Incomplete abortion refers to vaginal bleeding and/or pain in pregnant woman with dilated cervix and products of conception in uterine cavity or cervical canal on vaginal examination
► Abortion occurring before 12 weeks of gestation is commonly a complete abortion with scant vaginal bleeding and mild cramping
► After 12 weeks, membranes often rupture and the fetus passes, leaving significant amounts of retained placental tissue, leading to incomplete abortion; bleeding my lead to hypovolemic shock; painful cramps/contractions often present
► Ultrasound evaluation often nonspecific because RPOC and blood clots have overlapping sonographic appearance of intrauterine debris with or without Doppler flow; depends on viable versus necrotic tissue in RPOC
► RPOC clinically suspected with passage of an incomplete placenta or in patient with endometritis/prolonged postpartum hemorrhage
► Gestational trophoblastic disease in the first trimester can look like RPOC; classic "snowstorm pattern" usually seen in the second trimester

Management

► Can be managed surgically, medically, or expectantly
► Complete abortions theoretically do not require therapy, but incomplete abortions may be difficult to differentiate from complete abortions either clinically or ultrasonographically, thus leading to suction curettage
► Expectant management recommended for women with early pregnancy failure who have stable vital signs and no evidence of infection; if US shows an empty uterus and bleeding is minimal, no further action is needed

Further Reading

1. Durfee SM, Frates MC, Luong A, et al. The sonographic and color Doppler features of retained products of conception. *J Ultrasound Med.* 2005; 24(9): 1181–1186.
2. Sotiriadis A, Makrydimas G, Papatheodorou S, et al. Expectant, medical, or surgical management of first-trimester miscarriage: A meta-analysis. *Obstet Gynecol.* 2005; 105: 1104–1112.
3. Steinkeler J, Coldwell BJ, Warner MA. Ultrasound of the postpartum uterus. *Ultrasound Q.* 2012, 28: 97–103.

Case 35

History

- 19-Year-old gravida 3 para 1 with previous history of molar gestation presents with suspicion of molar pregnancy on initial office US (Figs. 35.1–35.4); last menstrual period unknown

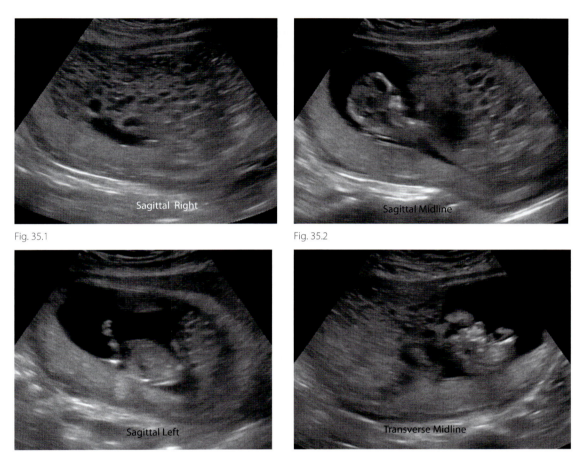

Fig. 35.1

Fig. 35.2

Fig. 35.3

Fig. 35.4

Case 35 Coexistent Molar Gestation With Intrauterine Pregnancy

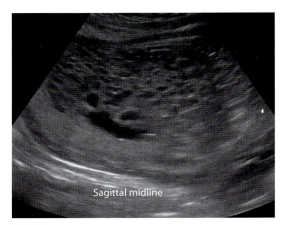

Fig. 35.5

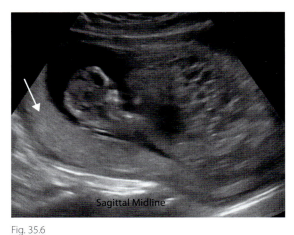

Fig. 35.6

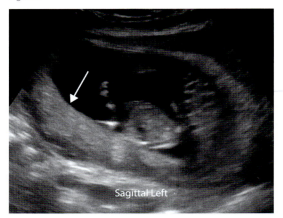

Fig. 35.7

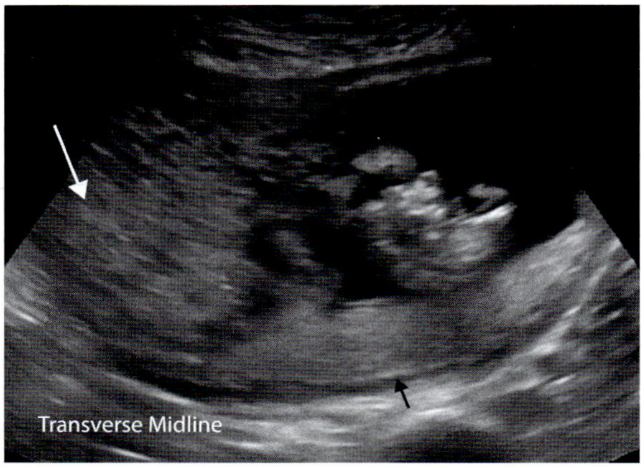

Fig. 35.8

Imaging Findings

▶ Uterine cavity is filled with a mass that contains both solid and cystic elements (Fig. 35.5) along the right lateral wall of the uterus

▶ Longitudinal midline image shows a normal echogenic, crescentic placenta (arrows in Figs. 35.6 and 35.7) with a normal-appearing fetus. Crown–rump length corresponded to 13 weeks' gestational age (not shown)

▶ Transverse image shows relationship of complete mole (white arrow in Fig. 35.8) occupying the right half of the endometrial cavity and the coexisting normal gestation to the left. The placenta is posterior and to the left (black arrow)

Differential Diagnosis

▶ Invasive mole
▶ Partial mole
▶ Choriocarcinoma
▶ Hydropic degeneration of the placenta

Teaching Points

▶ The spectrum of gestational trophoblastic disease (GTD) includes complete hydatidiform mole (CHM), partial mole, invasive mole, and choriocarcinoma
▶ The incidence of CHM is 1/2000 pregnancies
▶ Clinical presentation
  ▪ Vaginal bleeding
  ▪ Hyperemesis
  ▪ Preeclampsia

- Rapid uterine enlargement
- Markedly elevated serum hCG levels
▶ Twin pregnancy may be complicated by GTD and present as either a mole (partial or complete) and one viable fetus or two moles
  - Incidence of 1/22,000–100,000 pregnancies
▶ In a singleton pregnancy, the following entities may be further considered
  - Complete moles are always 46XX without the presence of a fetus
  - Partial moles are 69XXY and may occur with an abnormal fetus or fetal demise
  - Invasive moles, which account for 10% of all gestational trophoblastic disease, may penetrate or perforate the uterine wall
  - Choriocarcinoma is a rare, highly aggressive and vascular tumor, tends to metastasize, accounts for approximately 1% of all GTD
  - Hydropic degeneration of the placenta is a benign condition that results in few cystic areas in an otherwise normal placenta

A 34-year-old pregnant patient presented with hyperemesis and the typical US features of a partial mole. Note the molar degeneration with numerous anechoic cystic areas of part of the placenta (arrows in Figs. 35.9 and 35.10) with an adjacent abnormal hydropic fetus (arrowhead in Fig. 35.9) proven to have triploidy.

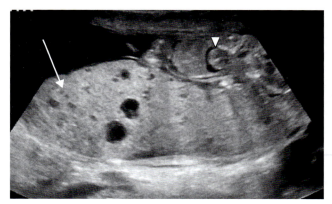

Fig. 35.9

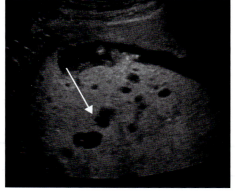

Fig. 35.10

Management

▶ Maternal counseling regarding risks
▶ Vaginal hemorrhage resulting in pregnancy termination or preterm delivery is a common complication if continuation of the pregnancy is elected.
▶ Conservative management not recommended in the presence of choriocarcinoma or fetal aneuploidy
▶ Postpartum, the placenta should be sent for evaluation by a pathologist experienced in the evaluation of GTD, and routine post-GTD surveillance initiated
▶ If termination is elected, treatment usually consists of uterine suction and curettage with close monitoring of serum hCG levels; concluded when levels decline to undetectable level
▶ In cases of invasive mole and choriocarcinoma, a course of chemotherapy, usually methotrexate, is recommended along with surveillance of hCG levels

Further Reading

1. Lurain, J. Gestational trophoblastic disease II: Classification and management of gestational trophoblastic neoplasia. *Am J Obstet Gynecol.* January 2011; 204: 11–18.
2. Green C, Angtuaco T, Shah H, et al. Gestational trophoblastic disease: A spectrum of radiologic diagnosis. *RadioGraphics.* 1996; 16: 1371–1384.
3. Steller MA, Genest DR, Bernstein MR, et al. Clinical features of multiple conception with partial or complete molar pregnancy and coexisting fetuses. *J Reprod Med.* 1994; 39: 147–154.
4. Sebire NJ, Foskett M, Paradinas FJ, et al. Outcome of twin pregnancies with complete hydatidiform mole and healthy co-twin. *Lancet.* 2002; 359: 2165–2171.

Case 36

History

► 35-Year-old gravida 4 para 3 presents with positive maternal serum screening test (Fig. 36.1)

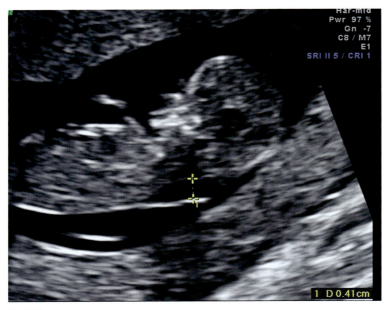

Fig. 36.1

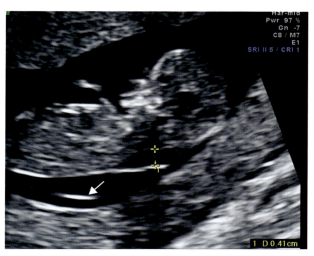

Fig. 36.2

Imaging Findings

▶ Midsagittal view of a 12-week fetus showing a nuchal translucency (NT) measurement of 4.1 mm (calipers in Fig. 36.2)
▶ Diagnosed with trisomy 21
▶ Separate amniotic membrane (arrow in Fig. 36.2) may normally be seen at this time

Differential Diagnosis

▶ Normal amniotic membrane mistaken for the nuchal translucency on improperly obtained image
▶ Neural tube defects, such as an occipital cephalocele or cervical meningocele

Teaching Points

▶ NT refers to the hypoechoic to anechoic region along the posterior portion of the fetal neck
▶ Technique for measurement
  ▪ Scans may be performed transabdominally between 11 and 14 weeks of gestation (crown–rump length (CRL) = 45–84 mm)
  ▪ Image used for measurement should be obtained in the midsagittal plane at the level of the neck
  ▪ Fetus should occupy at least 75% of the image so movement of the cursor produces less than a 0.1-mm change in the measurement
  ▪ Nuchal fluid space measured from inner-to-inner borders
  ▪ Widest area of lucency should be measured
  ▪ NT should be perpendicular to US beam
▶ Measurement of < 3 mm is normal (arrow in Fig. 36.3)
▶ Whether an NT measurement between 3 and 4 mm is normal or abnormal depends on the exact CRL

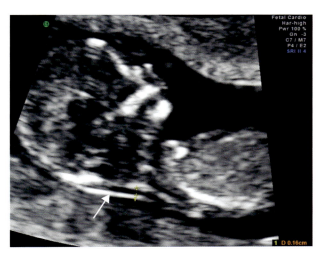

Fig. 36.3

- Pitfalls
  - Care must be taken to avoid mistaking the unfused amnion for the fetal skin line, leading to overestimation of NT, because the amnion and chorion are not completely fused until approximately 16 weeks of gestation
  - The amnion can be followed as it surrounds the fetus, whereas NT thickening is limited only to the posterior neck
  - Excessive extension of the fetal head can lead to overestimation of NT measurement
  - Extreme flexion of the fetus can attenuate the NT and lead to underestimation of measurement
  - If the measurement is obtained obliquely, it is possible to visualize the thickened NT as a cystic structure and mistake it for a cystic mass such as a cervical meningocele or occipital cephalocele
    - Observance of proper technique for measurement should resolve the issue
- NT commonly resolves spontaneously
  - If not resolved by the second trimester, higher likelihood of chromosomal abnormality
- An abnormally thick NT is related to dilated lymphatic channels in the neck resulting in cystic hygroma or mesenchymal edema (increased nuchal translucency)
  - Associated with 15% risk of aneuploidy overall
  - Trisomy 21 most commonly associated aneuploidy
  - Increased risk of structural abnormalities
  - Also seen with fetal cardiac abnormalities, diaphragmatic hernia, abdominal wall defects, skeletal dysplasias, and other fetal syndromes
  - Possibly associated with viral infection or early twin transfusion syndrome
- Fetus showing NT measurement of 4.8 mm (arrow in Fig. 36.4) and diffuse hydropic changes (Fig. 36.5) with irregular skin thickening around the neck and abdomen (arrows in Fig. 36.5)

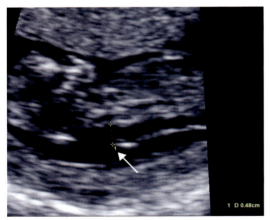

Fig. 36.4

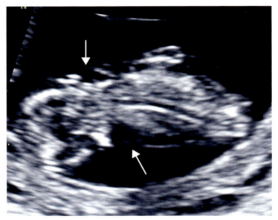

Fig. 36.5

- Further prediction of aneuploidy can be made by adding maternal age and first-trimester biochemical markers to the analysis

Management

- Fetal karyotyping (chorionic villus sampling or amniocentesis)
- Comprehensive fetal anatomic survey including fetal nuchal fold at 15–21 weeks
- Fetal echocardiography (18–20 weeks)
- Serial assessment of fetal status
- Supportive care for parents

Further Reading

1. Souka AP, Snijders RJ, Novakov A, et al. Defects and syndromes in chromosomally normal fetuses with increased nuchal translucency thickness at 10–14 weeks of gestation. *Ultrasound Obstet Gynecol.* 1998; 11: 391.
2. Scholl J, Durfee SM, Russell MA, et al. First-trimester cystic hygroma: Relationship of nuchal translucency thickness and outcomes. *Obstet Gynecol.* 2012; 120: 551.
3. Zoppi MA, Ibba RM, Floris M, et al. Changes in nuchal translucency thickness in normal and abnormal karyotype fetuses. *BJOG.* 2003; 110: 584.

Section III

Second and Third Trimester

History

▶ 23-Year-old gravida 4 para 0 at 19 weeks gestational age presents with abdominal cramping and vaginal bleeding with a history of three prior spontaneous abortions (Figs. 37.1–37.4)

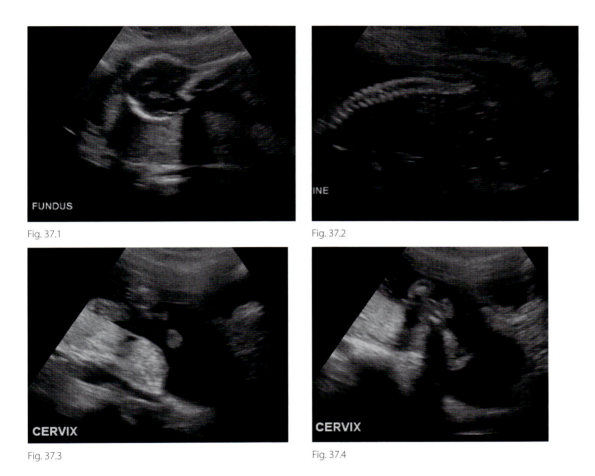

Fig. 37.1

Fig. 37.2

Fig. 37.3

Fig. 37.4

Case 37 Cervical Incompetence With Hourglass Membranes

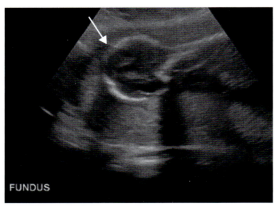

Fig. 37.5

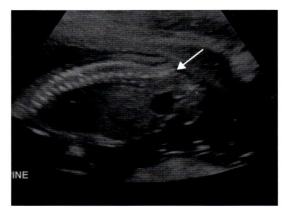

Fig. 37.6

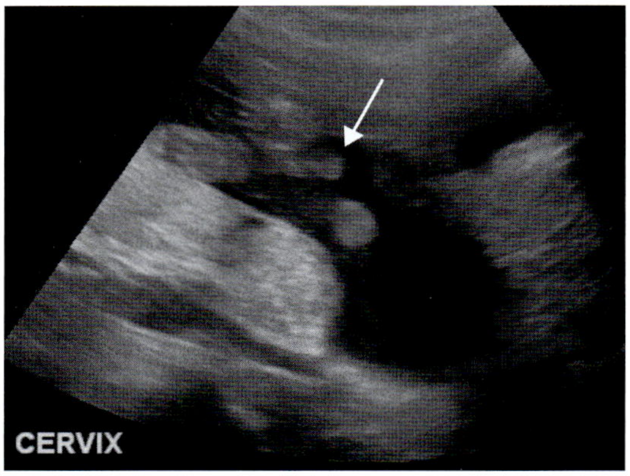

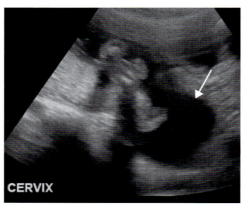

Fig. 37.7

Fig. 37.8

Imaging Findings

▶ The fetus is in breech presentation with the fetal head (arrow in Fig. 37.5) in the fundus of the uterus and the rump (arrow in Fig. 37.6) in the lower uterine segment

▶ Figures 37.7 and 37.8, taken seconds apart in the region of the cervix, demonstrate that the fetal lower extremities freely pass between the intrauterine cavity (arrow in Fig. 37.7) and the wide-open endocervical canal and upper vagina (arrow in Fig. 37.8)

Differential Diagnosis

▶ Normal cervical effacement during labor
▶ Abortion in progress

Teaching Points

▶ Cervical incompetence is defined as cervical length < 30 mm and/or widening of the internal os > 10 mm
  ▪ Incidence: approximately 1% of pregnant patients
  ▪ Responsible for 15% of second- and third-trimester abortions
▶ Normal median cervical length is 40 mm before 22 weeks, 35 mm at 22–32 weeks, and 30 mm after 32 weeks
▶ Cervical length below the 10th percentile (25 mm) is consistently associated with an increased risk of spontaneous preterm birth
  ▪ However, there is no threshold value below which a preterm delivery is inevitable
▶ Etiology: cause of preterm cervical shortening is often unclear but associated with the following
  ▪ DES exposure
  ▪ Congenital uterine malformations
  ▪ Cervical trauma
  ▪ Has also been attributed to biological variation, uterine overdistention, decidual hemorrhage, and infection or inflammation

- "Hourglass membranes": bulging of amniotic membranes through the cervical canal and into the vagina, giving the appearance of an hourglass
- Imaging protocol
  - Bladder must be empty because a full bladder may cause elongation of the cervix and obscure an open internal os
  - Image for several minutes because changes in the cervix may occur in a short time
- Differentiated from abortion in progress in which the membranes have already ruptured and abortion is inevitable

Management

- Prolapsed fetal membranes are a relative contraindication to emergent cerclage placement because of the high risk (> 50%) of iatrogenic premature rupture of membranes
- If cerclage placement is attempted, the prolapsed membranes must first be returned into the uterine cavity
- Women with multiple second-trimester losses and/or preterm births due to cervical insufficiency are potential candidates for a "history-indicated" cerclage at 12–14 weeks of gestation
- Women with a singleton pregnancy and short cervix (e.g., < 25 mm) on transvaginal US or dilated cervix on digital or speculum examination at 16–23 weeks of gestation are potential candidates for an "ultrasound-indicated"/"physical exam-indicated" cerclage

Further Reading

1. Iams JD, Goldenberg RL, Meis PJ, et al. The length of the cervix and the risk of spontaneous premature delivery. *N Engl J Med*. 1996; 334: 567–572.
2. McGahan JP, Phillips HE, Bowen MS. Prolapse of the amniotic sac: Ultrasound appearance. *Radiology*. 1981; 140(2): 463–466.
3. Scheerer LJ, Lam F, Bartolucci L, et al. A new technique for reduction of prolapsed fetal membranes for emergency cervical cerclage. *Obstet Gynecol*. 1989; 74: 408–412.

Case 38

► 34-Year-old gravida 4 para 3 referred for fetal dating; no prior prenatal care; 19 weeks pregnant by menstrual history; asymptomatic (Figs. 38.1–38.3)

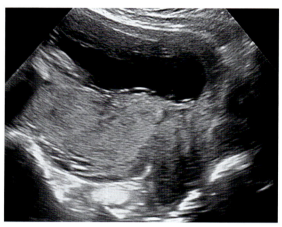

Fig. 38.1

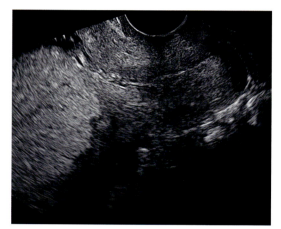

Fig. 38.2

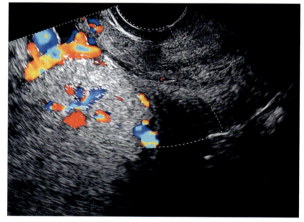

Fig. 38.3

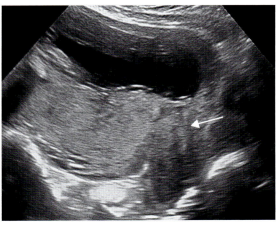

Fig. 38.4

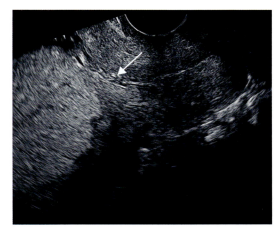

Fig. 38.5

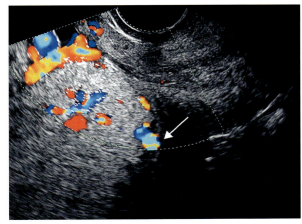

Fig. 38.6

Imaging Findings

► Midsagittal transabdominal image of the cervix shows a posterior placenta that partially covers internal os (arrow in Fig. 38.4)
► Confirmatory transvaginal ultrasound shows a portion of the echogenic placenta crossing internal os (arrow in Fig. 38.5)
► Color Doppler image showing intact retroplacental vessels (arrow in Fig. 38.6), thus excluding placenta increta

Differential Diagnosis

► False-positive findings due to poor technique, focal myometrial contraction, or full maternal bladder
► Early diagnosis of placenta previa prior to the physiologic "migration" of the placenta

Teaching Points

► Diagnosis based on identification of placental tissue covering or close to the internal cervical os on transvaginal ultrasound examination
► Suspected in women beyond 20 weeks of gestation with painless vaginal bleeding (70–80%)
► Prevalence is 3.5–4.6 per 1000 births
► Complications
  ▪ 5% associated with placenta accreta/percreta, vasa previa
  ▪ Potential for severe bleeding and preterm birth
  ▪ Need for cesarean delivery
► Risk factors
  ▪ Previous placenta previa

- Previous cesarean delivery
- Multiple gestations
- Multiparity
- Advanced maternal age
- Infertility treatment
- Previous abortion
- Previous intrauterine surgical procedure
► Classification
  - Low-lying—edge of the placenta within 2 cm but not abutting internal os
  - Marginal—placenta reaches the margin but does not cover internal os
  - Partial—placenta crosses midline and partially covers internal os
  - Complete—placenta completely covers internal os (arrow in Fig. 38.7)

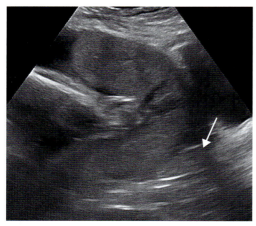

Fig. 38.7

► False-positive diagnosis is avoided by follow-up US examination if placenta previa (arrow in Fig. 38.8) is diagnosed early (14 weeks)
  - Third-trimester US (28 weeks) may show a normal examination with the placenta "migrating" superiorly (arrow in Fig. 38.9) as the uterus grows

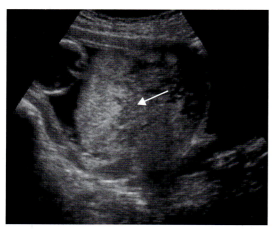

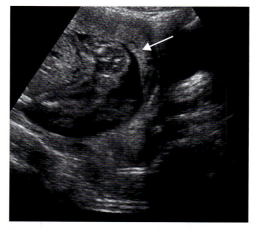

Fig. 38.8

Fig. 38.9

Management

► When diagnosed in second trimester: follow-up transvaginal US in the third trimester
► When diagnosed in third trimester
  - Low-lying placenta—trial of vaginal delivery
  - Marginal previa—recent studies suggest trial of labor
    - 1–2 cm from os, 75% delivered vaginally

- less than 1 cm from os, 30% rate of vaginal delivery
- Complete placenta previa in asymptomatic patients > 34 weeks—bed rest to decrease incidence of bleeding and cesarean section
- Bleeding placenta previa—bed rest, hospitalization if necessary, maternal transfusion, cesarean section

Further Reading

1. Dashe JS, Mcintire DD, Ramus RM, et al. Persistence of placenta previa according to gestational age at ultrasound detection. *Obstet Gynecol*. 2002; 99(5 Pt 1): 692–697.
2. Elsayes KM, Trout AT, Friedkin AM, et-al. Imaging of the placenta: A multimodality pictorial review. *RadioGraphics*. 2009; 29(5): 1371–1391.
3. Oyelese Y, Smulian JC. Placenta previa, placenta accreta, and vasa previa. *Obstet Gynecol*. 2006; 107: 927.

Case 39

History

▶ 32-Year-old multigravida with three previous cesarean sections presents for follow-up examination of placental abnormality prior to 32 weeks; she is asymptomatic (Figs. 39.1–39.3)

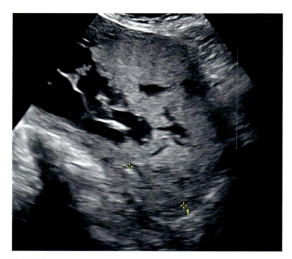

Fig. 39.1

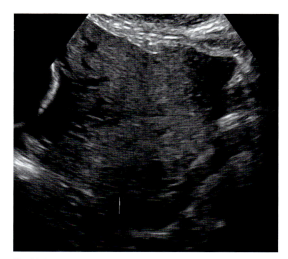

Fig. 39.2

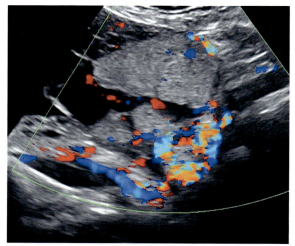

Fig. 39.3

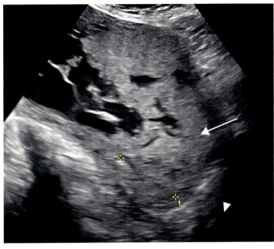

Fig. 39.4

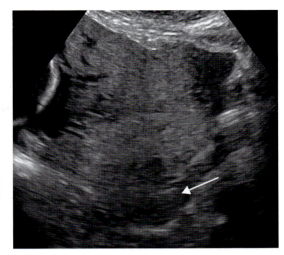

Fig. 39.5

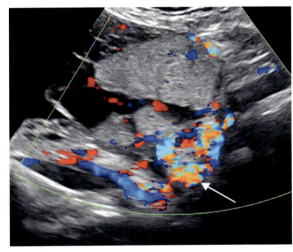

Fig. 39.6

Imaging Findings

► Transabdominal midsagittal image shows complete placenta previa (arrow in Fig. 39.4) with indistinct interface with the cervix (arrowhead in Fig. 39.4)
► Right parasagittal image shows irregular contour to the posterior placenta and invasion of the adjacent myometrium (arrow in Fig. 39.5)
► Color Doppler image shows increased vascularity to the posterior placenta and myometrium (arrow in Fig. 39.6)

Differential Diagnosis

► Placenta accreta
► Placenta increta
► Placenta previa
► Suboptimal scanning technique that simulates placental extension outside uterus

Teaching Points

► Sequela of morbidly adherent placenta can be classified into the following
  ▪ Placenta accreta—abnormality of placental implantation in which anchoring placental villi attach to myometrium rather than decidua
  ▪ Placenta increta—chorionic villi penetrate into myometrium
  ▪ Placenta percretachorionic villi penetrate through the myometrium to the uterine serosa or adjacent organs

- ▶ Pathogenesis primarily attributed to defective decidualization of implantation site
- ▶ Placenta accreta much more common than placenta increta and percreta (accreta, 79%; increta, 14%; percreta, 7%)
- ▶ Incidence increased from 1 in 30,000 deliveries in the 1950s to 1 in 2510 deliveries
  - Marked increase attributed to increasing prevalence of cesarean sections
- ▶ Major risk factor is placenta previa with previous cesarean section that increases with repeated frequency
- ▶ US findings: sensitivity 77–87%, specificity 96–98%
  - Loss of the normal retroplacental hypoechoic zone (arrow in Fig. 39.7)
  - Loss of the bladder and uterine wall interface (arrow in Fig. 39.8)
  - Presence of placenta previa or basal placental lakes
  - Vascularity extending into or beyond the myometrium
  - Bulging exophytic placental mass into the bladder

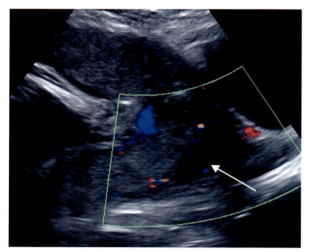

Fig. 39.7

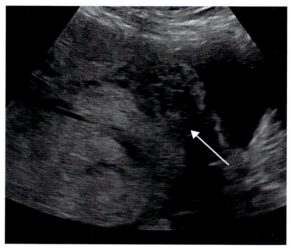

Fig. 39.8

- ▶ MRI can be helpful in confirmation and determination of extent of invasion. Note irregularity of the posterior margin of the placenta and bulging consistent with extension into the attenuated myometrium or increta (short arrows in Fig. 39.9). In addition, the high signal intensity of the placental tissue extends to the bladder lumen (long arrow in Fig. 39.9) without a fat plane between placenta and bladder and loss of the normal low signal intensity of the bladder wall, most consistent with percreta

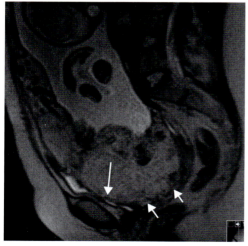

Fig. 39.9

- ▶ The degree of invasion of the myometrium in placenta accreta and increta is not easily distinguished by ultrasound, especially if the placenta is posterior. The interface between the thin myometrium and the posterior border of the placenta is not easy to see, especially late in gestation

- Placenta previa, especially when complete, can obscure the underlying myometrium and can be mistaken for placenta increta/percreta
- Poor technique and resolution can mimic placental invasion of the myometrium and should be confirmed on multiple views or rescanned with a higher frequency transducer

Management

- Careful evaluation of placental location and assessment for invasion in patients with previous cesarean section
- Confirmation of the diagnosis with preoperative MRI may be helpful
- Timing of delivery at 34 or 35 weeks preferred, with steroids to improve fetal lung maturity administered prior to delivery
- Planned delivery in tertiary care center and management by multidisciplinary team including surgeons, urogynecologists, and interventional radiologists, who may place prophylactic balloon catheters into the internal iliac arteries preoperatively to help control hemorrhage
- Abdominal hysterectomy and blood replacement products when necessary

Further Reading

1. Calì G, Giambanco L, Puccio G, et al. Morbidly adherent placenta: Evaluation of ultrasound diagnostic criteria and differentiation of placenta accreta from percreta. *Ultrasound Obstet Gynecol.* 2013; 41: 406–410.
2. Chou MM, Ho ES, Lee YH. Prenatal diagnosis of placenta previa accreta by transabdominal color Doppler ultrasound. *Ultrasound Obstet Gynecol.* 2000; 15: 28–30.
3. O'Brien JM, Barton JR, Donaldson ES. The management of placenta percreta: Conservative and operative strategies. *Am J Obstet Gynecol.* 1996; 175: 1632–1635.

Case 40

► 23-Year-old gravida 5 para 4 presenting with vaginal bleeding at 24 weeks of gestation (Figs. 40.1–40.3)

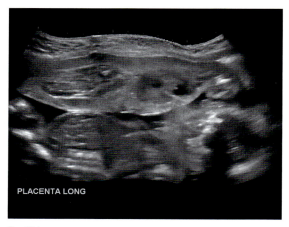

Fig. 40.1

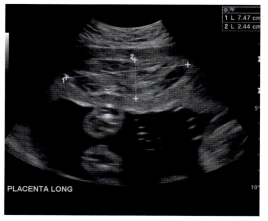

Fig. 40.2

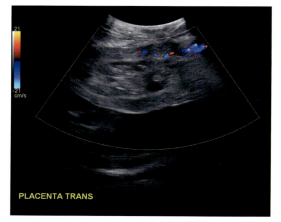

Fig. 40.3

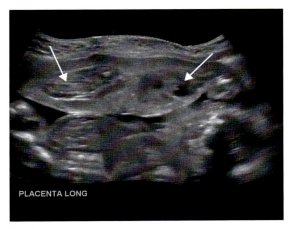

Fig. 40.4

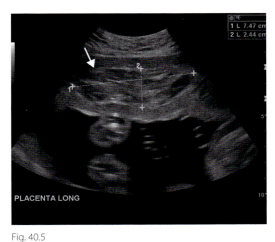

Fig. 40.5

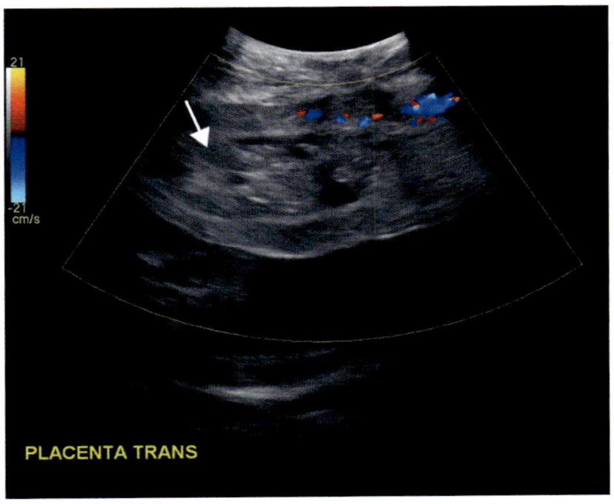

Fig. 40.6

Imaging Findings

▶ Longitudinal image using extended field of view showing multiple hypoechoic areas within the placental substance (arrows in Fig. 40.4)

▶ Heterogeneous predominantly hypoechoic hematoma corresponding to placental abruption (arrow and calipers in Fig. 40.5) covers approximately 50% of the retroplacental space; confirmed at delivery

▶ Color Doppler image of area of abruption showing the absence of flow in hematoma occupying space between myometrium and placenta (arrow in Fig. 40.6)

Differential Diagnosis

▶ Leiomyoma
▶ Placental tumors

Teaching Points

▶ Placental abruption refers to premature separation of the placenta from the uterus after 20 weeks gestational age
  ▪ Severe form occurs in approximately 1 out of 800–1600 pregnancies
▶ Location: The hematoma may be marginal and attached to the edge of the placenta (arrow in Fig. 40.7), retroplacental, or preplacental between the amnion and placental mass (can be subamnionic or subchorionic)

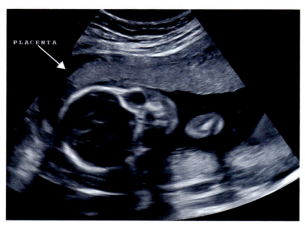

Fig. 40.7

- ► Size is variable
- ► Risk factors
  - Cause is often unknown
  - Trauma
  - Cocaine use, alcohol consumption (> 14 drinks per week), cigarette smoking
  - Blood clotting disorders
  - High blood pressure
  - Retroplacental leiomyoma
  - Diabetes
  - Increased uterine distention (including multiple gestations and multiparity)
  - Advanced maternal age
  - History of prior placental abruption
- ► Clinical presentation
  - May be completely asymptomatic
  - Sudden onset of vaginal bleeding, pelvic pain, nearly continuous contractions, fetal distress
  - Should always be considered as a potential cause of vaginal bleeding in the second or third trimester
- ► US appearance
  - The clot, if remote and resolving, appears hypoechoic and may reach the echogenicity of amniotic fluid
  - Recent clots appear echogenic and may appear solid or have mixed echogenicity
  - Absence of detectable Doppler blood flow is very helpful in making diagnosis
- ► Sensitivity of ultrasound is reported to be 25–50%, but positive predictive value (PPV) once detected is 88%
- ► Perinatal death likely (50% risk) if abruption undermines more than 50% of the placenta
- ► Other ultrasound findings
  - Large placenta due to intraplacental bleed
  - Echogenic debris in the amniotic fluid (due to blood traversing the amnion, resolving clot protein diffusing into the amniotic fluid)
  - Echogenic fetal bowel (due to swallowing of debris)
- ► Uterine leiomyomas posterior to the placenta may appear hypoechoic relative to the surrounding myometrium, but they distort the outer border of the uterus, unlike placental hematomas, which are limited to the placental substance
- ► Chorioangiomas of the placenta are usually well-defined and demonstrate some internal vascularity

Management

- ► Vaginal bleeding of unknown origin in pregnancy can be due to abruption, but ultrasound may be negative with an acute or small bleed
- ► Disseminated intravascular coagulation (DIC) screen may be normal in patients with mild and moderate abruptions
  - Fibrinogen levels ≤ 200 mg/dl have been reported to have a 100% PPV for severe postpartum hemorrhage
- ► Delivery depends on maternal and fetal status as well as gestational age
  - Continuous fetal monitoring recommended until maternal and fetal status determined
  - Transfuse to correct or prevent DIC
  - Deliver if severe abruption and non-reassuring maternal or fetal status at any gestational age
  - Lesser degrees of abruption may be monitored until 37 or 38 weeks at the risk of sudden progression to severe abruption

- Vaginal delivery may be attempted if access to cesarean section and blood products readily available
- Pregnancies complicated by intrauterine growth restriction or preeclampsia will require earlier delivery

Further Reading

1. Ananth CV, Wilcox AJ. Placental abruption and perinatal mortality in the United States. *Am J Epidemiol*. 2001; 153(4): 332.
2. Nyberg DA, Mack LA, Benedetti TJ, et al. Placental abruption and placental hemorrhage: Correlation of sonographic findings with fetal outcome. *Radiology*. 1987; 164(2): 357.
3. Tuuli MG, Norman SM, Odibo AO, et al. Perinatal outcomes in women with subchorionic hematoma: A systematic review and meta-analysis. *Obstet Gynecol*. 2011; 117(5): 1205.

Case 41

History

▶ 25-Year-old primigravida referred for fetal dating (Figs. 41.1 and 41.2)

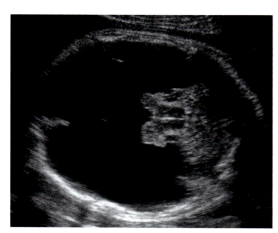

Fig. 41.1

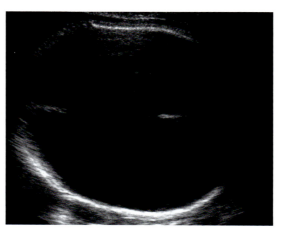

Fig. 41.2

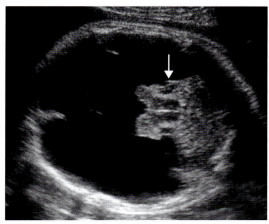

Fig. 41.3

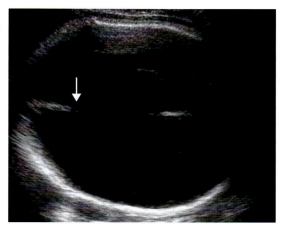

Fig. 41.4

Imaging Findings

► Axial image at level of midbrain (Fig. 41.3) shows no cerebral tissue; intact cerebral peduncle and cerebellum (arrow in Fig. 41.3)
► Axial image at parietal region (Fig. 41.4) shows no brain tissue; falx (arrow in Fig. 41.4) is present

Differential Diagnosis

► Severe hydrocephalus
► Holoprosencephaly

Teaching Points

► Congenital brain defect in which fluid-filled cavities replace the cerebral hemispheres
► Proposed etiologies include the following
  ▪ Infarction (bilateral carotid occlusion, placental abruption)
  ▪ Primary agenesis of neural wall
  ▪ Diffuse hypoxic–ischemic brain necrosis (carbon dioxide poisoning, toxins)
  ▪ Infection (TORCH)
  ▪ Hemorrhage (coagulation disorders, thrombocytopenia)
► Cerebellum, midbrain, thalami, and basal ganglia usually preserved
► Prenatal MRI is confirmatory for identification of the intact falx (arrow in Fig. 41.5) and posterior fossa (arrow in Fig. 41.6)

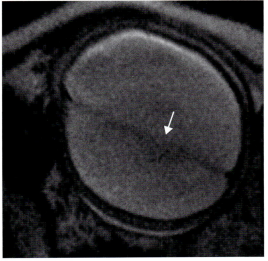

Fig. 41.5

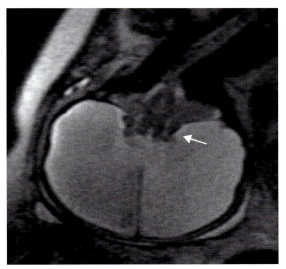

Fig. 41.6

- ▸ Sonographic findings vary according to time course
  - ▪ Macrocephaly
  - ▪ Large fluid-filled intracranial cavity; echogenicity variable, representing liquefied brain and blood (arrows in Fig. 41.7)

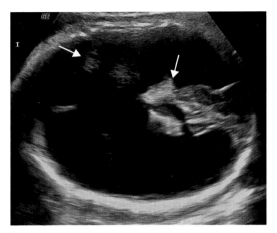

Fig. 41.7

- ▸ Cerebral hemispheres initially echogenic in hemorrhagic areas, becoming cystic as brain becomes necrotic
- ▸ Amount of cerebral cortex decreases over time and is replaced with fluid and debris
  - ▪ Eventually no cerebral cortex visible
  - ▪ Optimally demonstrated on MRI, on which relative volume of fluid and brain remnants (arrows in Fig. 41.8) are best seen

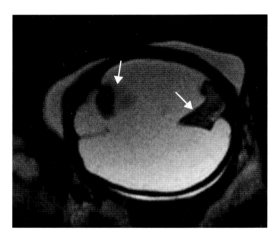

Fig. 41.8

- ▸ Polyhydramnios usually present by the end of second trimester because brain abnormality leads to poor fetal swallowing
  - ▪ Fetal movement, including breathing and sucking motions, preserved
- ▸ Results in microcephaly if insult occurs early with no cerebral cortex anteriorly, but portions of occipital lobe, midbrain, and basal ganglia variably preserved
- ▸ Alobar holoprosencephaly characterized by absence of midline echo
  - ▪ In hydranencephaly some midline structures (falx cerebri, interhemispheric fissure, third ventricle) are present, but they are absent in holoprosencephaly
  - ▪ Cerebral cortex absent in hydranencephaly but displaced in holoprosencephaly
  - ▪ Face usually normal in hydranencephaly, whereas midline facial dysmorphism is common in holoprosencephaly
  - ▪ Severe hydrocephalus will demonstrate massive enlargement of the ventricles, but a peripheral rim of brain will be present, although severely thinned, and the falx will be intact

Management

- ▶ Infant may appear normal at birth, but not compatible with prolonged life
  - Most infants deceased prior to 1 year of age
- ▶ Consider fetal MR for anatomic clarification and to distinguish between hydranencephaly and hydrocephalus
- ▶ Infection/coagulation screen, consider karyotyping
- ▶ If pregnancy progresses, no fetal monitoring during labor and no resuscitation

Further Reading

1. Greene MF, Benacerraf B, Crawford JM. Hydranencephaly: US appearance during in utero evolution. *Radiology.* 1985; 156: 779–782.
2. Lam YH, Tang MH. Serial sonographic features of a fetus with hydranencephaly from 11 weeks to term. *Ultrasound Obstet Gynecol.* 2000; 16(1): 77–79.
3. Sepulveda W, Cortes-Yepes H, Wong AE, et al. Prenatal sonography in hydranencephaly: Findings during the early stages of disease. *J Ultrasound Med.* 2012; 31: 799–802.

Case 42

History

▶ 27-Year-old gravida 4 para 3 presents for routine dating ultrasound (Figs. 42.1–42.4)

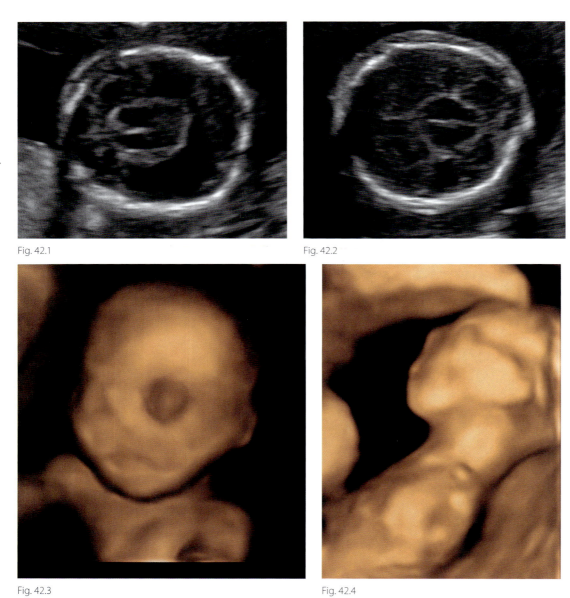

Fig. 42.1

Fig. 42.2

Fig. 42.3

Fig. 42.4

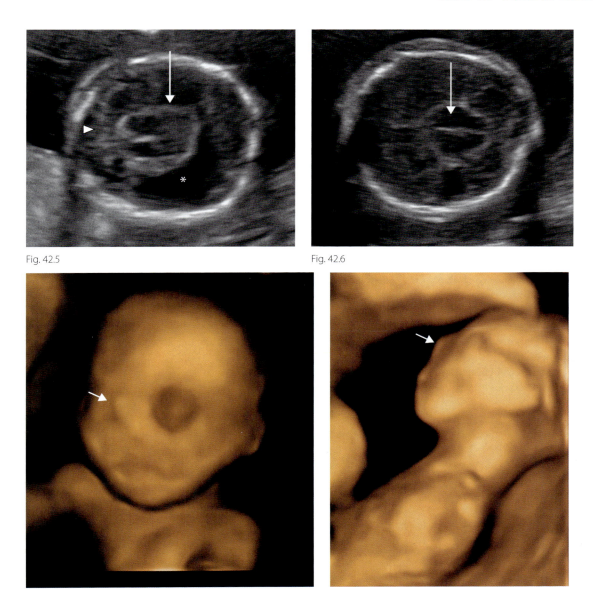

Fig. 42.5

Fig. 42.6

Fig. 42.7

Fig. 42.8

Imaging Findings

▶ Axial images of the brain demonstrate fused thalami (arrows in Figs. 42.5 and 42.6), small cerebellum (arrowhead in Fig. 42.5), monoventricle (asterisk in Fig. 42.5), and absence of a falx
▶ Coronal and sagittal three-dimensional surface rendered images show short proboscis (arrows in Figs. 42.7 and Fig. 42.8) instead of a nose
▶ One eye was well seen but the other eye cannot be defined, raising the suspicion of unilateral anophthalmia

Differential Diagnosis

▶ Encephalomalacia
▶ Hydrocephaly
▶ Isolated craniofacial defect

Teaching Points

▶ Holoprosencephaly develops from failure of the prosencephalon (forebrain) to differentiate into two cerebral hemispheres and lateral ventricles

- Developmental abnormality occurs at approximately 4–8 weeks gestational age, resulting in partial to complete fusion of the cerebral hemispheres and lateral ventricles that may communicate across the midline
- Incidence higher in abortuses than live births (0.4 vs. 0.06 per 1000 pregnancies)
- Prognosis is poor
- Three main types of holoprosencephaly in decreasing order of severity: alobar, semilobar, and lobar
- Alobar holoprosencephaly: lethal anomaly characterized by complete failure of cleavage of the prosencephalon
  - Cerebral hemispheres are fused with a single large midline fluid collection (ventricle)
  - Absent corpus callosum and falx cerebri
  - Thalami usually completely fused
- Semilobar holoprosencephaly: similar to alobar holoprosencephaly but with more cerebral tissue preserved
  - Typically has rudimentary occipital horns and separated occipital lobes
- Lobar holoprosencephaly: cerebral hemispheres and lateral ventricles better separated
  - Hemispheres fused anteriorly
  - Absent cavum septi pellucidi
  - Corpus callosum may be present or absent
  - Thalamus may be fused or separated
- "The face predicts the brain"—the most severe brain malformations are associated with the most severe dysmorphisms, such as cyclopia (single eye with proboscis located above the eye, nose absent), ethmocephaly (hypotelorism, micro-ophthalmia, interorbital proboscis, nose absent), or cebocephaly (hypotelorism, micro-ophthalmia, small flat single-nostril nose)
  - Less severe facial dysmorphisms include hypertelorism and cleft lip and/or palate
- Diagnosis cannot be made before the 10th week of pregnancy because the falx normally does not become sonographically apparent until 9 postmenstrual weeks
- Karyotypes reported in alobar holoprosencephaly: trisomy 13, euploidy, triploidy, trisomy 21, and trisomy 18
- Encephalomalacia and hydrocephalus may be mistaken for holoprosencephaly, but in both these entities, the falx will be present and two separate ventricles can be distinguished
- Unrelated defects such as porencephaly or encephalomalacia can occur independently from other facial defects such as clefts and hyper-/hypotelorism and can be mistaken for related abnormalities such as those seen in holoprosencephaly

Management

- Severe cases are not compatible with life and generally do not survive beyond early infancy
- Milder forms are more compatible with life
- Genetic counseling and karyotype testing recommended for afflicted family to discuss nature of the condition, possibility of recurrence (6%), and to rule out syndromic association

Further Reading

1. Blaas H-GK, Eriksson AG, Salvesen N, et al. Brains and faces in holoprosencephaly: Pre- and postnatal description of 30 cases. *Ultrasound Obstet Gynecol.* 2002; 19: 24–38.
2. Filly RA, Chinn DH, Callen PW. Alobar holoprosencephaly: Ultrasonographic prenatal diagnosis. *Radiology.* 1984; 151: 455–459.
3. McGahan JP, Nyberg DA, Mack LA. Sonography of facial features of alobar and semilobar holoprosencephaly. *Am J Roentgenol.* 1990; 154: 143–148.

History

▶ 27-Year-old gravida 3 para 2 referred for fetal tachycardia (Figs. 43.1–43.3)

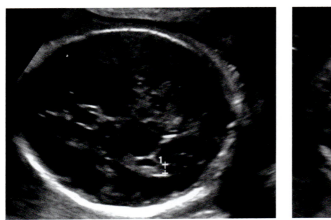

Fig. 43.1

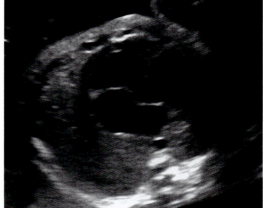

Fig. 43.2

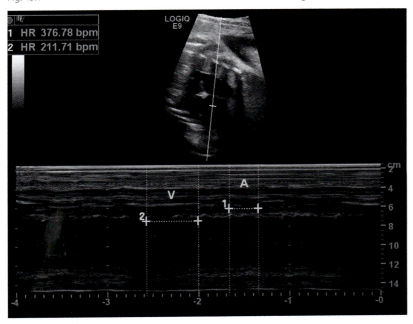

Fig. 43.3

Case 43 Vein of Galen Malformation

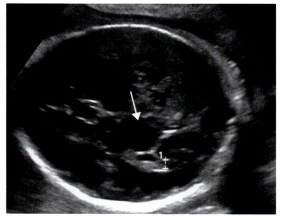

Fig. 43.4

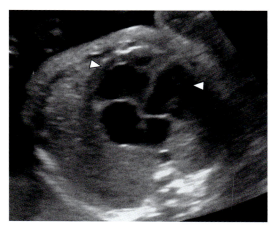

Fig. 43.5

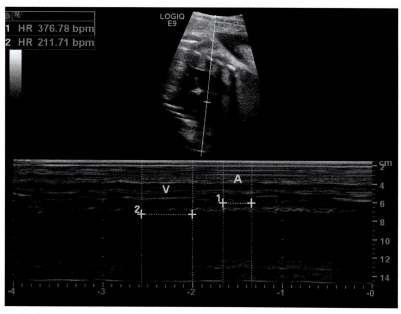

Fig. 43.6

Imaging Findings

▶ Initial fetal ultrasound of the head shows cystic structure (arrow in Fig. 43.4) medial to a normal ventricular atrium (cursors in Fig. 43.4)
▶ Four-chamber heart view shows cardiomegaly (arrowheads in Fig. 43.5); note that the heart occupies more than half of the chest circumference
▶ Fetal heart rate = 376 beats per minute (bpm) atrial rate and 211 bpm ventricular rate (Fig. 43.6)

Differential Diagnosis

▶ Enlarged third ventricle
▶ Arachnoid cyst
▶ Vascular tumor

Teaching Points

▶ A vein of Galen malformation is a congenital ateriovenous malformation (AVM) between major branches of the carotid/vertebrobasilar system and venous plexus resulting in marked dilation of the vein of Galen
▶ Develops at 6–11 weeks of gestation

- ▶ Extremely rare, affecting between 1 in 100,000 to 1 in 1 million newborns; no gender predilection
- ▶ Cause unknown; majority of cases sporadic with no hereditary risk
- ▶ Complications from arteriovenous shunting may result in the following
  - ▪ High-output cardiac failure soon after birth
  - ▪ Significant neurological problems within the first year of life
  - ▪ Kidney and liver failure
- ▶ If not treated within the first 6 months of life, can result in serious brain damage
- ▶ Can be detected on an ultrasound during the third trimester but often not diagnosed until after birth
- ▶ Ultrasound findings
  - ▪ Anechoic cystic structure in the midline posteriorly that fills in with color
- ▶ May be associated with the following
  - ▪ Cardiomegaly and tachycardia
  - ▪ Fetal hydrops
  - ▪ Obstruction of the aqueduct of Sylvius by the malformation can lead to hydrocephalus
- ▶ When seen early in the second trimester, may be missed or misdiagnosed as suprasellar arachnoid cyst that becomes manifest in the third trimester as an AVM when verified with color Doppler (arrows in Fig. 43.7 and Fig. 43.8)

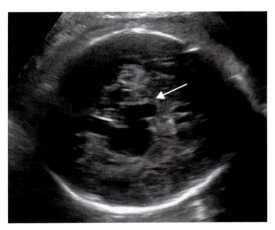 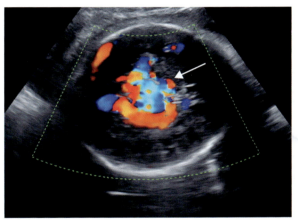

Fig. 43.7   Fig. 43.8

- ▶ A dilated third ventricle in cases of agenesis of the corpus callosum or aqueductal stenosis may manifest as a central anechoic cystic lesion but can usually be distinguished by other associated findings and the absence of flow on Doppler ultrasound
- ▶ Vascular brain tumors are exceedingly rare and usually have solid components and peripheral vascularity rather than being completely replaced by large vessels

Management

- ▶ Best treatment option in most cases is endovascular
- ▶ Treatment typically delayed until 6 months of age to allow for maturation of the cavernous sinus
- ▶ If cardiac failure is refractory to medical management, embolization can be performed at a younger age
- ▶ Both venous and arterial embolization may be necessary, depending on the number of feeders
- ▶ Hydrocephalus should not be shunted because this may exacerbate cerebral ischemia and increase risk of intracerebral hemorrhage

Further Reading

1. Nuutila M, Saisto T. Prenatal diagnosis of vein of Galen malformation: A multidisciplinary challenge. *Am J Perinatol.* 2008; 25(4): 225–227.
2. Jones BV, Ball WS, Tomsick TA, et al. Vein of Galen aneurysmal malformation: Diagnosis and treatment of 13 children with extended clinical follow-up. *Am J Neuroradiol.* 2002; 23(10): 1717–1724.
3. Raybaud CA, Strother CM, Hald JK. Aneurysms of the vein of Galen: Embryonic considerations and anatomical features relating to the pathogenesis of the malformation. *Neuroradiology.* 1989; 31: 109–128.

Case 44

History

▶ 28-Year-old gravida 2 para 1 referred for enlarged fetal head on initial US (Figs. 44.1–44.3)

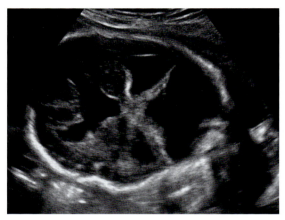

Fig. 44.1

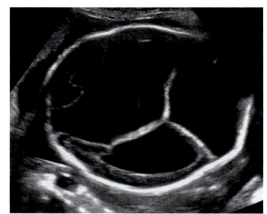

Fig. 44.2

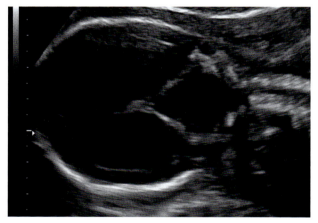

Fig. 44.3

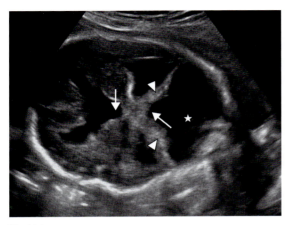

Fig. 44.4

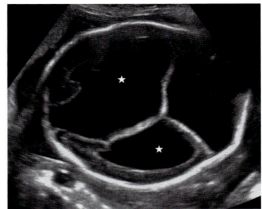

Fig. 44.5

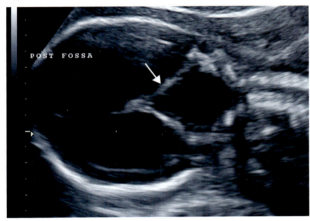

Fig. 44.6

Imaging Findings

► Axial image through base of brain shows large posterior fossa cyst (star in Fig.44.4) with compression of the cerebellar hemispheres (arrowheads in Fig.44.4) against the tentorium; the vermis not identified; the fourth ventricle (long arrow in Fig.44.4) communicates with the posterior fossa cyst; the third ventricle (short arrow in Fig.44.4) is dilated
► Contiguous axial image superior to Fig.44.4 demonstrates severe asymmetric bilateral ventriculomegaly (stars in Fig.44.5)
► Coronal image shows tentorium (arrow in Fig.44.6) separating the large posterior fossa cyst and severe bilateral ventriculomegaly

Differential Diagnosis

► Mega cisterna magna
► Arachnoid cyst
► Dandy–Walker variant

Teaching Points

► Complex developmental anomaly of the fourth ventricle occurring at during postmenstrual week 6 or 7
  ▪ Incidence is 1 in 30,000 births
► Symptoms: seizures, hypotonia, delayed or abnormal motor development
► 40% mortality in infancy/early childhood
► Normal intelligence in 35–50% of cases
► US findings
  ▪ Dilatation of the fourth ventricle
  ▪ Large posterior fossa cyst extending from the cisterna magna to the fourth ventricle

- Hypoplasia or complete agenesis of the cerebellar vermis
- Elevated tentorium
- Dilatation of the third and lateral ventricles

▶ Confirmation with prenatal MRI shows the elevated tentorium (arrow in Fig.44.7) and severe ventriculomegaly (arrowheads in Fig.44.8)

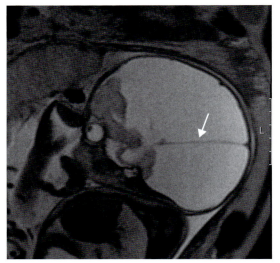

Fig. 44.7

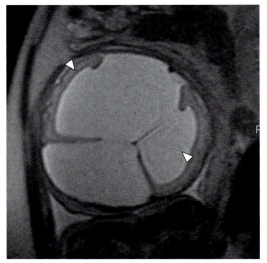

Fig. 44.8

▶ Hydrocephaly present in 75% of cases of Dandy–Walker malformation (DWM)
▶ Cerebellar hemispheres are often flattened and separated due to compression by the large DW cyst
▶ Corpus callosum may be absent
▶ Differentiation between DWM and an arachnoid cyst of the posterior fossa depends on demonstration of the hypoplastic vermis and connection of the DW cyst with the fourth ventricle
▶ DW variant: a small defect in the cerebellar vermis without dilatation of the cisterna magna
▶ Megacisterna magna: term utilized when the cisterna magna is enlarged (> 10 mm on oblique transverse plane) but the cerebellar hemispheres and vermis are normal

Management

▶ Combined shunting of the cyst and lateral ventricles is the initial procedure for patients with DWM

Further Reading

1. Robinson AJ, Blaser S, Toi A, et al. The fetal cerebellar vermis: Assessment for abnormal development by ultrasonography and magnetic resonance imaging. *Ultrasound Q.* 2007; 23(3): 211–223.
2. Kollias SS, Ball WS Jr, Prenger EC. Cystic malformations of the posterior fossa: Differential diagnosis clarified through embryologic analysis. *RadioGraphics.* 1993; 13(6): 1211–1231.
3. Osenbach RK, Menezes AH. Diagnosis and management of the Dandy–Walker malformation: 30 years of experience. *Pediatr Neurosurg.* 1992; 18(4): 179–183.

History

▶ 28-Year-old gravida 2 para 1 referred for fetal dating (Figs. 45.1 and 45.2)

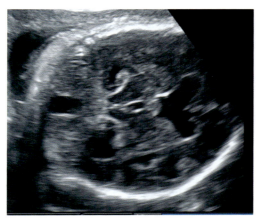

Fig. 45.1

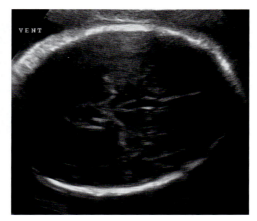

Fig. 45.2

Case 45 Agenesis of the Corpus Callosum

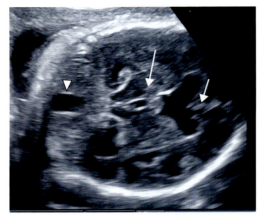

Fig. 45.3

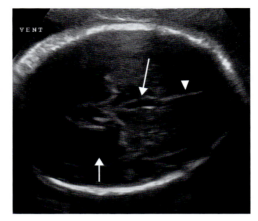

Fig. 45.4

Imaging Findings

► Axial image at the level of the cerebellum (Fig. 45.3) shows a posterior fossa cyst (arrowhead) that communicates with the fourth ventricle (Dandy–Walker variant), dilated third ventricle (long arrow), and anterior falx (short arrow)
► At the level of the thalamus (Fig. 45.4), the dilated third ventricle (long arrow) is high-riding and touches the anterior falx (arrowhead) due to the absence of the corpus callosum; the occipital horn of the lateral ventricle (short arrow) is also markedly dilated (colpocephaly)

Differential Diagnosis

► Obstructive hydrocephalus
► Dysgenesis of the corpus callosum
► Lobar holoprosencephaly

Teaching Points

► The corpus callosum connects the left and right cerebral hemispheres
► Agenesis of the corpus callosum (ACC) can be complete or partial, depending on the stage of development when growth was arrested
► Most cases are sporadic, but ACC may be associated with several genetic and chromosomal disorders, including Chiari malformation, Dandy–Walker syndrome, schizencephaly, lissencephaly, pachygyria, and midline facial defects
► Outcome dependent on the presence or absence of associated anomalies
► US findings
   ▪ With complete ACC, the gyri and sulci radiate perpendicular to the dilated third ventricle in a sunburst pattern; the frontal horns appear narrow and laterally displaced; the atria and occipital horns are dilated (colpocephaly); the cavum septi pellucidi is absent
   ▪ In partial agenesis, the posterior portion of the corpus callosum is usually absent or dysmorphic
► MRI studies are done when US studies are equivocal and will show the US findings in better detail
   ▪ Axial MRI image (Fig. 45.5) shows dilated third ventricle (long arrow) and colpocephaly (short arrows)
   ▪ Coronal MRI image at the level of the posterior fossa (Fig. 45.6) shows the posterior fossa cyst (arrow) and colpocephaly
   ▪ Midsagittal MRI image (Fig. 45.7) shows absence of a low signal corpus callosum at the expected location (arrows) above the cavum septi pellucidi et vergae

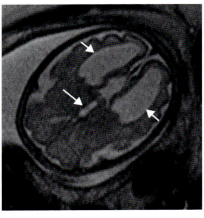

Fig. 45.5

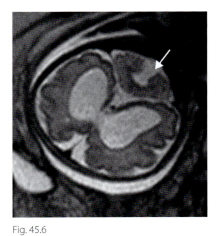

Fig. 45.6

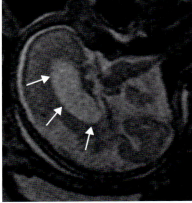

Fig. 45.7

- ▶ Obstructive hydrocephalus usually manifests as diffuse ventricular dilation, more severe than that seen in ACC
- ▶ Dysgenesis of the corpus callosum may show significant thinning (diffuse or partial) leading to false-positive diagnosis of ACC
- ▶ Lobar holoprosencephaly may not be easily diagnosed in utero because of very subtle findings
  - ▪ Fusion of the frontal horns that communicate with the third ventricle
  - ▪ Absence of the cavum septi pellucidi
  - ▪ The falx is present and the thalami are not fused
  - ▪ Best evaluated with MRI

Management

- ▶ Fetal MRI can be helpful to assess for associated anomalies and enhance prognostic counseling
- ▶ Karyotype recommended even in isolated cases

Further Reading

1. Warren ME, Cook JV. Agenesis of the corpus callosum. *Br J Radiol*. 1993; 66(781): 81–85.
2. Bertino RE, Nyberg DA, Cyr DR, et al. Prenatal diagnosis of agenesis of the corpus callosum. *J Ultrasound Med*. 1988; 7(5): 251–260.
3. Barkovich AJ, Norman D. Anomalies of the corpus callosum: Correlation with further anomalies of the brain. *Am J Roentgenol*. 1988; 151(1): 171–179.

Case 46

History

▶ 30-Year-old gravida 3 para 2 presents for genetic screening due to family history of fetal anomalies (Figs. 46.1–46.4)

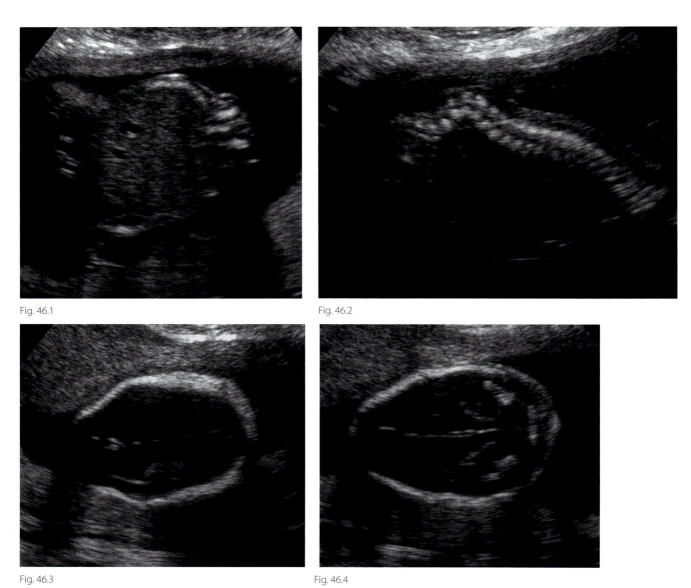

Fig. 46.1

Fig. 46.2

Fig. 46.3

Fig. 46.4

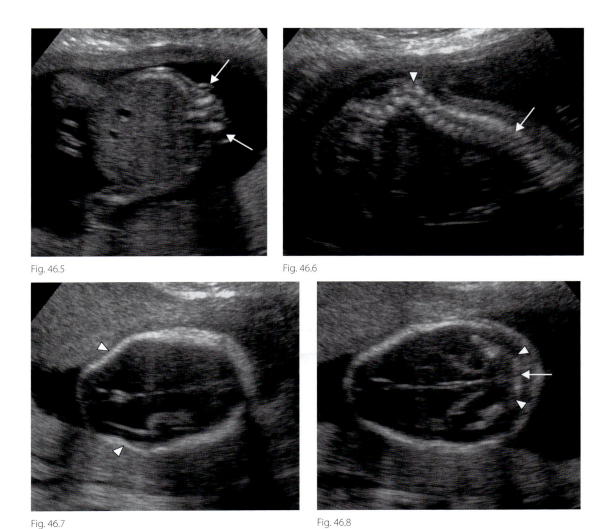

Fig. 46.5

Fig. 46.6

Fig. 46.7

Fig. 46.8

Imaging Findings

▶ Axial image at the level of the upper abdomen shows splaying of the posterior vertebral ossification centers (arrows in Fig. 46.5)
▶ Longitudinal image of spine shows relatively normal alignment of ossification centers of the cervical and thoracic spine (arrow in Fig. 46.6) but long segment of spinal deformity demonstrated in lumbosacral spine (arrowhead in Fig. 46.6)
▶ Axial image obtained high in the cerebral convexities shows indentation of both frontal bones (arrows in Fig. 46.7)—the "lemon sign"
▶ Axial image taken at level of cerebellum shows abnormal appearance of cerebellar hemispheres (arrows in Fig. 46.8) with obliteration of the cisterna magna—the "banana sign"

Differential Diagnosis

▶ Normal spine with oblique views
▶ Hemivertebrae with abnormal spinal curvature
▶ False-positive lemon sign
▶ False-negative lemon sign

Teaching Points

▶ Neural tube defects (NTDs) are the second most prevalent congenital anomaly, after cardiac malformations
▶ Prenatal maternal serum screening programs for α-fetoprotein (AFP), instituted in the 1970s and 1980s, combined with periconceptional folic acid supplementation and food fortification (instituted in the 1990s) have led to a decrease in the prevalence of NTDs where these interventions are practiced

- Multiple causes
  - Genetic
  - Teratogenic
  - Folate deficiency
  - Maternal diabetes
  - However, cause generally unknown
- Fetus can be born with ventriculomegaly or develop it postnatally, necessitating shunt placement
- Often have associated anatomic abnormalities such as deformities and limited motion of the lower extremities
- Symptoms: range from mild to life-threatening
  - Children < 2 years can have cranial nerve/brain stem signs/symptoms including respiratory symptoms; can be neurosurgical emergency
  - > 2 years: cervical myelopathy, headache
  - Most develop hydrocephalus
- Screening for NTDs recommended with maternal serum AFP and US
- Normal US of spine
  - Three ossification centers in the transverse view with normal orientation of the posterior elements (arrowheads in Fig. 46.9)
  - Intact skin covering spine
  - Longitudinal US of spine shows normal alignment of ossification centers and intact covering skin (arrow in Fig. 46.10)

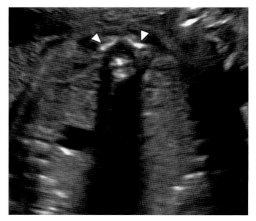 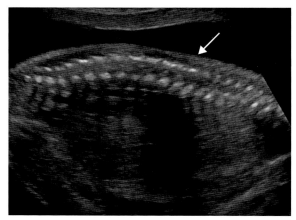

Fig. 46.9

Fig. 46.10

- US of open NTD demonstrates vertebral bony defect exposing the meninges and neural tissue on axial image (arrow in Fig. 46.11) and coronal image of sacrococcygeal spine (arrow in Fig. 46.12)
- Exiting neural tissue differentiates meningomyelocele from meningocele

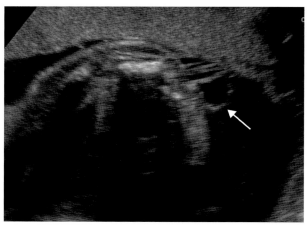 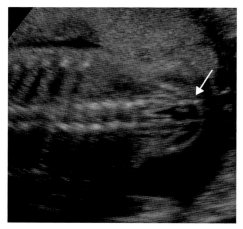

Fig. 46.11

Fig. 46.12

- The lemon and banana signs are markers for Chiari II malformation seen on second- or early third-trimester axial images of the fetal brain
  - Thought to be caused by downward shift of brain secondary to decreased intraspinal pressure indirectly transmitted to intracranial structures

156

- Lemon sign: flattened/concave frontal bones giving the cranial vault the shape of a lemon
  - Secondary to response of malleable frontal bones to drop in intracranial pressure triggered by distal opening in the spine
- Banana sign: cerebellum appears thin and wraps around the brain stem, giving it a curved banana-like appearance; small posterior fossa; cisterna magna obliterated secondary to herniation of the midbrain through the foramen magnum
  - It is believed that as the intraspinal pressure decreases due to the neural tube defect, intracranial pressure decreases causing the midbrain to herniate into the foramen magnum and obliterate the cisterna magna, resulting in the "banana" shape of the cerebellum
▶ Fetus with a myelomeningocele imaged at 33 weeks
- Banana sign present (arrows in Fig. 46.13 and Fig. 46.14)
- However, lemon sign is not seen and configuration of frontal bones appears normal (arrowheads in Fig. 46.13)
- Comparison image of a normal fetus with normal dumbbell shape of cerebellum (arrows in Fig. 46.15)

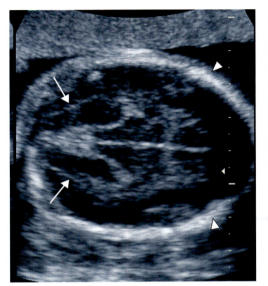

Fig. 46.13

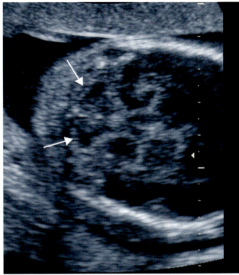

Fig. 46.14

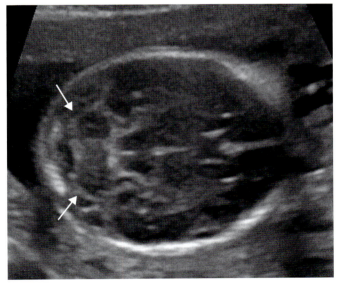

Fig. 46.15

▶ False-positive lemon sign: images taken at the level of the temporal bones may show false indentation of the skull due to the flattened shape of the bones compared to the convexities
▶ False-negative lemon sign: not seen in late third trimester once the frontal bones ossify and become resistant to changes in intracranial pressure (Fig. 46.13)

Management

► Screening for NTDs recommended for all pregnant women; two approaches
  ▪ Measurement of maternal serum AFP at 16–18 weeks
  ▪ Ultrasound examination at 18–20 weeks; ultrasound used as both a screening and a diagnostic test
► Surgical closure in neonate
► Intrauterine myelomeningocele repair controversial; however, performed at tertiary fetal surgery centers
► Neonatal shunt placement for hydrocephalus
► Cervical spine surgery including laminectomies and establishment of cerebrospinal fluid flow

Further Reading

1. Biggio JR, Wenstrom KD, Owen J. Fetal open spina bifida: A natural history of disease progression in utero. *Prenat Diagn.* 2004; 24: 287–289.
2. Mitchell LE, Adzick NS, Melchionne J, et al. Spina bifida. *Lancet.* 2004; 364: 1885–1895.
3. Copp AJ, Stanier P, Greene ND. Neural tube defects: Recent advances, unsolved questions, and controversies. *Lancet Neurol.* 2013; 12: 799–805.
4. Roche CJ, O'Keeffe DP, Lee WK, et al. Selections from the buffet of food signs in radiology. *RadioGraphics.* 2002; 22: 1369–1384.
5. Stevenson KL. Chiari type II malformation: Past, present, and future. *Neurosurg Focus.* 2004; 16: 1–7.
6. Thomas M. The lemon sign. *Radiology.* 2003; 228: 206–207.

History

▶ 37-Year-old gravida 4 para 3 referred for fetal anomaly screening due to advanced maternal age (Figs. 47.1–47.3)

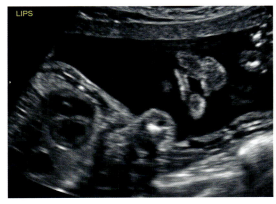

Fig. 47.1

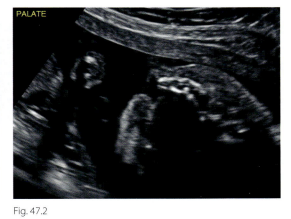

Fig. 47.2

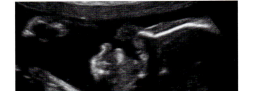

Fig. 47.3

Case 47 Cleft Lip and Palate

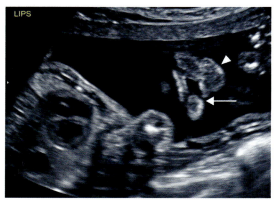
Fig. 47.4

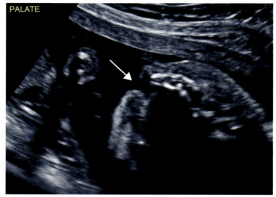
Fig. 47.5

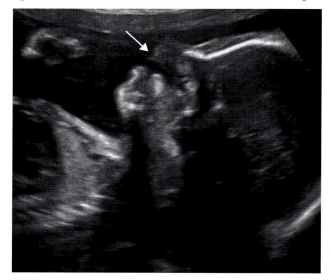
Fig. 47.6

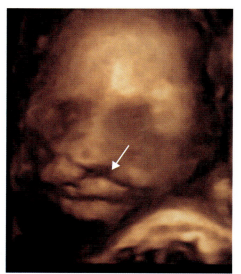
Fig. 47.7

Imaging Findings

▶ Coronal image of face shows midline cleft lip (arrow in Fig. 47.4) just inferior to tip of nose (arrowhead)
▶ Axial image of maxilla shows cleft palate (arrow in Fig. 47.5)
▶ Midsagittal view shows premaxillary protrusion (arrow in Fig. 47.6) highly suggestive of cleft lip and associated cleft palate
▶ Three-dimensional (3D) surface rendered image confirms midline location of clefts (arrow in Fig. 47.7)

Differential Diagnosis

▶ Facial mass lesion that can be confused with combined cleft lip and palate
▶ Deep normal philtrum can mimic a cleft

Teaching Points

▶ Orofacial clefts are the most common craniofacial anomaly and the second most common congenital malformation
  ▪ Incidence: 16/10,000 births
  ▪ 70% nonsyndromic
  ▪ 39% combined cleft lip and palate (CL/P)
  ▪ 34% isolated cleft lip (CL)
  ▪ 27% isolated cleft palate (CP)

- ► Diagnosed after 12 weeks when soft tissues of face are visualized
  - ▪ Detection rate highest if associated with other anomalies
  - ▪ For isolated clefts, detection rate is approximately 50%
- ► Can involve any part of the face, but most commonly presents as cleft between each nostril and central portion of posterior palate
- ► Imaging can be performed in angled coronal, axial, and sagittal views to evaluate the presence of an abnormality
  - ▪ CL without CP is best seen on anterior coronal view
  - ▪ CP is better seen on the axial views as a defect within the alveolar ridge
- ► Bilateral CL/CP presents as a premaxillary pseudo-mass
  - ▪ Visualization of the clefts more difficult on the sagittal and axial views
- ► Facial teratomas may mimic premaxillary mass on sagittal view but usually diagnosed on coronal and axial images
- ► Unilateral cleft lip is best seen on coronal view (arrow in Fig. 47.8) and 3D surface rendered image (arrow in Fig. 47.9)

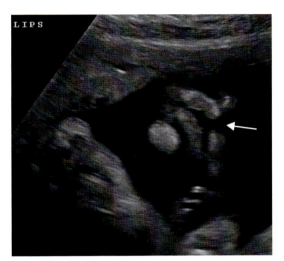

Fig. 47.8

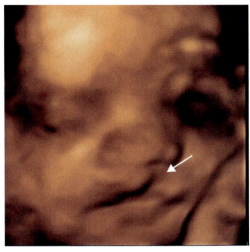

Fig. 47.9

- ► Correlative images of normal face with intact upper lip (arrow in Fig. 47.10) and normal palate (arrow in Fig. 47.11) on axial image of maxilla are helpful for comparison

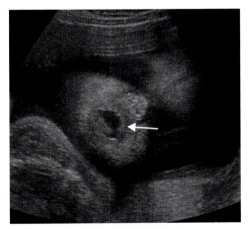

Fig. 47.10

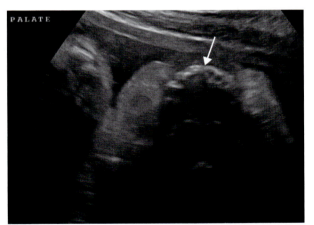

Fig. 47.11

Management

- ► 3D ultrasound and fetal MRI for confirmation
- ► Assess for additional structural anomalies, which are found in 50% of newborns with CP, 20% with CL/P, and 8% with isolated CL
- ► Karyotype offered if associated anomalies
- ► Excellent prognosis with surgical repair if an isolated abnormality

Further Reading

1. Maarse W, Bergé SJ, Pistorius L, et al. Diagnostic accuracy of transabdominal ultrasound in detecting prenatal cleft lip and palate: A systematic review. *Ultrasound Obstet Gynecol.* 2010; 35: 495–499.

2. Johnson CY, Honein MA, Hobbs CA, et al. Prenatal diagnosis of orofacial clefts, National Birth Defects Prevention Study, 1998–2004. *Prenat Diagn.* 2009; 29: 833–837.

3. Gillham JC, Anand S, Bullen PJ. Antenatal detection of cleft lip with or without cleft palate: Incidence of associated chromosomal and structural anomalies. *Ultrasound Obstet Gynecol.* 2009; 34: 410–414.

History

▶ 25-Year-old gravida 3 para 2 referred for suspicion of fetal chest mass (Figs. 48.1 and 48.2)

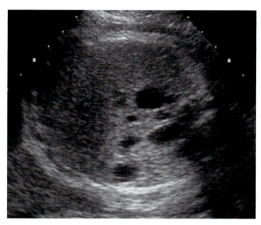 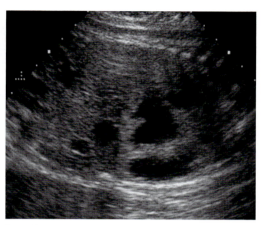

Fig. 48.1   Fig. 48.2

Case 48 Congenital Pulmonary Airway Malformation

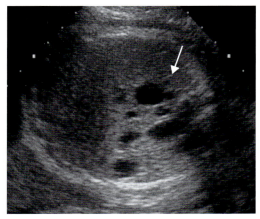
Fig. 48.3

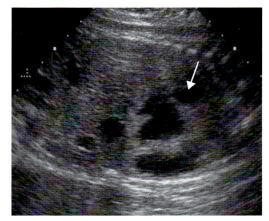
Fig. 48.4

Imaging Findings

▶ Multicystic mass (arrows) in posterior hemithorax on axial (Fig. 48.3) and sagittal (Fig. 48.4) images of the fetal chest

Differential Diagnosis

▶ Bronchopulmonary sequestration
▶ Congenital lobar emphysema
▶ Congenital diaphragmatic hernia

Teaching Points

▶ Previously known as congenital cystic adenomatoid malformation (CCAM)
▶ Hamartomatous lesion composed of cystic and adenomatous elements arising from tracheal, bronchial, bronchiolar, or alveolar tissue
  ▪ Regresses in late pregnancy
  ▪ May appear as a predominantly solid mass in the second trimester (arrows in Figs. 48.5 and 48.6)
  ▪ Regresses in the late third trimester (arrows in Figs. 48.7 and 48.8)

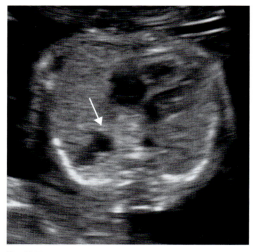
Fig. 48.5

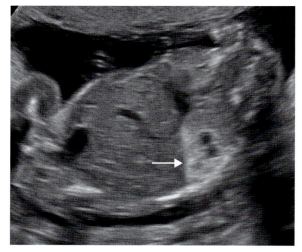
Fig. 48.6

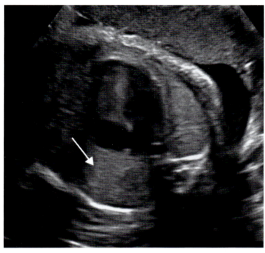

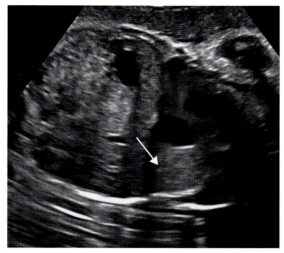

Fig. 48.7   Fig. 48.8

► New classification
- Type 0—rarest form (1–3%); small cysts < 0.5 cm, involves entire lung; gas exchange severely impaired; affected infants die at birth
- Type 1—most common (60–70%); cysts 2–10 cm; single or multiloculated; malignant potential
- Type 2—15–20%; cysts 0.5–2 cm in diameter with solid areas blending into adjacent normal tissue; no risk for malignancy
- Type 3—5–10%; often very large, can involve entire lobe or several lobes; cystic and solid tissue versus entirely solid; numerous small cysts < 0.5 cm in diameter; no risk for malignancy
- Type 4—10–15%; cysts maximum diameter of 7 cm; associated with malignancy, especially pleuropulmonary blastoma

► Bronchopulmonary sequestration usually extralobar and distinguished by direct arterial supply from aorta on color Doppler
► Congenital lobar emphysema may not be distinguishable in utero but characteristic hyperinflation of affected lung on postnatal chest X-ray
► Diaphragmatic hernia differentiated by herniated stomach and associated dextroposition of heart

Management

► Fetuses with large congenital pulmonary airway malformations and hydrops may be candidates for fetal surgery
► Symptomatic patients best managed by surgical resection
- Resected cysts carefully examined for malignancy
► Asymptomatic neonates evaluated with CXR; CT at 4–6 weeks of age
- Lesion will regress within first few months of life in minority of infants
► Surgical resection at 3–6 months of age, or soon after diagnosis is established in older patients

Further Reading

1. Stocker JT. Congenital pulmonary airway malformation—A new name for and an expanded classification of congenital cystic adenomatoid malformation of the lung. *Histopathology*. 2002; 41: 424–430.
2. De Santis M, Masini L, Noia G, et al. Congenital cystic adenomatoid malformation of the lung: Antenatal ultrasound findings and fetal–neonatal outcome. Fifteen years of experience. *Fetal Diagn Ther*. 2000; 15: 246.
3. Shanmugam G, MacArthur K, Pollock JC. Congenital lung malformations—Antenatal and postnatal evaluation and management. *Eur J Cardiothorac Surg*. 2005; 27: 45–52.

Case 49

History
▶ 20-Year-old gravida 1 para 0 with a history of aortic valve stenosis s/p balloon valvuloplasty as an infant presents at 22 weeks of gestation for further evaluation after 20-week obstetric US was concerning for possible congenital heart defect (Figs. 49.1–49.4)

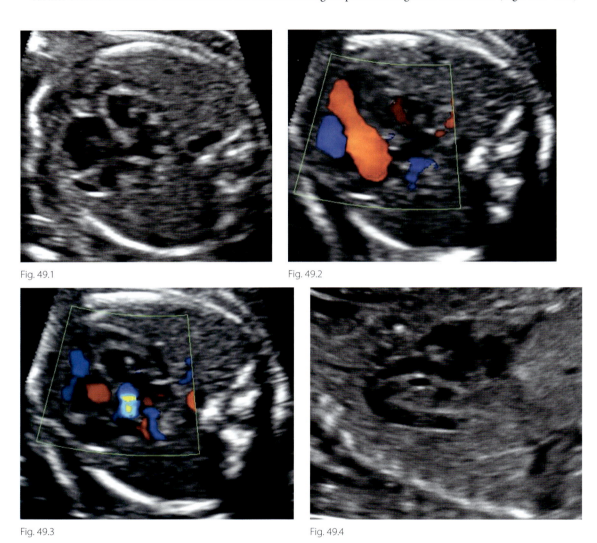

Fig. 49.1

Fig. 49.2

Fig. 49.3

Fig. 49.4

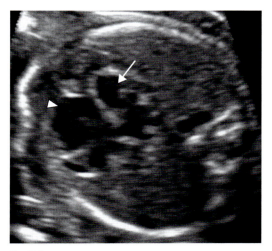

Fig. 49.5

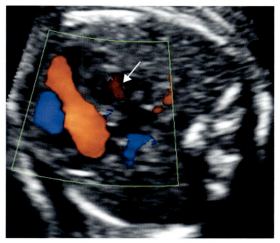

Fig. 49.6

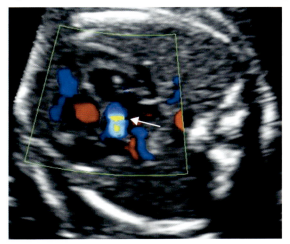

Fig. 49.7

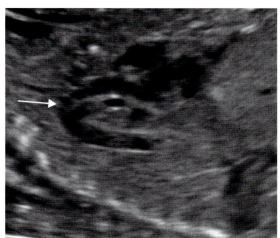

Fig. 49.8

Imaging Findings

► Hypoplastic left ventricle with mitral and aortic valve stenosis
► Four-chamber view demonstrates hypoplastic left ventricle (arrow in Fig. 49.5) that is not apex-forming. The apex of the heart is predominantly formed by the right ventricle (arrowhead in Fig. 49.5)
► Color Doppler image shows prograde flow through the mitral valve; limited left ventricular inflow (arrow in Fig. 49.6)
► Five-chamber view demonstrates obstruction to aortic outflow with flow acceleration across the hypoplastic aortic valve (arrow in Fig. 49.7)
► Longitudinal view of the aortic arch demonstrates moderate transverse arch hypoplasia with prominent pulmonary trunk and ductal arch (arrow in Fig. 49.8)

Differential Diagnosis

► Aortic valve stenosis
► Coarctation of the aorta
► Shone's complex

Teaching Points

► Hypoplastic left heart syndrome (HLHS) accounts for 3–4% of all congenital cardiac anomalies and is one of the most commonly diagnosed heart defects
► This diagnosis should be suspected in any fetus in whom a four-chamber view does not demonstrate an apex-forming left ventricle

- HLHS encompasses a wide spectrum of left ventricular hypoplasia depending on the degree of mitral and aortic valve obstruction
- Aortic root structures may be difficult to visualize, particularly in patients with aortic valve atresia
- Significant tricuspid valve insufficiency and a restrictive interatrial shunt are associated with poorer prognosis; color Doppler of atrial septum demonstrates left-to-right shunting at atrial level (arrow in Fig. 49.9)

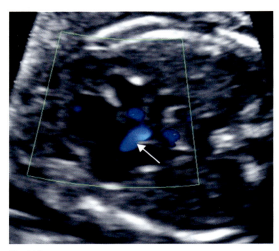

Fig. 49.9

- Chronically elevated left ventricular wall stress results in endocardial fibroelastosis demonstrated as hyperechogenicity in left ventricle (arrow in Fig. 49.10) demonstrated in a short-axis view

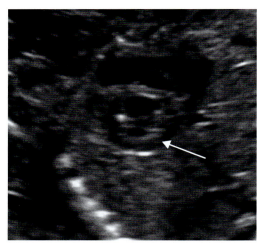

Fig. 49.10

- Coarctation of the aorta and aortic stenosis are difficult structural abnormalities to directly visualize, but they can be suspected using Doppler interrogation of the outflow tracts in utero. A small left ventricle may suggest the diagnosis that could trigger referral for fetal echocardiography
- Another complex cardiac anomaly mimicking HLHS is Shone's syndrome, which is a rare congenital heart disease consisting of four left-sided defects: supravalvular mitral membrane, parachute mitral valve, subaortic stenosis, and coarctation of the aorta

Management

- Serial prenatal ultrasounds should be performed to follow fetal growth, right heart function, and assess flow across the foramen ovale
- If available, fetal echocardiography by a pediatric cardiologist with expertise in this field is beneficial to coordinate postnatal care as well as to provide counseling to the mother
- Prostaglandin infusion should be initiated at birth, and the neonate should be immediately transferred to a tertiary care pediatric facility with access to pediatric cardiology and cardiovascular surgery
- Once considered a universally fatal condition, currently surgical outcomes have greatly improved with widespread experience with single ventricle palliation

► Pediatric cardiac transplantation is considered in cases of right ventricular failure, significant tricuspid valve insufficiency, or other forms of failed single ventricle palliation. In rare cases, it is offered as an option to neonates with this diagnosis

Acknowledgment

Images courtesy of the fetal echocardiography program at Arkansas Children's Hospital.

Further Reading

1. Kipps AK, Feuille C, Azakie A, et al. Prenatal diagnosis of hypoplastic left heart syndrome in current era. *Am J Cardiol*. 2011; 108(3): 421.
2. Mahle WT, Clancy RR, McGaurn SP, et al. Impact of prenatal diagnosis on survival and early neurologic morbidity in neonates with the hypoplastic left heart syndrome. *Pediatrics*. 2001; 107(6): 1277.

Case 50

History

▶ 27-Year-old gravida 1 para 0 mother with no significant past medical history presents at 24 weeks of gestation for further evaluation after obstetric US was concerning for possible congenital heart defect (Figs. 50.1–50.4)

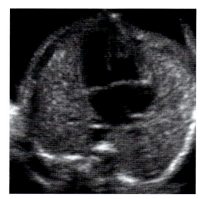

Fig. 50.1

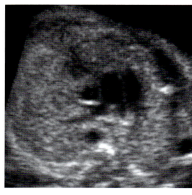

Fig. 50.2

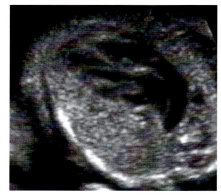

Fig. 50.3

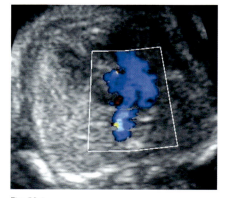

Fig. 50.4

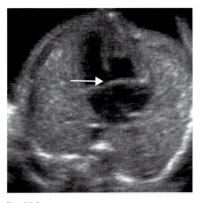

Fig. 50.5

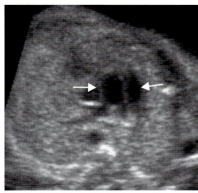

Fig. 50.6

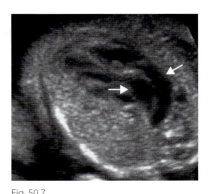

Fig. 50.7

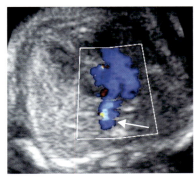

Fig. 50.8

Imaging Findings

► Four-chamber view of the heart is normal without evidence of septal defect (arrow in Fig. 50.5). Thin membranous portion of ventricular septum mimics ventricular septal defect

► Superior sweep from the four-chamber view demonstrates the great arteries to be in parallel relationship rather than crossing each other (arrows in Fig. 50.6)

► Oblique view demonstrates course of great arteries more clearly, again showing their courses to be parallel (arrows in Fig. 50.7)

► Oblique color Doppler view demonstrates blood flowing into the aorta (arrow in Fig. 50.8) from the anterior right ventricle

Differential Diagnosis

► Double-outlet right ventricle

Teaching Points

► Transposition of the great arteries is frequently missed on screening obstetric ultrasound when a normal four-chamber view alone is obtained
  ▪ Population-based studies show detection rate 3%

► In dextro-transposition of the great arteries (d-TGA), there is atrioventricular concordance and ventriculoarterial discordance
  ▪ The right atrium is connected to the right ventricle, which is connected to the aorta
  ▪ The left atrium provides flow into the left ventricle, which in turn flows into the pulmonary arteries

► Postnatal survival depends on adequacy of atrial level shunt, which provides the only source of oxygenated blood flow to systemic circulation

► Associated cardiac defects may include ventricular septal defect and pulmonary valve stenosis

► Distinction between TGA and double-outlet right ventricle is made by the demonstration of the separate origins of the vessels from their respective ventricles
  ▪ A cross section of the base of the heart showing the crossing of the aorta and pulmonary artery is also diagnostic

Management

▶ Although d-TGA is well tolerated in utero, special attention should be paid to the foramen ovale and ductus arteriosus as the fetus nears term

▶ Prostaglandin infusion initiated at birth to maintain ductal patency and provide effective pulmonary blood flow

▶ Restriction at atrial level is associated with poorer prognosis and often requires transcatheter balloon atrial septostomy soon after birth in order to relieve cyanosis

▶ Prognosis is excellent if postnatal care is provided at a tertiary care pediatric facility with pediatric cardiac intensive care available

▶ Definitive surgical repair usually performed within the first few weeks of life and involves an arterial switch operation, which restores ventriculoarterial concordance

  ▪ Procedure also involves translocation of the coronary arteries to the new aortic root

Acknowledgment

Images courtesy of the fetal echocardiography program at Arkansas Children's Hospital.

Further Reading

1. Friedberg MK, Silverman NH, Moon-Grady AJ, et al. Prenatal detection of congenital heart disease. *J Pediatr*. 2009; 155(1): 26.

2. Shipp TD, Bromley B, Hornberger LK, et al. Levorotation of the fetal cardiac axis: A clue for the presence of congenital heart disease. *Obstet Gynecol*. 1995; 85(1): 97.

History

► 30-Year-old gravida 2 para 1 referred for further evaluation of a fetal abdominal mass discovered on initial prenatal ultrasound (Fig. 51.1)

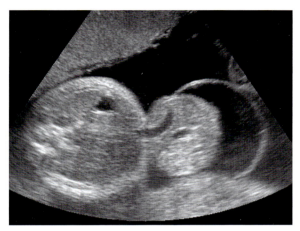

Fig. 51.1

Case 51 Omphalocele

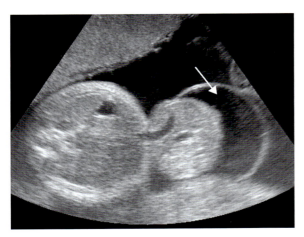

Fig. 51.2

Imaging Findings

▶ Transverse view of abdomen at cord insertion shows herniated liver with ascites (arrow in Fig. 51.2) covered by membrane
▶ Cord insertion cannot be seen on this image

Differential Diagnosis

▶ Umbilical hernia
▶ Gastroschisis
▶ Amniotic band syndrome
▶ Limb–body wall complex

Teaching Points

▶ Fetal abdominal wall defects occur in 1 in 2000–4000 live births
▶ Suspect when a normal cord insertion (arrows in Fig. 51.3) is not seen

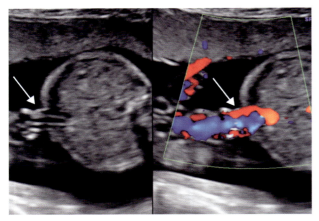

Fig. 51.3

▶ Omphalocele
  ▪ Midline abdominal wall defect into which the abdominal contents herniate
  ▪ Defect covered by amnion and peritoneum
  ▪ Occurs at the base of the umbilical cord
  ▪ Cord inserts at its apex
  ▪ May be confirmed by three-dimensional surface rendered image (arrow in Fig. 51.4), in which the extent of defect is best demonstrated

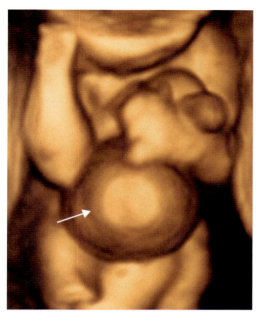

Fig. 51.4

▶ Categorized as either liver-containing (termed giant omphalocele if > 5 cm) or non-liver-containing, which will contain only bowel (arrow in Fig. 51.5)

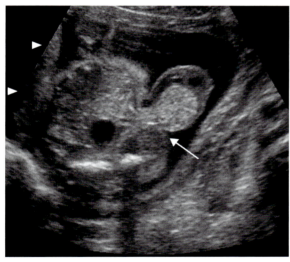

Fig. 51.5

▶ Chromosomal abnormalities, particularly aneuploidies such as trisomy 18, 21, or 13, are present in 40–60% of fetuses with omphaloceles that do not contain liver
▶ The sonographic diagnosis of a liver-containing omphalocele can be made before postmenstrual week 12 because herniated liver is never a normal developmental finding
  ▪ Fetuses with this type of omphalocele typically have normal karyotype
▶ Associated anomalies
  ▪ Aneuploidy (especially trisomies 13, 18, and 21)
  ▪ Congenital heart defects accompany omphalocele in as many as 50% of cases

- Pentalogy of Cantrell when associated with ectopia cordis (arrow in Fig. 51.6 demonstrating the heart protruding outside the thoracic cavity), amniotic band syndrome, OEIS syndrome (omphalocele, exstrophy of the bladder, imperforate anus, spinal defects), and Beckwith–Wiedemann syndrome

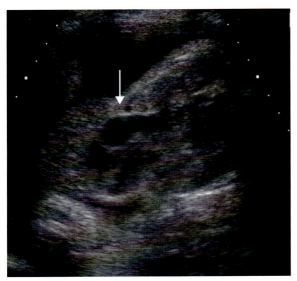

Fig. 51.6

- ▶ An umbilical hernia is covered by skin and usually has a much smaller size and thickened wall
- ▶ Distinguished from gastroschisis by the central location of the defect that involves the cord insertion versus a normal cord insertion found in gastroschisis
  - Herniated small bowel loops are more commonly seen in gastroschisis
- ▶ Complex abdominal wall defects such as amniotic band syndrome and limb–body wall complex are distinguished by larger defects that allow other organs besides the liver and small bowel to herniate
  - Also, the umbilical cord is difficult to define
  - Other associated defects can be seen, such as limb deformities and amputations in amniotic band syndrome; limb–body wall complex usually involves limb and spinal abnormalities

Management

- ▶ Amniocentesis for fetal karyotype
- ▶ Cesarean section for giant omphalocele to prevent dystocia or rupture; vaginal delivery for remainder
- ▶ Sac covered to prevent fluid and heat loss, stabilized to prevent rupture; urgent repair not indicated unless sac ruptures
- ▶ Goal of repair: return viscera to abdomen with skin, fascial coverage
- ▶ Abdominal compartment syndrome
  - Develops if viscera returned too quickly
  - Causes elevated intra-abdominal pressures with impaired visceral
  blood flow, hypotension, and respiratory distress
- ▶ Small/minor omphalocele: synthetic graft, skin-only closure, silo reduction
- ▶ Giant omphalocele: gradual reduction by silo with gravity versus synthetic graft plus increasing compression
  - For unstable patients: topical agents to promote epithelization of the sac, which gradually incorporates to abdominal cavity
  - Subsequent hernia repair required

Further Reading
1. Emanuel PG, Garcia GI, Angtuaco TL. Prenatal detection of anterior abdominal wall defects with US. *RadioGraphics*. 1995; 15(3): 517–530.
2. Getachew MM, Goldstein RB, Edge V, et al. Correlation between omphalocele contents and karyotypic abnormalities: Sonographic study in 37 cases. *Am J Roentgenol*. 1992; 158(1): 133–136.
3. Blazer S, Zimmer EZ, Ger A, et al. Fetal omphalocele detected early in pregnancy: Associated anomalies and outcomes. *Radiology*. 2004; 232(1): 191–195.

Case 52

History

- 26-Year-old primigravida referred for elevated α-fetoprotein (AFP) on maternal serum screening (Figs. 52.1–52.4)

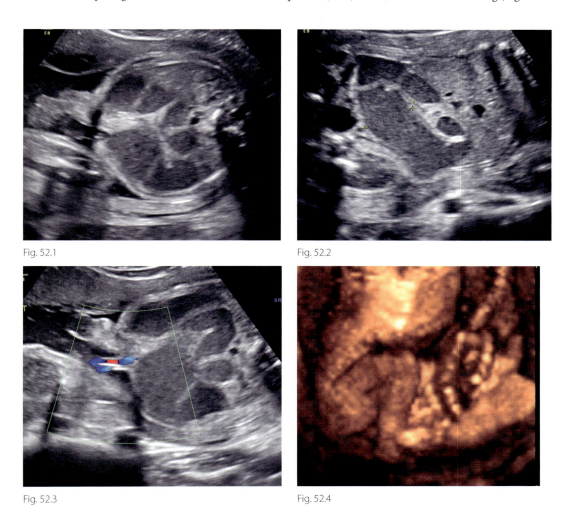

Fig. 52.1

Fig. 52.2

Fig. 52.3

Fig. 52.4

Case 52 Gastroschisis

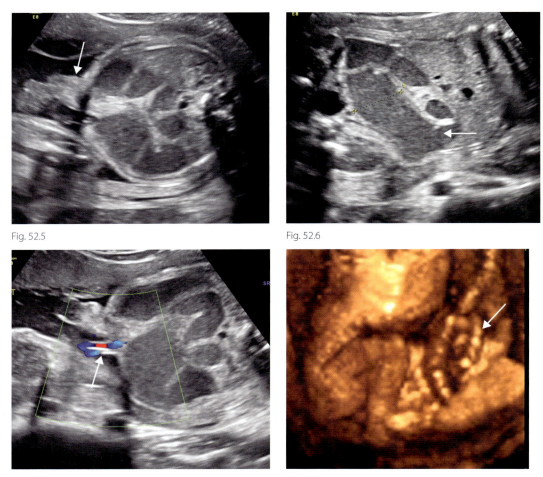

Fig. 52.5

Fig. 52.6

Fig. 52.7

Fig. 52.8

Imaging Findings

▶ Axial image of fetal abdomen at the level of the cord insertion shows right paramedian defect with herniated nondilated loops of bowel (arrow in Fig. 52.5)
▶ Markedly dilated intra-abdominal small bowel loops (arrow in Fig. 52.6) suggest obstruction at exit point of herniated bowel
▶ Color Doppler confirms normal cord insertion (arrow in Fig. 52.7) into anterior fetal abdomen
▶ Three-dimensional rendered surface image of the anterior abdominal wall shows normal-caliber herniated bowel loops (arrow in Fig. 52.8)

Differential Diagnosis

▶ Bowel-containing omphalocele
▶ Body stalk anomaly
▶ Amniotic band syndrome

Teaching Points

▶ Gastroschisis is a full-thickness defect in the anterior abdominal wall through which evisceration of the intestines occurs
  ▪ Reported in 1 in 2000–4000 live births
▶ Pathogenesis: vascular compromise of either the umbilical vein or the omphalomesenteric artery leading to abdominal wall defect
  ▪ Usually to the right of the cord insertion
  ▪ Generally small (< 2 cm)
  ▪ Occasionally occurs on the left

- Herniated contents do not have an overlying membrane
- Cord insertion is normally placed
▸ Early in pregnancy, bowel loops appear nondilated
▸ Late in pregnancy, eviscerated bowel often appears thickened, matted, and mildly dilated due to chronic exposure to amniotic fluid
  - Intra-abdominal bowel can dilate if exiting bowel is obstructed
▸ No increase in incidence of chromosomal aneuploidy and has fewer associated defects than omphalocele (32% vs. 80%)
▸ Coexistent bowel abnormalities include bowel malrotation, atresia, stenosis, and ischemia
▸ Associated abnormalities include exstrophy of the urinary bladder, fetal growth restriction, and minor cardiac anomalies
▸ Exposure of fetal bowel loops to amniotic cavity causes rise in maternal serum AFP
▸ Bowel-containing omphalocele can mimic appearance, but differentiated by the abnormal cord insertion at apex of the defect of an omphalocele
▸ Limb–body wall complex and amniotic band syndrome are severe abdominal wall defects in which the cord insertion is involved in the large opening of the anterior abdominal wall. The normal cord insertion is therefore not visualized. Both usually have amniotic bands floating in the amniotic cavity, and other associated anomalies may involve deformities of the extremities and spine

Management

▸ Planned timing of delivery at a tertiary care center and immediate surgical correction to decrease risk of sepsis and metabolic acidosis
▸ Moisture of herniated bowel needs to be maintained prior to surgery
▸ Staged surgical closure has overall good results, but complications are not uncommon and include malrotation, long- and short-segment small bowel atresias, stenosis, peritonitis, and short gut syndrome
▸ Prognosis is dependent on degree of intestinal damage

Further Reading

1. Christison-Lagay E, Kelleher C, Langer JC. Neonatal abdominal wall defects. *Semin Fetal Neonatal Med.* (2011); 16(3): 164–172.
2. Durfee S, Downard C, Benson CB, et al. Postnatal outcome of fetuses with the prenatal diagnosis of gastroschisis. *J Ultrasound Med.* March 1, 2002; 21: 269–274.
3. Hoyme HE, Jones MC, Jones KL. Gastroschisis: Abdominal wall disruption secondary to early gestational interruption of the omphalomesenteric artery. *Semin Perinatol.* 1983; 7: 294–298.

Case 53

► 31-Year-old primigravida with family history of fetal anomalies (Figs. 53.1–53.3)

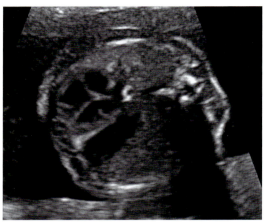

Fig. 53.1

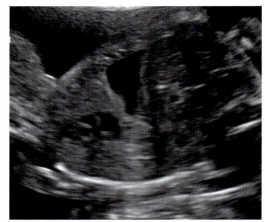

Fig. 53.2

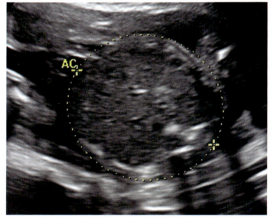

Fig. 53.3

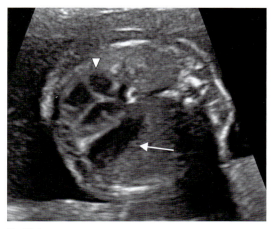

Fig. 53.4

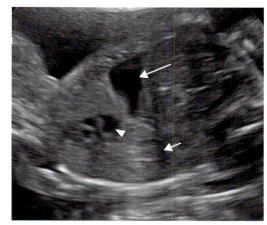

Fig. 53.5

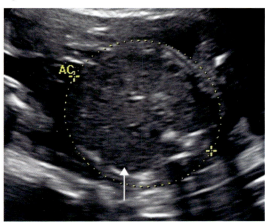

Fig. 53.6

Imaging Findings

► Axial image of fetal chest shows the heart (arrowhead in Fig. 53.4) displaced into the right hemithorax and the stomach (arrow in Fig. 53.4) in the left chest
► Sagittal image of chest shows the stomach (long arrow in Fig. 53.5) above the diaphragm (short arrow in Fig. 53.5), displacing heart (arrowhead in Fig. 53.5)
► Axial image at the level of abdominal circumference measurement shows no fluid-filled stomach at expected location (arrow in Fig. 53.6)

Differential Diagnosis

► Congenital pulmonary airway malformation (CPAM)
► Pulmonary sequestration
► Teratoma
► Bronchogenic/pericardial cyst

Teaching Points

► Developmental defect in diaphragm allowing abdominal viscera to herniate into the chest, interfering with normal lung development
  ▪ Incidence is 1/3000 births
► Pulmonary hypoplasia and pulmonary arterial hypertension can result in life-threatening respiratory compromise
► Prenatal MRI (see T2-weighted images below) can demonstrate the extent of small bowel herniation (arrows in Figs. 53.7 and 53.8) and estimate degree of pulmonary hypoplasia

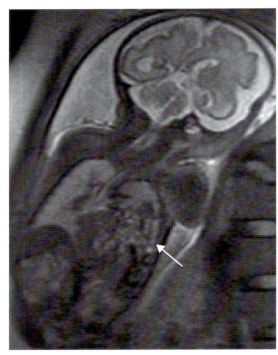

Fig. 53.7

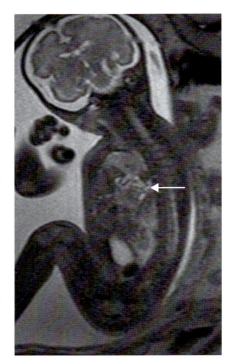

Fig. 53.8

► Prenatal US findings
  ▪ Chest mass
  ▪ Mediastinal shift, displacement of heart
  ▪ Malposition of stomach and/or liver
► Chromosomal abnormalities and structural malformations in other major organ systems often associated
► Worse prognosis if associated with abnormal karyotype, severe associated anomalies, right-sided defect, liver herniation, and lower fetal lung volume
► Absence of liver herniation is a strong predictor of postnatal survival
► CPAM and pulmonary sequestration appear on US as predominantly echogenic posterior thoracic masses without associated displacement of the heart
► Teratomas are usually anterior mediastinal masses and may compress the heart posteriorly or slightly to left
► Bronchogenic and pericardial cysts are middle mediastinal masses with no known cardiac displacement

Management

► Prenatal assessment should include
  ▪ Fetal karyotype
  ▪ Ultrafast fetal MRI to search for liver herniation
  ▪ Echocardiography
  ▪ Serial US examinations
► Fetal surgery (endoscopic tracheal occlusion) is an investigational procedure for treatment of isolated severe congenital diaphragmatic hernia performed in fetal therapy centers
  ▪ Obstructs normal egress of lung fluid during pulmonary development resulting in increased transpulmonic pressure and large fluid-filled lungs, which can prevent abnormal development of lung parenchyma and pulmonary vasculature
► Planned induction of labor between 38 and 39 weeks of gestation and delivery at a tertiary center with extracorporeal membrane oxygenation (ECMO) capability because up to 50% of cases require ECMO

Further Reading

1. Enns GM, Cox VA, Goldstein RB, et al. Congenital diaphragmatic defects and associated syndromes, malformations, and chromosome anomalies: A retrospective study of 60 patients and literature review. *Am J Med Genet*. 1998; 79: 215–220.
2. Graham G, Devine PC. Antenatal diagnosis of congenital diaphragmatic hernia. *Semin Perinatol*. 2005; 29: 69–73.
3. Taylor GA, Atalabi OM, Estroff JA. Imaging of congenital diaphragmatic hernias. *Pediatr Radiol*. 2009; 39: 1–5.

History

▶ 25-Year-old primigravida referred for size larger than dates (Figs. 54.1–54.3)

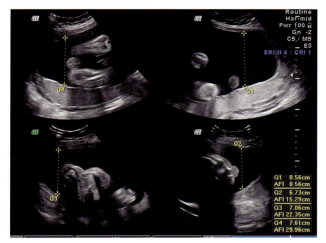

Fig. 54.1

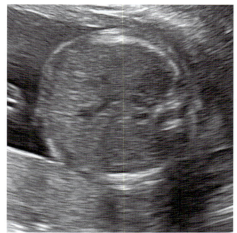

Fig. 54.2

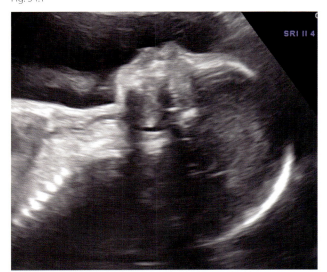

Fig. 54.3

Case 54 Esophageal Atresia

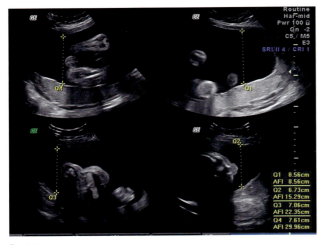

Fig. 54.4

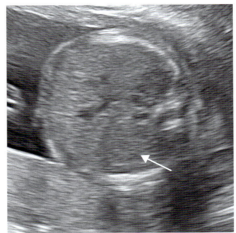

Fig. 54.5

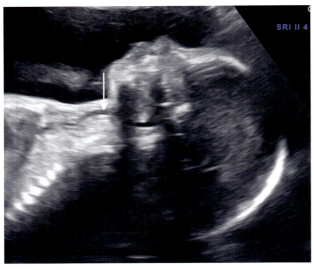

Fig. 54.6

Imaging Findings

► Amniotic fluid index elevated at 29 cm (Fig. 54.4)
► Stomach not observed in expected location (arrow in Fig. 54.5)
► Sagittal image of fetal neck shows a persistently fluid-filled esophagus (arrow in Fig. 54.6)

Differential Diagnosis

► Polyhydramnios secondary to other causes, including central nervous system anomalies, cleft lip/palate, duodenal atresia, and other intestinal atresias

Teaching Points

► Esophageal atresia is defined as a congenitally interrupted esophagus
  ▪ One or more tracheoesophageal fistulae (TEF) may be present
► Five types of tracheoesophageal anomalies
  ▪ Type A—esophageal atresia without TEF (10%)
  ▪ Type B—esophageal atresia with a TEF to proximal esophageal segment (< 1%)
  ▪ Type C—esophageal atresia with a TEF to distal esophageal segment (85%)

- Type D—esophageal atresia with TEF to both proximal and distal esophageal segments (< 1%)
  - Type E—TEF with no esophageal atresia (4%)
- Up to 50% of fetuses have additional anomalies
  - Cardiac malformations most common (25%) and result in highest morbidity and mortality
  - TEF often associated with VACTERL (vertebral, anal atresia, cardiac, tracheoesophageal fistula, renal, limb) association
- US findings
  - Isolated (type A) esophageal atresia readily diagnosed prenatally when polyhydramnios, absence of fluid-filled stomach, and dilated proximal esophageal pouch in neck or mediastinum are present
- Polyhydramnios defined as one of the following
  - Amniotic fluid volume subjectively more than expected for gestational age
  - Amniotic fluid index > 20–25 cm
  - Largest fluid pocket depth > 8 cm
  - Observed by third trimester in one-third of fetuses with esophageal atresia plus distal TEF and in 100% of fetuses with esophageal atresia without TEF
- Postnatal imaging of the chest shows a dilated proximal esophagus (arrow in Fig. 54.7) with inability to pass a nasogastric (NG) tube into the distal esophagus (arrow in Fig. 54.8 demonstrating end of NG tube in upper mediastinum)

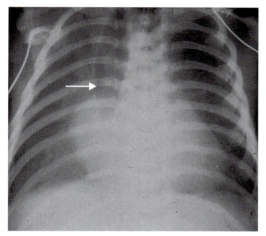

Fig. 54.7

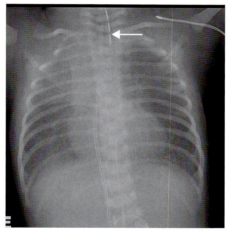

Fig. 54.8

- Double-contrast examination of the esophagus (arrow in Fig. 54.9) and stomach (arrowhead in Fig. 54.9) can delineate the length of the atretic segment

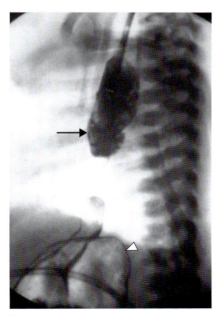

Fig. 54.9

Management

► Assess for associated anomalies
  ▪ Sonographic evaluation for VACTERL
  ▪ Echocardiography due to prevalence of cardiac malformations
► Fetal karyotyping
  ▪ 6–10% risk of chromosomal abnormalities, including trisomy 21 and 18
► Delivery at a center with appropriate neonatal support
► Esophageal abnormalities alone are not an indication for altering the route of delivery

Further Reading

1. Shulman A, Mazkereth R, Zalel Y, et al. Prenatal identification of esophageal atresia: The role of ultrasonography for evaluation of functional anatomy. *Prenat Diagn*. 2002; 22: 669–672.
2. Estroff JA, Parad RB, Share JC, et al. Second trimester prenatal findings in duodenal and esophageal atresia without tracheoesophageal fistula. *J Ultrasound Med*. 1994; 13: 375–379.
3. Kalache KD, Wauer R, Mau H, et al. Prognostic significance of the pouch sign in fetuses with prenatally diagnosed esophageal atresia. *Am J Obstet Gynecol*. 2000; 182: 978–981.

History

▶ 26-Year-old gravida 2 para 1 referred for evaluation of an abnormal fetal mass (Figs. 55.1 and 55.2)

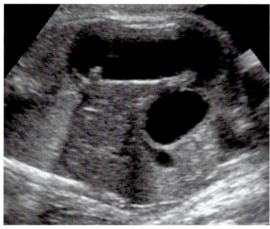

Fig. 55.1

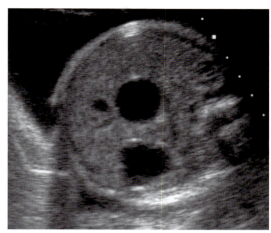

Fig. 55.2

Case 55 Duodenal Atresia

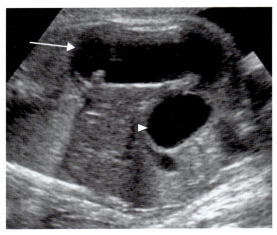

Fig. 55.3

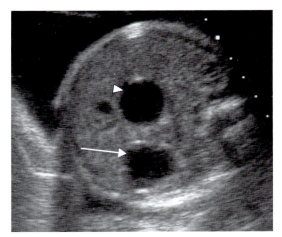

Fig. 55.4

Imaging Findings

▶ Coronal image of the fetal abdomen showing two cystic structures; the larger corresponds to the dilated stomach (arrow in Fig. 55.3), and the smaller represents the duodenum (arrowhead in Fig. 55.3)
▶ Axial image of the abdomen showing the same two cystic structures; the lateral one is the stomach (arrow in Fig. 55.4), and the medial one is the duodenum (arrowhead in Fig. 55.4)

Differential Diagnosis

▶ Duodenal web
▶ Duodenal stenosis
▶ Annular pancreas
▶ Ladd's bands
▶ Proximal jejunal obstruction

Teaching Points

▶ Duodenal atresia (DA) is due to failure of recanalization of the bowel after portions of the intestinal tract become occluded secondary to endodermal epithelium proliferation, which occurs at 6 or 7 weeks gestational age
  ▪ Recanalization normally occurs during weeks 8–10, restoring patency
▶ Incidence: 1/10,000–40,000 births
▶ Approximately 30% of infants with DA have chromosomal anomalies
  ▪ Primarily Down syndrome; approximately 2.5% of patients with Down syndrome have DA or duodenal stenosis
▶ Isolated finding in one-third to one-half of cases but often associated with other malformations, including gastrointestinal (biliary atresia, agenesis of the gallbladder), cardiac, renal, and vertebral anomalies
▶ US findings
  ▪ Two fluid collections (double-bubble) representing distended, fluid-filled stomach and enlarged duodenum that may exchange fluid between them
  ▪ No distal fluid-filled bowel
▶ On plain abdominal radiograph, air-filled stomach and proximal duodenum comprise the "double-bubble" sign (arrows in Fig. 55.5) that strongly suggests DA; with rare exceptions, distal gas is absent

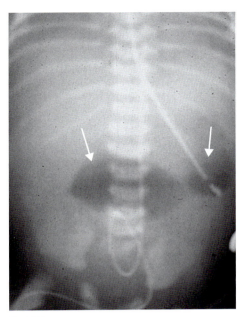

Fig. 55.5

► Duodenal web/stenosis and annular pancreas are not distinguishable by US findings of dilated stomach and proximal duodenum but may have fluid distally in the small bowel due to varying degrees of incomplete obstruction

► Jejunal obstruction, if severe as in jejunal atresia, may manifest as a large cystic mass in the mid-abdomen that does not have a "double-bubble" configuration; if incomplete, may also show fluid in distal bowel

Management

► Contrast radiographs to confirm and better define the anomaly

► Laboratory studies to assess infant's clinical condition

► Evaluate for associated conditions: echocardiogram, renal US, chest X-ray to assess for vertebral anomalies

► Preoperative management includes withholding feedings and placement of nasogastric or orogastric tube to continuous suction; parenteral fluids should be provided; abnormalities in fluid and electrolyte balance should be corrected

► Surgery is curative; approach depends on site of atresia

► The possibility of a second or multiple atresias should be considered

Further Reading

1. Escobar MA, Ladd AP, Grosfeld JL, et al. Duodenal atresia and stenosis: Long-term follow-up over 30 years. *J Pediatr Surg*. 2004; 39: 867–871.

2. Corteville JE, Gray DL, Langer JC. Bowel abnormalities in the fetus—Correlation of prenatal ultrasonographic findings with outcome. *Am J Obstet Gynecol*. 1996; 175: 724–731.

3. Brantberg A, Blaas HG, Salvesen KA, et al. Fetal duodenal obstructions: Increased risk of prenatal sudden death. *Ultrasound Obstet Gynecol*. 2002; 20: 439–442.

Case 56

► 31-Year-old gravida 4 para 5 referred for suspected fetal abdominal mass (Figs. 56.1–56.3)

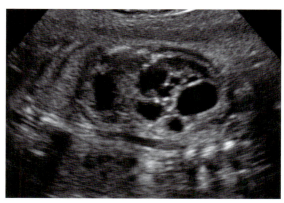

Fig. 56.1

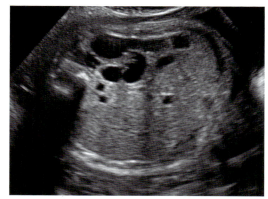

Fig. 56.2

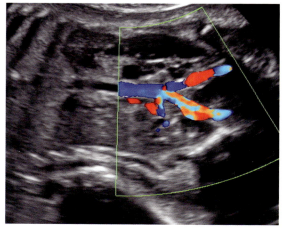

Fig. 56.3

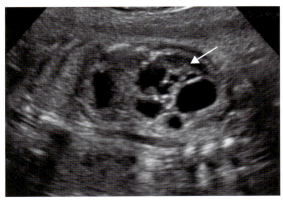

Fig. 56.4

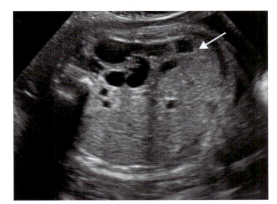

Fig. 56.5

Fig. 56.6

Imaging Findings

► Coronal view of the fetal abdomen shows enlarged kidney (arrow in Fig. 56.4) with multiple noncommunicating cysts of varying sizes
► Axial view shows enlarged kidney (arrow in Fig. 56.5) occupying entire anteroposterior diameter of the fetal abdomen
► Coronal color Doppler image of abdominal aorta shows normal renal artery (arrow in Fig. 56.6) to the other kidney; no renal artery seen on side of multicystic dysplastic kidney (MCDK)

Differential Diagnosis

► Hydronephrosis
► Ureteropelvic junction (UPJ) obstruction
► Multilocular cystic kidney

Teaching Points

► Severe form of renal dysplasia
  ▪ Kidney consists of multiple noncommunicating cysts of varying sizes separated by dysplastic parenchyma
  ▪ Enlarged kidney with irregular and non-reniform shape
► Most cases unilateral, prevalence of 1:4300 births
  ▪ More common in left kidney and in males
  ▪ Bilateral MCDK less common, prevalence of 1:10,000 live births
► Affected kidney nonfunctional, frequently involutes as cysts shrink due to lack of urine production resulting in picture similar to renal agenesis
► Associated with vesicoureteral reflux (20%) and UPJ obstruction
► US findings

- Multiloculated abdominal mass with multiple cysts distributed randomly
- No normal renal parenchyma or renal pelvis visible
- Typical appearance (arrows in Fig. 56.7) even when in abnormally low location in pelvis

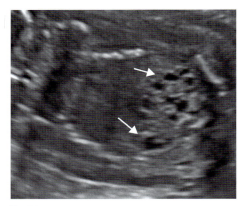

Fig. 56.7

- Main renal artery small or absent
- Amniotic fluid volume normal in unilateral disease
- Oligohydramnios with pulmonary hypoplasia and no bladder filling due to absent urine production if bilateral MCDK
- Kidneys enlarged early in pregnancy, decrease in size as pregnancy progresses; severely shrunken in terminal bilateral cases, which mimics renal agenesis and is fatal
- ▶ UPJ obstruction and severe hydronephrosis show cystic areas that communicate
- ▶ Multilocular cystic renal disease will demonstrate functional renal parenchyma with blood flow detected on Doppler US

Management

- ▶ Unilateral: conservative management with periodic US assessment
  - If normal contralateral kidney, good long-term outcomes with normal renal function, infrequent urinary tract infections, and compensatory contralateral renal hypertrophy
- ▶ Routine removal of MCDK no longer recommended
  - Risk of hypertension and infection low
  - Risk of malignancy not increased
- ▶ 60% of MCDKs atrophy and disappear over 5 years
- ▶ Infants with complex disease, bilateral MCDKs, or contralateral urological abnormalities have worse outcome with high incidence of chronic renal insufficiency or renal failure
- ▶ Bilateral disease with anhydramnios: poor prognosis
  - Option for pregnancy termination should be discussed

Further Reading

1. Schreuder MF, Westland R, van Wijk JA. Unilateral multicystic dysplastic kidney: A meta-analysis of observational studies on the incidence, associated urinary tract malformations and the contralateral kidney. *Nephrol Dial Transplant*. 2009; 24: 1810–1815.
2. Lin CC, Tsai JD, Sheu JC, et al. Segmental multicystic dysplastic kidney in children: Clinical presentation, imaging finding, management, and outcome. *J Pediatr Surg*. 2010; 45: 1856–1859.
3. Aslam M, Watson AR. Unilateral multicystic dysplastic kidney: Long-term outcomes. *Arch Dis Child*. 2006; 91(10): 820–823.

History

▶ 19-Year-old primigravida with unknown last menstrual period (Figs. 57.1–57.3)

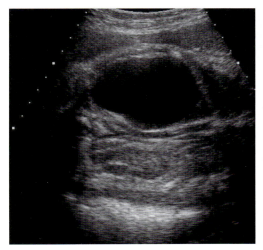

Fig. 57.1

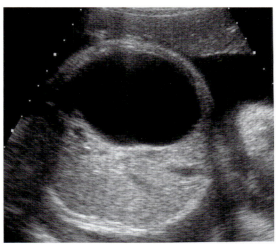

Fig. 57.2

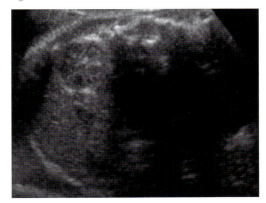

Fig. 57.3

Case 57 Ureteropelvic Junction Obstruction

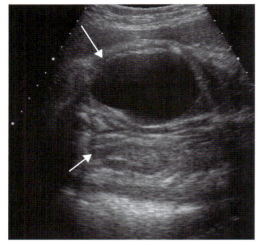

Fig. 57.4

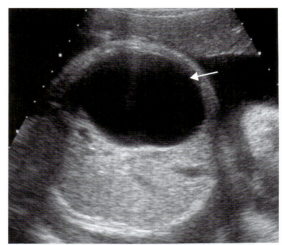

Fig. 57.5

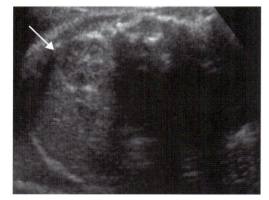

Fig. 57.6

Imaging Findings

► Coronal image of the fetal abdomen shows large cystic mass in the left renal fossa (long arrow in Fig. 57.4)
► The right kidney is normal (short arrow in Fig. 57.4)
► Axial image showing the large cystic mass (arrow in Fig. 57.5) occupying the whole left hemiabdomen
► Axial image of the right renal fossa demonstrates a normal kidney (arrow in Fig. 57.6)

Differential Diagnosis

► Obstructed stomach or bowel
► Unilocular renal cyst
► Mesenteric or duplication cyst

Teaching Points

► Partial or total blockage of the flow of urine occurring where the ureter enters the kidney results in hydronephrosis
► Ureteropelvic junction (UPJ) obstruction is the most common pathologic cause of antenatally detected hydronephrosis
  ▪ Incidence of up to 1 in 500 fetuses screened by antenatal US
► Etiology: both a congenital and an acquired condition; congenital causes more common
  ▪ Usually caused by intrinsic stenosis of the proximal ureter
  ▪ Less commonly caused by extrinsic compression of the UPJ by an aberrant or accessory renal artery
  ▪ Rarely due to an intraluminal fold or web

- ► US findings
  - ▪ Mild form: dilated renal pelvis may be visible medial to normal renal parenchyma
  - ▪ Moderate to severe form: renal parenchyma may not be visible
  - ▪ Normal bladder in unilateral cases
  - ▪ Contralateral kidney may be involved with mild pelvic dilation due to ureteral compression from large renal pelvis
- ► When enlarged enough to fill the hemiabdomen, may be difficult to differentiate from other fluid collections or cystic masses
- ► Follow-up neonatal US confirmed the diagnosis, showing a normal right kidney (arrow in Fig. 57.7) and markedly dilated left renal pelvis with minimal residual renal cortex (arrow in Fig. 57.8)

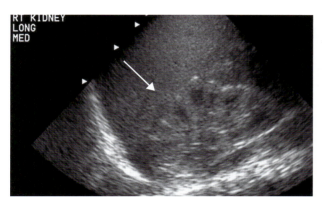

Fig. 57.7

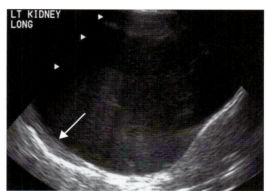

Fig. 57.8

- ► When the pelvic dilation is so severe as to occupy almost the entire hemiabdomen, it can be difficult to find a normal fluid-filled stomach to exclude gastric obstruction
- ► Likewise, finding a normal portion of the kidney to make the diagnosis of a large unilocular cyst may be problematic
- ► Enteric duplication or mesenteric cysts usually do not reach the dimensions of a severe UPJ obstruction but would be difficult to exclude. These diagnoses will be based on finding normal kidneys bilaterally

Management

- ► There are no randomized trials that provide conclusive evidence for the optimal management of congenital UPJ obstruction
- ► Imaging studies (e.g., diuretic renography, serial US, and voiding cystourethrogram) are useful to differentiate UPJ from other causes of hydronephrosis, including vesicoureteral reflux, transient and functional hydronephrosis, and other urological anomalies
- ► Prenatal intervention or early delivery in fetuses with unilateral UPJ obstruction not routinely recommended
  - ▪ In extremely rare cases, decompression of an enormously dilated renal pelvis may be considered to prevent dystocia or fetal pulmonary compression
- ► In symptomatic patients, surgical intervention may be performed to relieve the obstruction
- ► In asymptomatic patients with unilateral UPJ, observation and monitoring with serial US and diuretic renography recommended
- ► Indications for surgical intervention include increasing hydronephrosis and a decrease in split renal function

Further Reading

1. Corteville JE, Gray DL, Crane JP. Congenital hydronephrosis: Correlation of fetal ultrasonographic findings with infant outcome. *Am J Obstet Gynecol*. 1991; 165: 384–388.
2. González R, Schimke CM. Ureteropelvic junction obstruction in infants and children. *Pediatr Clin North Am*. 2001; 48: 1505–1515.
3. Flake AW, Harrison MR, Sauer L, et al. Ureteropelvic junction obstruction in the fetus. *J Pediatr Surg*. 1986; 21: 1058–1065.

Case 58

History

▶ 31-Year-old gravida 3 para 1 referred for suspected fetal abdominal mass (Figs. 58.1 and 58.2)

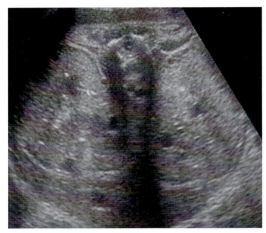

Fig. 58.1

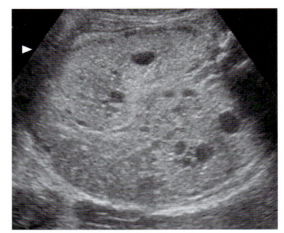

Fig. 58.2

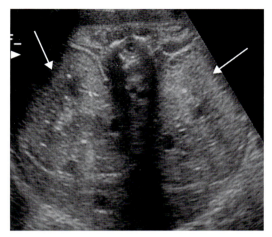

Fig. 58.3

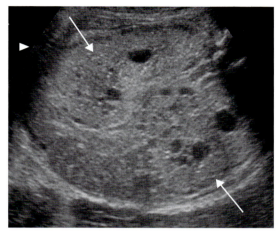

Fig. 58.4

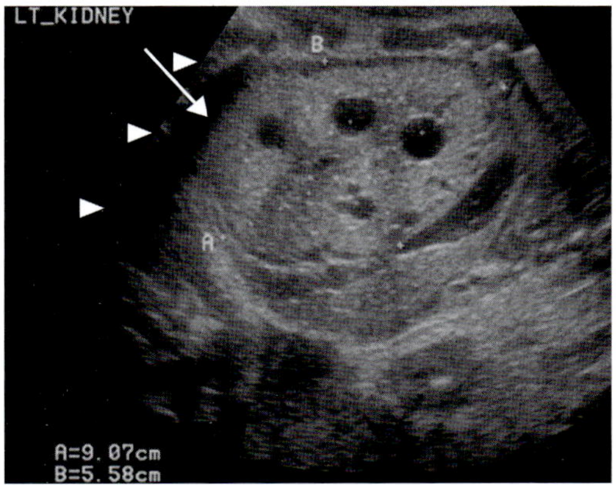

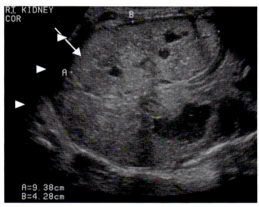

Fig. 58.5

Fig. 58.6

Imaging Findings

▶ Axial and coronal images of the fetal abdomen show huge kidneys (arrows in Fig. 58.3 and Fig. 58.4) filling the whole abdomen and pelvis
▶ Left kidney (arrow in Fig. 58.5) and right kidney (arrow in Fig. 58.6) each measure 9 cm in long axis

Differential Diagnosis

▶ Bilateral multicystic dysplastic kidney
▶ Autosomal dominant polycystic kidney disease
▶ Meckel–Gruber syndrome

Teaching Points

▶ Autosomal recessive (infantile) polycystic kidney disease (ARPKD) is a recessively inherited disorder characterized by cystic dilation of the renal collecting ducts and congenital hepatic fibrosis
  ▪ Mutations in the *PKHD1* gene located on chromosome 6
  ▪ Incidence of 1:10,000 to 1:40,000
  ▪ However, true incidence may be higher because severely affected infants may die as newborns without a diagnosis, and patients with mild disease may not be diagnosed until adulthood
▶ Always associated with biliary dysgenesis with some degree of congenital hepatic fibrosis, malformation of the biliary system, and dilatation of the intrahepatic bile ducts (Caroli disease)
▶ Other organ systems (lung and lower extremity deformities) secondarily involved as a result of kidney and/or liver disease
  ▪ Severe oligohydramnios results in musculoskeletal abnormalities secondary to fetal packing and pulmonary hypoplasia

- ▶ Fetal presentation
  - ▪ Enlarged kidneys with microcysts (usually < 3 mm)
  - ▪ Majority detected at gestational age greater than 24 weeks because most kidneys look normal until the late second trimester with delayed development of oligohydramnios after 28 weeks
  - ▪ Marked nephromegaly may cause dystocia at birth
  - ▪ Majority are stillborn or neonatal death
- ▶ Outcome dependent on the degree of renal and hepatic involvement, reflected in age at presentation
- ▶ Mortality rate greatest for patients who present as neonates with severe renal disease
- ▶ Perinatal form: severe renal disease, pulmonary hypoplasia, minimal hepatic fibrosis, worst prognosis, high mortality in first month of life
- ▶ Juvenile form: milder renal disease, more severe hepatic fibrosis, survival rate approximately 82% at 3 years and 79% at 15 years
- ▶ Classic multicystic dysplastic kidneys may be bilateral and enlarged but are usually distinguished by the presence of large cysts of varying sizes; other variants of multicystic renal dysplasia do not enlarge to the degree seen in ARPKD
- ▶ Autosomal dominant polycystic kidney disease does not usually present until adulthood
- ▶ Meckel–Gruber syndrome includes encephalocele, large polycystic kidneys, and polydactyly

Management

- ▶ No specific interventions prevent or delay the progression of ARPKD
- ▶ Supportive therapy: management of respiratory distress and renal replacement therapy if progression to end-stage renal diseases
- ▶ Counseling regarding prenatal genetic testing for interested family members
- ▶ Autopsy confirmation due to 25% risk of recurrence in subsequent pregnancies

Further Reading

1. Traubici J, Daneman A. High-resolution renal sonography in children with autosomal recessive polycystic kidney disease. *Am J Roentgenol*. 2005; 184(5): 1630–1633.
2. Guay-Woodford LM, Desmond RA. Autosomal recessive polycystic kidney disease: The clinical experience in North America. *Pediatrics*. 2003; 111: 1072–1075.
3. Gunay-Aygun M, Avner ED, Bacallao RL, et al. Autosomal recessive polycystic kidney disease and congenital hepatic fibrosis: Summary statement of a first National Institutes of Health/Office of Rare Diseases conference. *J Pediatr*. 2006; 149: 159–162.

History

► 28-Year-old gravida 3 para 2 referred for suspected cyst in the fetal abdomen (Figs. 59.1–59.4)

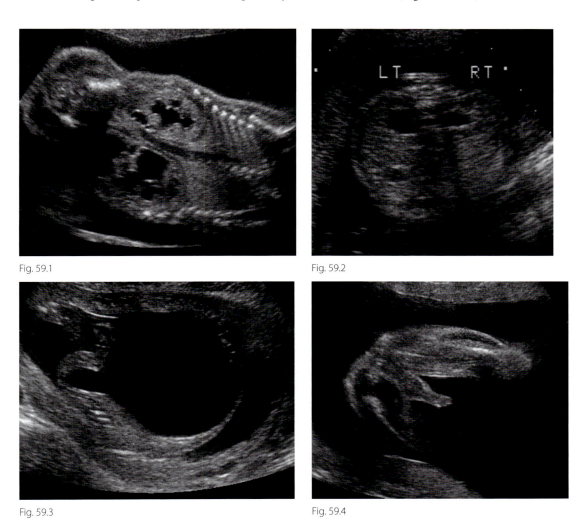

Fig. 59.1

Fig. 59.2

Fig. 59.3

Fig. 59.4

Case 59 Posterior Urethral Valves

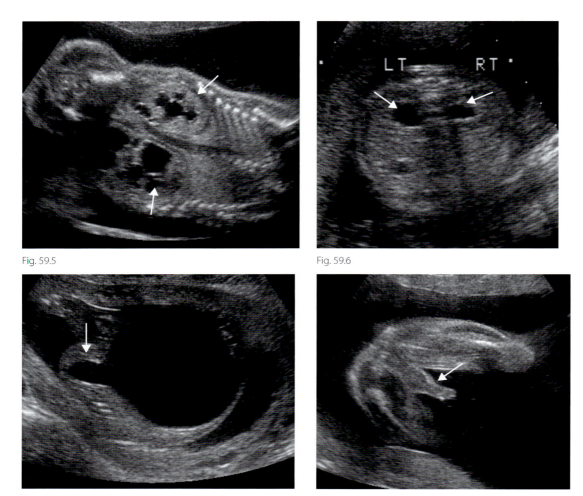

Fig. 59.5

Fig. 59.6

Fig. 59.7

Fig. 59.8

Imaging Findings

► Coronal image through the kidneys (arrows in Fig. 59.5) shows bilateral hydronephrosis
► Axial image confirms bilateral pyelectasis (arrows in Fig. 59.6) measuring > 4 mm
► Coronal image of the urinary bladder shows the typical "keyhole" appearance of the dilated posterior urethra (arrow in Fig. 59.7)
► Confirmatory image of male fetal genitalia (arrow in Fig. 59.8)

Differential Diagnosis

► Prune belly syndrome
► Urethral atresia
► Megalourethra, megacystis, microcolon syndrome (MMMS)

Teaching Points

► Obstructing membranous folds within the lumen of the posterior urethra
  ▪ Caused by disruption in normal embryologic development of the male urethra
► Estimated incidence is 1 in 10,000–25,000 live births
  ▪ Higher incidence in utero
  ▪ Vast majority are sporadic occurrences
  ▪ Rare cases of familial and genetic linkage reported

- ► Prenatal US findings
  - ▪ Bilateral hydronephrosis
  - ▪ Dilated bladder and dilated posterior urethra (keyhole sign)
  - ▪ Male fetus
  - ▪ Bladder wall may be thickened (> 3 mm)
  - ▪ Direct sonographic visualization of the posterior urethral valves (PUVs) not possible because of their small size
- ► Additional findings in severe cases
  - ▪ Oligohydramnios
  - ▪ Urinary ascites or perinephric urinoma due to rupture of fornix or calyx in the kidney secondary to increased pressure
  - ▪ Bladder diverticula or patent urachus
- ► Increased renal echogenicity and cortical cysts suggest renal dysplasia
- ► Risk of perinatal mortality and postnatal chronic kidney disease increased if diagnosed before 24 weeks
- ► Perinatal mortality can be as high as 90–95% with severe bilateral hydronephrosis, oligohydramnios, or findings consistent with renal dysplasia
- ► May be difficult to differentiate from prune belly syndrome in utero
- ► Urethral atresia and MMMS more common in female fetuses and have no keyhole bladder

Management

- ► Prenatal US not highly reliable in differentiating fetuses with urinary obstruction from those without obstruction. Therefore, fetal intervention based on US findings must be considered cautiously
- ► Diagnosis made postnatally on voiding cystourethrogram (VCUG)
  - ▪ Hallmark findings: dilated and elongated posterior urethra during the voiding phase when the urethral catheter is no longer present
  - ▪ One-third to one-half of patients will have either unilateral or bilateral vesicoureteral reflux
- ► Based on the VCUG findings, cystoscopy is performed to confirm the diagnosis and ablate the PUV

Further Reading

1. Berrocal T, Lopez-Pereira P, Arjonilla A, et al. Anomalies of the distal ureter, bladder, and urethra in children: Embryologic, radiologic, and pathologic features. *RadioGraphics*. 2002; 22: 1139–1164.
2. Krishnan A, de Souza A, Konijeti R, et al. The anatomy and embryology of posterior urethral vales. *J Urol.* 2006; 175(4): 1214–1220.
3. Hutton KA, Thomas DF, Davies BW. Prenatally detected posterior urethral valves: Qualitative assessment of second trimester scans and prediction of outcome. *J Urol.* 1997; 158: 1022–1029.

Case 60

History

▶ 33-Year-old gravida 2 para 1 presents with suspected small for dates gestation (Figs. 60.1–60.4)

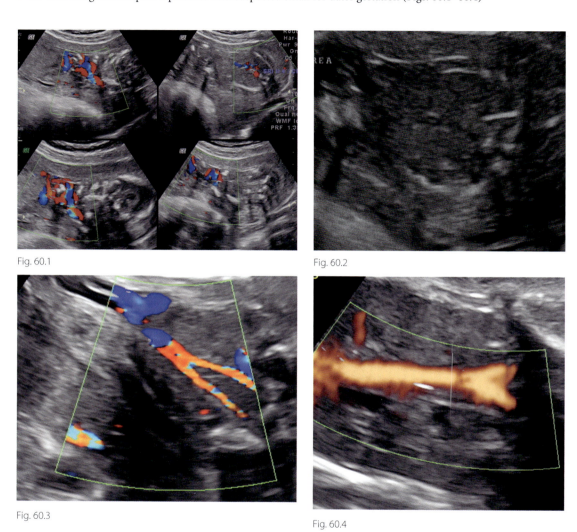

Fig. 60.1

Fig. 60.2

Fig. 60.3

Fig. 60.4

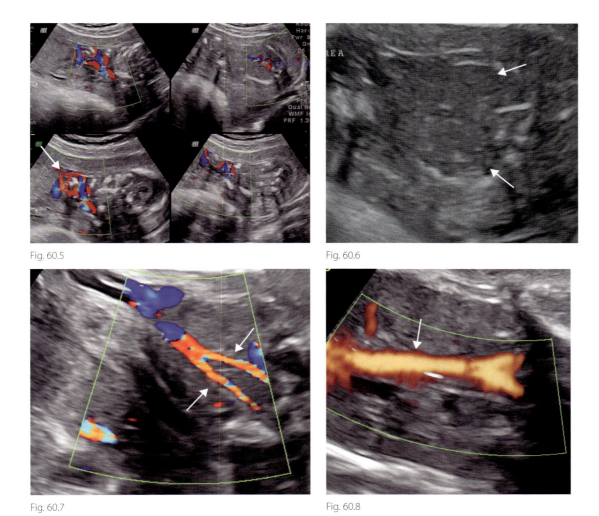

Fig. 60.5

Fig. 60.6

Fig. 60.7

Fig. 60.8

Imaging Findings

► Amniotic fluid index determination shows no measurable fluid (anhydramnios)
► Color Doppler images reveal that the umbilical cord with its vessels (arrow in Fig. 60.5) fills the amniotic space between fetus and uterine wall
► Transverse scan at the expected level of the kidneys (arrows in Fig. 60.6) shows no renal tissue
► Coronal color Doppler view of the pelvis shows no fluid in the urinary bladder, which should be located between the two umbilical arteries (arrows in Fig. 60.7)
► Coronal image of the abdominal aorta (arrow in Fig. 60.8) using power Doppler shows no evidence of the main renal arteries, which should branch laterally from the mid abdominal aorta

Differential Diagnosis

► Severe oligohydramnios secondary to premature rupture of membranes
► Post dates pregnancy
► Various maternal systemic problems, such as hypertension, diabetes, and preeclampsia

Teaching Points

▶ Renal agenesis refers to congenital absence of the kidney and ureter, which may be either unilateral or bilateral
▶ Most cases of bilateral renal agenesis are sporadic
  ▪ Risk of occurrence of bilateral renal agenesis in a subsequent pregnancy is 3–6%, but it may reach 8% in cases associated with multiple congenital abnormalities
  ▪ 9–14% of first-degree relatives of patients with bilateral renal agenesis or dysgenesis have renal abnormalities
▶ Associated with increased risk of other structural abnormalities and chromosomal abnormalities
▶ Diagnosis of bilateral renal agenesis is based on sonographic nonvisualization of the fetal kidneys, ureters, and bladder, accompanied by oligohydramnios, usually after 16 weeks of gestation
▶ Confirmation of the presence of normal renal arteries on color Doppler (arrows in Fig. 60.9) helps to exclude the diagnosis when the kidneys are difficult to delineate in the early second trimester

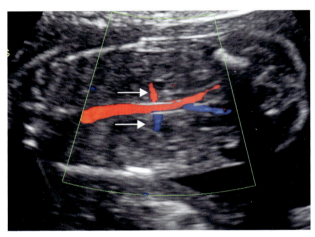

Fig. 60.9

▶ Unilateral renal agenesis more difficult to diagnose and depends on accurately excluding the presence of a second kidney in the renal fossa or in an ectopic location
▶ Other conditions that lead to severe oligohydramnios/anhydramnios listed in the differential diagnosis are usually suggested by maternal history and differentiated from renal agenesis by Doppler detection of the renal arteries

Management

▶ Bilateral renal agenesis is always fatal in the newborn period
▶ For pregnancies with unilateral renal agenesis, thorough screening for other structural defects (especially of the reproductive tract) should be performed
  ▪ If additional anomalies are detected, there is an increased risk of chromosomal abnormality
▶ Amniocentesis to determine the fetal karyotype should be offered
▶ There are no indications for early delivery

Further Reading

1. Bronshtein M, Amit A, Achiron R, et al. The early prenatal sonographic diagnosis of renal agenesis: Techniques and possible pitfalls. *Prenat Diagn*. 1994; 14: 291–293.
2. Chow JS, Benson CB, Lebowitz RL. The clinical significance of an empty renal fossa on prenatal sonography. *J Ultrasound Med*. 2005; 24: 1049–1051.
3. Sepulveda W, Stagiannis KD, Flack NJ, et al. Accuracy of prenatal diagnosis of renal agenesis with color flow imaging in severe second-trimester oligohydramnios. *Am J Obstet Gynecol*. 1995; 173: 1788–1791.

History

▶ 24-Year-old primigravida presents for fetal dating; last menstrual period unknown (Figs. 61.1–61.4)

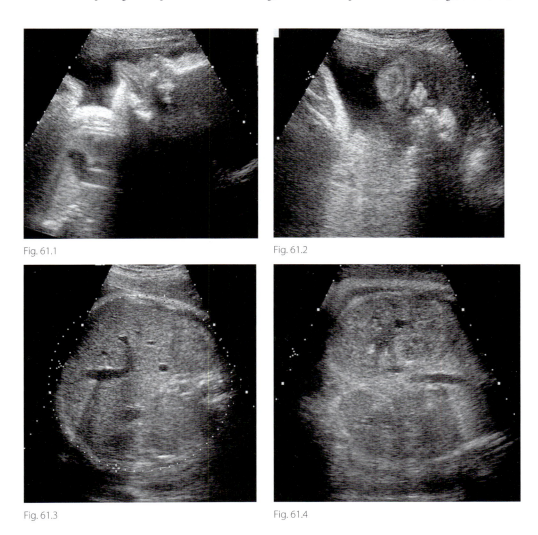

Fig. 61.1

Fig. 61.2

Fig. 61.3

Fig. 61.4

Case 61 Beckwith–Wiedemann Syndrome

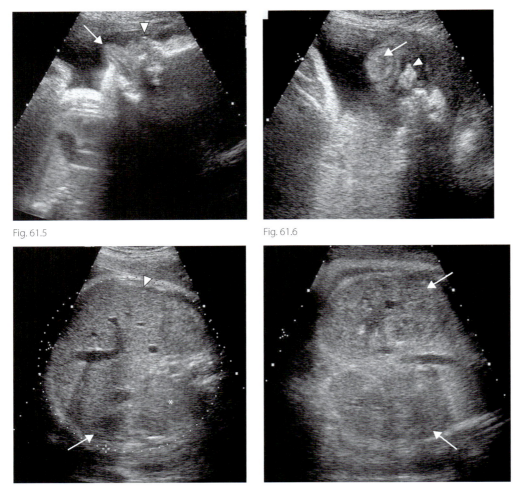

Fig. 61.5

Fig. 61.6

Fig. 61.7

Fig. 61.8

Imaging Findings

▶ Sagittal (Fig. 61.5) and coronal (Fig. 61.6) views of the face show fetal tongue (arrows in Figs. 61.5 and 61.6) protruding through the open mouth during the whole exam; nose is directly superior to tongue (arrowheads in Figs. 61.5 and 61.6)

▶ Markedly enlarged liver (arrowhead in Fig. 61.7) and spleen (asterisk in Fig. 61.7); stomach (arrow in Fig. 61.7) is compressed in front of the spleen

▶ Axial view (Fig. 61.8) of the lower abdomen shows markedly enlarged kidneys filling the abdominal cavity (arrows)

Differential Diagnosis

▶ Endocrine disorders and overgrowth syndromes, including maternal diabetes mellitus and congenital hypothyroidism

Teaching Points

▶ Pediatric overgrowth disorder with predisposition to tumor development
  ▪ Panethnic disorder with prevalence of 1 in 13,700
  ▪ Equal incidence in males and females
  ▪ 85% of cases sporadic, but familial transmission in approximately 5% of cases
  ▪ 50% are born preterm
▶ Hallmark features: omphalocele, macroglossia, and macrosomia (gigantism) with significant clinical heterogeneity
▶ Most common features of Beckwith–Wiedemann Syndrome observed prenatally are macrosomia (90%) and polyhydramnios (50%)

- Common findings: hemihyperplasia, macroglossia, omphalocele/umbilical hernia/diastasis recti, anterior linear ear lobe creases/posterior helical ear pits, visceromegaly involving one or more intra-abdominal organs, embryonal tumors (e.g., Wilms tumor, hepatoblastoma, neuroblastoma, rhabdomyosarcoma)
- Prognosis: increased risk for mortality mainly due to complications of prematurity, macroglossia, hypoglycemia, tumors, and, rarely, cardiomyopathy
  - Generally favorable after childhood

Management

- Assessment of airway sufficiency in the presence of macroglossia; may be done prenatally with MRI and EXIT (ex utero intrapartum treatment) procedure done at delivery if needed
- Evaluation by a feeding specialist if macroglossia causes significant feeding difficulties in immediate postnatal period
- Assess neonates for hypoglycemia
- Abdominal neonatal US to assess for organomegaly, structural abnormality, and tumors postnatally
- α-Fetoprotein assay at initial diagnosis to screen for hepatoblastoma
- Comprehensive cardiac evaluation including electrocardiogram prior to any surgical procedures or when a cardiac abnormality is suspected on clinical evaluation

Further Reading

1. Weksberg R, Shuman C, Beckwith JB. Beckwith–Wiedemann syndrome. *Eur J Hum Genet.* 2010; 18: 8–13.
2. Wiedemann HR. Familial malformation complex with umbilical hernia and macroglossia—A "new syndrome"? *J Genet Hum.* 1964; 13: 223–226.

Case 62

► 38-Year-old gravida 4 para 3 with positive serum screen (Figs. 62.1–62.3)

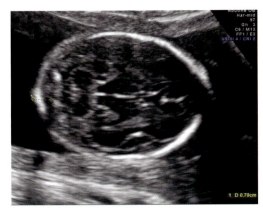

Fig. 62.1

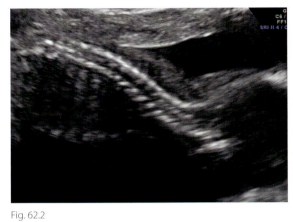

Fig. 62.2

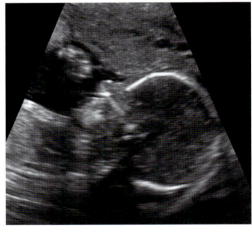

Fig. 62.3

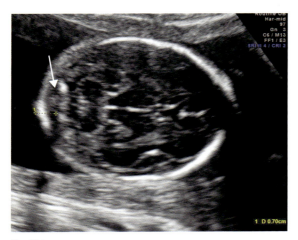

Fig. 62.4

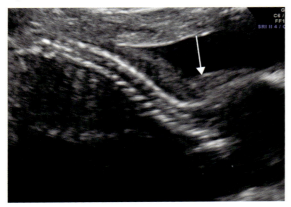

Fig. 62.5

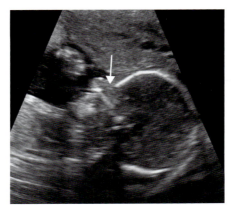

Fig. 62.6

Imaging Findings

► Axial image of the fetal head at the level of the cerebellum showing abnormal thick nuchal fold measuring 7 mm (arrow and calipers in Fig. 62.4)
► Sagittal view of the cervicothoracic spine showing redundant skin behind the neck (arrow in Fig. 62.5)
► Profile image demonstrating absence of the nasal bone (arrows in Fig. 62.6)

Differential Diagnosis

► Turner syndrome
► Trisomy 13
► Trisomy 18
► Normal nuchal skin in third trimester
► Incorrect measurement due to wrong plane of image

Teaching Points

► Thickening of the nuchal fold is due to skin edema posterior to the occiput
► It may be a remnant of a cystic hygroma that can also be seen in cases of Turner syndrome, but in these cases no other anomalies are usually demonstrated
► Overlap in the manifestations of trisomies 13, 18, and 21 has been reported, although nuchal fold thickening has been described to be more characteristic of trisomy 21
► The nuchal fold, in contrast to the nuchal translucency, is measured in the second trimester
► The nuchal fold should not be measured in the third trimester, in which the normal increase in nuchal fat can result in an abnormal measurement

- Meticulous technique will avoid pitfalls due to wrong plane of imaging or incorrect measurement
- The measurement (cursors in Fig. 62.7) is made from the outer edge of the occipital bone to the outer margin of the skin in the axial plane at the level of the cavum septi pellucidi, cerebellum, and thalami

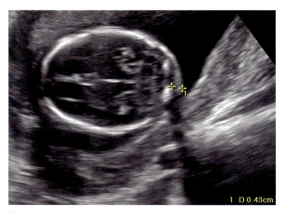

Fig. 62.7

- 40–50% of fetuses with Down syndrome have a thickened nuchal fold of ≥ 6 mm between 15 and 20 weeks of gestation
  - There is a < 1% false-positive rate
  - Can revert to normal later in pregnancy
- A thickened nuchal fold is the most sensitive (40–50%) and specific (99%) single US marker for Down syndrome in the second trimester (15–20 weeks), but not later
- Sensitivity of thickening of the nuchal translucency for the detection of Down syndrome may vary between laboratories and is higher in the first trimester (70–80% at 10–14 weeks of gestation)
  - However, there is also a higher false-positive rate of approximately 5%
- Trisomy 21 (Down syndrome)
  - 1 of every 700 live births
  - Associated with advanced maternal age; 35% of infants with trisomy 21 born to mothers > 35 years old
  - Mean IQ: 50–60
  - Mean survival is 20 years; survival associated with severity of cardiac anomalies
  - Cardiac defects common, affecting 40% of infants with Down syndrome
  - 20-fold increase in incidence of leukemias
  - Absence of the nasal bone (arrow in Fig. 62.8) at approximately 13 weeks of gestation is another reliable sign used to corroborate the diagnosis of trisomy 21; useful adjunct to screening, especially when other studies such as the quad screen show a borderline or high risk of Down syndrome

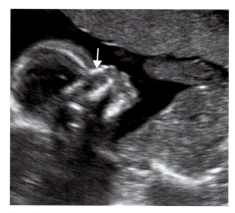

Fig. 62.8

Management

To assist in the care of children with Down syndrome the Committee on Genetics of the American Academy of Pediatrics (AAP) provide the following recommendations:

▶ Monitor for disturbances of growth and excessive weight gain
▶ Evaluation by pediatric cardiologist for congenital heart disease in the newborn
▶ Cardiac monitoring in adolescence and adulthood for mitral valve prolapse and aortic regurgitation
▶ Hearing screen in newborn and throughout childhood
▶ Monitor for otitis media which is a common cause of heating loss
▶ Ophthalmologic assessment before six months of age and then annually to screen for ophthalmologic disorders
▶ Thyroid function testing in the newborn period, 6 months, 12 months of age, and then yearly thereafter
▶ Monitor for celiac disease beginning at one year of age or if signs or symptoms develop
▶ Blood tests to evaluate for myeloproliferative disorders, polycythemia, leukemia and iron deficiency anemia
▶ Neurologic evaluation which may include MRI for spinal cord injury
▶ Monitor for symptoms related to sleep apnea

Further Reading

1. Bethune M. Literature review and suggested protocol for managing ultrasound soft markers for Down syndrome: Thickened nuchal fold, echogenic bowel, shortened femur, shortened humerus, pyelectasis and absent or hypoplastic nasal bone. *Australas Radiol*. 2007; 51: 218–222.
2. Bromley B, Lieberman E, Shipp TD, et al. The genetic sonogram: A method of risk assessment for Down syndrome in the second trimester. *J Ultrasound Med*. 2002; 21: 108–112.
3. Nicolaides KH, Snijders RJ, Gosden CM, et al. Ultrasonographically detectable markers of fetal chromosomal abnormalities. *Lancet*. 1992; 340: 704–706.

Case 63

History

▶ 42-Year-old gravida 5 para 4 with vaginal spotting; known diabetic; has a previous child with Down syndrome (Figs. 63.1–63.4)

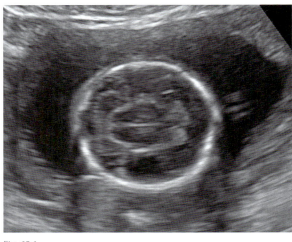

Fig. 63.1

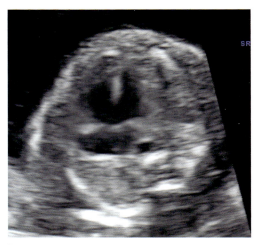

Fig. 63.2

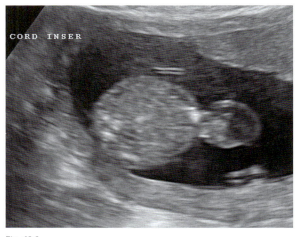

Fig. 63.3

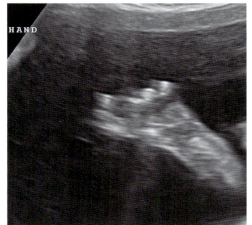

Fig. 63.4

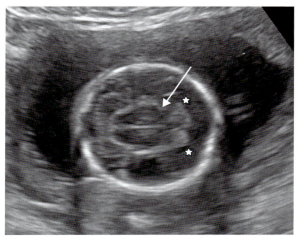

Fig. 63.5

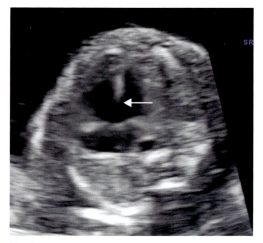

Fig. 63.6

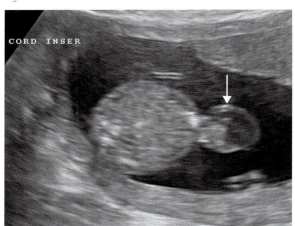

Fig. 63.7

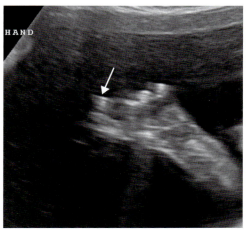

Fig. 63.8

Imaging Findings

▶ Axial image through the brain demonstrates fused thalami (arrow in Fig. 63.5), monoventricle (stars), and lack of a falx—all characteristics of holoprosencephaly
▶ Four-chamber view of the heart shows a large ventricular septal defect (arrow in Fig. 63.6)
▶ Axial image of the abdomen shows a bowel-containing omphalocele (arrow in Fig. 63.7)
▶ Deformed hand showing fused thumb and index finger (arrow in Fig. 63.8) with flexion of the remaining fingers

Differential Diagnosis

▶ Trisomy 21
▶ Trisomy 13
▶ Pena–Shokeir syndrome (pseudo-trisomy 18)

Teaching Points

▶ Trisomy 18 (Edward syndrome) occurs in approximately 1 in 6000 births; more prevalent in older mothers
▶ Prevalence is three- to fivefold higher in the first and second trimesters than at birth because many affected fetuses spontaneously abort
▶ Suspected in the first trimester when increased nuchal translucency (> 3 mm) is demonstrated (also seen in trisomy 21)
▶ Multiple anomalies detected later in the second trimester overlap with those seen in other trisomies (including trisomy 21), namely cardiac defects, spina bifida, cerebellar dysgenesis, micrognathia, diaphragmatic hernia, omphalocele, clenched hands, radial aplasia, clubbed feet, cystic hygroma choroid plexus cysts, and brachycephaly

► Should be differentiated from Pena–Shokeir syndrome, which is a rare autosomal recessive disease that is not associated with aneuploidy and presents with similar limb anomalies

Management

► Once the diagnosis is suspected from the US findings, genetic counseling and work-up may include chorionic villous sampling, amniocentesis, or cell-free fetal DNA testing depending on gestational age at the time of discovery
► Poor prognosis
  ▪ Two-thirds of fetuses alive at 16 weeks die before term
  ▪ 95% of affected infants die within the first year of life
  ▪ 50% die within the first week
► Infants who survive have severe mental and physical retardation

Further Reading

1. Driscoll DA, Gross SJ; Professional Practice Guidelines Committee. Screening for fetal aneuploidy and neural tube defects. *Genet Med*. 2009; 11(11): 818–821.
2. Yonehara T, et al. Three-dimensional sonography in diagnosing trisomy 18. *Am J Roentgenol*. 1998; 1771(4): 1165–1166.

History

► 39-Year-old gravida 5 para 4 referred for genetic screening (Figs. 64.1–64.4)

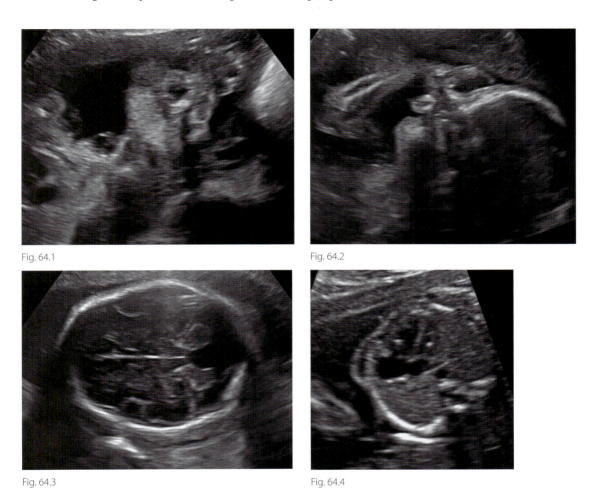

Fig. 64.1

Fig. 64.2

Fig. 64.3

Fig. 64.4

Case 64 Trisomy 13

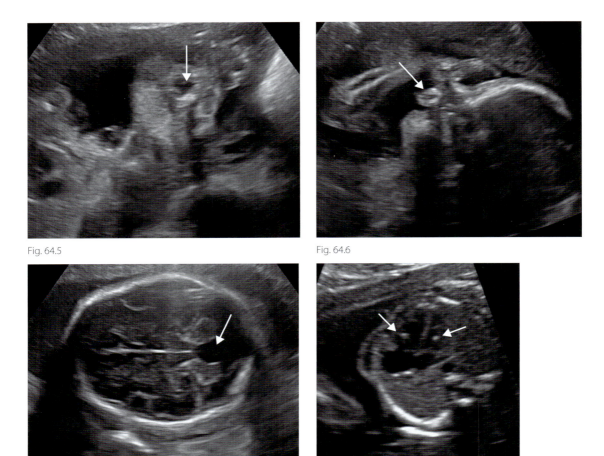

Fig. 64.5

Fig. 64.6

Fig. 64.7

Fig. 64.8

Imaging Findings

► Coronal image of face shows midline cleft lip (arrow in Fig. 64.5)
► Sagittal view of face shows premaxillary protrusion (arrow in Fig. 64.6) seen in cleft lip and palate
► Axial image of head shows a posterior fossa cyst consistent with a Dandy–Walker variant (arrow in Fig. 64.7)
► Four-chamber view of the heart shows bilateral echogenic intracardiac foci (arrows in Fig. 64.8)

Differential Diagnosis

► Many of the abnormal findings described previously are also associated with other trisomies and Turner syndrome

Teaching Points

► Trisomy 13 is the least common of the autosomal trisomies that can result in live birth
  ▪ Rare, with an incidence of 1/5000 to 1/20,000 births
  ▪ Associated with advanced maternal age (> 35 years)
  ▪ 1% of spontaneous abortions related to trisomy 13
  ▪ Associated with more severe structural malformations than trisomy 21 or 18, and therefore worse prognosis
► Sonographically detectable in > 90% of cases due to the presence of multiple, severe structural malformations, including the following
  ▪ Alobar holoprosencephaly
  ▪ Severe midline facial abnormalities (e.g., cyclopia, midline facial clefts, anophthalmia, and hypoplastic nose)
  ▪ Polycystic kidneys
  ▪ Posterior fossa anomalies
  ▪ Agenesis of the corpus callosum

- Ventriculomegaly
- Neural tube defects
- Cardiac defects (e.g., septal defects, tetralogy of Fallot, hypoplastic left ventricle, and echogenic intracardiac foci)
- Skeletal defects (e.g., polydactyly)
- Nuchal thickening
- Urogenital defects (e.g., enlarged echogenic kidneys and horseshoe kidney)
- Gastrointestinal defects (e.g., omphalocele and diaphragmatic hernia)

▶ Because several of these defects can be visualized at 11–14 weeks of gestation, first-trimester detection of trisomy 13 is quite high

▶ US combined with maternal biochemistries for aneuploidy will detect 90% of fetuses with trisomy 13 in the first trimester

Management

▶ Considered lethal condition; more than 75% of affected fetuses die in utero

▶ 49% stillbirth rate; median survival of 7 days

Further Reading

1. Lehman CD, Nyberg DA, Winter TC, et al. Trisomy 13 syndrome: Prenatal US findings in a review of 33 cases. *Radiology*. 1995; 194: 217–222.
2. Watson WJ, Miller RC, Wax JR, et al. Sonographic detection of trisomy 13 in the first and second trimesters of pregnancy. *J Ultrasound Med*. 2007; 26: 1209–1213.
3. Tongsong T, Sirichotiyakul S, Wanapirak C, et al. Sonographic features of trisomy 13 at midpregnancy. *Int J Gynaecol Obstet*. 2002; 76(2): 143–148.

Case 65

► 34-Year-old gravida 4 para 3 for assessment of growth of known twin gestation (Figs. 65.1–65.4)

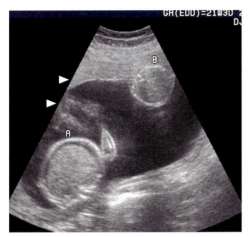

Fig. 65.1

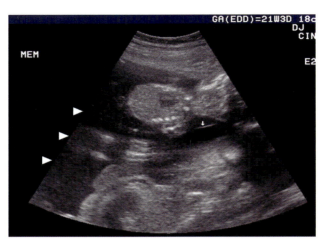

Fig. 65.2

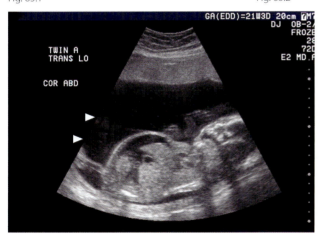

Fig. 65.3

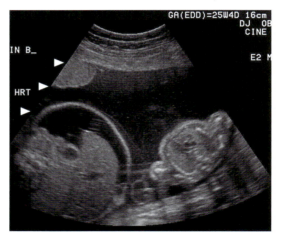

Fig. 65.4

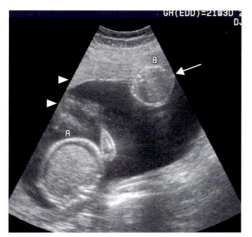

Fig. 65.5

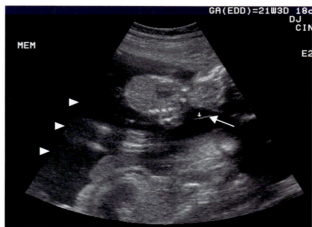

Fig. 65.6

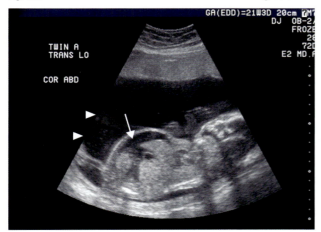

Fig. 65.7

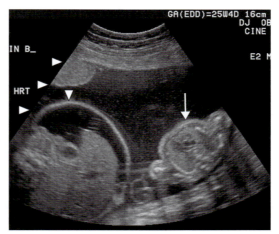

Fig. 65.8

Clinical Findings

▶ "Stuck twin" appearance of monochorionic diamniotic twin gestation with smaller donor twin (arrow in Fig. 65.5) appearing adherent to anterior uterine wall on transverse image
▶ Longitudinal image shows thin intertwin membrane (arrow in Fig. 65.6) surrounding the smaller donor twin documenting severe oligohydramnios in the sac of the donor twin at 21 weeks
▶ Longitudinal view of the larger recipient twin showing ascites (arrow in Fig. 65.7)
▶ Follow-up examination at 25 weeks (4 weeks later) shows increasing polyhydramnios and marked size discrepancy between the donor twin (arrow in Fig. 65.8) and the hydropic recipient twin who has increasing ascites (arrowhead in Fig. 65.8)

Differential Diagnosis

▶ Various entities have been grouped under the twin oligohydramnios/polyhydramnios sequence, under which twin transfusion syndrome (TTS) is also included
  ▪ Only two-thirds of twins with the "stuck twin" appearance are secondary to TTS
▶ For the donor twin
  ▪ Decreased urine output due to renal abnormalities
  ▪ Ruptured amnion
  ▪ Intrauterine growth restriction

- For the recipient twin
  - Neural tube defect
  - Gastrointestinal anomalies
  - Hydrops secondary to other causes

Teaching Points

- One of the most serious complications of monochorionic multifetal gestations
  - High risk of fetal/neonatal mortality
  - Surviving fetuses are at risk for severe cardiac, neurologic, and developmental disorders
- Unbalanced placental intertwin vascular anastomoses play a key role in the pathophysiology of TTS. One twin becomes hypovolemic (donor twin), and the other becomes hypervolemic (recipient twin)
  - Complications include preterm labor, placental abruption, embolic phenomenon, and coagulation problems
- US findings
  - Single monochorionic placenta
  - Polyhydramnios/oligohydramnios sequence
    - Before 20 weeks of gestation, maximum vertical amniotic fluid pockets for oligohydramnios and polyhydramnios are < 2 cm and > 8 cm, respectively
  - After 20 weeks, maximum vertical pocket for polyhydramnios should be > 10 cm
  - Severe oligohydramnios results in the "stuck twin" appearance of donor twin
  - Intertwin separating membrane that may be difficult to find
  - Fetuses of the same sex
  - Weight discordance ≥ 20%

Management

- Monitor monochorionic twin pregnancies for development of TTS with serial US examinations every 2 or 3 weeks
- Serial amniocentesis to drain the excess fluid may be performed
- Ablation of supplying vessels on the placental surface
- Close clinical monitoring is warranted to prevent complications

Further Reading

1. Lewi L, Jani J, Boes AS, et al. The natural history of monochorionic twins and the role of prenatal ultrasound scan. *Ultrasound Obstet Gynecol.* 2007; 30: 401–405.
2. Lutfi S, Allen VM, Fahey J, et al. Twin–twin transfusion syndrome: A population-based study. *Obstet Gynecol.* 2004; 104: 1289–1292.
3. Brown DL, Benson CB, Driscoll SG, et al. Twin–twin transfusion syndrome: Sonographic findings. *Radiology.* 1989; 170: 61–64.

History

▶ 29-Year-old pregnant female presents for US evaluation (Figs. 66.1 and 66.2)

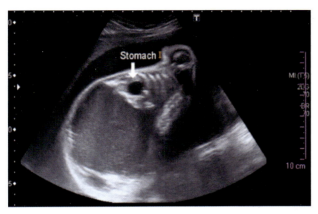

Fig. 66.1

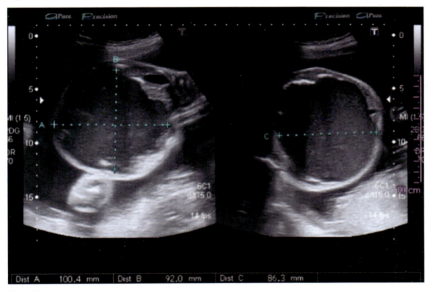

Fig. 66.2

Case 66 Meconium Pseudocyst

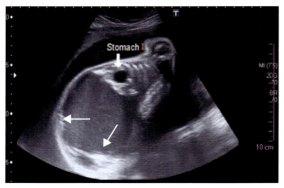

Fig. 66.3

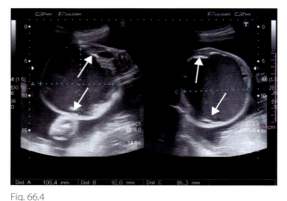

Fig. 66.4

Imaging Findings

▶ Large cystic structure containing low-level internal echoes, and curvilinear echogenic peripheral calcifications (arrows in Fig. 66.3 and Fig. 66.4) fill the abdominal cavity compressing and displacing the stomach and bowel

Differential Diagnosis

▶ Meconium peritonitis
▶ Enteric duplication cyst
▶ Ovarian cyst
▶ Viral infection

Teaching Points

▶ Meconium peritonitis occurs secondary to in utero small bowel perforation and extrusion of meconium into the peritoneal cavity, which causes an intense sterile inflammatory response
  ▪ If the extruded meconium becomes walled off, it is termed a meconium pseudocyst
▶ Risk factors or underlying causes: cystic fibrosis (~40%), bowel stenosis or atresia, infection, volvulus, and meconium ileus versus idiopathic or vascular compromise
▶ US findings
  ▪ Cyst with internal echoes and echogenic/calcified wall
  ▪ May be associated with ascites, polyhydramnios, intraperitoneal calcifications (linear or punctate), dilated bowel, and compression and displacement of bowel or other structures
▶ 20% associated with fetal anomalies
▶ Neonatal KUB (kidneys, ureters, and bladder) X-ray demonstrates a distended abdomen with peripheral thin arclike calcifications (arrows in Figs. 66.5 and 66.6). Note air in displaced and compressed descending colon lateral to the calcifications. The chest is dysplastic
▶ Neonatal contrast-enhanced CT scan demonstrating non-enhancing large homogeneous cystic structure filling the abdomen. There are peripheral calcifications (arrows in Fig. 66.6). The bowel is displaced and compressed to the left, and the kidneys are displaced and compressed posteriorly

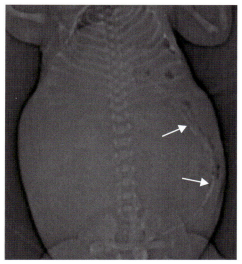

Fig. 66.5

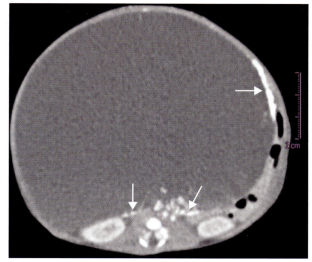

Fig. 66.6

▶ Enteric duplication or ovarian cyst: usually not as large, not calcified
▶ Viral infection: intra-abdominal calcifications but without cyst formation

Management

▶ Followed throughout pregnancy with serial US
▶ Delivery at tertiary care center with neonatal intensive care unit
▶ Postnatal surgery if large bowel perforation/obstruction and associated with bowel dilatation, ascites, and/or polyhydramnios

Further Reading

1. Foster MA, Nyberg DA, Mahony BS, et al. Meconium peritonitis: Prenantal sonographic findings and their clinical significance. *Radiology.* 1987; 165: 661.
2. Eckoldt F, Heling KS, Woderich R, et al. Meconium peritonitis and pseudo-cyst formation: Prenatal diagnosis and post-natal course. *Prenat Diagn.* 2003; 23: 904.

Case 67

History

▶ 33-Year-old gravida 2 para 1 for routine fetal dating (Figs. 67.1–67.4)

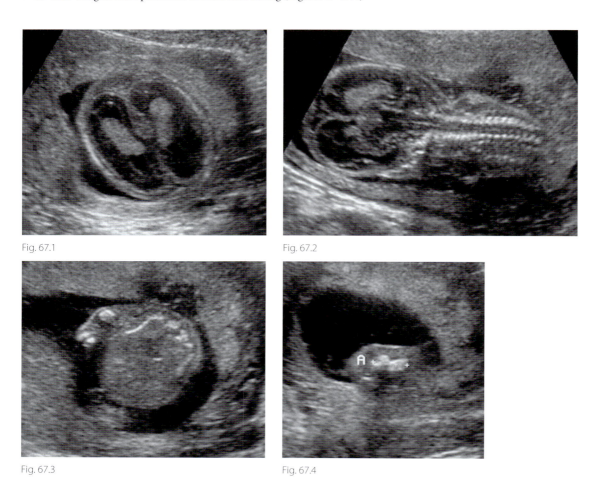

Fig. 67.1

Fig. 67.2

Fig. 67.3

Fig. 67.4

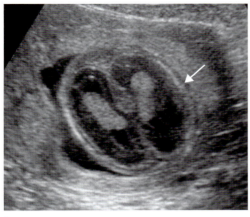

Fig. 67.5

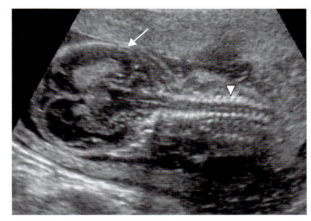

Fig. 67.6

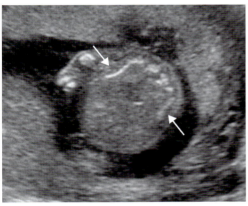

Fig. 67.7

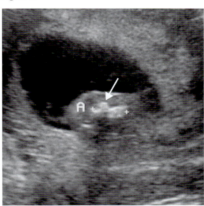

Fig. 67.8

Imaging Findings

▶ Axial image of the fetal head shows severe demineralization of the calvarium (arrow in Fig. 67.5) resulting in unusually clear visualization of the intracranial structures

▶ Coronal view of the cervicothoracic junction showing the difference in mineralization between the calvarium (arrow in Fig. 67.6) and the fetal spine (arrowhead in Fig. 67.6)

▶ Axial image of the chest shows outward flaring of the ribs (arrows in Fig. 67.7) due to previous fractures

▶ Severe shortening and fracture of the femur (arrow and calipers in Fig. 67.8)

Differential Diagnosis

▶ Thanatophoric dysplasia
▶ Achondrogenesis
▶ Hypophosphatasia

Teaching Points

▶ Osteogenesis imperfecta is a heterogeneous group of collagen disorders characterized by brittle bones prone to fracture
▶ Four major subtypes based on genetic, radiographic, and clinical considerations
  - Type I: osteogenesis imperfecta tarda
    • Most mild form
  - Type II: perinatal lethal
    • Most severe form—lethal
  - Type III: progressively deforming
    • Significantly shortened life span
    • Multiple fractures at birth, blue sclerae

- Type IV: delayed presentation
  - Spectrum between types I–III, normal to slightly decreased life span
- Key US features
  - Severe micromelia; femur length more than 3 standard deviations below mean for gestational age
  - Small thoracic circumference
  - Normal cranial size
  - Short trunk length
  - Decreased mineralization; bones deform with transducer pressure
  - Multiple bone fractures, including rib fractures with concave contour of thorax giving the appearance of outward flaring of the ribs
- Diagnosis made sonographically at 13–15 weeks
- Normal US examination after 17 weeks virtually excludes this diagnosis
- Normal reference images important for comparison
  - Equal mineralization of calvarium and spine (arrows in Fig. 67.9)
  - Normal orientation of ribs (arrow in Fig. 67.10)

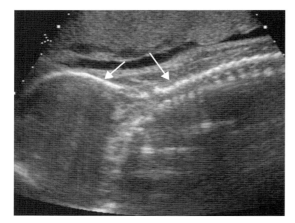 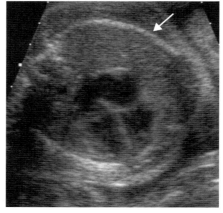

Fig. 67.9   Fig. 67.10

- Primary goal is to determine lethality; secondary goal is to determine the diagnosis or to narrow the differential diagnosis
  - Thanatophoric dwarfism has normal bone mineralization and no fractures
  - Achondrogenesis has patchy demineralization with occasional fractures
  - Hypophosphatasia shows patchy or diffuse demineralization with occasional fractures
- Postmortem radiograph of fetus can confirm healed fractures of the humeri, femurs, and ribs (arrows in Fig. 67.11)

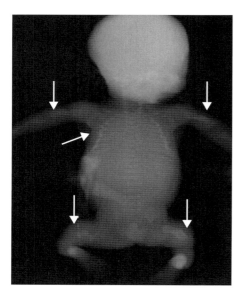

Fig. 67.11

Management

▶ Counseling of couples by a team that includes perinatal imaging specialists, medical geneticists, maternal–fetal medicine specialists, and neonatologists

▶ Parents with skeletal dysplasia should have their own diagnoses determined; discuss implications of diagnosis, including the mode of delivery and postnatal treatment

▶ After delivery or pregnancy termination, the diagnosis should be confirmed by clinical, radiographic, photographic, and histomorphic analysis

▶ Results and the implications of the final diagnosis on future reproductive plans should be discussed with the parents

Further Reading

1. DiMaio MS, Barth R, Koprivnikar KE, et al. First-trimester prenatal diagnosis of osteogenesis imperfecta type II by DNA analysis and sonography. *Prenat Diagn*. 1993; 13: 589.

2. Sillence DO, Barlow KK, Garber AP, et al. Osteogenesis imperfecta type II delineation of the phenotype with reference to genetic heterogeneity. *Am J Med Genet*. 1984; 17: 407.

3. Munoz C, Filly RA, Golbus MS. Osteogenesis imperfecta type II: Prenatal sonographic diagnosis. *Radiology*. 1990; 174: 181.

History

▸ 56-Year-old woman with metastatic small-cell lung cancer and history of low-grade fevers (Figs. 68.1 and 68.2)

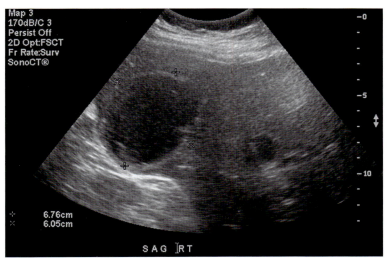

Fig. 68.1

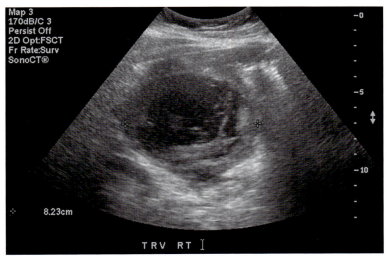

Fig. 68.2

Case 68 Pyogenic Liver Abscess

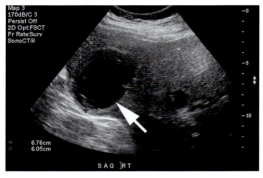

Fig. 68.3

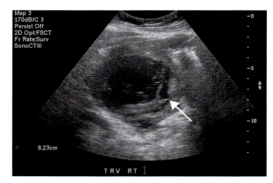

Fig. 68.4

Imaging Findings
► Thick-walled anechoic fluid collection
► Internal septations and debris (arrows in Fig. 68.3 and Fig. 68.4)

Differential Diagnosis
► Hematoma
► Cystic or necrotic metastasis
► Biliary cystadenoma

Teaching Points
► Variable clinical presentation
  ▪ Acute presentation: high fever, rigors, right-sided abdominal pain
  ▪ Clinically occult "cold" abscess: Weight loss, vague abdominal pain
  ▪ Nonspecific elevations of liver enzymes and total bilirubin and decreased serum albumin
► Pyogenic liver abscesses are most often polymicrobial, with *Escherichia coli* the most commonly recovered pathogen. Sources include the following
  ▪ Biliary tract disease
  ▪ Hematogenous spread (from gastrointestinal infection via portal vein or from disseminated sepsis via hepatic artery (rare))
  ▪ Superinfection of necrotic tissue, hematoma, or preexisting cysts
  ▪ Idiopathic
► Classified as macroabscesses (> 2 cm) or microabscesses (< 2 cm)
► Pyogenic abscesses have wide range of US appearances
  ▪ Complex fluid collection with echogenic rim
  ▪ Variable degrees of internal echoes and debris
  ▪ Gas in the abscess can create echogenic foci with dirty shadowing
► Clinical history is helpful in distinguishing pyogenic abscesses from hematomas or cystic neoplasms, which may have a similar appearance
► US features that differentiate other entities in the differential diagnosis from abscess
  ▪ Hematoma
    • Acute hematoma usually echogenic
    • Subacute hematoma becomes more hypoechoic and cystic due to liquefaction and can mimic abscess
  ▪ Cystic or necrotic metastasis
    • Thick peripheral, often irregular echogenic rim with vascular flow
    • May have solid components
  ▪ Biliary cystadenoma
    • Rare neoplasm
    • Usually large when discovered
    • Often have septations

Management

▶ US is useful for image-guided percutaneous aspiration and abscess drainage

▶ Aspirated fluid can be sent for gram stain and culture to confirm diagnosis and guide antibiotic therapy

▶ Early diagnosis and image-guided percutaneous drainage have reduced mortality rate of pyogenic liver abscess from 40% to 2%

Further Reading

1. Li D, Hann LE. A practical approach to analyzing focal lesions in the liver. *Ultrasound Q.* 2005; 21(3): 187–200.
2. Mortelé KJ, Segatto E, Ros PR. The infected liver: Radiologic–pathologic correlation. *RadioGraphics.* 2004; 24(4): 937–955.

Case 69

History

► 18-Year-old woman with history of right lower quadrant pain, nausea, and vomiting (Figs. 69.1–69.3)

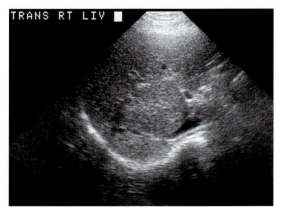

Fig. 69.1

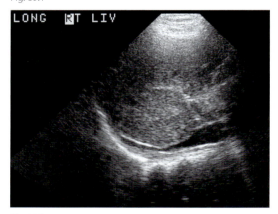

Fig. 69.2

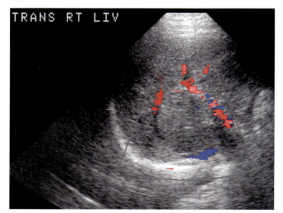

Fig. 69.3

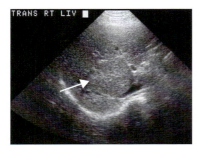

Fig. 69.4

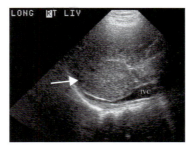

Fig. 69.5

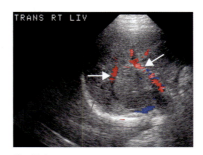

Fig. 69.6

Imaging Findings

▶ Subtle isoechoic mass (arrows in Figs. 69.4 and 69.5) in right hepatic lobe, compressing inferior vena cava (IVC)
▶ Blood vessels are displaced along periphery of mass (arrows in Fig. 69.6)

Differential Diagnosis

▶ Hepatic adenoma
▶ Fibrolamellar hepatocellular carcinoma
▶ Hepatocellular carcinoma
▶ Metastatic disease
▶ Cavernous hemangioma

Teaching Points

▶ Second most common benign liver tumor after cavernous hemangioma; prevalence of 0.9%; 20% multiple
▶ Female:male ratio = 8:1; typically third to fourth decade
▶ Hepatocyte nodules surrounded by radiating fibrous septa originating from central scar
▶ Mostly asymptomatic; incidental imaging finding
▶ US features
  ▪ Slightly hypoechoic or isoechoic. Very rarely echogenic
  ▪ Some only detected because of mass effect and displacement of surrounding vessels
  ▪ Hypoechoic halo may be present
  ▪ Echogenic central scar usually not well visualized on US
  ▪ Color Doppler: central feeding artery with "spoke-wheel" pattern of radiating arteries; best seen on contrast-enhanced US (CEUS)
  ▪ CEUS: central vascular supply with centrifugal filling to periphery on early arterial phase; homogeneous enhancement on late arterial phase; remains slightly echogenic or isoechoic in late portal venous phase
  ▪ Adenoma
    • Heterogeneous echotexture, if large
    • Difficult to differentiate from focal nodular hyperplasia (FNH) on grayscale images
    • Stellate enhancement pattern seen on CEUS
    • Sustained portal venous phase enhancement less common
  ▪ Hepatocellular carcinoma
    • Background of cirrhotic liver
    • CEUS: hypervascularity during arterial phase; washout during portal venous and delayed phases
  ▪ Metastatic disease
    • Commonly multifocal
    • Variable echogenicity depending on primary tumor
  ▪ Cavernous hemangioma
    • Classically homogeneously echogenic; however, 30–40% have variable grayscale appearance
    • CEUS: peripheral nodular enhancement with progressive centripetal filling

Management

▶ Most patients asymptomatic; require no specific treatment
▶ CEUS features: improve differentiation of FNH from other benign and malignant liver masses
▶ Multiphase contrast-enhanced CT or MRI helpful for confirmation of diagnosis
▶ Follow-up CT or MRI in 6–12 months to ensure stability
▶ Atypical FNH requires US-guided percutaneous biopsy for diagnosis

Further Reading

1. Hussain SM, Terkivatan T, Zondervan PE, et al. Focal nodular hyperplasia: Findings at state-of-the-art MR imaging, US, CT, and pathologic analysis. *RadioGraphics*. 2004; 24(1): 3–17.
2. Strobel D, Seitz K, Blank W, et al. Contrast-enhanced ultrasound for the characterization of focal liver lesions—Diagnostic accuracy in clinical practice. *Ultraschall Med*. 2008; 29(5): 499–505.

History

► 23-Year-old man with markedly elevated liver function tests and acute liver failure secondary to hepatitis C (Figs. 70.1 and 70.2)

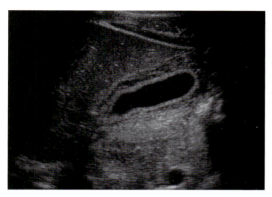

Fig. 70.1

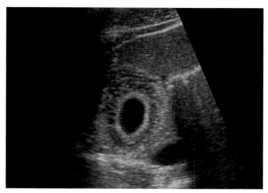

Fig. 70.2

Case 70 Gallbladder Wall Thickening Due to Hepatitis

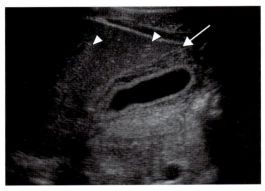

Fig. 70.3

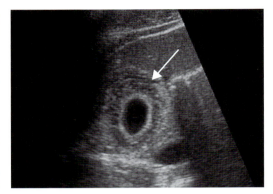

Fig. 70.4

Findings

▶ Marked circumferential thickening of the gallbladder wall with a striated appearance (arrows in Figs. 70.3 and 70.4)
▶ Gallbladder lumen is not distended
▶ Echogenic prominent periportal echoes (arrowheads in Fig. 70.3)

Differential Diagnosis

▶ Pseudo-gallbladder wall thickening in contracted postprandial gallbladder
▶ Diffuse gallbladder wall thickening
  ▪ Acute cholecystitis
  ▪ Chronic cholecystitis
  ▪ Acute pancreatitis, perforated duodenal ulcer, colitis
  ▪ Hypoalbuminemia
  ▪ Cirrhosis and portal hypertension
  ▪ Congestive heart failure
  ▪ Chronic renal failure
  ▪ Graft-versus-host disease
  ▪ Veno-occlusive disease after bone marrow transplant

Teaching Points

▶ Normal gallbladder wall: 3 mm or less
▶ Mechanisms implicated in gallbladder wall thickening in patients with acute hepatitis
  ▪ Inflammation of mucosal and submucosal layers of the gallbladder associated with hepatitis
  ▪ Inflammation caused by hepatocyte necrosis
  ▪ Decreased bile production by injured hepatocytes
▶ US findings in acute cholecystitis
  ▪ Distention of gallbladder lumen; impacted stone in cystic duct or distended gallbladder filled with echogenic material representing sludge, blood, or pus; hyperemia of gallbladder wall on color or power Doppler US
▶ Focal tenderness over the gallbladder (sonographic Murphy's sign): helpful if present
▶ Presence of gallstones and positive sonographic Murphy's sign: positive predictive value 92%
▶ Critically ill patients in intensive care units demonstrate abnormalities of the gallbladder, especially wall thickening. Patients are at risk for acalculous cholecystitis. A specific diagnosis is often difficult on ultrasound due to other conditions associated with gallbladder wall thickening. Clinical context is important in determining etiology of gallbladder wall thickening and exclude other causes in the differential diagnosis list.
▶ Lack of distension of the gallbladder is an important differential feature

Management

► Unless the clinical or sonographic picture suggests acute cholecystitis, diffuse gallbladder wall thickening is often a secondary finding. Management focuses on the primary underlying condition

► In equivocal cases, nuclear medicine hepatobiliary study is often recommended

Further Reading

1. Suk KT, Kim CH, Baik SK, et al. Gallbladder wall thickening in patients with acute hepatitis. *J Clin Ultrasound*. 2009; 37: 144–148.
2. Boland GW, Slater G, Lu DS, et al. Prevalence and significance of gallbladder abnormalities seen on sonography in intensive care unit patients. *Am J Roentgenol*. 2000; 174: 973–977.

Case 71

History

▶ 64-Year-old male with abnormal liver function tests (Figs. 71.1–71.3)

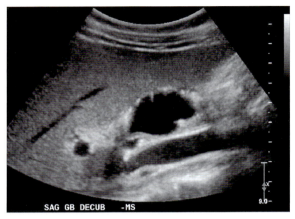

Fig. 71.1

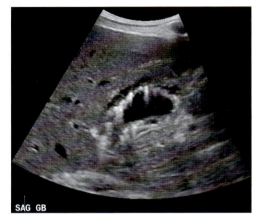

Fig. 71.2

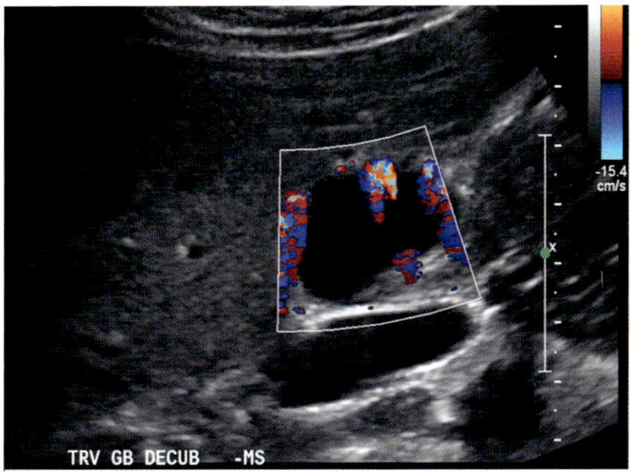

Fig. 71.3

240

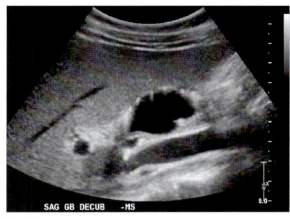

Fig. 71.4

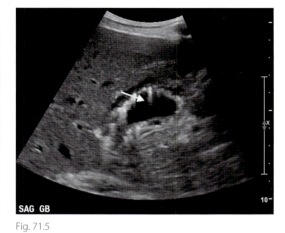

Fig. 71.5

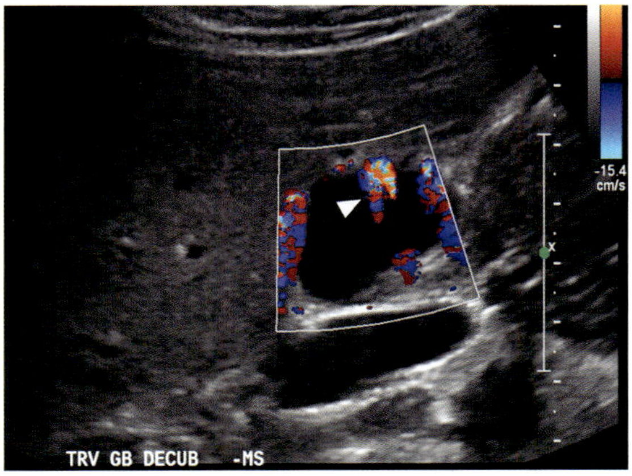

Fig. 71.6

Imaging Findings

▶ Multiple echogenic foci within the wall of the gallbladder (Fig. 71.4) causing "comet tail" artifact (arrow in Fig. 71.5)
▶ On color Doppler, these foci show "twinkle" artifact (arrowhead in Fig. 71.6)
▶ Absent sonographic Murphy's sign

Differential Diagnosis

▶ Cholelithiasis
▶ Gallbladder polyp or carcinoma
▶ Emphysematous cholecystitis
▶ Porcelain gallbladder

Teaching Points

▶ Adenomyomatosis is one of the hyperplastic cholecystoses (cholesterolosis and gallbladder polyp are the others) and results from hyperplasia of the layers of the gallbladder walls and the formation of intramural diverticular or sinuses, called Rokitansky–Aschoff sinuses, in which cholesterol crystals deposit
▶ Cholesterol crystals are thought to account for the "comet tail" artifact.
▶ Twinkle artifact may result from the cholesterol crystals or from associated intramural calcifications
▶ It can be diffuse or focal and most commonly involves the fundus of the gallbladder
▶ Rarely, anechoic cystic spaces within the gallbladder wall may be seen corresponding to the Rokitansky–Aschoff sinuses
▶ It is important to distinguish twinkle artifact from blood flow in the stalk of a polyp, mural mass, or focal thickening of the gallbladder wall, which would indicate gallbladder carcinoma

- Both cholelithiasis and porcelain gallbladder would produce posterior acoustic shadowing rather than the "comet tail" artifact. Although "floating" gallstones can occur, gallstones are typically in a dependent location
- Air within the gallbladder wall in emphysematous cholecystitis will produce "dirty shadowing" rather than the "comet tail" artifact. The sonographer should also evaluate for additional signs of inflammation, such as gallbladder wall thickening or pericholecystic fluid. A sonographic Murphy's sign may be present

Management

- Adenomyomatosis is a benign condition
- If there is doubt regarding the diagnosis, MRI can be performed

Further Reading

1. Boscak AR, Al-Hawary M, Ramsburgh SR. Best cases from the AFIP: Adenomyomatosis of the gallbladder. *RadioGraphics*. 2006; 26: 941–946.
2. Ghersin E, Soudack M, Gaitini D. Twinkling artifact in gallbladder adenomyomatosis. *J Ultrasound Med*. 2003; 22: 229–231.

History

► 21-Year-old male with abdominal pain (Figs. 72.1–72.3)

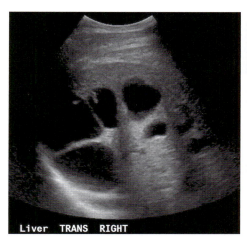

Fig. 72.1

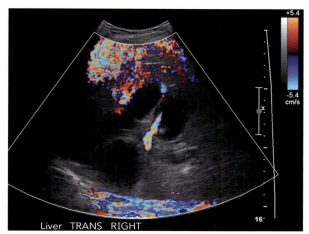

Fig. 72.2

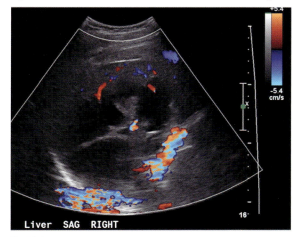

Fig. 72.3

Case 72 Caroli Disease

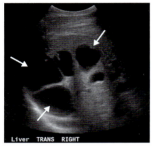
Fig. 72.4

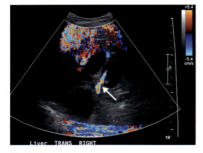
Fig. 72.5

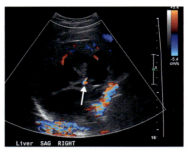
Fig. 72.6

Imaging Findings

▶ Multiple intrahepatic anechoic fluid-filled spaces (arrows in Fig. 72.4) separated by intervening septations
▶ Note color flow within central portion of the septations (arrow in Fig. 72.5), "central dot sign" (arrow in Fig. 72.6)

Differential Diagnosis

▶ Polycystic liver disease
▶ Biliary cystadenoma/cystadenocarcinoma
▶ Echinococcal cyst

Teaching Points

▶ Rare congenital disorder secondary to abnormal ductal plate formation (a layer of cells surrounding the portal veins and a precursor to the formation of the intrahepatic bile ducts) resulting in nonobstructive dilatation of the intrahepatic bile ducts
▶ Autosomal recessive without gender predilection
▶ Caroli syndrome, the more common form, presents in children or young adults (< 30 years) with cirrhosis and portal hypertension secondary to congenital periportal hepatic fibrosis
▶ Caroli disease, the less common "classic" or "simple" variety, is associated with recurrent episodes of cholangitis (fever, RUQ pain, jaundice, and liver abscess) and stone formation in the intrahepatic bile ducts due to stasis
▶ Increased risk of cholangiocarcinoma (~7%)
▶ Associated with medullary sponge kidney and autosomal recessive polycystic kidney disease
▶ Imaging findings
  ▪ Saccular, occasionally fusiform, dilatation of the intrahepatic bile ducts
  ▪ Diffuse involvement more common than focal
  ▪ Extrahepatic bile ducts often spared
  ▪ "Central dot sign" (portal vein radicals engulfed by the dilated intrahepatic bile ducts)
  ▪ Echogenic septa coursing through the lumen of the dilated bile ducts ("intraductal bridging")
  ▪ Stones/sludge in intrahepatic bile ducts
  ▪ Signs of portal hypertension
▶ Differentiation from multiple simple hepatic cysts, polycystic liver disease, or other causes of complex cystic masses may be difficult on US or CT
  ▪ Cholangiography (conventional or MR) may be required to confirm communication with the biliary tree
▶ Biliary cystadenomas and cystadenocarcinomas: multiseptated intrahepatic masses; more likely to have solid, vascular nodules; septations often irregular; no central dot sign
▶ Echinoccocal cysts: more likely unilocular with the "floating membrane sign" or multiple daughter cysts, no central blood flow

Management

▶ Segmentectomy or hepatic lobectomy for segmental form
▶ Liver transplantation may be required for diffuse form

Further Reading

1. Vachha B, et al. Cystic lesions of the liver. *Am J Roentgenol*. 2011; 196: W355–W366.
2. Santiago I, Loureiro R, Curvo-Semedo L, et al. Congenital cystic lesions of the biliary tree. *Am J Roentgenol*. 2012: 19: 825–835.

History

▶ 61-Year- old male with past medical history of alcohol abuse presents with nausea, vomiting, and abdominal pain for 1 day (Figs. 73.1 and 7.32)

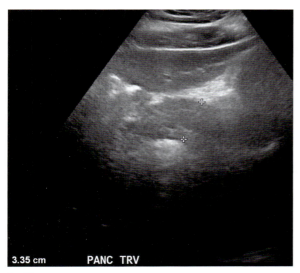

Fig. 73.1

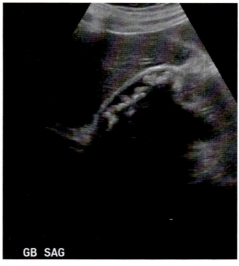

Fig. 73.2

Case 73 Acute Pancreatitis

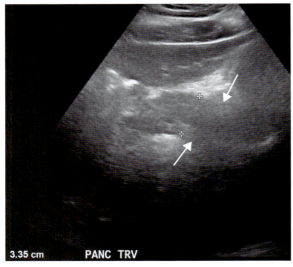

Fig. 73.3

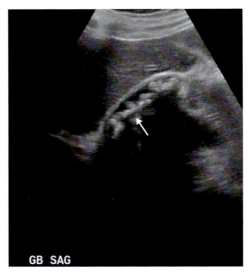

Fig. 73.4

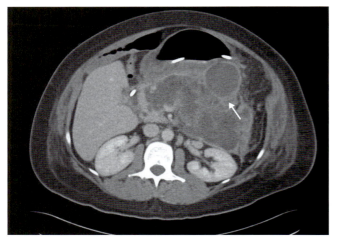

Fig. 73.5

Imaging Findings

▶ Enlarged, hypoechoic pancreas body and tail (calipers in Fig. 73.3)
▶ Blurred pancreatic margins (arrows in Fig. 73.3) indicate inflammation
▶ Multiple gallstones (arrow in Fig. 73.4)
▶ CT shows markedly necrotic pancreas with a pseudocyst (arrow in Fig. 73.5)

Differential Diagnosis

▶ Infiltrating pancreatic carcinoma
▶ Lymphoma

Teaching Points

▶ Presenting symptoms: sudden-onset epigastric pain, nausea, vomiting, and fever
▶ Diagnosis made by elevated serum amylase and lipase
▶ Young and middle-aged patients, males > females
▶ Most common causes: alcohol abuse and gallstones (40% each)
▶ Other causes: congenital anomalies, hereditary pancreatitis, metabolic etiologies, infection, trauma, iatrogenic, and drugs/medications
▶ Visualization of the pancreas on US often impaired by bowel gas from ileus in the setting of acute abdominal pain

- US findings may be normal or subtle
  - Normal pancreas is typically greater in echogenicity compared to the liver
  - Thickness of normal pancreatic body is 10.1 ± 3.8 mm
  - > 23 mm (3 standard deviations above the mean) is suggested as an appropriate criterion for enlargement
- US does not have a primary role in the diagnosis of suspected acute pancreatitis
- Primary roles of US in the evaluation of the patient with acute pancreatitis include the following
  - Identification of gallstones as a causal factor
  - Detection of bile duct dilatation, suggesting obstruction
  - Color duplex ultrasonography can aid in the diagnosis of vascular complications such as hepatic artery pseudoaneurysm and splenic vein thrombosis
- CT: more sensitive than US for diagnosis of acute pancreatitis; used to grade severity, detect necrosis/complications, and predict clinical outcome
- Infiltrating carcinoma and lymphoma are unlikely diagnoses given the clinical scenario

Management

- CT: modality of choice for evaluation/staging
- Treatment is based on disease severity
- Conservative treatment strategy includes nothing by mouth, gastric tube decompression, and analgesics
- Antibiotics are indicated in cases complicated by pancreatic necrosis
- Surgery and/or image-guided drainage may be necessary with infected pancreatic necrosis or infected pseudocysts

Further Reading

1. Gandolfi L, Torresan F, Solmi L, et al. The role of ultrasound in biliary and pancreatic diseases. *Eur J Ultrasound*. 2003; 16(3): 141–159.
2. Finstad TA, Tchelepi H, Ralls PW. Sonography of acute pancreatitis: Prevalence of findings and pictorial essay. *Ultrasound Q*. 2005; 21(2): 95–104.

Case 74

History

▶ 24-Year-old female with fever and 2-day history of initially crampy periumbilical and now constant, sharp, right lower quadrant abdominal pain and nausea (Figs. 74.1–74.3)

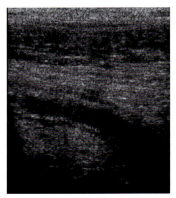

Fig. 74.1

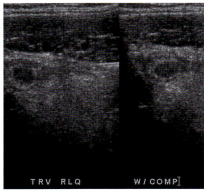

Fig. 74.2

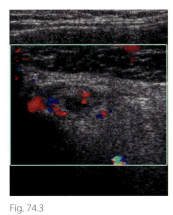

Fig. 74.3

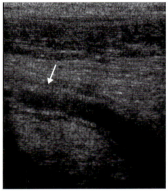

Fig. 74.4

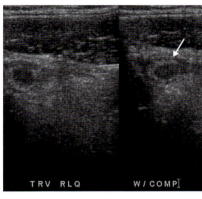

Fig. 74.5

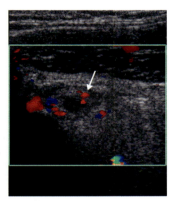

Fig. 74.6

Imaging Findings

▶ Noncompressible, enlarged (< 6 mm), blind-ending, fluid-filled tubular structure (arrows in Figs. 74.4 and 74.5) with hyperemic wall and increased vascularity in surrounding fat on color Doppler US (arrow in Fig. 74.6)

Differential Diagnosis

▶ Mesenteric adenitis
▶ Ileitis and ileocolitis
▶ Pelvic inflammatory disease

Teaching Points

▶ Most frequently suspected cause of acute right lower quadrant pain; most common indication for emergency abdominal surgery
▶ Graded compression US: primary diagnostic test in the young, female, and slender patients
▶ Normal appendix: blind-ended, aperistaltic tubular structure with typical striated gut signature originating from the base of the cecum with a diameter ≤ 6 mm.
▶ Threshold 6-mm diameter of the appendix with lack of compression is the most accurate US finding for appendicitis. 7 mm increases specificity
▶ Additional findings: hyperemia of the wall and surrounding tissues, echogenic periappendiceal fat, appendicolith and nonspecific lymphadenopathy
▶ Given an enlarged, hyperemic appendix and right lower quadrant tenderness, the other differential diagnoses are much less likely
▶ Predominate feature of terminal ileitis is bowel wall thickening centered on the inner layers with a normal appendix. Terminal ileum is peristaltic, compressible, and lacks haustra, helping to differentiate it from the cecum
▶ Hallmark of Crohn's disease: bowel wall thickening ileocecal in location. In more severe Crohn's disease, bowel wall stratification becomes ill-defined with reduced or absent peristalsis
▶ Enlarged mesenteric lymph nodes are appreciated in mesenteric adenitis with possible focal thickening of adjacent colonic wall, which should not be circumferentially thickened
▶ Pelvic inflammatory disease involves ovaries and fallopian tubes with thickening of endosalpingeal folds (cogwheel sign), incomplete septation sign, simple or complex fluid in the in the endometrial cavity and/or cul-de-sac, and ovarian enlargement with ill-defined borders ± abscess formation

Management

▶ CT or MRI if US examination is equivocal. MRI only if patient is pregnant and US equivocal
▶ Surgery if nonperforated or minimal perforation
▶ Percutaneous drainage if well-localized abscess > 3 cm is seen
▶ Antibiotic therapy if periappendiceal soft tissue inflammation and no abscess

Further Reading

1. Chan L, Shin LK, Pai RK, et al. Pathologic continuum of acute appendicitis: Sonographic findings and clinical management implications. *Ultrasound Q.* 2011; 27(2): 71–79.

Case 75

History

► 7-Month-old boy with a 1-day history of irritability, vomiting, intermittent crying, bloody stools, and a palpable mass in the right lower abdominal quadrant (Figs. 75.1–75.3)

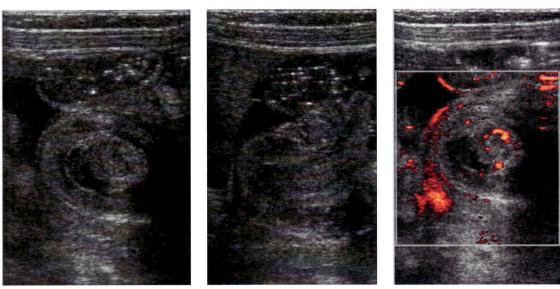

Fig. 75.1   Fig. 75.2   Fig. 75.3

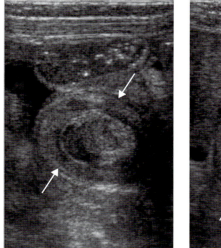
Fig. 75.4

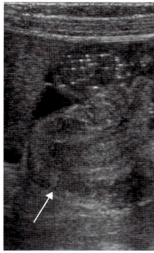
Fig. 75.5

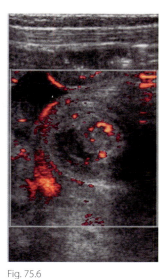
Fig. 75.6

Imaging Findings

► Target or doughnut sign of bowel within bowel on transverse view (arrows in Fig. 75.4)
► Pseudo-kidney appearance with outer hypoechoic intussuscipiens and inner intussusceptum on sagittal view (arrow in Fig. 75.5)
► Mural and mesenteric vascularity on power Doppler image. No pathologic lead point identified (Fig. 75.6)

Differential Diagnosis

► Small bowel obstruction
► Meckel diverticulum
► Bowel duplication cyst
► Lymphoma

Teaching Points

► Most common cause of small bowel obstruction in children
► 75% occur before the age of 2 years; 95% are pediatric; male > female (2–4:1)
► 90% of cases in children do not have a pathologic lead point and are most frequently ileocolic
  ▪ Thought to be due to lymphoid hyperplasia, a benign reactive process, likely related to recent infection, acting as benign lead point
  ▪ Most common pathological lead points in children are Meckel diverticulum, bowel duplication cysts, and lymphoma
► Pathological lead point: in approximately 80% of adults; most cases involve small bowel, commonly associated with malignancy or lipoma
► Classic US appearance: bowel within bowel producing a target, doughnut, or pseudo-kidney sign without a lead point
► Proximal, inner (inverting) segment of bowel is the intussusceptum; outer distal (receiving) segment is the intussuscipiens
► Intussusception may cause bowel obstruction; however, the diagnosis of small bowel obstruction alone would not be accurate in this case
► Diverticula or duplication cysts: more cystic lesions without internal bowel characteristics

Management

► Nonsurgical enema reduction: management of choice in pediatrics with absence of pathological lead point
  ▪ Risk: bowel perforation
  ▪ Contraindications: evidence of peritonitis (e.g., shock, sepsis, or free air on abdominal radiographs), no detectable blood flow in bowel wall on Doppler examination due to increased risk of ischemia with perforation
  ▪ Pneumoreduction preferred; performed with sonographic guidance or fluoroscopy, up to maximum limit of 120 mm Hg pressure
  ▪ If partial reduction and patient clinically stable, repeat attempt
  ▪ Reduction confirmed by resolution of the mass and air and fluid refluxing into terminal ileum
► Surgical reduction with evidence of pathological lead point or after failed enema reduction

Further Reading

1. Mandeville K, Chien M, Willyerd FA, et al. Intussusception: Clinical presentations and imaging characteristics. *Pediatr Emerg Care*. 2012; 28(9): 842–844.

Case 76

History

▶ 45-Year-old male with pelvic pain and sepsis. Transrectal images of the prostate (Figs. 76.1 and 76.2)

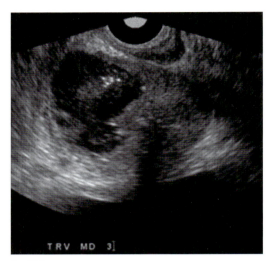

Fig. 76.1

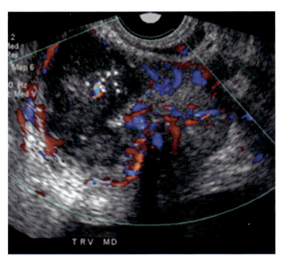

Fig. 76.2

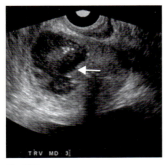

Fig. 76.3

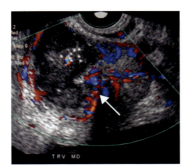

Fig. 76.4

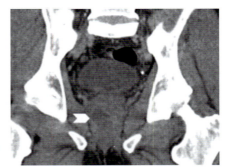

Fig. 76.5

Imaging Findings

▶ Hypoechoic complex avascular fluid collection with posterior acoustic enhancement in the right prostate lobe (arrow in Fig. 76.3)
▶ Small echogenic foci may represent tiny calcifications or air bubbles
▶ Color Doppler interrogation demonstrates no internal blood flow, but note hyperemia in the prostatic tissue surrounding the collection (arrow in Fig. 76.4)
▶ Coronal CT images confirm the presence of low-attenuation fluid collection in the right lobe of prostate (arrowhead in Fig. 76.5)
▶ Transrectal aspiration yielded purulent fluid with culture positive for methicillin-resistant *Staphylococcus aureus*

Differential Diagnosis

▶ Prostate cancer with necrosis
▶ Prostate retention cyst

Teaching Points

▶ Prostate abscesses are uncommon but can be seen in the setting of acute bacterial prostatitis, direct spread from adjacent organ (i.e., rectum), or hematogenous spread with sepsis
▶ Risk factors include instrumentation, diabetes, and immunodeficiency
▶ Coliform organisms are the most common cause (i.e., *Escherichia coli*)
▶ Transrectal US and CT are the preferred imaging modalities to evaluate for prostate abscess
  ▪ Clinical scenario (fever, dysuria, urinary hesitancy, pelvic pain) in combination with the sonographic appearance are diagnostic
▶ US has the additional value of being able to provide therapeutic aspiration as well as a specimen for culture/sensitivities in addition to the diagnosis
▶ Prostate cancer with necrosis: unlikely unless superinfected by prior biopsy. On US, most prostate cancers are hypoechoic with occasionally increased internal vascularity. The most common location of prostate cancer is in the peripheral zone of the gland
▶ Prostate retention cysts result from duct obstruction. They are small focal cysts usually located on the surface of the prostate

Management

▶ Empiric antibiotics with gram-negative coverage pending results of cultures
▶ Transrectal aspiration may be utilized to obtain sample for culture and can be therapeutic, decreasing the length of treatment/hospitalization time

Further Reading
1. Chou Y-H, Tiu C-M, Liu J-Y, et al. Prostatic abscess: Transrectal color Doppler ultrasonic diagnosis and minimally invasive therapeutic management. *Ultrasound Med Biol.* 2004; 30(6): 719.
2. Collado A, Palou J, García-Penit J, et al. Ultrasound-guided needle aspiration in prostatic abscess. *Urology.* 1999; 53(3): 548–552.

Case 77

History

► 34-Year-old female presenting with flank pain (Figs. 77.1 and 77.2)

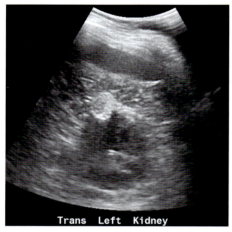

Fig. 77.1

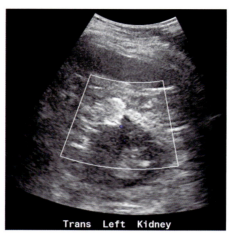

Fig. 77.2

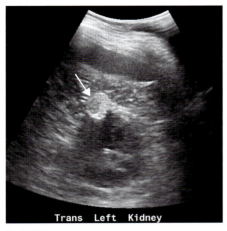

Fig. 77.3

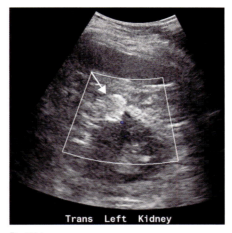

Fig. 77.4

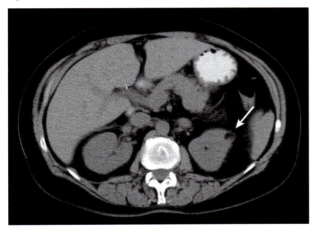

Fig. 77.5

Imaging Findings

▶ Heterogeneous echogenic exophytic mass arising from the upper pole of the left kidney (arrows in Figs. 77.3 and 77.4) without blood flow on color Doppler (Fig. 77.4)

▶ Axial non contrast-enhanced CT image confirms that the left renal mass (arrow in Fig. 77.5) has the same attenuation as retroperitoneal fat

Differential Diagnosis

▶ Renal cell carcinoma (RCC)

▶ Adrenal myelolipoma

▶ Juxtaglomerular tumor

Teaching Points

▶ Most common benign renal neoplasm
  ▪ Highest incidence in middle-aged women
  ▪ 4:1 female-to-male ratio
  ▪ 80–90% sporadic
  ▪ Found in approximately 80% of patients with tuberous sclerosis (often small, multiple, and bilateral), rarely in patients with Von Hippel–Lindau syndrome or neurofibromatosis type 1

▶ Histology: varying amounts of blood vessels, fat, and smooth muscle
  ▪ Abnormal blood vessels prone to aneurysm formation and hemorrhage
  ▪ The lipid-poor variant (angiomyolipomas (AMLs) with minimal fat) can mimic RCCs on imaging

- ► Usually asymptomatic and found incidentally
  - ▪ No malignant potential
  - ▪ AMLs > 4 cm may hemorrhage, presenting with flank pain ± hematuria
- ► US findings: homogeneous to heterogeneous, echogenic well-defined renal cortical mass
  - ▪ Similar in echogenicity to renal sinus fat
  - ▪ Echogenicity depends on fat content
  - ▪ Posterior attenuation due to fat
  - ▪ Typically no cystic components or calcifications
- ► Confirmation with CT or MR advised because up to one-third of small (< 2 cm) RCCs are echogenic on US
  - ▪ Bulk fat on CT or MRI in a renal lesion without calcifications confirms diagnosis of renal AML
  - ▪ RCCs with bulk fat reported, but often contain calcification, which is very rare in AMLs
- ► Adrenal myelolipoma: echogenic suprarenal mass with posterior attenuation ± speed propagation artifact
- ► Juxtaglomerular tumor: renin-secreting renal mass, occurs in young women with severe hypertension, may be echogenic

Management

- ► Imaging surveillance not required for confirmed AMLs < 4 cm
- ► For lesions approaching 4 cm, consider surveillance because prophylactic intervention for lesions > 4 cm may be warranted due to risk of hemorrhage
- ► Selective embolization or resection of lesions with intralesional hemorrhage, aneurysms, or abnormal vasculature

Further Reading

1. Wagner B, Wong-You-Cheong JJ, Davis CJ Jr. Adult renal hamartomas. *RadioGraphics*. 1997; 17: 155–169.

Case 78

History

► 58-Year-old female with cirrhosis. Right upper quadrant ultrasound was performed to evaluate for liver mass (Figs. 78.1–78.4).

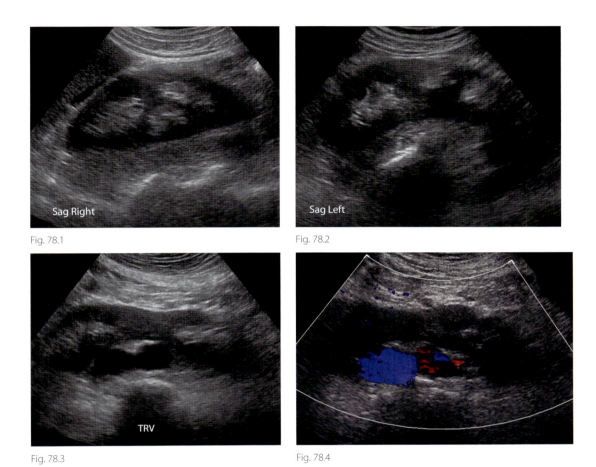

Fig. 78.1

Fig. 78.2

Fig. 78.3

Fig. 78.4

Case 78 Horseshoe Kidney

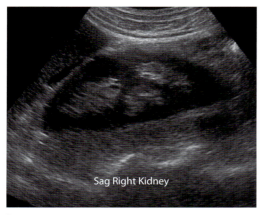

Fig. 78.5

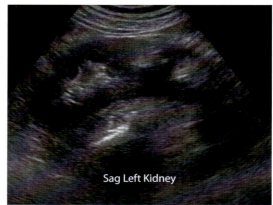

Fig. 78.6

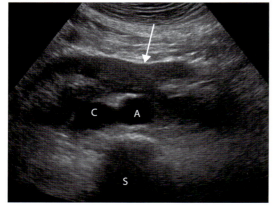

Fig. 78.7

Imaging Findings

▶ Right and left kidneys are medially rotated at the lower poles preventing a true midline sagittal view of either kidney (Figs. 78.5 and 78.6). Left kidney is more severely malrotated
▶ Renal tissue (arrow in Fig. 78.7) connects the lower poles of the kidneys anterior to the inferior vena cava (C), aorta (A), and spine (S) on transverse views

Differential Diagnosis

▶ Malrotation of kidneys
▶ Crossed fused renal ectopia
▶ Retroperitoneal fibrosis
▶ Lymphoma

Teaching Points

▶ Most common renal fusion anomaly, occurring in approximately 1/400 births
▶ Isthmus connecting the right and left lower poles can be fibrous tissue or normal renal parenchyma
▶ Isthmus prevents normal ascent of the kidneys into the upper abdomen from the pelvis because inferior mesenteric artery impedes its migration cephalad
▶ Presentation: often asymptomatic, but increased risk of infection, obstruction, stone formation, injury following trauma (seat belt injury), and tumors (i.e., Wilms tumor, transitional cell carcinoma, and renal carcinoid tumors)
▶ Patients may have additional congenital anomalies

- ► US findings
  - ▪ Difficulty obtaining a midline sagittal image that includes the lower pole due to their abnormal curved orientation
  - ▪ Low lying
  - ▪ Renal pelves positioned anteriorly
  - ▪ Band of tissue (isthmus) connecting the two lower poles anterior to aorta/inferior vena cava on transverse imaging
- ► Important to make the diagnosis so as not to confuse with abdominal mass, retroperitoneal fibrosis, or lymphadenopathy
- ► The presence of isthmus excludes bilateral renal malrotation or crossed fused ectopia
- ► Crossed fused renal ectopia: both kidneys on the same side of the abdomen and fused together. Ureters insert in normal location, confirmed by bilateral ureteral jets
- ► Retroperitoneal fibrosis: mass surrounding the aorta and common iliac arteries often resulting in medial displacement of ureters, causing ureteral obstruction and hydronephrosis
- ► Lymphoma: hypoechoic solid mass(es) in a paraoartic, aortocaval, or paracaval location

Management

- ► Treatment/prevention of complications such as infection and stone formation
- ► Evaluate for other congenital anomalies
- ► Patients should be made aware of diagnosis. They may have unusual symptoms of renal colic, etc., or may go to another facility and be diagnosed with an abdominal mass

Further Reading

1. Strauss S, Dushnitsky T, Peer A, et al. Sonographic features of horseshoe kidney: Review of 34 patients. *J Ultrasound Med.* 2000; 19: 27–31.

Case 79

History

▶ 35-Year-old asymptomatic male presents for hepatitis C screening (Figs. 79.1 and 79.2)

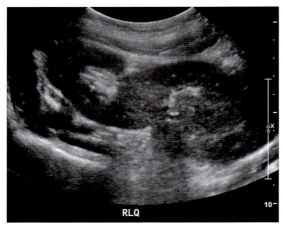

Fig. 79.1

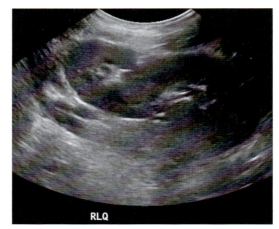

Fig. 79.2

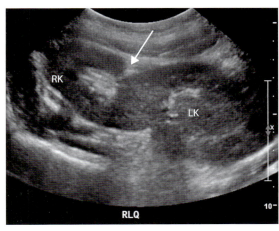

Fig. 79.3

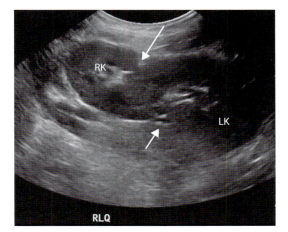

Fig. 79.4

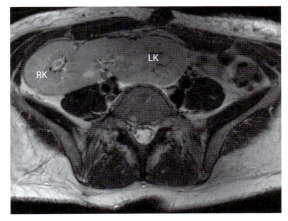

Fig. 79.5

Imaging Findings

► Both kidneys are located in the right lower quadrant, with the upper pole of the left kidney (LK) fused with the lower pole of the right kidney (RK)
► Note characteristic notch anteriorly between the fused kidneys (long arrows in Figs. 79.3 and 79.4)
► The ectopic left kidney is malrotated with the hilum facing posteriorly (short arrow in Fig. 79.4)
► T2-weighted axial MR image (Fig. 79.5) confirms that the two kidneys are fused and located in the right lower quadrant with the left kidney "crossing" the midline

Differential Diagnosis

► Asymmetric horseshoe kidney
► Ectopic pelvic kidney
► Unilateral renal agenesis

Teaching Points

► Congenital anomaly due to abnormal renal ascent during embryogenesis and fusion of the kidneys within the pelvis
  ▪ Both kidneys located on the same side of midline, usually in lower abdomen
  ▪ Fusion may be partial or complete
  ▪ Ectopic kidney usually malrotated
  ▪ Male-to-female ratio 2:1
► Arterial supply to both kidneys often anomalous
  ▪ Renal arteries may originate from iliac artery or lower abdominal aorta

- ► Ureters insert normally into bladder
- ► Several subtypes based on orientation of ectopic kidney and location of fusion
  - ▪ ~10% do not fuse but located on same side of abdomen: crossed unfused ectopia
- ► US findings
  - ▪ Both kidneys on same side of abdomen
  - ▪ Empty contralateral renal fossa
  - ▪ Characteristic "notch" between the two fused kidneys
  - ▪ Depend on degree of fusion and malrotation
  - ▪ Normal insertion of ureters into bladder with normal ureteral jets
- ► Associated with other anomalies: imperforate anus, skeletal or uterine anomalies
- ► Horseshoe kidney: fusion of lower poles of right and left kidneys in midline
- ► Pelvic kidney: single kidney in pelvis
  - ▪ Often malrotated
  - ▪ Empty ipsilateral renal fossa
- ► Renal agenesis: congenital absence of one kidney with empty renal fossa
  - ▪ Contralateral compensatory renal hypertrophy
  - ▪ Normal reniform shape preserved

Management

- ► No treatment necessary; however, advise patient of condition
- ► At risk for infection, calculi, and hydronephrosis (50% of cases)
- ► Because blood supply is usually anomalous, angiography or MR angiography recommended before regional surgical intervention

Further Reading

1. Muttarak M, Peh WC, Lerttumnongtum P. Clinics in diagnostic imaging: Crossed fused renal ectopia. *Singapore Med J*. 2001; 42(3): 139–141.

History

▶ 62-Year-old female status post renal transplant with fever and acute renal failure (figs. 80.1 and 80.2)

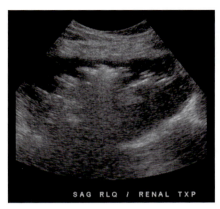

Fig. 80.1

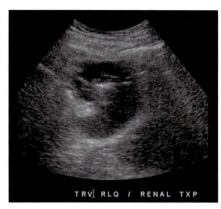

Fig. 80.2

Case 80 Emphysematous Pyelonephritis

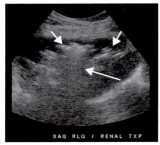 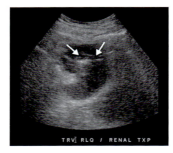 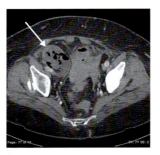

Fig. 80.3   Fig. 80.4   Fig. 80.5

Imaging Findings

▶ Linear echogenic foci (short arrows in Figs. 80.3 and 80.4) with dirty shadowing (long arrow in Fig. 80.3) are present throughout the transplanted kidney both centrally within the collecting system and also peripherally in the renal cortex consistent with air
▶ Axial contrast-enhanced CT image confirms the presence of air within the renal parenchyma (arrow in Fig. 80.5) and renal pelvis in right lower quadrant renal transplant

Differential Diagnosis

▶ Emphysematous pyelitis
▶ Reflux of air into the collecting system post instrumentation
▶ Nephrocalcinosis
▶ Multiple renal calculi
▶ Papillary necrosis

Teaching Points

▶ Renal parenchymal gas in the setting of a urinary tract infection is termed emphysematous pyelonephritis
  ▪ Necrotizing infection with gas forming organism, > 70% of cases due to *Escherichia coli*
  ▪ Most patients have diabetes mellitus (90%) and are severely ill
  ▪ Life-threatening
  ▪ Twice as common in women
▶ Urinary obstruction often present secondary to renal calculi, neoplasm, or sloughed papilla in nondiabetic patients
▶ US findings
  ▪ Linear echogenic foci in renal collecting system and parenchyma with dirty shadowing, consistent with air
  ▪ May dissect into retroperitoneum
▶ Emphysematous pyelitis: gas present only in collecting system
▶ Refluxed air in collecting system: gas present only in collecting system, history of prior instrumentation
▶ Nephrocalcinosis: echogenic foci in renal parenchyma, sharp shadowing (depending on size), not acutely ill
▶ Multiple renal calculi: round echogenic foci within renal sinus, sharp shadowing, no parenchymal abnormality, ± hydronephrosis
▶ Papillary necrosis: triangular echogenic foci in the collecting system representing the sloughed papilla, no shadowing, may have pain but not acutely ill

Management

▶ CT may be helpful in differentiating emphysematous pyelonephritis from emphysematous pyelitis
▶ Emphysematous pyelonephritis: radical nephrectomy may be required in poorly controlled diabetic patients. Antibiotics may be effective early or in stable nondiabetic patients
▶ Emphysematous pyelitis: urinary drainage and antibiotics

Further Reading

1. Grayson DE, Abbott RM, Levy AD, et al. Emphysematous infections of the abdomen and pelvis: A pictorial review. *RadioGraphics*. 2002; 22(3): 543–561.
2. Shokeir AA, El-Azab M, Mohsen T, et al. Emphysematous pyelonephritis: A 15-year experience with 20 cases. *Urology*. 1997; 49(3): 343–346.

History

► 67-Year old male with abdominal pain following renal biopsy (Figs. 81.1 and 81.2)

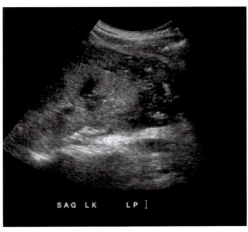

Fig. 81.1

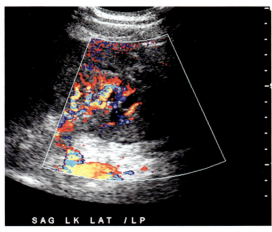

Fig. 81.2

Case 81 Perinephric Hematoma Following Renal Biopsy

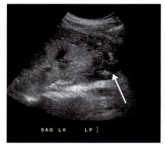

Fig. 81.3

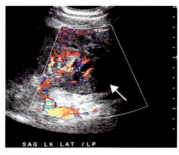

Fig. 81.4

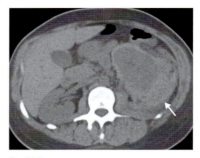

Fig. 81.5

Imaging Findings

▶ Heterogeneous, slightly hypoechoic tissue in the left perinephric space primarily surrounding the lower pole of the echogenic left kidney but not compressing the renal cortex (arrow in Fig. 81.3)
▶ Color Doppler image shows no flow within this perinephric tissue (arrow in Fig. 81.4)
▶ Axial CT image confirms high attenuation material compatible with hemorrhage surrounding left kidney (arrow in Fig. 81.5)

Differential Diagnosis

▶ Subcapsular hematoma
▶ Lymphoma
▶ Retroperitoneal sarcoma
▶ Metastases
▶ Perinephric abscess

Teaching Points

▶ Perinephric hematoma is an uncommon complication of percutaneous renal biopsy
  ▪ Predisposing factors include coagulopathy, large needle size, vascularity, and depth of the lesion, often in the setting of renal failure
▶ Other etiologies include trauma or underlying renal lesion/mass
  ▪ Hence, when spontaneous perinephric hemorrhage occurs, one must evaluate for underlying renal cell carcinoma or angiomyolipoma
▶ Renal/perirenal hematomas may be echogenic, hypoechoic, or heterogeneous on US, depending on the age of the bleed, and will change in appearance over time
▶ In the post biopsy setting, it is important to closely evaluate for underlying vascular complications, such as arteriovenous fistula (AVF) and pseudoaneurysm (PSA)
▶ Subcapsular hematoma: hyperechoic collection causing subcapsular flattening of the renal contour
▶ Renal and perirenal lymphoma, sarcoma, and metastases (most common from melanoma) are rare and usually due to hematogenous spread or direct extension and often located in the perinephric pace. Variable US appearance, although lymphoma is usually hypoechoic. Most often flow is identified within the lesion on color Doppler US
▶ Perinephric abscess: complication of pyonephrosis. Complex perinephric collections with coustic enhancement, internal debris, ± dirty shadowing from air

Management

▶ Typically a self-limiting process secondary to tamponade from Gerota's fascia, unless large bleed or underlying coagulopathy. Rarely requires transfusion and/or saline infusion
▶ Underlying PSA or AVF may require endovascular embolization
▶ If the hemorrhage is spontaneous, follow-up CT or MRI is performed to evaluate for underlying lesion as the source of the bleed

Further Reading

1. Helenon O, el Rody F, Correas JM, et al. Color Doppler US of renovascular disease in native kidneys. *RadioGraphics*. July 1995; 15: 833–854.
2. Uppot RN, Harisinghani MG, Gervais DA. Imaging-guided percutaneous renal biopsy: Rationale and approach. *Am J Roentgenol*. 2010; 194: 1443–1449.

History

▶ 40-Year-old female with past medical history of hematuria (Figs. 82.1 and 82.2)

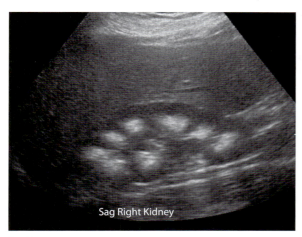

Fig. 82.1

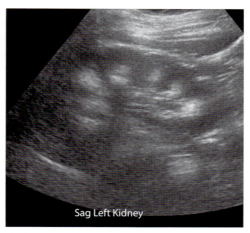

Fig. 82.2

Case 82 Medullary Nephrocalcinosis Caused by Medullary Sponge Kidneys

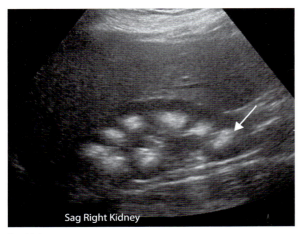

Fig. 82.3

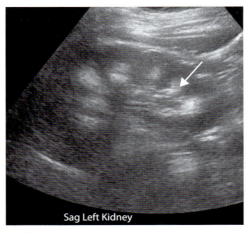

Fig. 82.4

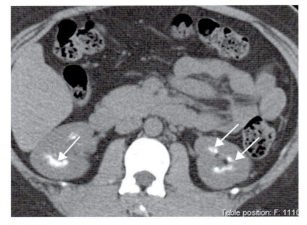

Fig. 82.5

Imaging Findings

▶ Markedly echogenic medullary pyramids in both kidneys (arrows in Figs. 82.3 and 82.4)
▶ Calcifications in medullary pyramids of both kidneys (arrows in Fig. 82.5) on axial noncontrast CT

Differential Diagnosis

▶ Echogenic medullary pyramids secondary to hyperuricemia, hypokalemia, or hyperparathyroidism
▶ Dystrophic renal calcifications
▶ Metastatic nephrocalcinosis

Teaching Points

▶ Deposition of calcium in the medullary pyramids. If the concentration of calcium in the renal tubules exceeds the capacity of the medullary lymphatics to remove it, calcium is deposited in the medullary pyramids, starting peripherally
▶ Medullary sponge kidney: malformation of the terminal collecting tubules, which dilate, predisposing patients to medullary nephrocalcinosis and renal stone formation. Dilated collecting tubules can be visualized on intravenous urography or excretory phase multidetector CT
▶ Early US appearance of medullary nephrocalcinosis: the presence of an echogenic rim around the medullary pyramids. As calcifications progress, the pyramids become diffusely echogenic and may develop punctate calculi with or without shadowing
▶ US is more sensitive than CT or plain film radiography in early stages of nephrocalcinosis

- ► Causes of medullary nephrocalcinosis
  - ▪ Infants and children
    - • Prolonged treatment with furosemide in infancy and treatment of hypophosphatemia rickets with phosphates and vitamin D
  - ▪ Adults
    - • Hyperparathyroidism (40%); proximal and distal renal tubular acidosis (20%); medullary sponge kidney; bone metastases; excess vitamin D; Wilson or Cushing disease; hyperoxalosis; sickle cell disease; hypercalciuric states and use of drugs such as amphotericin B, lithium, and analgesics
- ► Dystrophic renal calcifications
  - ▪ Due to deposition of calcium in devitalized tissues
  - ▪ Usually in tumors, hematomas, and abscesses; however, usually more focal and not diffuse and symmetrical as in medullary nephrocalcinosis
- ► Metastatic nephrocalcinosis
  - ▪ Most often in hypercalcemic states caused by renal tubular acidosis, hyperparathyroidism, and renal failure with calcium deposits in either cortex or medulla

Management

- ► Determine the underlying etiology, including detailed history (furosemide intake) and laboratory workup
- ► Alkaline medication (sodium bicarbonate, potassium citrate) to correct acidic conditions

Further Reading

1. Alon US. Nephrocalcinosis. *Curr Opin Pediatr*. 1997; 9: 160–165.
2. Jequier S, Kaplan BS. Echogenic renal pyramids in children. *J Clin Ultrasound*. 1991; 19: 85–92.
3. Koraishy FM, Ngo TT, Israel GM, et al. CT urography for the diagnosis of medullary sponge kidney. *Am J Nephrol*. 2014; 39: 165–170.

Case 83

History

▶ 31-Year-old woman with right upper quadrant pain, nausea, and vomiting (Figs. 83.1 and 83.2)

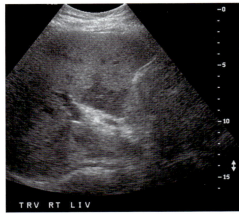

Fig. 83.1

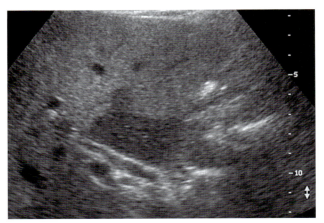

Fig. 83.2

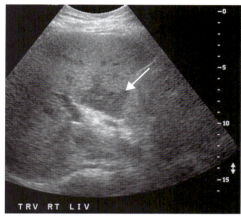

Fig. 83.3

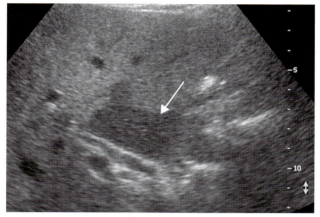

Fig. 83.4

Imaging Findings

▶ The liver parenchyma demonstrates diffusely increased echogenicity
▶ An area of focal fatty sparing appears hypoechoic relative to abnormal background liver echogenicity (arrows in Figs. 83.3 and 83.4)

Differential Diagnosis

▶ Hepatocellular carcinoma
▶ Metastasis
▶ Focal nodular hyperplasia
▶ Adenoma
▶ Lymphoma

Teaching Points

▶ Prevalence of hepatic steatosis in the general U.S. population is approximately 15%. Incidence is increased in patients with alcohol overuse, insulin resistance, obesity, and hyperlipidemia
▶ Less commonly associated with hepatitis B, hepatitis C, steroids, chemotherapeutic agents, radiation therapy, nutritional abnormality, and genetic metabolic disorders
▶ Patients are usually asymptomatic and present with abnormal liver function tests or as an incidental finding
▶ US appearance: focal or geographic areas that appear hypoechoic relative to abnormally echogenic background liver
▶ US can differentiate focal fatty sparing from liver masses based on the following
  ▪ Characteristic locations: near the falciform ligament, anterior to the porta hepatis, gallbladder fossa
  ▪ Small focal hypoechoic area of focal fatty sparing adjacent to the gallbladder (arrow in Fig. 83.5)

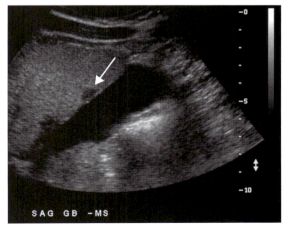

Fig. 83.5

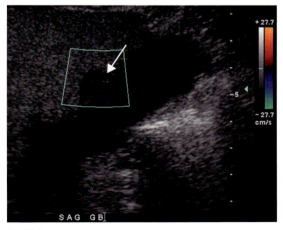

Fig. 83.6

- Geographic shape
- Absence of mass effect on normal structures, including vessels
- Absence of internal vascularity (arrow in Fig. 83.6)
▶ US features that help differentiate other entities from focal fatty sparing
  - Hepatocellular carcinoma
    - Background of cirrhotic liver
    - Mass effect
    - Internal vascularity
  - Metastasis
    - Commonly multifocal with target appearance
    - Can have diffusely infiltrative appearance that mimics diffuse liver disease
  - Focal nodular hyperplasia
    - Mass effect
    - Spoke wheel arterial pattern, rarely seen without intravenous contrast
    - Usually isoechoic, may have hypoechoic halo
  - Adenoma
    - Heterogeneous appearance due to mixture of intratumoral fat, hemorrhage, necrosis, and calcifications if large. Small adenomas usually homogeneous
  - Lymphoma
    - Homogeneous hypoechoic mass ± posterior acoustic enhancement
    - Can have target appearance
    - Often multifocal

Management

▶ CT and MRI can be used for confirmation in atypical cases, especially if there is a history of malignancy
▶ In equivocal cases, image-guided biopsy may be necessary
▶ Alcohol cessation and diet modification may slow progress and may reverse some changes of hepatic steatosis

Further Reading

1. Bhatnagar G, Sidhu HS, Vardhanabhuti V, et al. The varied sonographic appearances of focal fatty liver disease: Review and diagnostic algorithm. *Clin Radiol.* 2012; 67(4): 372–379.
2. Hamer OW, Aguirre DA, Casola G, et al. Fatty liver: Imaging patterns and pitfalls. *RadioGraphics.* 2006; 26(6): 1637–1653.

History

▶ 46-Year-old woman with postprandial abdominal pain (Figs. 84.1 and 84.2)

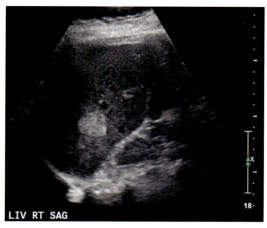

Fig. 84.1

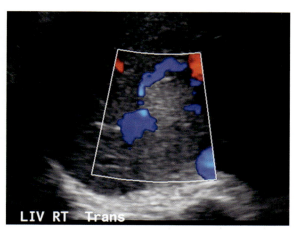

Fig. 84.2

Case 84 Cavernous Hemangioma—Classic Type

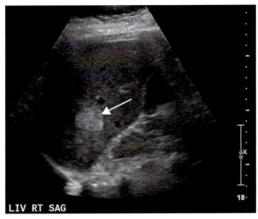

Fig. 84.3

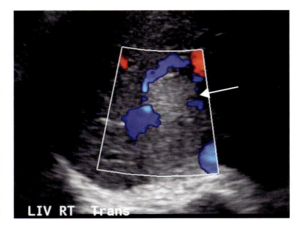

Fig. 84.4

Imaging Findings

▶ Homogeneous echogenic well-marginated round mass (arrow in Fig. 84.3) demonstrating minimal increased through-transmission
▶ Color Doppler shows flow in vessels adjacent to the mass (arrow in Fig. 84.4) but no flow within the mass

Differential Diagnosis

▶ Atypical/nonclassic cavernous hemangioma
▶ Hepatocellular carcinoma
▶ Metastasis
▶ Hepatic adenoma
▶ Focal nodular hyperplasia
▶ Focal fatty infiltration

Teaching Points

▶ Estimated prevalence of 0.4–20% based on autopsy studies; more common in women, with a 5:1 female-to-male ratio
▶ Most found incidentally
▶ Composed of multiple, large vessels lined by a single layer of endothelial cells within a thin fibrous stroma
▶ Classic US features of cavernous hemangiomas, accounting for 60–80%
  ▪ Homogeneous echogenic liver mass, 10% multiple
  ▪ Round or slightly lobulated mass with smooth margins
  ▪ Increased through-transmission
  ▪ Flow in vessels adjacent to the mass but no internal flow detected on Doppler US
  ▪ Remains stable over time
  ▪ Nodular, peripheral contrast enhancement initially with centripetal fill-in following intravenous contrast administration
  ▪ Similar enhancement pattern on contrast-enhanced US and MRI
▶ US features of atypical/nonclassic cavernous hemangioma
  ▪ Internal isoechoic or hypoechoic texture with peripheral hyperechoic border due to internal thrombosis or scarring—reversed target sign (arrow in Fig. 84.5)
  ▪ Large heterogeneous hemangioma may have central scar (myxomatous degeneration, thrombosis, or fibrosis) or appear mildly echogenic with indistinct margins (arrow in Fig. 84.6)
  ▪ Liver capsule retraction (peripheral fibrotic changes)
  ▪ Pedunculated hemangioma
  ▪ Calcifications, central or peripheral

▶ Typical hemangioma may appear hypoechoic and "atypical" in the presence of diffuse fatty liver
▶ Atypical hemangioma is a difficult diagnosis on US

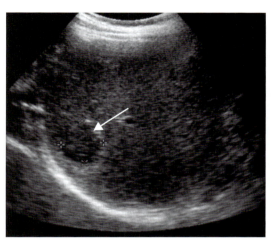

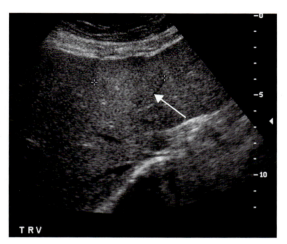

Fig. 84.5   Fig. 84.6

▶ US features that differentiate other entities in the differential diagnosis
  ▪ Hepatocellular carcinoma
    • Background of cirrhotic liver
    • Small tumors tend to be hypoechoic rather than echogenic
    • Portal vein and hepatic vein invasion
  ▪ Metastasis
    • Variable echogenicity
    • Target lesion with peripheral hypoechoic halo most common
    • Multifocal
  ▪ Hepatic adenoma
    • Heterogeneous appearance due to mixture of intratumoral fat, hemorrhage, necrosis, and calcification depending on size
  ▪ Focal nodular hyperplasia
    • Usually isoechoic rather than echogenic
    • The presence of central feeding artery with stellate or spoke wheel pattern
  ▪ Focal fatty infiltration
    • Focal echogenic region relative to the normal or echogenic background of fatty liver
    • Absence of mass effect

Management

▶ No treatment required unless large; large hemangiomas can lead to bleeding and are therefore sometimes prophylactically resected
▶ In the absence of cirrhosis or risk factors for malignancy, no further evaluation is necessary if the mass demonstrates sonographic features of a typical hemangioma, especially in the younger age group
▶ In the older age group or in the presence of cirrhosis or risk factors for malignancy, confirmation with CT, MRI, or contrast-enhanced US is recommended to confirm presumed diagnosis of hemangioma
▶ Atypical hemangioma currently requires multiphase contrast-enhanced CT or MRI for confirmation and to exclude potentially malignant liver masses
▶ Contrast-enhanced US also holds promise for the diagnosis
▶ Image-guided biopsy may be necessary in equivocal cases
▶ Large hemangiomas can lead to bleeding, compression effect on adjacent structures, and torsion
▶ Surgical management may be considered in symptomatic patients

Further Reading

1. Caseiro-Alves F, Brito J, Araujo AE, et al. Liver haemangioma: Common and uncommon findings and how to improve the differential diagnosis. *Eur Radiol.* 2007; 17(6): 1544–1554.
2. Kim KW, Kim TK, Han JK, et al. Hepatic hemangiomas: Spectrum of US appearances on grayscale, power Doppler, and contrast-enhanced US. *Korean J Radiol.* 2000; 1(4): 191–197.
3. Vilgrain V, et al: Imaging of atypical hemangiomas of the liver with pathologic correlation. *RadioGraphics.* 2000; 20(2): 379–397.

Case 85

History

▶ 51-Year-old female with history of breast cancer and increasing bilirubin (Figs. 85.1 and 85.2)

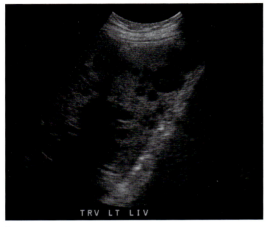

Fig. 85.1

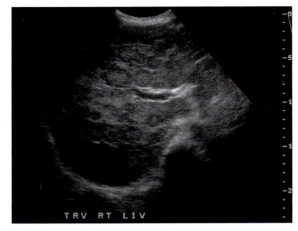

Fig. 85.2

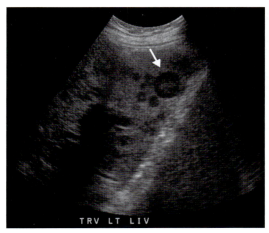

Fig. 85.3

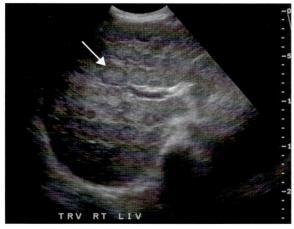

Fig. 85.4

Imaging Findings

▶ Numerous hepatic masses of varying size with hypoechoic rims giving the lesions a target-like appearance (arrow in Figs. 85.3 and 85.4)

Differential Diagnosis

▶ Multifocal hepatocellular carcinoma
▶ Lymphoma
▶ Abscesses

Teaching Points

▶ Metastasis is the most common type of malignant lesion in a noncirrhotic liver and multifocal in more than 90% of patients
▶ Most common malignancies to metastasize to the liver are lung, colon, breast, pancreas, and stomach
▶ The sonographic appearance of metastases can be variable with either focal nodules or a diffusely infiltrative appearance. Focal liver metastases may be hypo-, iso-, or echogenic and are most often multiple and of varying sizes
▶ Examples of the variety of sonographic appearances
  ▪ Classic appearance: target lesion with echogenic or isoechoic center with hypoechoic halo (arrows in Figs. 85.3–85.5)
  ▪ Can present as heterogeneous or homogeneous echogenic (arrows in Fig. 85.6), isoechoic, or hypoechoic masses
  ▪ Peripheral and diffuse infiltrative masses can result in a nodular appearance of the liver mimicking cirrhosis (arrows in Fig. 85.7)
  ▪ Cystic metastases are rare, although metastases can be necrotic (arrow in Fig. 85.8)
    ▪ Mural nodularity, thick rim, and blood flow along peripheral are suspicious features
  ▪ Occasionally metastases can calcify (arrows in Figs. 85.9 and 85.10)
  ▪ Internal blood flow on Doppler US may be present or absent

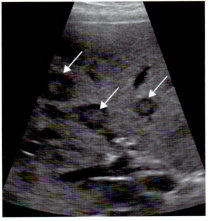

Fig. 85.5

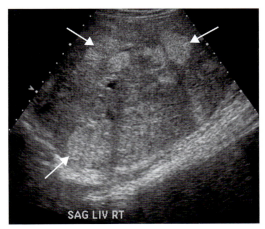

Fig. 85.6

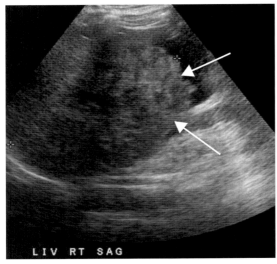

Fig. 85.7

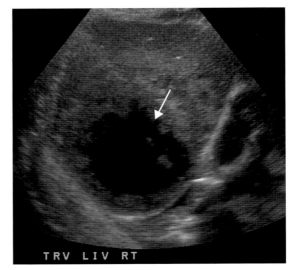

Fig. 85.8

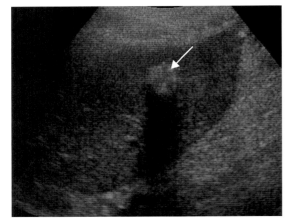

Fig. 85.9

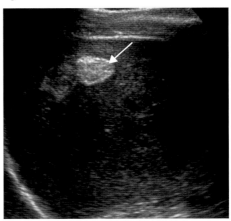

Fig. 85.10

- ▶ US features of liver metastases can suggest source of primary malignancy
  - Hypoechoic metastases: lung, breast, stomach, esophagus, pancreas, lymphoma
  - Echogenic metastases: colorectal, renal cell, neuroendocrine, choriocarcinoma, Kaposi sarcoma
  - Cystic metastases: squamous cell, sarcoma, melanoma, neuroendocrine
  - Calcified liver metastases: mucin-producing neoplasms such as colon, ovarian, breast, and stomach
  - Infiltrative pattern: lung, breast, melanoma
- ▶ US features that differentiate other entities in the differential diagnosis from metastatic disease
  - Multifocal hepatocellular carcinoma
    - Background of cirrhotic liver
    - Portal vein and hepatic vein invasion
  - Lymphoma
    - Homogeneous hypoechoic masses can mimic metastases
    - Target appearance can mimic metastatic disease
    - Often occurs in the setting of advanced disease
  - Liver abscess
    - Clinical signs of infection
    - Immunocompromised patient

Management

▶ Patients with liver metastases identified on US are usually referred to CT, MRI, and/or fluorodeoxyglucose–positron emission tomography for complete cancer staging or to search for underlying primary tumor

▶ US-guided fine needle aspiration biopsy should be performed to confirm the diagnosis of liver metastases in order to guide therapy

▶ Treatment of underlying primary malignancy, which may include radiofrequency ablation or chemoembolization

Further Reading

1. Tchelepi H, Ralls PW. Ultrasound of focal liver masses. *Ultrasound Q*. 2004; 20: 155–169.
2. Li D, Hann LE. A practical approach to analyzing focal lesions in the liver. *Ultrasound Q*. 2005; 21(3): 187–200.

Case 86

History

► 53-Year-old man with abdominal pain and elevated bilirubin (Figs. 86.1–86.4)

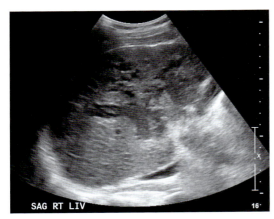

Fig. 86.1

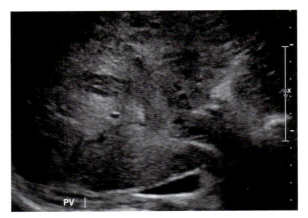

Fig. 86.2

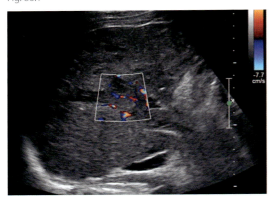

Fig. 86.3

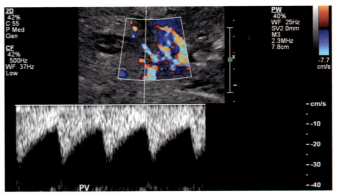

Fig. 86.4

Case 86 Hepatocellular Carcinoma With Portal Vein Tumor Thrombus

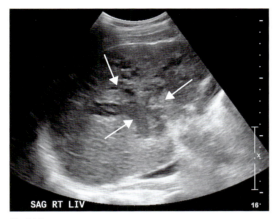

Fig. 86.5

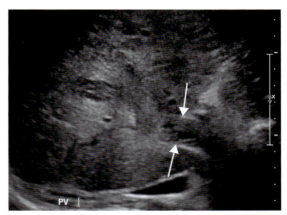

Fig. 86.6

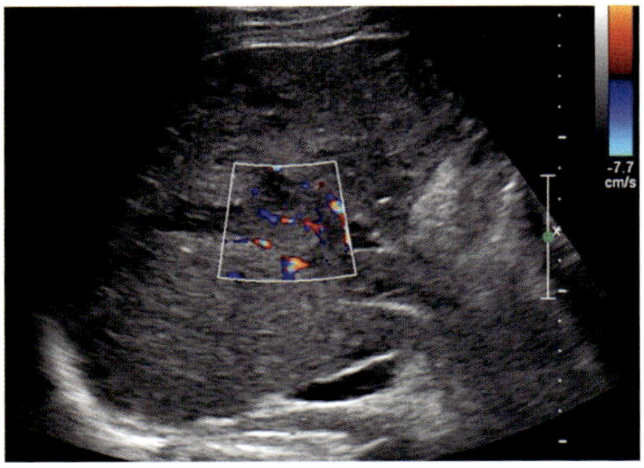

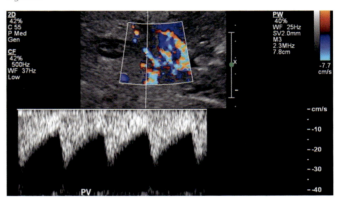

Fig. 86.7

Fig. 86.8

Imaging Findings

- Diffusely heterogeneous echotexture with a mass extending into the portal vein (arrows in Figs. 86.5 and 86.6)
- Echogenic mass distending and filling main portal vein (arrows in Fig. 86.6)
- Color and spectral Doppler image shows vascularity with an arterial waveform within the portal vein tumor thrombus (PVT) (Figs. 86.7 and 86.8)

Differential Diagnosis

- Bland PVT
- Cavernous transformation of the portal vein
- Cholangiocarcinoma

Teaching Points

- Hepatocellular carcinoma (HCC) is the most common primary malignancy of the liver, and it is strongly associated with underlying cirrhosis and chronic hepatitis B and hepatitis C infection
- US is less sensitive than CT or MR for the diagnosis of HCC. However, because it is noninvasive and less costly to perform, US is a good screening modality for HCC. The American Association for the Study of Liver Diseases (AASLD) 2010 practice guidelines recommend surveillance US screening every 6 months for patients with cirrhosis and chronic hepatitis B and C infection
- HCC can present as a solitary liver mass, multiple liver masses, or as a diffuse infiltrative process
- US findings
  - Hypoechoic, isoechoic, echogenic, or a target appearance
  - Most small (< 5 cm) HCCs are hypoechoic
  - Margins can be well circumscribed or infiltrative

- Larger tumors tend to be more heterogeneous due to hemorrhage, fibrosis, or focal fat
- Calcifications are uncommon; however, they are sometimes seen in fibrolamellar HCCs
► HCC has the propensity to invade the portal and hepatic veins
► Other causes of malignant PVT: pancreatic carcinoma, cholangiocarcinoma, metastatic disease
► US features useful in differentiating tumor thrombus versus bland thrombus
  - Arterial waveforms on spectral Doppler obtained from the thrombus
  - Internal flow within the PVT, although can be seen with partially recanalized bland thrombus
  - Expansion of portal vein (although acute bland thrombus may also expand the portal vein)
  - In bland PVT, echogenic material will be seen in the PV with no flow on color or power Doppler US (arrows in Figs. 86.9 and 86.10)

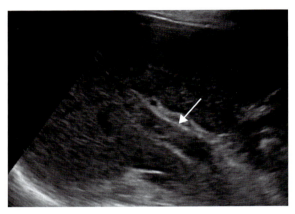 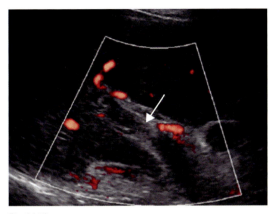

Fig. 86.9   Fig. 86.10

► Cavernous transformation of the portal vein may develop as early as 2 weeks following PVT. Multiple, tortuous collateral vessels will be observed in the hepatoduodenal ligament and/or wall of the PV in the porta hepatis demonstrating venous flow
► Cholangiocarcinoma can cause PVT; however, it usually would also cause associated biliary ductal dilatation, especially centrally

Management

► Patients with low tumor burden may be candidates for surgical resection or radiofrequency ablation and/or liver transplantation, with potential cure of the disease
  - Single HCC < 5 cm *or*
  - Up to three HCCs, each < 3 cm
► Most patients present with more advanced stage disease and are treated with transarterial chemoembolization (TACE)
► Patients with PVT have poorer prognosis compared to patients without PVT
► PVT has traditionally been a contraindication to TACE; recent studies have shown that TACE can be performed safely in patients with PVT
► Specificity and positive predictive value of Doppler US for PVT are close to 98%, although false positives may occur secondary to slow flow. Attempt to augment flow with abdominal compression or Valsalva and release and consider confirmation with CEUS, CT, or MR
► Negative predictive value is close to 98%, although color blooming may obscure non-occlusive thrombus. Therefore, always look with both grayscale and color Doppler
► Treated medically with anticoagulation therapy
► If variceal bleeding occurs, sclerotherapy, transjugular intrahepatic portacaval shunt, or surgical shunt may be necessary

Further Reading

1. Anis M, Irshad A. Imaging of hepatocellular carcinoma: Practical guide to differential diagnosis. *Clin Liver Dis*. 2011; 15(2): 335–352.
2. McNaughton DA, Abu-Yousef MM. Doppler US of the liver made simple. *RadioGraphics*. 2011; 31(1): 161–188.
3. Parvey HR, Raval B, Sandler CM. Portal vein thrombosis: Imaging findings. *Am J Roentgenol*. 1994; 162: 77–81.
4. Sobhonslidsuk A, Reddy KR. Portal vein thrombosis: A concise review. *Am J Gastroenterol*. 2002; 97: 535–541.
5. Taratino L, Francica G, Sordelli I, et al. Diagnosis of benign and malignant portal vein thrombosis in cirrhotic patients with hepatocellular carcinoma: Color Doppler US, CE US, and fine needle biopsy. *Abdom Imaging*. 2006; 31: 537–544.

History

▶ 56-Year-old female from South Africa presents with chronic right upper quadrant abdominal pain. Ultrasound images of the liver were obtained (Figs. 87.1–87.4).

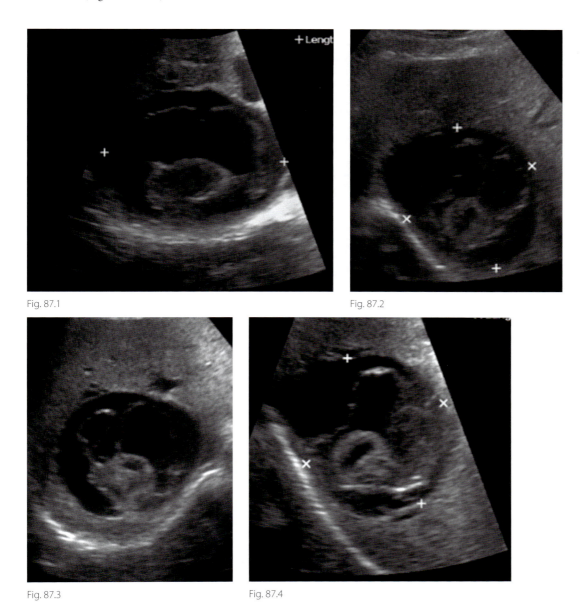

Fig. 87.1

Fig. 87.2

Fig. 87.3

Fig. 87.4

Case 87　Hydatid Disease

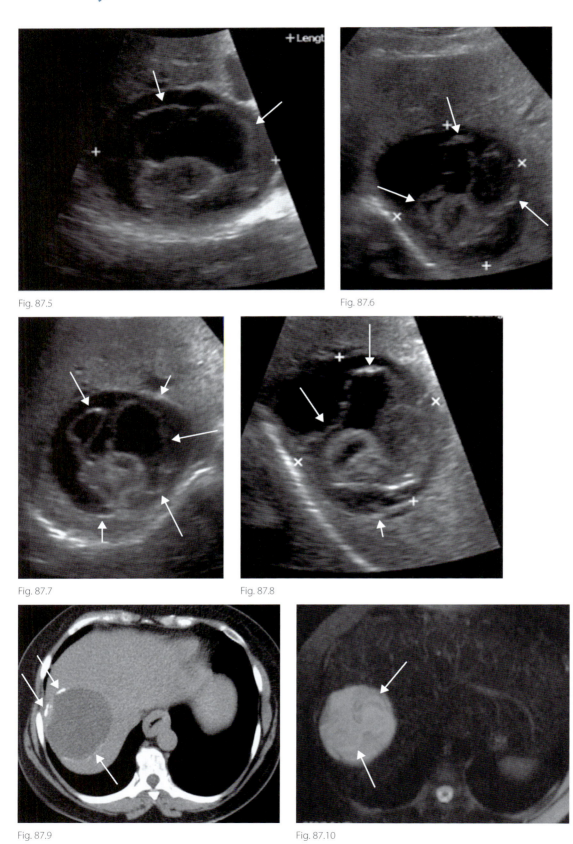

Fig. 87.5

Fig. 87.6

Fig. 87.7

Fig. 87.8

Fig. 87.9

Fig. 87.10

Imaging Findings

▶ Large (7.3-cm) unilocular cyst (calipers in Figs. 87.5, 87.6, and 87.8) in the right lobe of the liver that contains internal floating membranes (water lily sign) or endocyst (long arrows in Figs. 87.5–87.8)

▶ The wall of the cyst appears slightly more echogenic in several focal areas, suggesting mural calcification, although no posterior shadowing is seen (short arrows in Figs. 87.7 and 87.8)

▶ Noncontrast axial CT image of the liver demonstrates calcification in the cyst wall (arrows in Fig. 87.9). Note that the internal membranes are not well visualized on the CT scan

▶ T2-weighted fat sat axial MR image of the liver demonstrating the internal membranes within the cyst (arrows in Fig. 87.10)

Differential Diagnosis

▶ Pyogenic hepatic abscess
▶ Cyst with internal hemorrhage
▶ Biliary cystadenoma or carcinoma
▶ Cystic metastasis

Teaching Points

▶ Infection from the dog tapeworm, *Echinococcus granulosus*
  ▪ Most commonly occurs in the liver (50–70%)
  ▪ Less common sites of infection include lungs (20–30%), spleen, bones, central nervous system
▶ Most common in sheep- and cattle-raising areas: South America, northern or eastern Africa, Middle East, Mediterranean, Australia
  ▪ Transmitted by domestic dogs in livestock-raising areas
▶ Pathophysiology
  ▪ Canines are the definitive host
  ▪ Humans, sheep, goats, camels, cattle, and horses are intermediate hosts that become infected by ingesting egg-infested plants and vegetables
  ▪ Reaches the liver via the portal vein developing into slowly growing cysts
  ▪ External membrane (ectocyst) may calcify
  ▪ Host response leads to formation of a dense connective tissue capsule surrounding the cyst (pericyst)
  ▪ Inner germinal layer (endocyst) gives rise to the brood capsules
▶ Presentation
  ▪ Patients often asymptomatic even in advanced stages, often detected incidentally on imaging studies, self-limited
  ▪ Likely that only 10% become symptomatic
  ▪ Mass effect (compression of biliary tree can cause obstructive jaundice), right upper quadrant pain, eosinophilia
▶ Complications
  ▪ Rupture into biliary tree, peritoneal cavity, or bloodstream (may cause anaphylaxis)
  ▪ Superinfection (may result in sepsis)
▶ US the primary means of diagnosis, staging, and follow-up
▶ US appearance depends on stage of disease
▶ World Health Organization Informal Working Group on Echinococcosis 2003 US classification used to characterize hepatic hydatid cysts into active, transitional, or inactive status based on their sonographic appearance
  ▪ More common in right lobe of the liver
  ▪ CL: unilocular anechoic cyst, wall may calcify

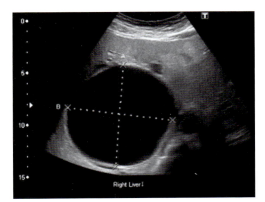

Fig. 87.11

Note large unilocular simple cyst in the right lobe of the liver (calipers and dotted lines in Fig. 87.11). The cyst is anechoic with increased through-transmission and a smooth imperceptible wall. There are no internal echoes or septations. Same patient as in Figs. 87.5–87.10, 4 months previously.

- CE 1: unilocular cyst with fine internal shifting echoes (hydatid sand or snowflake sign) due to separation of "brood capsules" from wall

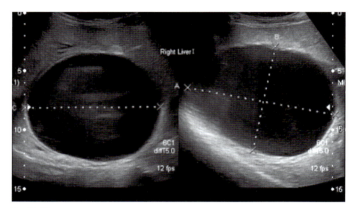

Fig. 87.12

Same patient as in Figs. 87.5–87.11. Note low-level internal echoes, which moved and swirled with change in patient position. These images were obtained 2 months after Fig. 87.11 was obtained.

- CE 2 (active stage): multivesicular cyst with multiple septations arranged like rosette or honeycomb appearance
- CE 3 (transitional stage): unilocular cyst with detachment of internal membranes (water lily sign) (Figs. 87.5–87.8) due to detachment of endocyst or multiple daughter cysts; fluid in cyst has variable echogenicity
- CE 4 (degenerative): cyst with heterogeneous hypoechoic or hyperechoic contents (ball of wool sign); no daughter cysts
- CE 5 (inactive and infertile): cyst with thick calcified wall
► Different stages could mimic a simple or hemorrhagic hepatic cyst, abscess, or biliary cystadenoma
► Simple hepatic cyst: most often unilocular and anechoic with smooth wall and increased through-transmission. Hence, indistinguishable on US from CL appearance of hydatid disease. High level of epidemiological suspicion and serologic testing necessary to make diagnosis
- May contain low-level or layering internal echoes (CE 1 mimic) or septations
► Pyogenic hepatic abscess: complex cystic liver mass with internal echoes, ± thick vascular wall, variable echogenicity, might demonstrate central echogenic foci with dirty shadowing consistent with air, unlikely to calcify, no daughter cysts or water lily sign
► Hemorrhagic hepatic cyst: thin wall, sometimes calcifies, unilocular, variable pattern of internal echoes—diffuse, layering, clumped, strandlike
► Biliary cystadenoma: unilocular cyst
► Biliary cystadenocarcinoma and cystic metastasis: complex cystic appearance, but more likely to demonstrate solid vascular components

Management

► Infection confirmed by serologic testing (80–100% sensitivity and 88–96% specificity for liver disease)
► Treatment dependent on stage, location, and symptoms
► Definitive therapy is surgical
► US-guided percutaneous aspiration with alcohol injection is a good alternative to surgery in selected cases
- Anaphylaxis post aspiration is very rare, despite initial concerns
► Medical therapy with albendazole, mebendazole
► Follow-up with serial US post treatment to assess for adequacy of treatment and/or local relapse

Further Reading

1. World Health Organization Informal Working Group. International classification of ultrasound images in cystic echinococcosis for application in clinical and field epidemiological settings. *Acta Trop*. 2003; 85(2): 253–261.
2. Polat P, Kantarci M, Alper F, et al. Hydatid disease from head to toe. *RadioGraphics*. 2003; 23(2): 475–494.

History

► 67-Year-old male with cirrhosis of the liver and abnormal MRI (Figs. 88.1–88.3)

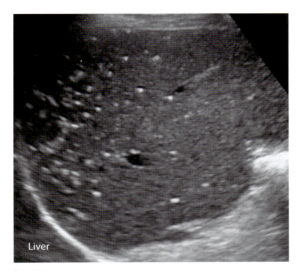

Fig. 88.1

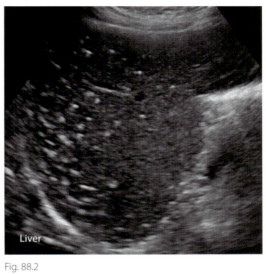

Fig. 88.2

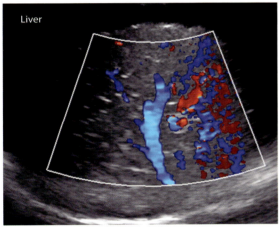

Fig. 88.3

Case 88 Biliary Hamartomas

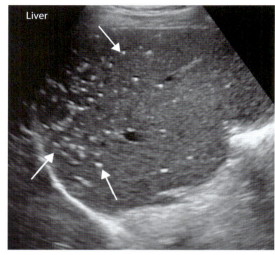

Fig. 88.4

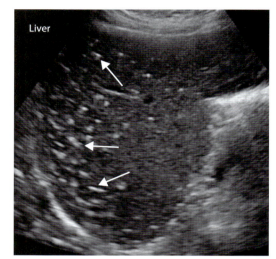

Fig. 88.5

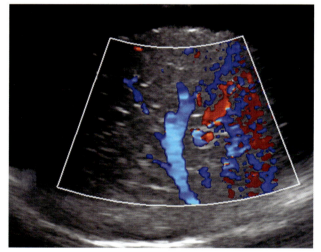

Fig. 88.6

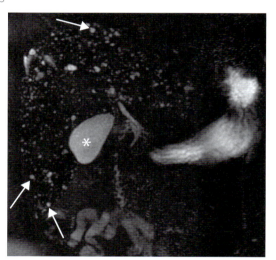

Fig. 88.7

Imaging Findings

- ▶ Innumerable tiny echogenic foci are present throughout the liver parenchyma (arrows in Figs. 88.4 and 88.5), some of which demonstrate comet tail artifact
- ▶ No communication with the biliary ducts; no abnormal vascularity on color Doppler (Fig. 88.6); no intrahepatic biliary ductal dilatation
- ▶ Coronal magnetic resonance cholangiopancreatography image reveals multiple punctate fluid signal lesions throughout the liver compatible with biliary hamartomas (arrows in Fig. 88.7) (asterisk, gallbladder)

Differential Diagnosis

- ▶ Granulomas
- ▶ Multiple liver microabscesses
- ▶ Multiple liver metastases
- ▶ Portal venous air
- ▶ Pneumobilia

Teaching Points

▶ Biliary hamartomas (Von Meyenburg complexes) are benign hepatic lesions
  ▪ Prevalence at autopsy is approximately 3%, although prevalence on imaging is < 1% because these are difficult to detect due to their small size (< 5 mm)
  ▪ Female predilection of 3:1
  ▪ Associated with autosomal dominant polycystic kidney disease and polycystic liver disease
▶ Composed of disorganized clusters of dilated cystic bile ducts that generally do not communicate with the biliary tree
  ▪ Believed to arise from embryonic bile duct remnants that have failed to involute
▶ Presentation: asymptomatic, incidentally discovered
▶ US findings: innumerable tiny foci in liver
  ▪ Most common in subcapsular location
  ▪ Usually echogenic due to fibrotic foci within walls
  ▪ No posterior shadowing
  ▪ Occasionally hypoechoic or mixed echogenicity
  ▪ Well circumscribed, uniform in size, measuring 1 to 15 mm, usually < 5 mm
  ▪ No communication with the biliary tree; not associated with intrahepatic biliary ductal dilatation
  ▪ Diffusely heterogeneous liver echotexture if the cysts are too small to discriminate individually (rare)
  ▪ Large solitary hamartomas are typically echogenic solid lesions that may be vascular
▶ Hepatic granulomas: similar appearance of multiple punctate echogenic foci
  ▪ Posterior acoustic shadowing likely unless very small
  ▪ Usually not so numerous and slightly larger than the echogenic foci in this case
  ▪ Might also involve the spleen
▶ Liver microabscesses: more often hypoechoic
  ▪ Treated microabscesses, especially fungal, more likely to be echogenic
▶ Multiple miliary liver metastases: more commonly hypoechoic, less regular
▶ Portal venous air or pneumobilia: in a single projection could possibly appear as multiple discrete echogenic round foci, with air in the portal vein more peripheral and air in the biliary tree more central
  ▪ However, turning the transducer 90° should demonstrate linearity of the echogenic foci
  ▪ Expect to see dirty posterior shadowing from air

Management

▶ CT and MRI best imaging modalities for definitive diagnosis
▶ Incidental finding, no treatment or follow-up necessary

Further Reading

1. Markhardt BK, Rubens DJ, Huang J, et al. Sonographic features of biliary hamartomas with histopathologic correlation. *J Ultrasound Med.* 2006; 25: 1631–1633.
2. Tohmé-Noun C, Cazals D, Noun R, et al. Multiple biliary hamartomas: Magnetic resonance features with histopathologic correlation. *Eur Radiol.* 2008; 18: 493–499.
3. Mortelé B, Mortelé K, Seynaeve P, et al. Hepatic bile duct hamartomas (von Meyenburg complexes): MR and MR cholangiography findings. *J Comput Assist Tomogr.* 2002; 26(3): 438–443.

Case 89

History

► 50-Year-old hospitalized female with history of liver cirrhosis, increasing ascites, and right upper quadrant pain (Figs. 89.1–89.4)

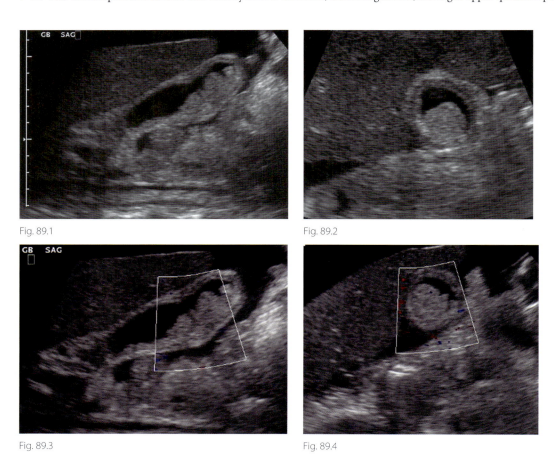

Fig. 89.1

Fig. 89.2

Fig. 89.3

Fig. 89.4

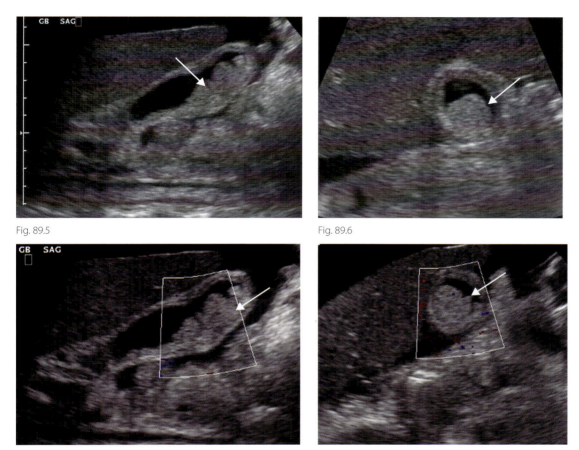

Fig. 89.5

Fig. 89.6

Fig. 89.7

Fig. 89.8

Imaging Findings

► Polypoid mass within the gallbladder on sagittal and transverse views (arrow in Figs. 89.5 and 89.6)
► Avascular on color Doppler ultrasound (CDUS) (arrow in Figs. 89.7 and 89.8)

Differential Diagnosis

► Gallbladder polyp
► Gallbladder carcinoma
► Focal adenomyomatosis
► Hemobilia

Teaching Points

► Biliary sludge
  ▪ First recognized with advent of sonography
  ▪ Prevalence unknown
► Precursor to stone formation, acalculous cholecystitis, biliary colic, and pancreatitis
► Predisposing factors
  ▪ Pregnancy
  ▪ Prolonged fasting
  ▪ Critical illness
  ▪ Prolonged total parenteral nutrition
  ▪ Sickle cell disease

▶ US findings
- ▪ Amorphous, low-level echoes within the gallbladder, some variability of echogenicity
- ▪ May completely fill the gallbladder
- ▪ May mimic polypoid tumors, thus called tumefactive sludge
- ▪ Usually no acoustic shadowing
- ▪ Avascular on CDUS (arrow in Fig. 89.9)
- ▪ Change with position and movement on left lateral decubitus view (arrow in Fig. 89.9)
- ▪ May be associated with crystals or stones

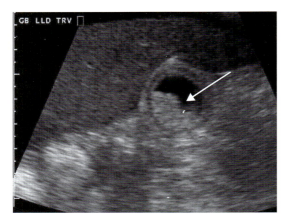

Fig. 89.9

▶ Gallbladder polyp: echogenic soft tissue mass(es)/nodule(s) attached to gallbladder wall; nonmobile; may show central vascularity
▶ Gallbladder carcinoma: focal irregular asymmetric gallbladder wall thickening, intraluminal mass (least common), or mass within the gallbladder bed. Vascular on CDUS
▶ Focal adenomyomatosis: benign gallbladder condition due to hypertrophy of the smooth muscle and epithelium. May contain bile and cholesterol crystals giving "comet tail" artifact—more common in the fundus of the gallbladder. "Twinkle artifact " on CDUS
▶ Hemobilia: usually caused by iatrogenic trauma, mainly percutaneous procedures or liver biopsy. Could mimic US appearance of tumefactive sludge in early echogenic phase of blood. Clinical history is essential

Management

▶ Demonstrate movement of sludge on decubitus views
▶ Repeat exam after 1 or 2 weeks or after eating
▶ Obtain contrast-enhanced CT or MRI in equivocal cases

Further Reading

1. Ko CW, Sekiimja JH, Lee SP: Bliary sludge. *Ann Intern Med.* 1999; 130: 301–311.
2. Fakhry J. Sonography of tumefactive biliary sludge. *Am J Roentgenol.* 1982; 139: 717–719.

History

▶ 61-Year-old diabetic female with right upper quadrant abdominal pain and fever (Figs. 90.1–90.4)

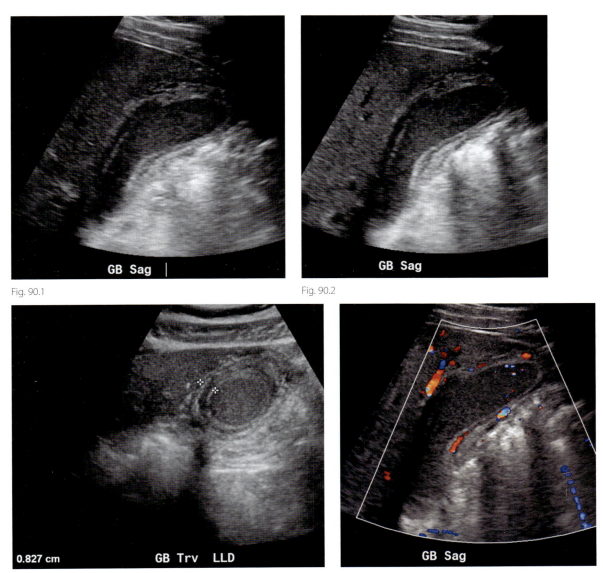

Fig. 90.1

Fig. 90.2

Fig. 90.3

Fig. 90.4

Case 90 Acute Cholecystitis With Focal Necrosis of Gallbladder Wall

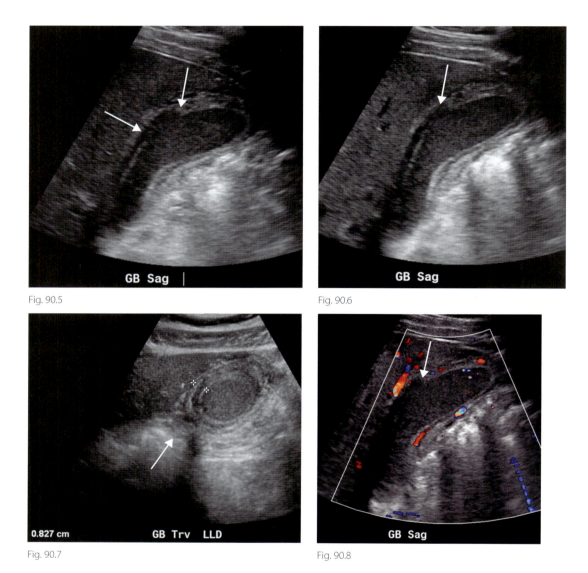

Fig. 90.5

Fig. 90.6

Fig. 90.7

Fig. 90.8

Imaging Findings

▶ The gallbladder wall is thick (8 mm) (calipers in Fig. 90.7) with focal disruption of the echogenic mucosa (arrows in Figs. 90.5, 90.6, and 90.8) and a small amount of complex pericholecystic fluid (arrow in Fig. 90.7) consistent with pericholecystic abscess or inflammation

▶ Note low-level echoes within the gallbladder lumen consistent with sludge

▶ Much of the gallbladder wall is hypervascular on color Doppler imaging (Fig. 90.8), consistent with inflammation

Differential Diagnosis

▶ Uncomplicated acute cholecystitis

▶ Acalculous cholecystitis

▶ Wall edema secondary to low albumin, congestive heart failure (CHF), or liver disease

Teaching Points

▶ Acute cholecystitis is a common cause of right upper quadrant (RUQ) pain

▶ Presentation: RUQ pain, tenderness, nausea, vomiting, anorexia, fever, leukocytosis, elevated serum bilirubin, alkaline phosphatase

■ Three times more common in women

- ► Pathophysiology
  - ▪ In > 90–95% of patients, a gallstone impacted in the neck of the gallbladder or cystic duct results in obstruction and distention leading to inflammation, ischemia, and superinfection
  - ▪ 5–10% of cases occur in the absence of gallstones, termed "acalculous" cholecystitis
- ► US first-line imaging modality of choice
- ► US findings of acute cholecystitis
  - ▪ Gallstones, especially if impacted
  - ▪ Sonographic Murphy's sign (focal tenderness over the gallbladder)
    - • High positive predictive value
    - • However, absence does not exclude acute cholecystitis, especially if the patient has received analgesia, steroids, or has altered mental status
  - ▪ Distended gallbladder
  - ▪ Nonspecific secondary signs: wall thickening (> 3 mm) and pericholecystic fluid

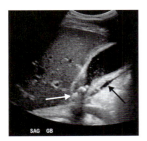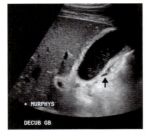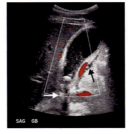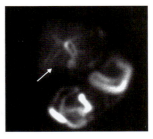

Fig. 90.9   Fig. 90.10   Fig. 90.11   Fig. 90.12

This 46-year-old female presented with right upper quadrant abdominal pain and fever. The gallbladder is distended and contains low-level echogenic material consistent with sludge as well as several echogenic shadowing gallstones, one of which is impacted in the neck of the gallbladder (white arrows in Figs. 90.9 and 90.11). The gallbladder wall is thick, and there was a positive sonographic Murphy's sign (Fig. 90.10). There is a small amount of pericholecystic fluid (black arrows in Figs. 90.9–90.11), and increased vascularity is noted in the wall (red in Fig. 90.11) on color Doppler. Hepatobiliary scintigraphy demonstrated no filling of the gallbladder (arrow in Fig. 90.12).

- ► Gangrenous cholecystitis
  - ▪ Disruption of echogenic mucosal layer of gallbladder wall

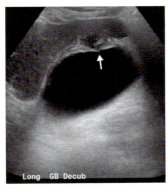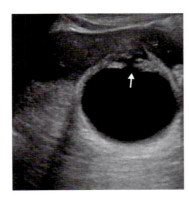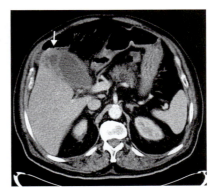

Fig. 90.13   Fig. 90.14   Fig. 90.15

Note focal disruption of gallbladder wall (arrows in Figs. 90.13 and 90.14) with adjacent pericholecystic fluid collection indicating gallbladder perforation and pericholecystic abscess. Axial contrast-enhanced CT scan confirms the presence of complex pericholecystic fluid collection (arrow in Fig. 90.15).

- ▪ Ulceration of wall, cystic spaces within wall
- ▪ Focal bulge of gallbladder wall
- ▪ Sloughed mucosal membranes

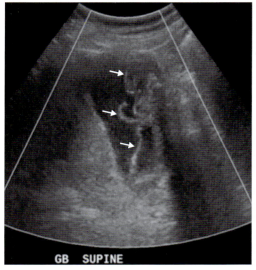

Fig. 90.16

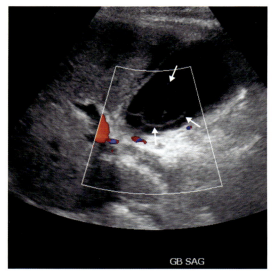

Fig. 90.17

Two different patients with curvilinear echogenic strands (arrows in Figs. 90.16 and 90.17) within the gallbladder lumen suggestive of sloughing of the gallbladder mucosa. Surgery confirmed gangrenous cholecystitis in both cases.

- Focal disruption/perforation of gallbladder wall
  - May lead to pericholecystic biloma or abscess
  - May cause adjacent liver abscess
  - The gallbladder may become decompressed if perforated

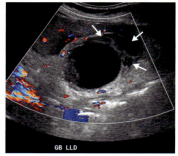

Fig. 90.18

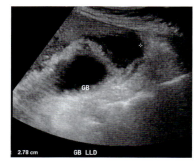

Fig. 90.19

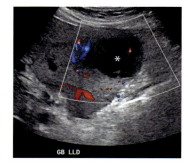

Fig. 90.20

In this elderly patient with right upper quadrant pain and fever, the gallbladder wall is thick with several focal cystic areas (arrows in Fig. 90.18) consistent with gangrenous changes. Note complex fluid collection (calipers in Fig. 90.19) superior to the fundus of the gallbladder (GB). In addition, there is a complex cystic area within the adjacent liver (asterisk in Fig. 90.20) consistent with a liver abscess.

- Absence of vascularity in gallbladder wall
- Murphy's sign may be absent if gangrene has occurred
▶ Acalculous cholecystitis
- Occurs in the setting of bile stasis or extreme systemic illness, including patients in intensive care, trauma or burn victims, patients on hyperalimentation, and following major surgery
- Rarely seen in outpatients
- Distended gallbladder (> 4 cm in transverse dimension), wall thickening, positive Murphy's sign, no gallstones

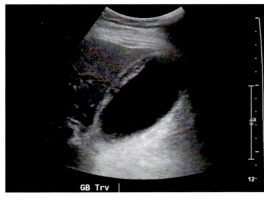

Fig. 90.21

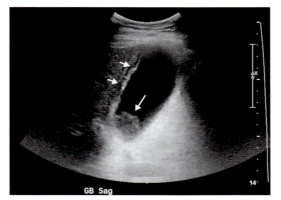

Fig. 90.22

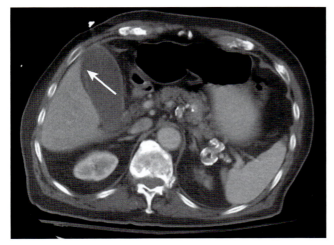

Fig. 90.23

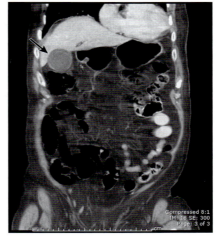

Fig. 90.24

This intensive care unit trauma patient developed an elevated white blood cell count and worsening liver function tests. The gallbladder is distended with a small amount of sludge (long arrow in Fig. 90.22), thick striated wall (Fig. 90.21), and a small amount of pericholecystic fluid (short arrows in Fig. 90.22). No gallstones were identified.

Axial (Fig. 90.23) and coronal (Fig. 90.24) CT scans demonstrate pericholecystic inflammation/fluid with focal absence of mucosal enhancement (arrows) indicative of mucosal necrosis that was not identified on US.

▶ There are multiple causes of diffuse gallbladder wall thickening, including hepatitis, CHF, hypoproteinemia, and pancreatitis
  ▪ Patients are usually afebrile, no leukocytosis
  ▪ Wall may be striated and edematous
  ▪ Not associated with disruption of mucosa, focal bulge in wall, or pericholecystic abscess

Management

▶ If US is equivocal, nuclear cholescintigraphy (hepatobiliary iminodiacetic acid (HIDA) scan) can assess patency of cystic duct
▶ Antibiotics and cholecystectomy (urgent if concern for gangrene, perforation, pericholecystic abscess)
▶ Percutaneous cholecystostomy for poor operative candidates

Further Reading

1. O'Connor O, Maher M. Imaging of cholecystitis. *Am J Roentgenol.* 2011; 196: 367–374.
2. Ralls PW, Colletti PM, Lapin SA, et al. Real-time sonography in suspected acute cholecystitis: Prospective evaluation of primary and secondary signs. *Radiology.* 1985; 155: 767–771.

Case 91

► 68-Year-old diabetic female with right upper quadrant (RUQ) pain, fever, and gram-negative bacteremia (Figs. 91.1–91.3)

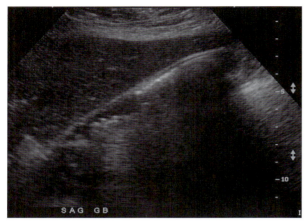

Fig. 91.1

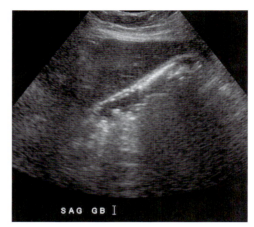

Fig. 91.2

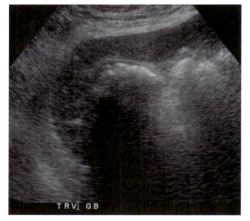

Fig. 91.3

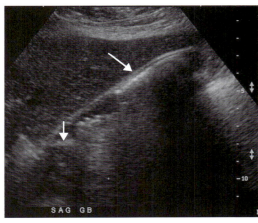

Fig. 91.4

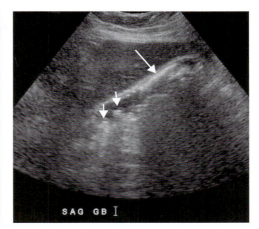

Fig. 91.5

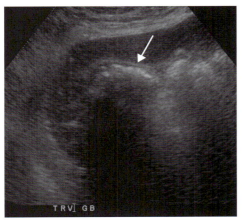

Fig. 91.6

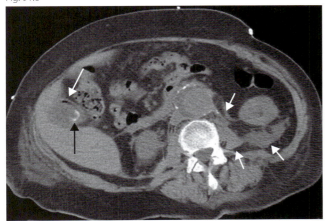

Fig. 91.7

Imaging Findings

▶ Moderately distended gallbladder with linear echogenic area (long arrows in Figs. 91.4–91.6) in the gallbladder wall near the fundus with dirty shadowing consistent with air in the nondependent wall

▶ Note sludge and echogenic foci with dirty shadowing (short arrows in Figs. 91.4 and 91.5) consistent with intraluminal air bubbles

▶ Non contrast-enhanced axial CT scan demonstrating air within the wall of the gallbladder (long white arrow in Fig. 91.7) and gallstone (black arrow in Fig. 91.7). Incidentally noted is free fluid in the left posterior pararenal space (short arrows in Fig. 91.7)

Differential Diagnosis

► Porcelain gallbladder
► Gallbladder filled with gallstones (wall–echo–shadow complex or WES sign)
► Adenomyomatosis
► Air in biliary tree refluxing secondary to biliary–enteric anastomosis, sphincterotomy, or cholecystoduodenal fistula
► Gas-filled duodenum

Teaching Points

► Uncommon form of acute cholecystitis (< 1%) secondary to ischemia of the gallbladder wall with subsequent superinfection by gas-forming bacteria
► Presentation
  ▪ Patients are extremely ill: severe RUQ pain, fever, sepsis, elevated white blood cell count
  ▪ Elderly, sixth and seventh decades
  ▪ More common in males (~70% of cases)
  ▪ 30–50% of patients do not have gallstones
  ▪ High mortality rate, approximately 15%
  ▪ Increased incidence of gallbladder gangrene and perforation
► Risk factors: diabetes (up to 50%) and peripheral vascular disease
► US findings
  ▪ Punctate or linear echogenic mural foci with dirty shadowing due to gas in nondependent gallbladder wall
  ▪ Ring-down artifact may be present
  ▪ Mobile echogenic intraluminal foci with dirty shadowing due to air bubbles floating in bile: will change with patient position
  ▪ If the lumen is filled with air, it will collect in the nondependent portion of the gallbladder

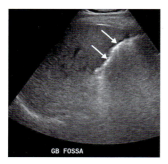 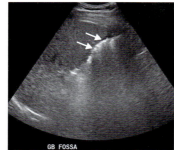 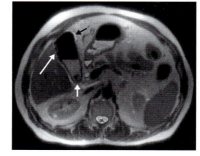

Fig. 91.8   Fig. 91.9   Fig. 91.10

79-Year-old male presenting with RUQ pain and fever. Note echogenic curvilinear area (arrows in Figs. 91.8 and 91.9) with dirty shadowing in the gallbladder fossa. The dirty shadowing from the air obscures visualization of the far wall of the gallbladder and intraluminal contents, mimicking the US appearance of a loop of bowel. T2-weighted axial MR image (Fig. 91.10) demonstrates an air (black contents)–fluid (white contents) level in the gallbladder. Note gallstones (short white arrow in Fig. 91.10), high signal intensity free fluid (black arrow in Fig. 91.10) in the soft tissues near the fundus, as well as multiple tiny round low signal intensity foci aligned along the gallbladder wall consistent with a small amount of mural air (long white arrow in Fig. 91.10) confirming the diagnosis of emphysematous cholecystitis.

► Porcelain gallbladder: echogenic gallbladder wall due to mural calcification
  ▪ Circumferential or interrupted
  ▪ Shadowing denser and sharper
  ▪ No intraluminal air
  ▪ Patients usually asymptomatic
► Gallbladder full of stones (WES sign): echogenic gallbladder wall
  ▪ Two echogenic arcs separated by hypoechoic arc
  ▪ Sharp, dense posterior shadowing from gallstones
► Adenomyomatosis: multiple echogenic mural foci
  ▪ Comet tail artifact rather than dirty shadowing
  ▪ More common in fundus, can be confluent
  ▪ No intraluminal air

► Reflux of air into the biliary tree can occur following manipulation of the common bile duct (CBD), passage of a CBD stone, or in patients with a biliary–enteric anastomosis or fistula , but would not cause air in the gallbladder wall
  ■ Patients often asymptomatic
► An air-filled loop of bowel could create an echogenic curvilinear structure with dirty shadowing near the gallbladder fossa mimicking a gallbladder filled with air
  ■ Clinical presentation, imaging in orthogonal planes, peristalsis, or water intake can help differentiate an air-filled loop of bowel from the gallbladder, if the gallbladder is not identifiable separately

Management

► CT more sensitive than US
  ■ Can be useful to distinguish between emphysematous cholecystitis, porcelain gallbladder, and a gallbladder filled with stones
► Urgent cholecystectomy or cholecystostomy with antibiotic therapy

Further Reading

1. Parulekar SG. Sonographic findings in acute emphysematous cholecystitis. *Radiology*. 1982; 145(1): 117–119.
2. O'Connor OJ, Maher MM. Imaging of cholecystitis. *Am J Roentgenol*. 2011; 196(4): W367–W374.
3. Grayson DE, Abbott RM, Levy AD, et al. Emphysematous infections of the abdomen and pelvis: A pictorial review. *RadioGraphics*. 2002; 22(3): 543–561.

Case 92

▶ 53-Year-old male with right upper quadrant pain (Figs. 92.1 and 92.2)

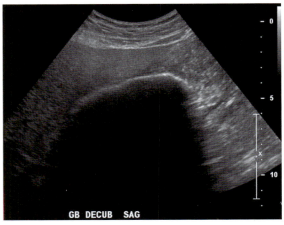

Fig. 92.1

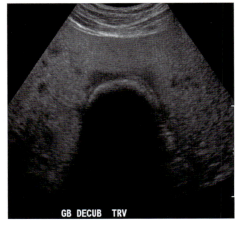

Fig. 92.2

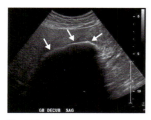

Fig. 92.3

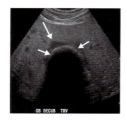

Fig. 92.4

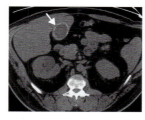

Fig. 92.5

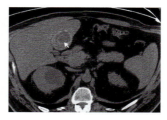

Fig. 92.6

Imaging Findings

► Curvilinear echogenic structure with sharp, dense posterior acoustic shadowing in the region of the gallbladder fossa (short arrows in Figs. 92.3 and 92.4) indicative of diffuse calcification in the gallbladder wall. Due to the dense posterior shadowing, the contents of the gallbladder cannot be visualized

► Note increased echogenicity of the liver parenchyma with a geographic hypoechoic area near the gallbladder (long arrow in Fig. 92.4) consistent with hepatic steatosis and focal fatty sparing

► Non-contrast-enhanced axial CT scan demonstrates thin peripheral calcification in the gallbladder wall (arrow in Fig. 92.5). The mural calcification appears slightly less regular and less continuous on the CT scan in comparison to the US images. Note large gallstone with high attenuation calcified rim (arrow in Fig. 92.6) that was obscured on US by shadowing from the mural calcification

Differential Diagnosis

► Emphysematous cholecystitis
► Gallbladder filled with gallstones (wall–echo–shadow complex or WES sign)
► Calcified hepatic or renal cyst

Teaching Points

► Porcelain gallbladder is the term used to describe calcification of the gallbladder wall
  ▪ Most commonly an incidental finding
  ▪ Strongly associated with chronic gallbladder inflammation, although most patients are asymptomatic
  ▪ 90–95% of patients have gallstones
  ▪ Significant risk of developing adenocarcinoma of the gallbladder (20–30%)
► CT is the most sensitive imaging modality for the detection of associated gallbladder carcinoma
► Three sonographic patterns have been described
  ▪ Type I: circumferential, curvilinear increased echogenicity of the gallbladder wall with sharp, dense posterior acoustic shadowing (as in this case). Creates single echogenic arc in gallbladder fossa with distal shadowing
  ▪ Type II: thinner echogenic wall with less posterior shadowing, such that the curvilinear echogenic posterior wall of the gallbladder may also be visualized
  ▪ Type III: discontinuous areas of echogenic mural calcification with shadowing
► Emphysematous cholecystitis
  ▪ Air in the gallbladder wall can also produce a curvilinear echogenic pattern
  ▪ Dirty rather than sharp posterior shadowing
  ▪ Air may be present in the gallbladder lumen
  ▪ Clinically, patients with emphysematous cholecystitis are typically extremely ill
► A gallbladder filled with gallstones may demonstrate the WES sign (Figures 92.7 and 92.8)

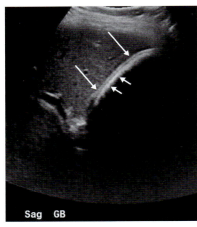

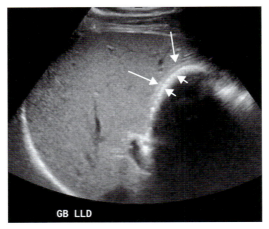

Fig. 92.7   Fig. 92.8

18-year-old female presented with abdominal pain. The sonographic Murphy's sign was negative. Note two parallel echogenic curvilinear lines with an intervening hypoechoic line in the gallbladder fossa. The more superficial or superior echogenic arc (long arrows in Figs. 92.7 and 92.8) likely represents pericholecystic fat and/or the interface between the gallbladder wall and the surface of the liver; the hypoechoic middle line represents the gallbladder wall; the second inner or inferior echogenic arc (short arrows in Figs. 92.7 and 92.8) is created by the gallstone(s) that causes the dense posterior acoustic shadowing. With a porcelain gallbladder, only a single echogenic arc will be observed.

➤ Occasionally, a thin rim of anechoic bile (arrows in Figs. 92.9 and 92.10) can be seen to layer on top of echogenic gallstones filling the gallbladder lumen (Figs. 92.9 and 92.10) mimicking the WES sign

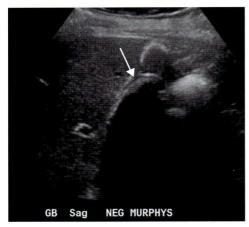

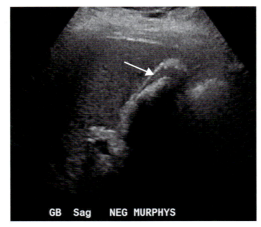

Fig. 92.9   Fig. 92.10

58-Year-old male presenting with right upper quadrant pain. Note that the anechoic layer (arrows in Figs. 92.9 and 92.10) separating the two echogenic arcs likely represents bile surrounding the gallstones rather than the gallbladder wall because it is so thick on a slightly lateral image (Fig. 92.10).

➤ Calcified cysts may have a thin, curved echogenic wall with distal shadowing and can be distinguished from a porcelain gallbladder by demonstrating attachment to the kidney or liver

Management

➤ Look carefully for evidence of gallbladder carcinoma
➤ Most studies recommend prophylactic cholecystectomy due to risk of gallbladder carcinoma
   ■ However, recent studies suggest that the risk of gallbladder carcinoma is lower than previously reported and recommend observation unless the patient is symptomatic or the mural calcification is incomplete or discontinuous, which is believed to pose a higher risk

Further Reading

1. Kane RA, Jacobs R, Katz J. Porcelain gallbladder: Ultrasound and CT appearance. *Radiology*. 1984; 152: 137–141.
2. Shimizu M, Miura J, Tanaka T, et al. Porcelain gallbladder: Relation between its type by ultrasound and incidence of cancer. *J Clin Gastroenterol*. 1989; 11: 471–476.
3. Kim JH, Kim WH, Yoo BM, et al. Should we perform surgical management in all patients with suspected porcelain gallbladder? *Hepatogastroenterology*. 2009; 56: 943–945.

History

▶ 62-Year-old female presents with right upper quadrant pain (Figs. 93.1–93.6)

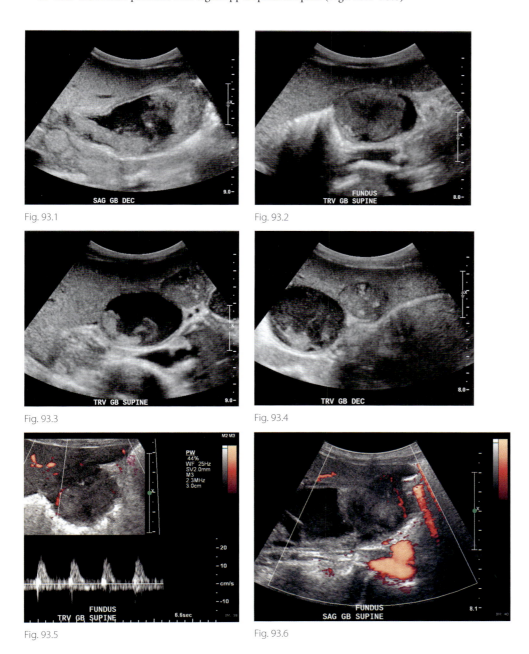

Fig. 93.1

Fig. 93.2

Fig. 93.3

Fig. 93.4

Fig. 93.5

Fig. 93.6

Case 93 Gallbladder Adenocarcinoma

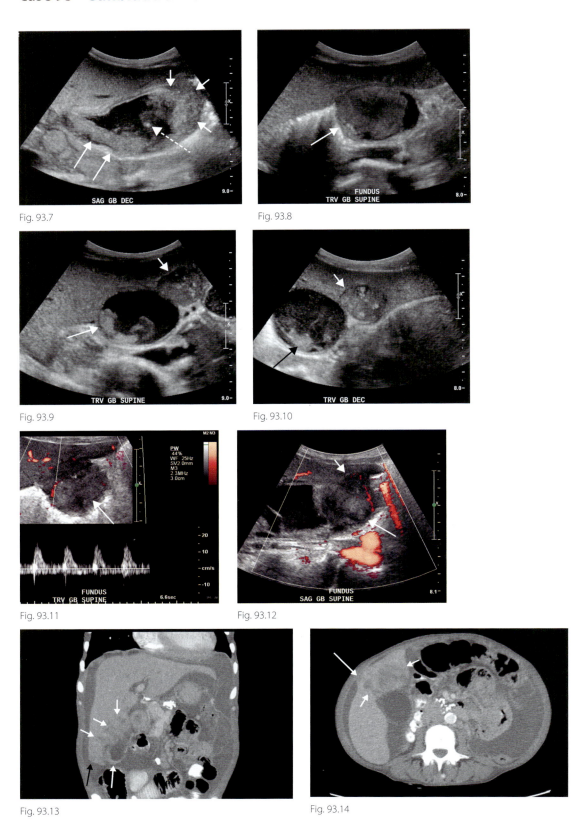

Fig. 93.7

Fig. 93.8

Fig. 93.9

Fig. 93.10

Fig. 93.11

Fig. 93.12

Fig. 93.13

Fig. 93.14

Imaging Findings

▶ Large polyploid fundal gallbladder mass (short arrows in Fig. 93.7; arrows in Figs. 93.8 and 93.11; long arrow in Fig. 93.12) and mural-based mass (long arrows in Figs. 93.7 and 93.9; black arrow in Fig. 93.10) as well as small gallstone (dashed arrow in Fig. 93.7) and sludge

▶ Adjacent heterogeneous hepatic mass (short white arrows in Figs. 93.9 and 93.10)

▶ Note direct hepatic invasion (short arrow in Fig. 93.12) by the fundal gallbladder mass (long arrow in Fig. 93.12), which demonstrates minimal vascularity on power Doppler (Figs. 93.11 and 93.12)

▶ Coronal (Fig. 93.13) and axial (Fig. 93.14) contrast-enhanced CT images demonstrate focal gallbladder wall thickening (long white arrow in Fig. 93.13) corresponding to the smaller mural-based mass and invasion of the liver (short arrows in Figs. 93.13 and 93.14) by the large fundal mass. Focal invasion through the liver capsule (black arrow in Fig. 93.13 and long arrow in Fig. 93.14) is also present with moderate surrounding ascites concerning for peritoneal disease

Differential Diagnosis

▶ Tumefactive sludge
▶ Metastatic disease
▶ Hepatocellular carcinoma invading gallbladder

Teaching Points

▶ Rare entity; most are adenocarcinomas
  ▪ Most common in elderly women, with 3:1 female-to-male ratio
▶ Chronic inflammation from gallstone disease leading to dysplasia within gallbladder wall is most common etiology
▶ Prognosis: poor, with a 10–15% 5-year survival
  ▪ Usually presents at an advanced stage
▶ Risk factors: cholelithiasis, chronic cholecystitis (especially typhoid), obesity, porcelain gallbladder, primary sclerosing cholangitis
▶ Presentation: right upper quadrant pain, jaundice, weight loss, fever
  ▪ Signs and symptoms may overlap with acute cholecystitis
  ▪ Most do not become symptomatic until late stage
  ▪ May be found incidentally at cholecystectomy
▶ US limited sensitivity in detecting early stage
▶ Three classic US imaging patterns
  1. Mass nearly filling gallbladder lumen (most common)
     • ± Gallstones visualized within mass ("trapped gallstone" engulfed by mass) or direct invasion of liver
  2. Focal or diffuse asymmetric thickening of gallbladder wall
  3. Polypoid intraluminal mural based mass > 1 cm (least common)
▶ Tumefactive sludge: may mimic US appearance of gallbladder carcinoma, especially patterns 1 and 3
  ▪ Echogenic polypoid mass-like conglomeration of intraluminal echoes
  ▪ Often associated with or containing gallstones
  ▪ No blood flow or invasion of liver
  ▪ Will change in configuration or size on follow-up US
▶ Metastases: may mimic pattern 3 of gallbladder cancer
  ▪ Polypoid mural-based vascular lesions
  ▪ Multiple more common than single
  ▪ Melanoma most common primary followed by lung
  ▪ Other primaries: liver, non-Hodgkin lymphoma, gastrointestinal, pancreas, renal, and breast
  ▪ Usually evidence of metastatic disease elsewhere
▶ Hepatocellular carcinoma invading gallbladder: may mimic gallbladder cancer pattern 1
  ▪ Epicenter of mass will be within the hepatic parenchyma rather than in the gallbladder lumen

Management

▶ MRI and CT for assessing local extent of disease and staging
▶ Positron emission tomography can also be used in staging or follow-up
▶ Extended surgical resection
▶ If imaging findings equivocal, the surgeon should obtain frozen section to allow extended resection/nodal dissection if necessary

Further Reading

1. Furlan A, Ferris JV, Hosseinzadeh K, et al. Gallbladder carcinoma update: Multimodality imaging evaluation, staging, and treatment options. *Am J Roentgenol.* 2008; 191: 1440–1447.
2. Rooholamini SA, Tehrani NS, Razavi MK, et al. Imaging of gallbladder carcinoma. *RadioGraphics.* 1994; 14: 291–306.

Case 94

History

► 45-Year-old female with right upper quadrant pain (Figs. 94.1–94.4)

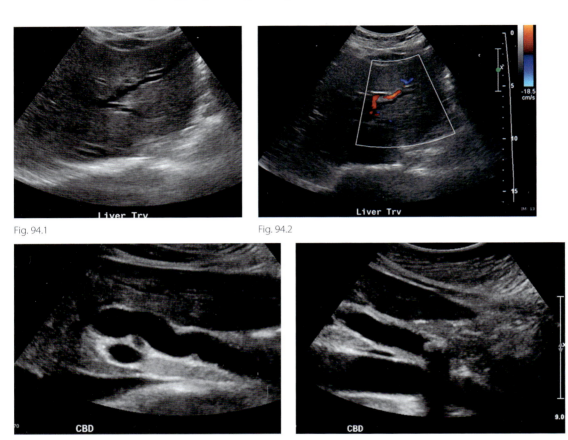

Fig. 94.1

Fig. 94.2

Fig. 94.3

Fig. 94.4

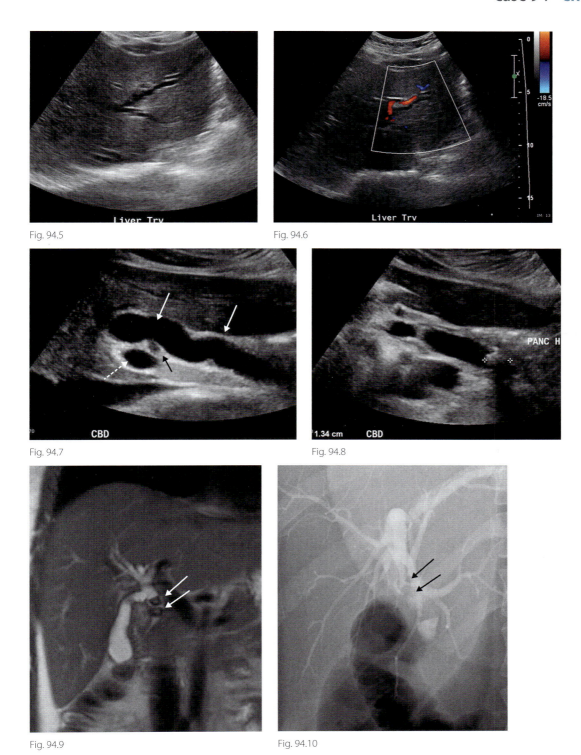

Fig. 94.5

Fig. 94.6

Fig. 94.7

Fig. 94.8

Fig. 94.9

Fig. 94.10

Imaging Findings

▶ Grayscale image (Fig. 94.5) of the liver demonstrating tubular anechoic structures that do not fill in with color on color Doppler image (Fig. 94.6), consistent with intrahepatic biliary ductal dilatation

▶ The common bile duct (CBD) is markedly dilated, measuring 14 mm (long white arrows in Fig. 94.7). Hepatic artery (black arrow in Fig. 94.7). Portal vein (dashed white arrow in Fig. 94.7)

- Note 13 mm echogenic stone (calipers in Fig. 94.8) with posterior acoustic shadowing in the distal CBD near the head of the pancreas
- T2 HASTE (half-Fourier acquisition single-shot turbo spin-echo) coronal MR image demonstrates two low-signal filling defects (arrows in Fig. 94.9) in the distal CBD consistent with choledocholithiasis. The proximal CBD and intrahepatic biliary ducts are also dilated
- Filling defects confirmed on endoscopic retrograde cholangiopancreatography (ERCP) (arrows in Fig. 94.10)

Differential Diagnosis

- Distal common bile duct stricture
- Ampullary cancer
- Cholangiocarcinoma
- Primary sclerosing cholangitis with pneumobilia

Teaching Points

- Primary bile duct stones (5%) form directly within the bile ducts
  - Associated with Caroli disease, chronic hemolytic disease, recurrent cholangitis, biliary stasis, and parasites
- Secondary CBD stones (95%) migrate from the gallbladder
  - Risk factors include obesity, elevated triglycerides, hyperalimentation, and small bowel surgery
- Clinical presentation of CBD stones: biliary colic, pruritus, jaundice, pancreatitis, elevated alkaline phosphatase, and/or elevated direct bilirubin levels
- Complications: cholangitis, obstructive jaundice, and pancreatitis
- US is approximately 75% sensitive for the diagnosis of choledocholithiasis
- US findings
  - Echogenic focus in the CBD
  - ± Posterior acoustic shadowing depending on size
  - Twinkle artifact on color Doppler
  - Intrahepatic biliary ductal and/or CBD dilatation present if stone is large enough to obstruct duct
  - Abrupt cutoff of the CBD without tapering may be observed if the duct is completely obstructed
  - Findings should be confirmed on two orthogonal imaging planes to exclude partial volume artifact from air in adjacent bowel or adjacent fat
  - Right posterior oblique positioning will improve visualization of the distal CBD
- Ampullary cancer, cholangiocarcinoma, distal CBD stricture, or sclerosing cholangitis can all cause biliary ductal dilatation
  - An intraluminal tumor would not be as echogenic or cause shadowing
  - Stones or sludge can be seen above a CBD stricture due to stasis
  - Air in the CBD secondary to infection or reflux would be more likely to be multifocal, more linear, and demonstrate "dirty shadowing" rather than dense, sharp posterior shadowing as in this case

Management

- If no cause for the obstruction is found on US in a patient with biliary ductal dilatation, magnetic resonance cholangiopancreatography may help differentiate choledocholithiasis from tumor, stricture, or extrinsic compression
- CBD stones are almost always removed via ERCP

Further Reading

1. Kim YJ, Kim MJ, Kim KW, et al. Preoperative evaluation of common bile duct stones in patients with gallstone disease. *Am J Roentgenol.* 2005; 184: 1854–1859.
2. Kondo S, Isayama H, Akahane M, et al. Detection of common bile duct stones: Comparison between endoscopic ultrasonography, magnetic resonance cholangiography, and helical-computed-tomographic cholangiography. *Eur J Radiol.* 2005; 54: 271–275.

History

▶ 64-Year-old male presents with painless jaundice (Figs. 95.1 and 95.2)

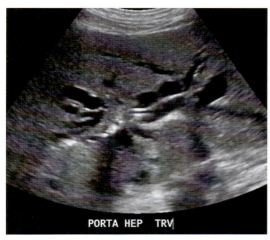

Fig. 95.1

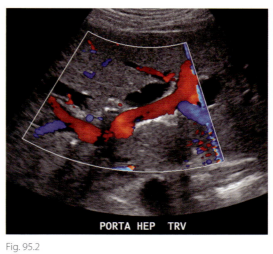

Fig. 95.2

Case 95 Cholangiocarcinoma

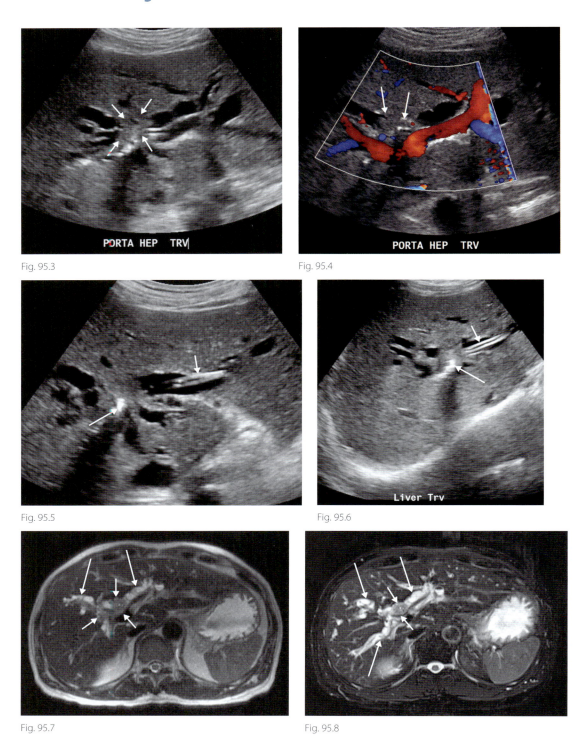

Fig. 95.3

Fig. 95.4

Fig. 95.5

Fig. 95.6

Fig. 95.7

Fig. 95.8

Imaging Findings

► Note tubular anechoic structures in both the right and left lobes of the liver that do not fill in with color on color Doppler imaging (Fig. 95.4), indicating marked intrahepatic biliary ductal dilatation

► The dilated ducts converge toward the porta hepatis but end abruptly without joining together and are separated by an ill-defined, irregular mass that is slightly hypoechoic relative to the liver parenchyma (arrows in Figs. 95.3 and 95.4)

- The common bile duct (CBD) was not dilated (not shown)
- Later images demonstrate an echogenic stent with shadowing (long arrows in Figs. 95.5 and 95.6) in the center of the mass at the confluence of the right and left intrahepatic bile ducts. The peripheral end of the stent is located in the left intrahepatic bile duct (short arrows in Figs. 95.5 and 95.6).
- T2-weighted HASTE (half-Fourier acquisition single-shot turbo spin-echo; Fig. 95.7) and T2-weighted TSE (turbo spin-echo) fat-suppressed (Fig. 95.8) MR images demonstrate the fluid-filled high signal intensity dilated intrahepatic ducts (long arrows) in both the right and left lobes of the liver. The tumor mass (short arrows) at the expected confluence of the right and left intrahepatic bile ducts is higher in signal intensity than the liver parenchyma and is more easily seen than on US

Differential Diagnosis

- Liver metastases
- Periportal lymphadenopathy
- Hepatocellular carcinoma
- Distal CBD stricture
- Sclerosing cholangitis

Teaching Points

- Cholangiocarcinoma is a malignant tumor arising from the biliary tree
  - Most common in Southeast Asia
  - More common in elderly: seventh and eighth decades
  - 90% are adenocarcinomas, with squamous cell carcinoma being the next most common histology
  - Extremely poor prognosis: 5-year survival of 10–44%
- Presentation: painless jaundice, pruritis, abnormal liver function tests consistent with cholestasis
- Risk factors: chronic biliary stasis, biliary stones, and inflammation
  - Primary sclerosing cholangitis most common risk factor in Western world
  - Viral infection (HIV, hepatitis B and C, Epstein–Barr virus)
  - Recurrent pyogenic cholangitis
  - Liver flukes (*Opisthorchis viverrini, Clonorchis sinensis*)
  - Caroli disease
  - Choledochal cysts
  - Biliary toxins (dioxin, polyvinyl chloride, alcohol)
- Most commonly occur at the confluence of the right and left intrahepatic ducts, termed Klatskin tumors (60%)
  - Distal duct (30%)
  - Intrahepatic ducts (10%)
  - 5% are multifocal
- Pattern of metastasis
  - Intrahepatic vascular involvement will result in hepatic metastases
  - Regional lymph nodes
  - Hematogenous: lungs, bones (vertebrae), adrenal glands, brain
- US findings of Klatskin tumors
  - Dilated intrahepatic ducts in both right and left lobes of the liver abruptly terminating at the level of the tumor (i.e., converging but not joining at the porta hepatis)
  - Distal (i.e., closer to the head of the pancreas) CBD not dilated
  - Mass typically infiltrating and poorly marginated with similar echogenicity to liver parenchyma and, therefore, often not directly visualized on US despite frequent large size and hepatic invasion
  - Retraction of liver capsule
- Less common US appearance of cholangiocarcinomas
  - Focal thickening of bile duct wall
  - Intraluminal polypoid mass
  - Intrahepatic mass with distal ductal obstruction
- Metastases or periportal lymphadenopathy
  - Could cause bilobar obstruction and dilatation of the intrahepatic bile ducts with abrupt termination
  - Visualization of a focal discrete mass in the porta hepatis more likely
- Hepatocellular carcinoma
  - Could cause a poorly visualized perihilar liver mass
  - Less likely to cause distal ductal dilatation

- ▶ Distal CBD stricture
  - ▪ Dilatation of the entire biliary tree: the dilated right and left intrahepatic bile ducts will join at the porta hepatis
- ▶ Sclerosing cholangitis
  - ▪ Different clinical scenario: young to middle-aged men, history of inflammatory bowel disease (especially ulcerative colitis)
  - ▪ Tends to cause wall thickening of the bile ducts with multifocal strictures resulting in a beaded appearance rather than massive smooth ductal dilatation as in this case
  - ▪ May lead to portal hypertension and cirrhosis
  - ▪ Predisposes to cholangiocarcinoma, which should be considered if a liver mass, wall thickening > 5 mm, or a focal area of disproportionally dilated bile ducts are observed

Management

- ▶ Local staging usually performed with MR; CT used to assess for distant metastases
- ▶ Important features to assess include the following
  - ▪ Tumor size (> 3 cm)
  - ▪ Extent of biliary tree involvement
  - ▪ Presence of vascular invasion
  - ▪ Lymph node involvement
  - ▪ Multiplicity
- ▶ Most important determinant of prognosis is whether or not the tumor can be resected. However, even with resection, prognosis is poor
- ▶ Criteria precluding resection
  - ▪ Bilobar biliary involvement to level of secondary radicles (right anterior, right posterior, left medial, and left lateral intrahepatic ducts)
  - ▪ Metastases (hepatic, lymph node, or distant)
  - ▪ Invasion/encasement of main portal vein
  - ▪ Multiple lesions
  - ▪ Lobar atrophy with encasement of contralateral portal vein branch or involvement of secondary biliary radicle
- ▶ Liver transplantation now considered for small, unresectable hilar lesions

Further Reading

1. Chung YE, Kim MJ, Park YN, et al. Varying appearances of cholangiocarcinoma: Radiologic–pathologic correlation. *RadioGraphics*. 2009; 29: 683–700.
2. Vilgrain V. Staging cholangiocarcinoma by imaging studies. *HPB (Oxford)*. 2008; 10: 106–109.
3. Han JK, Choi BI, Kim AY, et al. Cholangiocarcinoma: Pictorial essay of CT and cholangiographic findings. *RadioGraphics*. 2002; 22: 173–187.

History

▶ 44-Year-old male with history of HIV and alcohol abuse presents with worsening chronic abdominal pain (Figs. 96.1–96.3)

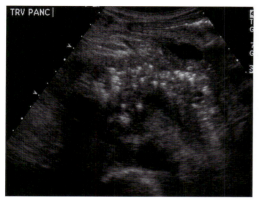

Fig. 96.1

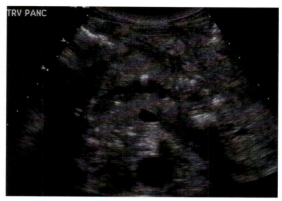

Fig. 96.2

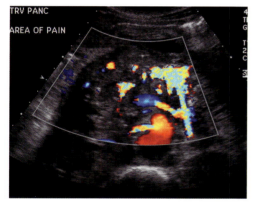

Fig. 96.3

Case 96 Chronic Pancreatitis

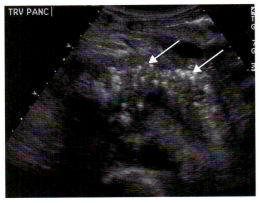

Fig. 96.4

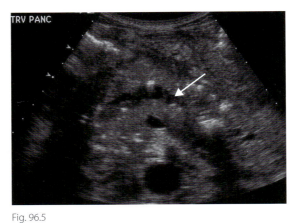

Fig. 96.5

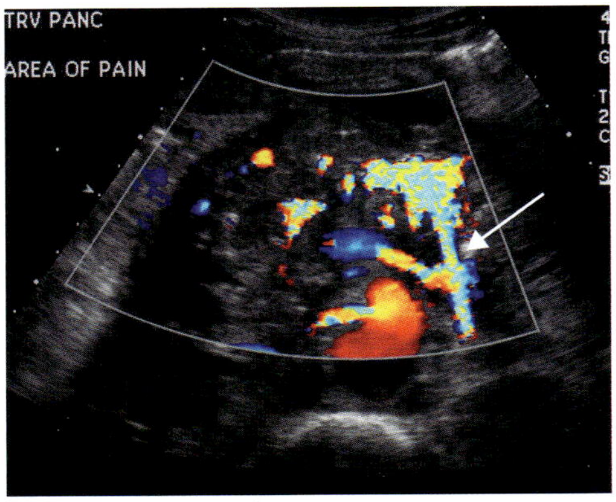

Fig. 96.6

Imaging Findings

► Enlarged pancreas with heterogeneous pancreatic parenchyma and multiple calcifications (arrows in Fig. 96.4)
► Dilated pancreatic duct (arrow in Fig. 96.5)
► Twinkle artifact making calcifications more conspicuous (arrow in Fig. 96.6)

Differential Diagnosis

► Acute pancreatitis
► Intraductal papillary mucinous neoplasm (IPMN)
► Pancreatic carcinoma

Teaching Points

► Chronic pancreatitis results from destructive and inflammatory change of the pancreas secondary to long-standing pancreatic injury
► Symptoms: chronic epigastric abdominal pain, weight loss, pancreatic insufficiency, and diabetes mellitus
► Most common cause in the United States is alcohol abuse
► Additional etiologies: congenital anomalies such as pancreatic divisum or annular pancreas, cystic fibrosis, hereditary pancreatitis, chronic biliary tract disease, hyperlipidemia, and hyperparathyroidism
► Autoimmune diseases such as Sjogren syndrome, lupus, and ulcerative colitis can lead to a subtype of chronic pancreatitis known as sclerosing pancreatitis
► Demographics: middle-aged population, males > females
► Poor prognosis with increased rate of pancreatic cancer
► Imaging plays a crucial role because clinical diagnosis can be difficult
► Visualization of the pancreas on US may be impaired by bowel gas or body habitus
► Advanced chronic pancreatitis can easily be visualized by US

- Calcifications are the most specific finding: hyperechoic foci with posterior acoustic shadowing, focal or diffuse causing twinkle artifact on color Doppler US
- Atrophy of the pancreatic gland with heterogeneous echotexture; however, if acute on chronic pancreatitis, gland is enlarged and edematous gland
- Dilated pancreatic duct
- Dilated common bile duct and portosplenic vein thrombosis are less common findings
▶ Pseudocysts are present in approximately 20% of patients
▶ CT is more sensitive to indicate acute on chronic pancreatitis

Contrast-enhanced CT in this patient shows an enlarged pancreas with decreased enhancement, likely due to edema from acute on chronic pancreatitis as well as pancreatic tail calcification confirming the chronic nature of the underlying disease (arrow in Fig. 96.7).

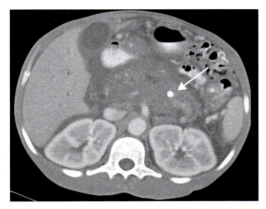

Fig. 96.7

▶ Acute pancreatitis: no calcifications, unless acute on chronic changes
▶ IPMN: cystic masses communicating with the ductal system
▶ Pancreatic carcinoma
- A focal hypoechoic mass may be seen in some patients with acute pancreatitis and may mimic pancreatic adenocarcinoma
- Presence of calcifications helps to exclude neoplasm
- When imaging is not specific, biopsy may be necessary

Management

▶ Conservative treatment with pain control for uncomplicated disease
▶ US or CT-guided aspiration for large or persistently symptomatic pseudocysts
▶ Surgical or image-guided intervention for complications of obstructive jaundice

Further Reading

1. Tchelepi H, Ralls PW. Color comet-tail artifact: Clinical applications. *Am J Roentgenol*. 2009; 192: 11–18.
2. Etemad B, Whitcomb DC. Chronic pancreatitis: Diagnosis, classification, and new generic developments. *Gastroenterology*. 2001; 120: 682–707.

Case 97

History

▶ 52-Year-old male with history of HIV and multiple prior admissions for acute on chronic pancreatitis presents with acute epigastric pain (Figs. 97.1–97.3)

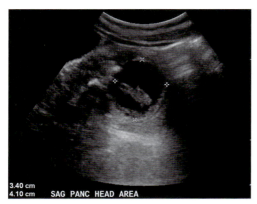

Fig. 97.1

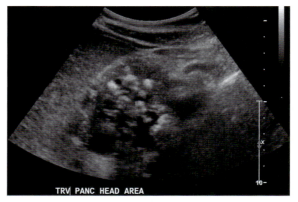

Fig. 97.2

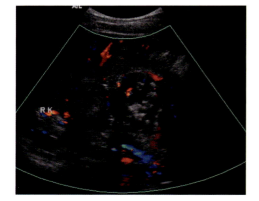

Fig. 97.3

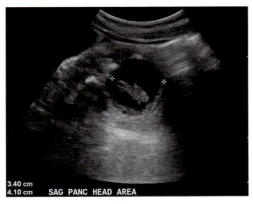

Fig. 97.4

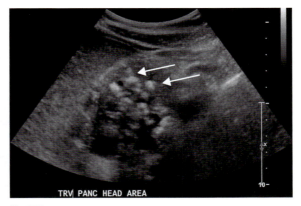

Fig. 97.5

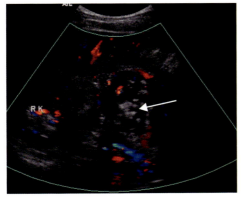

Fig. 97.6

Clinical Findings

► Well-defined complex fluid collection adjacent to the pancreatic head (between calipers in Fig. 97.4)
► Evidence of chronic pancreatitis with heterogeneous echotexture and numerous echogenic shadowing foci consistent with calcifications (arrows in Fig. 97.5)
► Internal avascular debris (arrow in Fig. 97.6)

Differential Diagnosis

► Intraductal papillary mucinous neoplasm (IPMN)
► Serous cystadenoma (SCA)
► Mucinous cystic tumor of the pancreas (MCA)
► Congenital cysts (CC)
► Pancreatic pseudoaneurysm (PSA)

Teaching Points

► Pseudocysts represent the most common cystic lesion of the pancreas
► They are sequelae of acute or chronic pancreatitis, more common in chronic pancreatitis (20–40% chronic vs. 5–16% acute)
► Pathogenesis involves disruption of the pancreatic duct with extravasation of pancreatic secretions
► Pseudocysts are rich in pancreatic enzymes such as amylase and have a wall of fibrous tissue without an epithelial lining
► Clinical presentation ranges from asymptomatic to abdominal pain/anorexia to major catastrophe secondary to complications
  ▪ Acute complications: infection, rupture, and bleeding (usually from splenic or gastroduodenal artery pseudoaneurysm)
  ▪ Chronic complications: biliary obstruction, gastric outlet obstruction, and splenic or portal vein thrombosis with resultant gastric varices and bleeding
  ▪ Less commonly, patients can present with sepsis secondary to an infected pseudocyst due to superinfection
► US plays an important role in initial diagnosis and follow-up imaging

- ▶ Major differential criteria include clinical history of acute or chronic pancreatitis, thick wall, and location
- ▶ Variable sonographic appearance
  - ▪ Well-defined anechoic or purely cystic structure (arrow in Fig. 97.7)
  - ▪ Avascular on color Doppler US (CDUS) (arrow in Fig. 97.8)
  - ▪ Adjacent pancreatic calcifications with twinkle artifact may be present (arrows in Fig. 97.10 and 97.11)
  - ▪ Internal echoes secondary to necrotic debris versus hemorrhage or infection (arrows in Fig. 97.12)
  - ▪ Hemorrhage, necrosis, or infection lead to a complex or even solid appearance

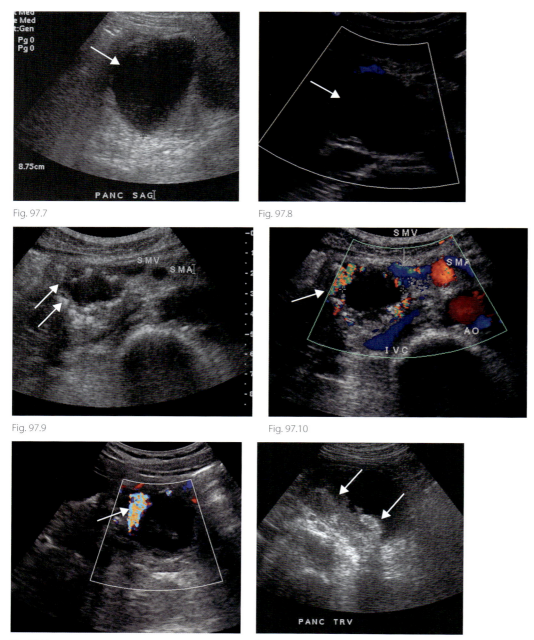

Fig. 97.7

Fig. 97.8

Fig. 97.9

Fig. 97.10

Fig. 97.11

Fig. 97.12

- ▶ IPMN presents as cystic lesion(s) with connection to the pancreatic ductal system
- ▶ Differentiation of pseudocyst from other cystic pancreatic neoplasms (SCA, MCA, CC) may be difficult. Major differential criteria include clinical history of acute and chronic pancreatitis
- ▶ Percutaneous or endoscopic US with fine needle aspiration biopsy may be helpful to distinguish pseudocysts from other cystic pancreatic neoplasms

- CDUS should be performed to exclude a pancreatic PSA
- Fluid in the lesser sac will be more anterior in location, echofree, and avascular on CDUS

Management

Most pseudocysts resolve spontaneously with supportive care alone, such as intravenous fluids, analgesics, antiemetics, and low-fat diet if patients can tolerate oral intake.

- Follow-up with serial imaging exams to monitor size
- Percutaneous, endoscopic, or surgical drainage may be indicated when
  - Size > 4–5 cm, compression of adjacent organs
  - Interval increase in size on follow-up exams
  - Patients become symptomatic and concern for infection

Further Reading

1. Habashi S, Draganov PV. Pancreatic pseudocyst. *World J Gastroenterol.* 2009; 15(1): 38–47.

Case 98

History

▶ 61-Year-old male with history of back pain for 3 months (Figs. 98.1–98.3)

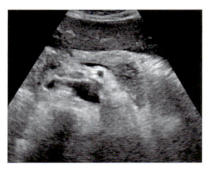

Fig. 98.1

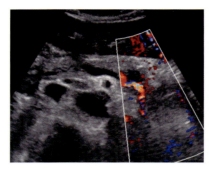

Fig. 98.2

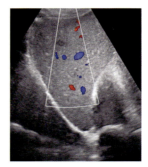

Fig. 98.3

322

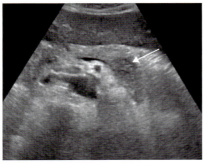

Fig. 98.4

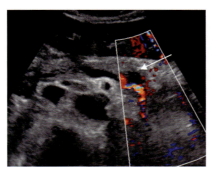

Fig. 98.5

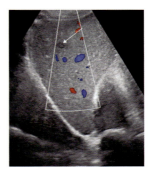

Fig. 98.6

Clinical Findings

► Irregular slightly hypoechoic mass in the pancreatic tail (arrows in Figs. 98.4 and 98.5)
► No significant vascularity on color Doppler US (CDUS) (arrow in Fig. 98.5)
► Hypoechoic liver metastasis (arrow in Fig. 98.6)

Differential Diagnosis

► Focal pancreatitis
► Neuroendocrine tumor
► Serous cystadenoma
► Mucinous cystic pancreatic tumor
► Lymphoma/metastatic disease

Teaching Points

► Pancreatic adenocarcinoma: fourth leading cause of cancer-related deaths in the United States
  ▪ < 20% present with localized, potentially resectable and curable tumors
  ▪ Location: 60–70% head, 25–35% body and tail, 3–5% diffuse
  ▪ Poor prognosis: overall 5-year survival rate is < 5%
► Risk factors: smoking, diabetes, chronic pancreatitis, and cancer-predisposing genetic syndromes
► Demographics: elderly population, males slightly > females
► Symptoms: vague abdominal discomfort, back pain, anorexia, and weight loss
  ▪ Tumors in the head of the pancreas cause obstructive cholestasis and jaundice
  ▪ Obstruction of the pancreatic duct can lead to pancreatitis and distal atrophy of the gland
  ▪ Deep or superficial thrombosis of extremity veins (Trousseau syndrome)
► US: often first modality used to assess patients with nonspecific abdominal pain and hepatobiliary symptoms. US findings include the following
  ▪ Hypoechoic or heterogeneous mass with distal glandular atrophy
  ▪ Double duct sign with pancreatic and common bile duct dilation if head lesion
  ▪ Hepatic metastases

- CDUS useful in tumor assessment
  - Tumor involvement of the celiac axis or superior mesenteric artery or vein or superior mesenteric vein thrombosis indicates unresectability
► Computed tomography
  - Heterogeneous pancreas tail mass on contrast-enhanced computed tomography (CECT) (arrow in Fig. 98.7)

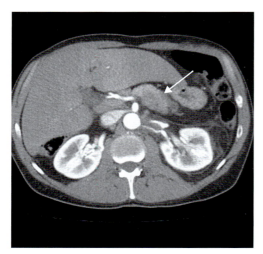

Fig. 98.7

► Positron emission tomography (PET) scan
  - Metabolic uptake in pancreatic mass (arrow in Fig. 98.8) and liver metastases on PET (arrows in Fig. 98.9)

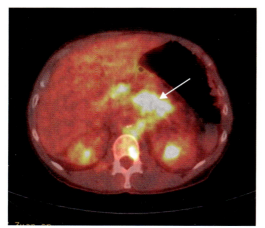

Fig. 98.8   Fig. 98.9

► Transabdominal or endoscopic ultrasound (EUS) used to guide biopsy of suspected tumor
► EUS, although invasive, is a useful modality for detection of even small pancreatic tumors with greater sensitivity/specificity than CT
► Focal pancreatitis may present as a hypoechoic mass; however, does not cause liver metastases
► Neuroendocrine tumors are usually vascular
► Serous or mucinous lesions have cystic component(s)
► Metastases and lymphoma suspected if the patient has a primary malignancy and widespread disease. Vascularity depends on the primary malignancy

Management

► The goal of imaging is staging and to determine potential for surgical resection
► CECT or MRI and PET are the modalities of choice for staging

- ▶ Pancreaticoduodenectomy (Whipple resection) is performed in cases amenable for surgical resection
- ▶ Palliative/adjuvant therapy includes radiation, chemotherapy, and endoscopic stenting to relieve obstruction of the biliary or pancreatic ducts

Further Reading

1. Shrikhande SV, Barreto SG, Goel M, et al. Multimodality imaging of pancreatic ductal adenocarcinoma: A review of the literature. *HPB (Oxford).* 2012; 14(10): 658–668.

Case 99

History

▶ 94-Year-old male with history of chronic lymphocytic leukemia presents with elevated liver function tests (Figs. 99.1–99.3)

Fig. 99.1

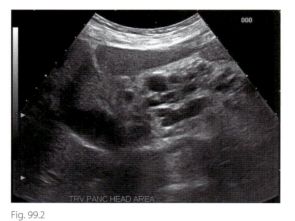

Fig. 99.2

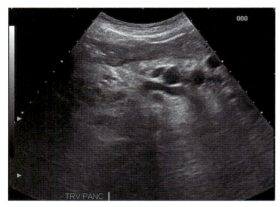

Fig. 99.3

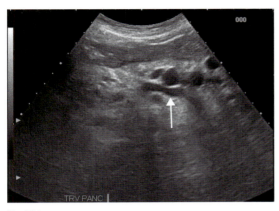

Fig. 99.4

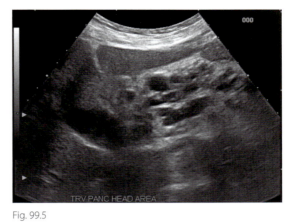

Fig. 99.5

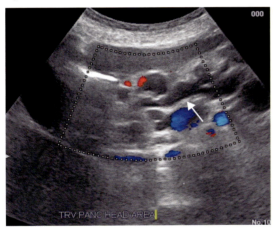

Fig. 99.6

Clinical Findings

▶ Dilated pancreatic duct (arrows in Figs. 99.4 and 99.6)
▶ Multiple cystic lesions throughout the pancreas, some communicating with the pancreatic duct (arrow in Figs. 99.4; Fig. 99.5)
▶ No flow on color Doppler US (Fig. 99.6)

Differential Diagnosis

▶ Pancreatic cysts
▶ Pancreatic pseudocyst
▶ Mucinous cystic pancreatic neoplasm (MCPN)
▶ Serous cystic pancreatic neoplasm (SCPN)

Teaching Points

▶ Intraductal papillary mucinous neoplasms arise in the pancreatic ducts, and they have slow growth rates and malignant potential. Peak incidence: 60–80 years, male > female
▶ Discovered incidentally due to nonspecific and indolent presentation; larger tumors may cause episodic epigastric pain
▶ Can occur in all segments of the pancreas, most commonly in the head, classified as main or side-branch pancreatic duct lesions
▶ Main duct lesions: diffuse ductal dilatation and gross mucin production and have a greater likelihood of malignancy
▶ Combined involvement of the main pancreatic duct and side branches may make it impossible to identify the primary site of origin
▶ US findings
  ▪ Unilocular or multilocular anechoic cysts
  ▪ Communication with duct difficult to see on US; however, it is possible

- Sometimes indistinguishable from surrounding pancreatic parenchyma due to echogenic mucin
- Heterogeneous cystic contents, thick walls/septae, and mural nodules are worrisome features for malignancy
▸ Endoscopic ultrasound (EUS) improves visualization and is used to guide biopsy or aspiration
▸ Communication with main pancreatic duct or a side-branch duct also demonstrated on CT or MR
- Multiple cystic lesions (long arrows in Fig. 99.7) communicating with the main pancreatic duct (short arrow in Fig. 99.7)

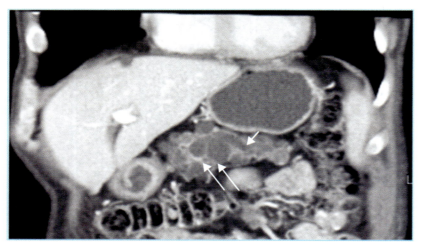

Fig. 99.7

▸ Simple pancreatic cysts
- In patients with adult polycystic disease and von Hippel–Lindau syndrome
▸ Pseudocysts
- Sequelae of chronic pancreatitis and may be associated with dilatation of the pancreatic duct and calcifications. May also occur outside the pancreas and demonstrate heterogeneous content and thick irregular walls
- Mucinous cystic pancreatic neoplasms
- Do not arise from the pancreatic ducts, often demonstrate internal loculations and have malignant potential
- Mostly in women (95%) aged 40-50 years
▸ Serous cystic pancreatic neoplasms
- May have many tiny cysts and central calcification and usually benign
- More common in women and most often in pancreatic head

Management

▸ EUS, CT, or MR best demonstrate communication with the pancreatic duct
▸ Surgical resection followed by surveillance imaging advised due to malignant potential
▸ Periodic monitoring in older patients/asymptomatic patients is an alternative approach

Further Reading

1. Prasad SR, Sahani D, Nasser S, et al. Intraductal papillary mucinous tumors of the pancreas. *Abdom Imaging*. 2003; 28(3): 357–365.

Case 100

History

► 68-Year-old woman presents with unexplained leukocytosis and left upper quadrant (LUQ) discomfort (Figs. 100.1–100.3)

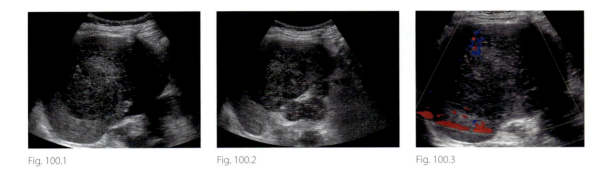

Fig. 100.1

Fig. 100.2

Fig. 100.3

Case 100 Diffuse B-Cell Lymphoma Involving the Spleen

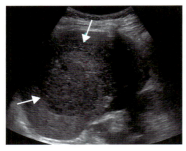

Fig. 100.4

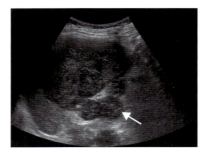

Fig. 100.5

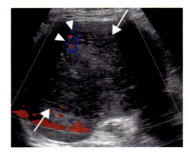

Fig. 100.6

Clinical Findings

▶ Large hypoechoic mass within the spleen (arrows in Fig. 100.4)
▶ Enlarged lymph nodes adjacent to the splenic hilum mimicking splenules (arrow in Fig. 100.5)
▶ Only minimal flow on color Doppler US (arrowheads in Fig. 100.6) and at the periphery of the mass (arrows in Fig. 100.6)

Differential Diagnosis

▶ Splenic hemangioma
▶ Splenic infarct
▶ Infectious processes including tuberculosis, atypical mycobacteria, fungal infections, and bacterial abscess
▶ Sarcoidosis
▶ Primary malignancies of the spleen such as angiosarcoma
▶ Metastases

Teaching Points

▶ Solid masses in the spleen are uncommon and often detected incidentally on cross-sectional imaging studies, although patients may present with left upper quadrant pain
▶ US appearance of splenic masses is generally nonspecific, and the etiology is best determined by the clinical context, history of known malignancy, and the presence of lesions in other organs
▶ Splenic lymphoma: four US patterns—typically hypoechoic and hypovascular
  ▪ Diffuse involvement with splenomegaly
  ▪ Small focal hypoechoic lesions < 3 cm
  ▪ Nodular focal large lesions > 3 cm
  ▪ Large bulky solid lesions
▶ CT
  ▪ Contrast-enhanced CT (CECT) shows the large splenic mass (arrowheads in Fig. 100.7) and additional adenopathy in the retroperitoneum, adjacent to the splenic hilum and the mediastinum (arrows in Fig. 100.7)

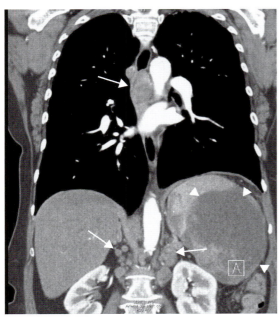

Fig. 100.7

- ▶ Hemangioma: common benign neoplasm of the spleen, often echogenic on US or of mixed echogenicity
- ▶ Splenic infarcts: wedge-shaped and peripheral in location and can mimic a focal mass
- ▶ Infectious processes: tuberculosis and atypical mycobacterial infections, as well as fungal infections, often affect immunocompromised patients and present as multiple, often small, lesions. Bacterial abscesses are more likely to result in single large debris containing cystic lesion. A reactive pleural effusion or ascites may be noted
- ▶ Sarcoidosis: calcified splenic granulomas; echogenic foci ± shadowing
- ▶ Splenic metastases: rarely isolated and are typically multiple. After leukemia and lymphoma, melanoma is the most common malignancy to involve the spleen
- ▶ Angiosarcoma: rare primary malignancy of the spleen with a heterogeneous US appearance and vascularity

Management

- ▶ Additional cross-sectional imaging such as CECT if the etiology of the splenic lesion is unclear, to determine if there are additional findings of malignancy or infection
- ▶ If masses are isolated to the spleen and tissue sampling is necessary, image-guided biopsy has been established as a safe method to obtain a definitive diagnosis without significant risk of bleeding

Further Reading

1. Goerg C, Schwerk WB, Goerg K. Sonography of focal lesions of the spleen. *Am J Roentgenol*. 1991; 156: 949–953.
2. Lucey BC, Boland GW, Maher MM, et al. Percutaneous nonvascular splenic intervention: A 10-year review. *Am J Roentgenol*. 2002; 179: 1591–1596.

Case 101

History

▶ 59-Year-old female with history of level 2 melanoma 5 years previously presents with abdominal pain and distension (Figs. 101.1–101.4)

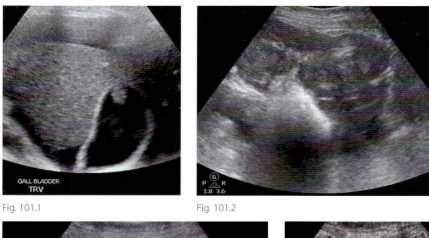

Fig. 101.1

Fig. 101.2

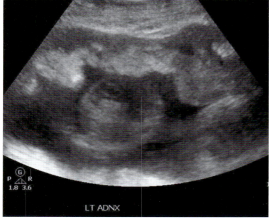

Fig. 101.3

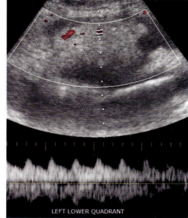

Fig. 101.4

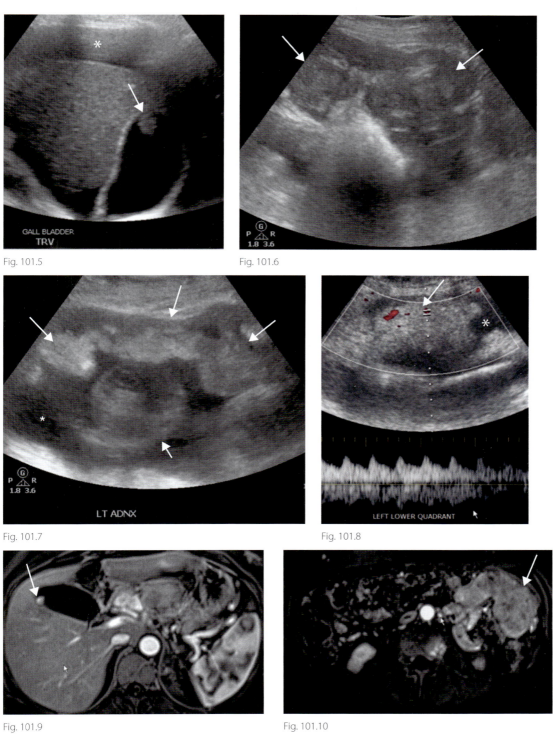

Fig. 101.5

Fig. 101.6

Fig. 101.7

Fig. 101.8

Fig. 101.9

Fig. 101.10

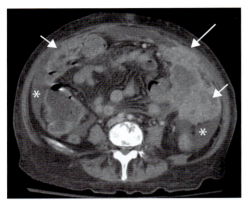

Fig. 101.11

Imaging Findings

▶ Nonmobile mural-based soft tissue nodule in gallbladder (arrow in Fig. 101.5)
▶ Multiple soft tissue masses along the anterior peritoneal surface (arrows in Fig. 101.6; long arrows in Fig. 101.7) as well as mesenteric masses (short arrow in Fig. 101.7; arrow in Fig. 101.8)
▶ Color and spectral Doppler image (Fig. 101.8) confirms arterial flow within the mesenteric mass
▶ Ascites with low-level internal echoes (asterisks in Figs. 101.5, 101.7, and 101.8)
▶ Axial T1-weighted fat sat contrast-enhanced MR images demonstrate enhancing mural nodule in gallbladder (arrow in Fig. 101.9) and left lower quadrant mass consistent with peritoneal carcinomatosis (arrow in Fig. 101.10)
▶ Axial contrast-enhanced CT scan demonstrating multiple peritoneal mestastases (short arrows in Fig. 101.11). The largest is invading the left anterior abdominal wall (long arrow). Ascites (asterisks)

Differential Diagnosis

▶ Primary peritoneal carcinoma including mesothelioma
▶ Chronic bacterial peritonitis
▶ Peritoneal tuberculosis

Teaching Points

▶ Most common primaries associated with intraperitoneal spread of malignancy include ovary, melanoma, gastrointestinal, lung, breast, and uterus
  ▪ Usually secondary to direct seeding or local invasion
  ▪ Can also occur from hematogenous or lymphatic spread of tumor
▶ Presentation: initially usually asymptomatic, but with progressive involvement and extensive disease, patients develop abdominal distention, pain, and bowel obstruction
▶ New onset of ascites in a cancer patient should prompt careful evaluation for peritoneal carcinomatosis
▶ US findings
  ▪ Ascites is very common in patients with peritoneal metastases: may be anechoic or contain low-level internal echoes due to proteinaceous material, debris, sloughed malignant cells, or hemorrhage; may be the only finding
  ▪ Peritoneal metastases are often so small that they are difficult to detect on imaging until > 1 cm
  ▪ Tumor implants on the visceral or parietal peritoneal surfaces generally appear as hypoechoic nodules or as sheet-like masses
  ▪ Peritoneal implants may be cystic in patients with cystic epithelial ovarian carcinomas
  ▪ May invade local structures (including the abdominal wall) and encase bowel
  ▪ Vascularity often detected on Doppler examination
  ▪ Tumor infiltrating the omentum generally appears as a plaque-like more echogenic mass, termed "omental cake," which may "float" in the ascites or become adherent to the anterior abdominal wall or bowel
  ▪ The pouch of Douglas is a common site for peritoneal deposits and is best evaluated with transvaginal US

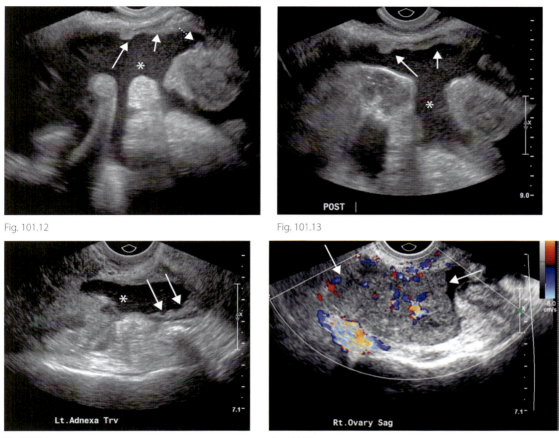

Fig. 101.12

Fig. 101.13

Fig. 101.14

Fig. 101.15

► Note nodular tumor implants along the anterior peritoneal surface (long arrows in Figs. 101.12 and 101.13) as well as on the surface of the bowel (dotted arrow in Fig 101.12).
► In addition, there are more plaque-like tumor implants along the anterior peritoneal surface (short arrows in Figs. 101.12 and 101.13) and in the pelvis (arrows in Fig. 101.14)
► Note large vascular tumor mass in the right adnexa (arrows in Fig. 101.15)
► Ascites with low-level echoes due to either malignant cells or hemorrhage is present (asterisks in Figs. 101.12–101.14)
► This patient had stage 3 ovarian carcinoma

In another patient with stage 3 ovarian carcinoma, both cystic (long arrows in Fig. 101.16) and solid (short arrows in Fig. 101.16) implants are demonstrated in the cul-de-sac on transvaginal imaging.

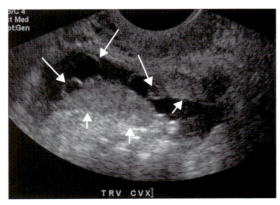

Fig. 101.16

- ▶ Mesothelioma: uncommon primary malignancy of peritoneum
  - ▪ Often history of asbestos exposure
  - ▪ Most common in middle-aged men
  - ▪ May mimic peritoneal carcinomatosis with plaque-like hypoechoic to echogenic peritoneal masses
  - ▪ Calcification rare (as opposed to pleural mesothelioma)
  - ▪ Variable amount of ascites, most prominent in patients with primary cystic peritoneal mesothelioma
- ▶ Peritoneal tuberculosis (TB): only 25% will have findings of TB on chest X-ray
  - ▪ Increased risk of peritoneal spread in patients with TB who have cirrhosis, HIV, diabetes, or underlying malignancy
  - ▪ May be indistinguishable from peritoneal carcinomatosis
  - ▪ Ascites
  - ▪ Cake-like omental/peritoneal thickening or masses
  - ▪ Intra-abdominal lymphadenopathy
- ▶ Chronic bacterial peritonitis: signs of infection, no history of malignancy
  - ▪ Ascites more likely to contain numerous septations and locules as well as low-level echoes
  - ▪ Less likely to be associated with peritoneal masses

Management

- ▶ US-guided peritoneal biopsy to confirm diagnosis because imaging appearance of peritoneal carcinomatosis, mesothelioma, and TB similar, especially if no known primary
- ▶ Treatment as per primary malignancy
- ▶ US guidance to drain ascites for symptomatic relief
- ▶ Peritoneal carcinomatosis portends poor prognosis with repeated bouts of symptomatic ascites and bowel obstruction

Further Reading

1. Levy AD, Shaw JC, Sobin LH. Secondary tumors and tumorlike lesions of the peritoneal cavity: Imaging features with pathologic correlation. *RadioGraphics*. 2009; 29(2): 347–373.
2. Savelli L, De Iaco P, Ceccaroni M, et al. Transvaginal sonographic features of peritoneal carcinomatosis. *Ultrasound Obstet Gynecol*. 2005; 26(5): 552–557.

History

► 69-Year-old male presents with abdominal pain and bloating (Figs. 102.1–102.4)

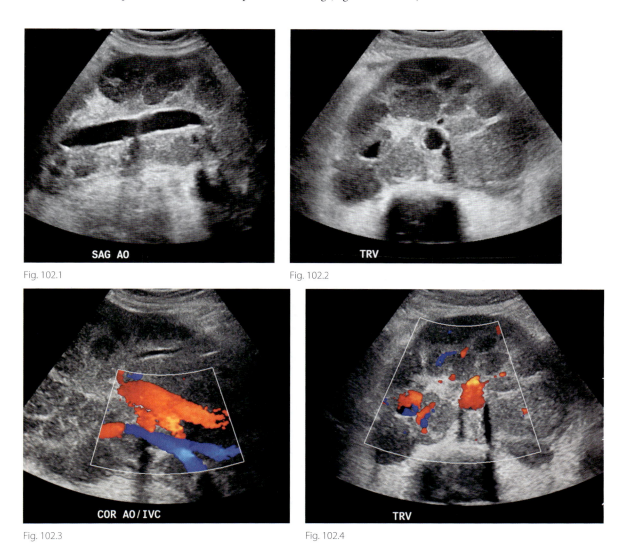

Fig. 102.1

Fig. 102.2

Fig. 102.3

Fig. 102.4

Case 102 Retroperitoneal Lymphadenopathy Secondary to Chronic Lymphocytic Leukemia

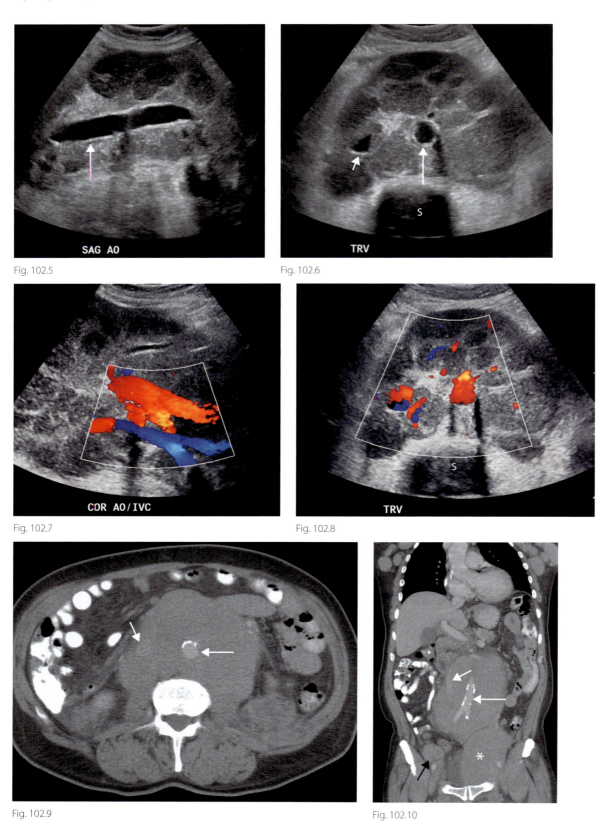

Fig. 102.5

Fig. 102.6

Fig. 102.7

Fig. 102.8

Fig. 102.9

Fig. 102.10

Imaging Findings

► Numerous hypoechoic round masses of varying sizes surround the aorta (arrow in Fig. 102.5 and long arrow in Fig. 102.6; red in Figs. 102.7 and 102.8) and inferior vena cava (IVC) (short arrow in Fig. 102.6; blue in Fig. 102.7; blue/red in Fig. 102.8) without compressing them, lifting the vessels off the spine (S in Figs. 102.6 and 102.8). This appearance has been termed the "sandwich sign" and "floating aorta sign" and is a classic appearance of retroperitoneal lymphadenopathy in lymphoma

► Axial (Fig. 102.9) and coronal (Fig. 102.10) contrast-enhanced CT images demonstrate a large mass encasing the IVC (short arrows) and calcified aorta (long arrows). Note extensive left iliac lymphadenopathy (asterisk in Fig. 102.10) and smaller right iliac lymph nodes (black arrow in Fig. 102.10). Individual lymph nodes are better delineated on the US images, appearing more homogeneous and confluent on the CT scan

Differential Diagnosis

► Retroperitoneal lymphadenopathy from metastatic carcinoma
► Infectious or inflammatory lymphadenopathy
► Retroperitoneal hemorrhage
► Retroperitoneal fibrosis
► Retroperitoneal mass, such as liposarcoma, leiomyosarcoma, or neurofibroma

Teaching Points

► Clinical presentation
  ■ Asymptomatic
  ■ Palpable mass (may be pulsatile due to encasement of aorta)
  ■ Back, abdominal, or flank pain
  ■ Renal failure due to ureteric obstruction
  ■ Abdominal distention or bloating
  ■ ± History of lymphoma or chronic leukemia
► US appearance of normal lymph nodes (LNs)
  ■ Ovoid or reniform shape
  ■ Smooth, thin, and regular hypoechoic peripheral cortex
  ■ Echogenic central hilum
  ■ Feeding vessels (single artery and vein) enter hilum with regular branching of distal vessels
► US appearance of abnormal LNs
  ■ Round, lobular, clustered, matted
  ■ May appear confluent as a homogeneous hypoechoic mass, but most often seen as multiple adjacent hypoechoic masses of varying sizes
  ■ Diffusely hypoechoic with obliteration of central echogenic hilum
  ■ Increased vascularity: numerous feeding vessels with irregular distal, asymmetric branching pattern
  ■ "Floating aorta" or "IVC sign": retroperitoneal LNs between aorta and IVC or between vessels and spine lift vessels off spine so that they appear to be floating in the abdomen
  ■ "Sandwich sign": lymphadenopathy surrounds vessels without compressing or narrowing them
  ■ Necrosis and calcification uncommon prior to treatment
► Overlap in US appearance of malignant, infectious, and inflammatory LNs
  ■ Large LN size and history of primary cancer favors malignancy
  ■ History of infection or inflammatory condition favors infectious or inflammatory etiology
► Retroperitoneal hemorrhage
  ■ Ill-defined or poorly marginated, avascular, heterogeneous mass usually lateral to aorta and IVC along psoas muscle
  ■ History of pain, hypotension, anticoagulation, decreasing hematocrit
  ■ Would not expect to see multiple distinct retroperitoneal masses
► Retroperitoneal fibrosis or chronic peri-aortitis
  ■ May present with renal obstruction or pain, often asymptomatic
  ■ Hypoechoic mass surrounding the aorta that may encase and displace ureters causing hydronephrosis
  ■ However, back wall of aorta usually spared and, therefore, does not lift aorta off spine
  ■ IVC usually spared
► Retroperitoneal masses, whether benign or malignant, are unlikely to be multiple or confluent, although they can grow quite large
  ■ Neurofibromas most likely to be multiple
  ■ Malignancies more likely to invade local structures
  ■ Such masses could lift aorta and IVC off spine, giving a similar "floating aorta" appearance

Management

► Retroperitoneal masses and/or lymphadenopathy should be fully evaluated with CT or MR to determine extent of disease, exclude invasion of adjacent structures, or search for a primary malignancy

  ▪ Scrotal US, especially in young males, is recommended to rule out testicular neoplasm

► In patients with lymphoma or chronic leukemia, positron emission tomography CT is performed to determine extent of disease and to follow response to treatment

► US is often used in the setting of renal failure to assess for hydronephrosis secondary to ureteral obstruction from retroperitoneal lymphadenopathy

Further Reading

1. Jing BS. Imaging of abdominal and pelvic lymph nodes in lymphoma. *Radiol Clin North Am*. 1990; 28: 801–831.
2. Sanyal R, Remer EM. Radiology of the retroperitoneum: Case based review. *Am J Roentgenol*. 2009; 192: S112–S117.
3. Moussavian B, Horrow MM. Retroperitoneal fibrosis. *Ultrasound Q*. 2009; 25: 89–91.
4. Rajiah P, Sinha R, Cuevas C, et al. Imaging of uncommon retroperitoneal masses. *RadioGraphics*. 2011; 31: 949–976.

History

▶ 67-Year-old female with right upper quadrant pain, anticoagulated with INR of 5 (Figs. 103.1–103.4)

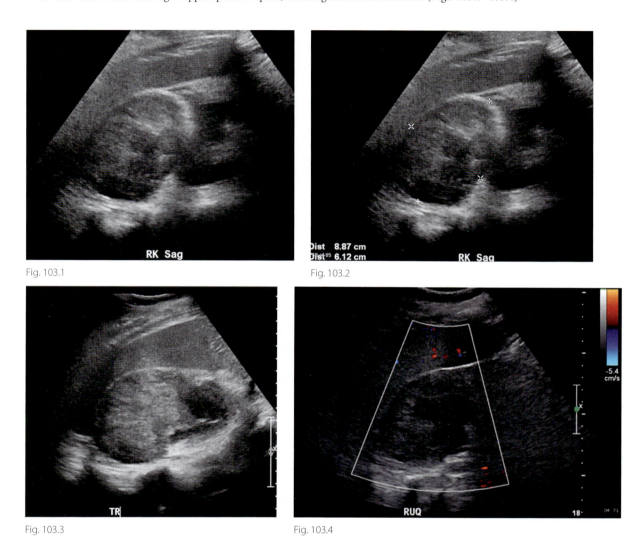

Fig. 103.1

Fig. 103.2

Fig. 103.3

Fig. 103.4

Case 103 Spontaneous Adrenal Hemorrhage

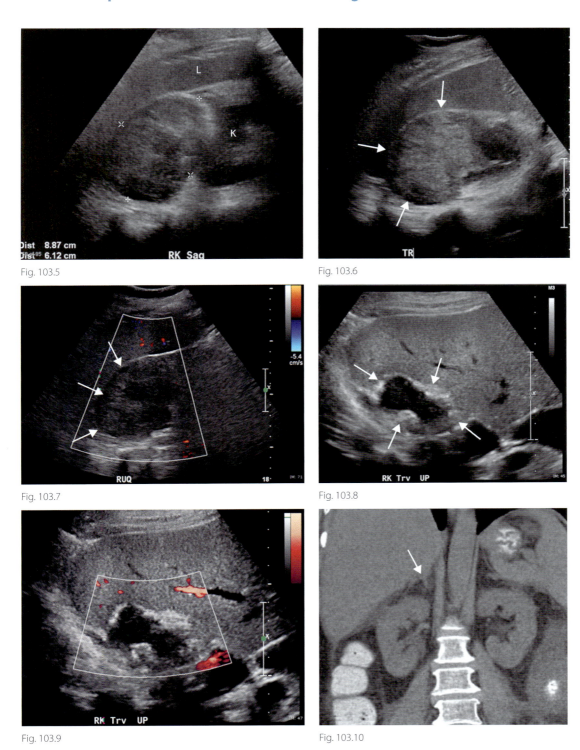

Fig. 103.5

Fig. 103.6

Fig. 103.7

Fig. 103.8

Fig. 103.9

Fig. 103.10

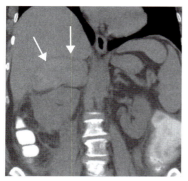

Fig. 103.11

Imaging Findings

▶ Large 8.9 × 6.1 cm heterogeneous predominantly echogenic mass (calipers in Fig. 103.5; arrows in Fig. 103.6) in the expected location of the right adrenal gland above the right kidney (K in Fig. 103.5) and inferior to the liver (L in Fig. 103.5). A thin echogenic fat plane separates the mass from the liver and most of the right kidney, which appears compressed and displaced inferiorly by the mass
▶ Color Doppler image demonstrates no detectable flow within the mass (arrows in Fig. 103.7)
▶ Findings are nonspecific but are consistent with adrenal hemorrhage
▶ Six-month follow-up US (Figs. 103.8 and 103.9) demonstrating evolution of the adrenal hematoma, which now appears centrally anechoic and cyst-like with an echogenic, irregular wall (arrows in Fig. 103.8) and no flow on power Doppler imaging (Fig. 103.9)
▶ Non contrast-enhanced coronal CT (NECT) scan of the abdomen 1 day prior to the initial US demonstrated a normal right adrenal gland (arrow in Fig. 103.10)
▶ Coronal NECT scan immediately following the initial US demonstrated a large oval well-circumscribed hyperattenuating mass in the location of the right adrenal gland (arrows in Fig. 103.11), consistent with acute adrenal hemorrhage

Differential Diagnosis

▶ Adrenal adenoma
▶ Adrenal metastases
▶ Adrenocortical carcinoma
▶ Adrenal myelolipoma

Teaching Points

▶ Adrenal hemorrhage is uncommon in adults
  ▪ Most common in neonates; incidence ranges from 1.7 to 3/1000 live births
  ▪ Male-to-female ratio of 2:1
▶ Presentation in adults: abdominal pain, palpable mass, adrenal insufficiency (if more than 90% of the gland is destroyed), may be asymptomatic
▶ Etiology
  ▪ Trauma
  ▪ Severe stress: surgery, sepsis, burns, hypotension, or steroids—possibly precipitated by adrenal vein thrombosis or spasm
  ▪ Anticoagulation therapy, disseminated intravascular coagulopathy, bleeding diathesis
  ▪ Neonatal stress
  ▪ Post liver transplantation
  ▪ Adrenal tumors
  ▪ Idiopathic
▶ Pathophysiology of nontraumatic adrenal hemorrhage: excessive production of ACTH increases adrenal arterial blood flow while venous drainage is limited due to venous spasm or thrombosis resulting in hemorrhage into the parenchyma
▶ US findings: Avascular adrenal mass, echogenicity depends on time course
  ▪ Acute: echogenic
  ▪ Subacute: more heterogeneous
  ▪ Chronic: anechoic and cyst-like areas ± mural calcifications
▶ Adrenal adenomas, metastases, pheochromocytomas: adrenal masses of variable echogenicity and heterogeneity, more likely to be vascular
  ▪ Adenomas most common adrenal mass: most often small (< 3 cm), hypoechoic or isoechoic to the liver, and asymptomatic, although may cause Cushing or Conn syndrome

- Metastases and pheochromocytomas more often larger and heterogeneous. Hemorrhagic metastases may be echogenic
- ▶ Adrenocortical carcinoma: rare, unilateral large (average > 6 cm) vascular mass that may invade into the adrenal/renal vein or inferior vena cava
- ▶ Adrenal myelolipoma: echogenic adrenal mass
  - May demonstrate posterior attenuation and distal speed propagation artifact due to fat content
  - Less echogenic if more myeloid tissue than fat

Management

- ▶ CT or MRI best imaging modalities for definitive diagnosis of adrenal masses, including adrenal hemorrhage
  - CT attenuation coefficients and signal intensity on MR sequences are specific for hemorrhage
- ▶ Prognosis dependent on cause rather than extent of adrenal hemorrhage, with overall mortality rate of 15%
- ▶ Follow-up imaging required to exclude underlying tumor as cause of bleed

Further Reading

1. Dunnick NR, Korobin M. Imaging of adrenal incidentalomas: Current status. *Am J Roentgenol*. 2002; 179: 559–568.
2. Mayo-Smith WW, Boland GW, Noto RB, et al. State-of-the-art adrenal imaging. *RadioGraphics*. 2001; 21: 995–1012.
3. Johnson PT, Horton KM, Fishman EK. Adrenal imaging with MDCT: Nonneoplastic disease. *Am J Roentgenol*. 2009; 193: 1128–1135.

History

▶ 51-Year-old female with abnormal liver function tests (Figs. 104.1–104.4)

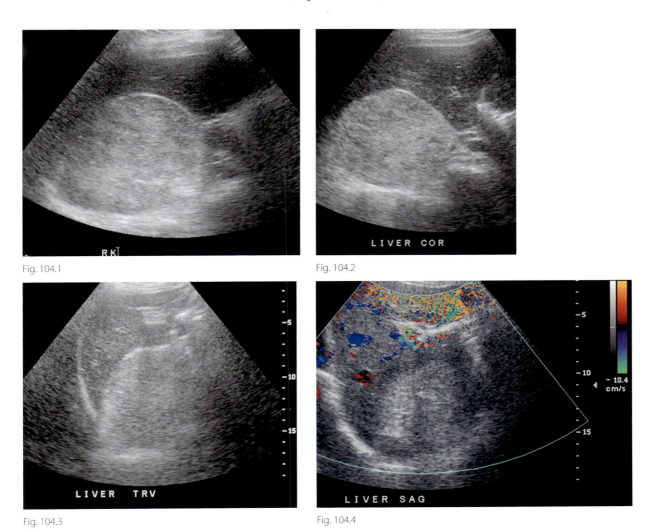

Fig. 104.1

Fig. 104.2

Fig. 104.3

Fig. 104.4

Case 104 Adrenal Myelolipoma

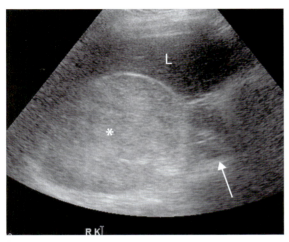

Fig. 104.5

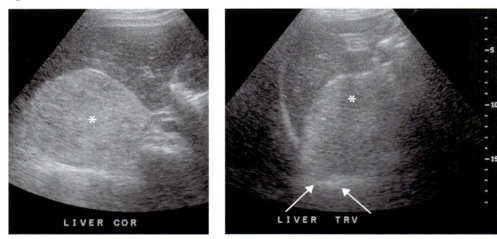

Fig. 104.6

Fig. 104.7

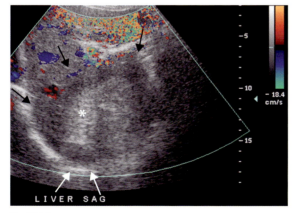

Fig. 104.8

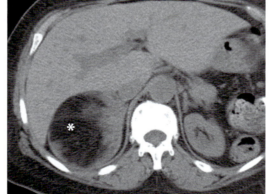

Fig. 104.9

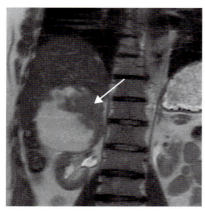

Fig. 104.10

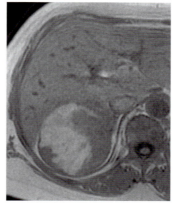

Fig. 104.11

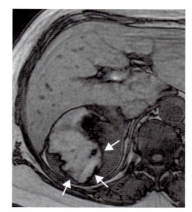

Fig. 104.12

Imaging Findings

▶ Large echogenic solid right adrenal mass (asterisks in Figs. 104.5–104.8) superior to the right kidney (arrow in Fig. 104.5) with echogenic fat plane separating the mass from the liver (L in Fig. 104.5)

▶ Medially, the mass is more hypoechoic (black arrows in Fig. 104.8)

▶ Note posterior attenuation as well as apparent disruption and posterior displacement of the diaphragm behind the mass due to "speed propagation artifact" (white arrows in Figs. 104.7 and 104.8). This artifact occurs because the sound waves propagate more slowly through fat (1450 m/s) than soft tissue (1540 m/s). Thus, it takes longer for the returning echoes to reach the transducer, causing the diaphragm to be displayed more posteriorly than its true position

▶ No significant vascularity is seen within the echogenic component of the mass on color Doppler US (Fig. 104.8)

▶ Axial non-contrast CT image reveals a large, well-defined, fat-containing right adrenal mass with more medial soft tissue component. The presence of fat is confirmed by the low attenuation of the mass (asterisk in Fig. 104.9) similar to the appearance of subcutaneous and retroperitoneal fat

▶ Coronal T2 HASTE (half-Fourier acquisition single-shot turbo spin-echo) MR image (Fig. 104.10) demonstrates the large right adrenal mass with both hyperintense and hypointense components. Bulk fat is hyperintense on T2-weighted images, and the more medial myeloid tissue is hypointense (arrow in Fig. 104.10). In (Fig. 104.11) and out (Fig. 104.12) of phase axial T1-weighted images demonstrating India ink artifact (black line at arrows in Fig. 104.12) at the boundary of the bulk fat and myeloid tissue

Differential Diagnosis

▶ Retroperitoneal lipoma/liposarcoma
▶ Adrenal hemorrhage
▶ Adrenal adenoma
▶ Adrenal metastases
▶ Adrenal carcinoma
▶ Pheochromocytoma

Teaching Points

▶ Adrenal myelolipomas are uncommon (< 0.2% prevalence), nonfunctioning benign tumors composed of mature adipocytes and myeloid elements
▶ Presentation
  ▪ Sixth and seventh decades
  ▪ No gender predilection
  ▪ Asymptomatic, often discovered incidentally
  ▪ Abdominal pain if complicated by hemorrhage/necrosis
▶ US findings consistent with the presence of fat in a suprarenal mass
  ▪ Markedly echogenic
  ▪ Posterior attenuation
  ▪ Speed propagation artifact: abrupt stepwise disruption and apparent posterior displacement of the diaphragm immediately behind the mass due to the slower propagation of sound through fat compared to soft tissue

- ► Additional US features
  - Usually homogeneous
  - However, echogenicity and heterogeneity variable depending on degree of myeloid (iso- or hypoechoic) and fatty (echogenic) tissue
  - Relatively avascular
  - Unilateral, 2–10 cm in size (most < 5 cm)
  - If large, may see cystic components, calcification, and hemorrhage
- ► Retroperitoneal lipoma or liposarcoma: echogenic retroperitoneal solid mass
  - Adrenal gland noted separately on MR or CT
  - Liposarcomas likely to be vascular and heterogeneous with infiltrative margins—variable depending on grade
- ► Adrenal hemorrhage: echogenic adrenal mass if hemorrhage acute
  - Subacute hemorrhage more heterogeneous
  - Avascular
  - No speed propagation artifact or posterior attenuation
- ► Adrenal adenoma: hypoechoic adrenal mass
  - Most common adrenal mass
  - Usually sharply marginated and isoechoic to liver
  - Contains intracellular rather than bulk fat, so unusual to be echogenic
- ► Adrenal metastases: echogenicity variable
  - Usually heterogeneous and isoechoic to liver; rarely homogeneously echogenic
  - Often bilateral
  - Fourth most common site of metastatic disease
- ► Adrenocortical carcinoma: large (> 4 cm) heterogeneous adrenal mass
  - Could be echogenic if complicated by hemorrhage, but unlikely to be homogeneous
  - Central necrosis and calcification common
  - Vascular
  - Associated with invasion of renal vein and inferior vena cava
  - No speed propagation artifact
- ► Pheochromocytoma: secretes catecholamines causing hypertension, tachycardia, and headache
  - Usually sharply marginated, vascular, heterogeneous, ± cystic areas
  - Unlikely to be homogeneously echogenic
  - Very high signal intensity on T2-weighted MR images

Management

- ► US findings of adrenal masses are generally nonspecific
- ► CT and MRI used to confirm location and to assess for fat within the lesion
- ► If imaging findings are indeterminate, percutaneous biopsy can be performed, unless there is clinical concern or biochemical evidence for pheochromocytoma
- ► Myelolipomas are surgically removed if symptomatic

Further Reading

1. Craig WD, Fanburg-Smith JC, Henry LR, et al. Fat-containing lesions of the retroperitoneum: Radiologic–pathologic correlation. *RadioGraphics*. 2009; 29: 261–290.
2. Cyran KM, Kenney PJ, Memel DS, et al. Adrenal myelolipoma. *Am J Roentgenol*. 1996; 166: 395–400.
3. Rao P, Kennedy PJ. Imaging and pathologic features of myelolipoma. *RadioGraphics*. 1997; 17: 1360–1371.

History

► 34-Year-old African American HIV-positive male with renal failure and right flank pain (Figs. 105.1–105.4)

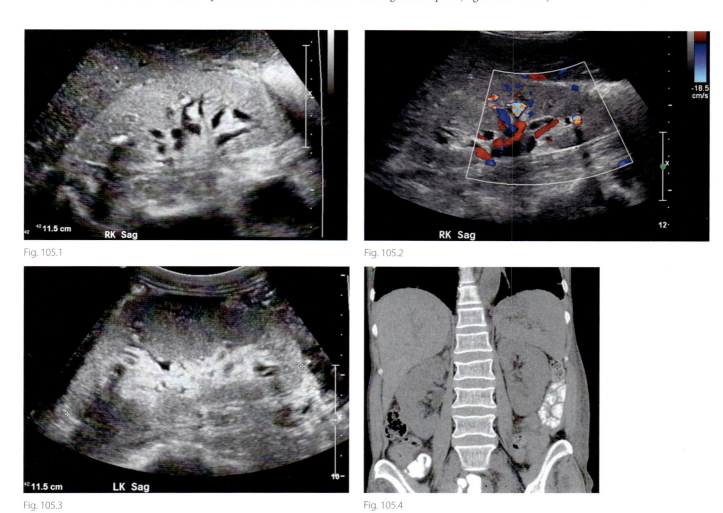

Fig. 105.1

Fig. 105.2

Fig. 105.3

Fig. 105.4

Case 105 Human Immunodeficiency Virus Nephropathy With Renal Calculi Secondary to Indinavir Antiviral Therapy

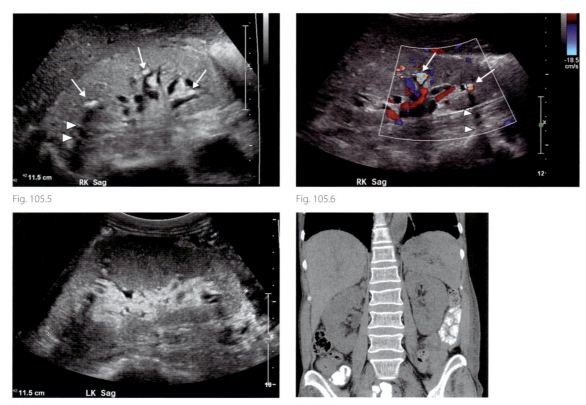

Fig. 105.5

Fig. 105.6

Fig. 105.7

Fig. 105.8

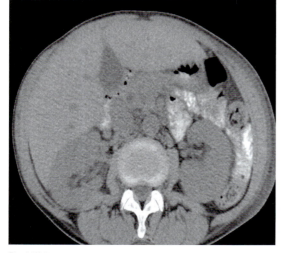

Fig. 105.9

Imaging Findings

▶ Both kidneys are normal to mildly enlarged (11.5 cm) in size for this small patient with diffusely increased cortical echogenicity (more echogenic than the liver parenchyma) and loss of corticomedullary differentiation (Figs. 105.5–105.7)

▶ Note several brightly echogenic nonobstructive right renal calculi (arrows in Fig. 105.5) some of which demonstrate posterior shadowing (arrowheads in Figs. 105.5 and 105.6) and twinkle artifact on color Doppler image (arrows in Fig. 105.6).

▶ There is mild dilatation of the right intrarenal collecting system due to obstruction from a stone in the right ureter (not shown)

▶ These stones are not calcified and are not radiopaque. Therefore, they are not visualized on nonenhanced CT scans (Figs. 105.8 and 105.9), consistent with stones secondary to indinavir antiviral therapy

Differential Diagnosis

▶ Medical renal disease
▶ Pyelonephritis
▶ Acute tubular necrosis (ATN)

Teaching Points

▶ Human immunodeficiency virus nephropathy (HIVAN): focal collapsing segmental glomerulosclerosis with microcystic tubular dilatation and interstitial inflammation
  ▪ More common in African American patients with advanced HIV infection
  ▪ 80% have CD4 count < 200
  ▪ More common in men than in women
  ▪ Increased mortality
  ▪ Incidence decreasing due to highly active antiretroviral therapy (HAART)
▶ Presentation: renal failure with nephrotic syndrome (proteinuria > 3.5 g/day)
▶ Protease inhibitors (antiviral medications) used to treat HIV infection may precipitate nephrolithiasis
  ▪ Indinavir has the highest incidence of crystalluria and nephrolithiasis, independent of renal function
  ▪ Stones secondary to indinavir and other protease inhibitors are not calcified or radiopaque and as such will not be identified on CT
  ▪ Best seen on US as echogenic foci with posterior shadowing on grayscale images and twinkle artifact on color Doppler imaging because echogenicity and posterior shadowing of renal calculi on US are not dependent on calcification
  ▪ Resolve after cessation of indinavir therapy
  ▪ Newer protease inhibitors have a significantly lower incidence of nephrolithiasis
▶ US findings of HIVAN: echogenic renal cortex (often patchy with echogenic bands)
  ▪ Normal sized to slightly enlarged kidneys
  ▪ Normal thickness of renal cortex
  ▪ Lack of decrease in renal size and cortical thickness helps differentiate HIVAN from other causes of chronic medical renal insufficiency, likely because renal failure develops relatively quickly
  ▪ Advanced: markedly echogenic renal cortex, loss of corticomedullary differentiation, obliteration of renal sinus fat, globular renal shape, pelvicaliceal thickening
▶ The renal cortex is considered echogenic if it is more echogenic than the liver, equal to or more echogenic than the spleen, or if there is increased corticomedullary differentiation with relatively hypoechoic renal pyramids (lost in advanced stages)
▶ Medical renal disease: increased renal cortical echogenicity
  ▪ Decreased renal size
  ▪ Thin renal cortex
  ▪ Decreased diastolic flow with elevated resistive indices (RIs) on spectral Doppler waveform
▶ Pyelonephritis: may see enlarged echogenic kidney
  ▪ More often heterogeneous or hypoechoic
  ▪ Rarely bilateral
  ▪ Associated with flank pain, pyuria, and fever
▶ ATN: kidneys are typically normal in size and echogenicity
  ▪ Decreased diastolic flow with elevated RIs on spectral Doppler waveform

Management

▶ Kidney biopsy is diagnostic in most cases
▶ HAART will prevent HIVAN and/or slow its progression

Further Reading

1. Atta MG, Longenecker JC, Fine DM, et al. Sonography as a predictor of human immunodeficiency virus-associated nephropathy. *J Ultrasound Med.* 2004; 23: 603–610.
2. Kalim S, Szczech LA, Wyatt CM. Acute kidney injury in HIV-infected patients. *Semin Nephrol.* 2008; 28: 556–562.
3. Symeonidou C, Standish R, Sahdev A, et al. Imaging and histopathologic features of HIV-related renal disease. *RadioGraphics.* 2008; 28: 1339–1354.

Case 106

History

▶ 62-Year-old female with psychiatric disorder presents with flank pain (Figs. 106.1–106.3)

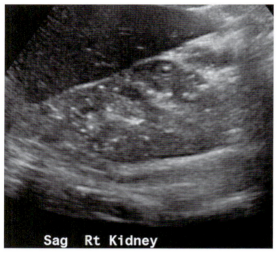

Fig. 106.1

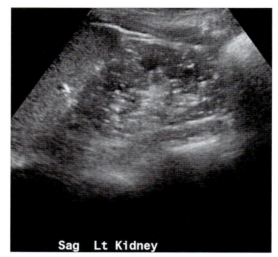

Fig. 106.2

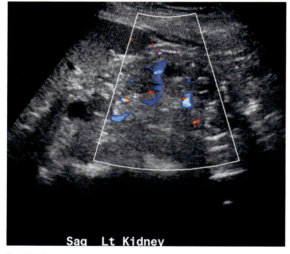

Fig. 106.3

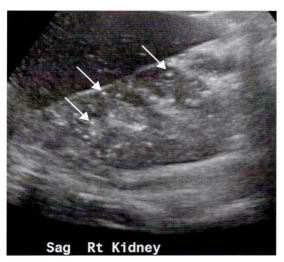

Fig. 106.4

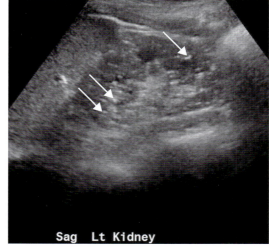

Fig. 106.5

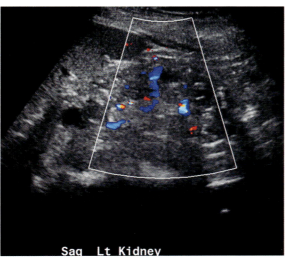

Fig. 106.6

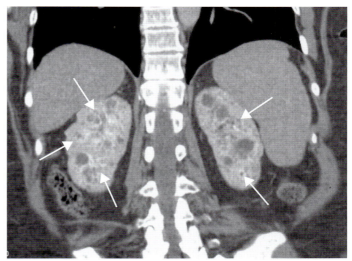

Fig. 106.7

Imaging Findings

► Both kidneys are normal in size
► There is no hydronephrosis
► The renal cortex is slightly echogenic (more echogenic than adjacent liver parenchyma), and several small anechoic renal cysts are noted bilaterally
► Color Doppler image of the left kidney (Fig. 106.6) reveals normal vascularity
► Note multiple bilateral tiny punctate brightly echogenic foci located in the renal cortex as well as in the renal pyramids (arrows in Figs. 106.4 and 106.5) that correspond to numerous tiny bilateral renal cysts on the corresponding coronal contrast-enhanced CT image (arrows in Fig. 106.7). Several larger cysts, but no calcifications, are also noted on the CT scan. Incidentally noted is splenomegaly

Differential Diagnosis

► Autosomal recessive polycystic kidney disease (ARPKD)
► Medullary cystic disease
► Vascular calcifications
► Renal calculi

Teaching Points

► Lithium-based medications are commonly used in treatment of bipolar disorder
► Nephrotoxicity is a well-known side effect of chronic lithium use
  ■ Mean time of onset is approximately 13 years; range, 2–25 years
  ■ Acute toxicity (rare)
  ■ Nephrogenic diabetes insipidus (NDI) (25–40%)
  ■ Chronic tubulointerstitial nephropathy (12%)
► In patients with NDI, the kidneys lose the ability to concentrate urine, and patients present with polyuria, nocturia, and polydipsia
► The hallmarks of lithium-induced chronic nephrotoxicity are tubular atrophy and interstitial fibrosis with the development of innumerable 1 to 2 mm cysts located primarily in the distal and collecting tubules
  ■ Cysts are found in both the cortex and the medulla
► US findings
  ■ Normal renal size and vascularity
  ■ Most other causes of chronic renal failure result in decreased renal size and cortical atrophy
  ■ Echogenic renal cortex
  ■ Multiple small cysts (usually < 2 cm in diameter)
  ■ Multiple punctate tiny nonshadowing bilateral echogenic foci involving both the medulla and the renal cortex likely due to specular reflections from tiny cortical cysts below the threshold for resolution with US and/or protein resorption granules within the tubules
    • May demonstrate ring-down artifact
    • Visualization requires a high-frequency transducer
  ■ Calcifications infrequently documented on correlative imaging studies or renal biopsy
► ARPKD: patients who live past infancy often present with manifestations of portal hypertension
  ■ Massively enlarged echogenic kidneys containing numerous small cysts
► Medullary cystic disease: patients present with salt-wasting nephropathy and renal failure
  ■ Small, echogenic kidneys with anechoic cysts < 1 cm in diameter in the renal pyramids and corticomedullary junction
► Vascular calcifications
  ■ Linear, occasionally punctate, echogenic foci located in the renal sinus as well as cortex
  ■ Less likely to be found in the renal pyramids
► Renal calculi
  ■ Round, punctate echogenic foci
  ■ Demonstration of posterior shadowing as well as twinkle artifact on color Doppler imaging dependent on size of calculi and placement of focal zone
  ■ Would not expect to see so many calculi or of such similarity in size
  ■ In addition, renal calculi would be expected to be found in the renal sinus and not in the renal cortex

Management

► NDI is reversible if the lithium is discontinued, and it may be managed by thiazide diuretics and nonsteroidal anti-inflammatory drugs
► Chronic renal disease is usually irreversible despite discontinuation of lithium therapy and is managed medically
  ■ Early detection is critical to prevent progression to end-stage renal disease
  ■ Lithium should be discontinued
  ■ However, only a minority of patients have been found to progress to end-stage renal disease

Further Reading

1. Di Salvo DN, Park J, Laing FC. Lithium nephropathy: Unique sonographic findings. *J Ultrasound Med*. 2012; 31: 637–644.
2. Karaosmanoğlu AD, Butros SR, Arellano R. Imaging findings of renal toxicity in patients on chronic lithium therapy. *Diagn Interv Radiol*. 2013; 19: 299–303.
3. Tuazon J, Casalino D, Syed E, et al. Lithium-associated kidney microcysts. *ScientificWorldJournal*. 2008; 8: 828–829.
4. van Melick EJ, Meinders AE, Hoffman TO, et al. Renal effects of long-term lithium therapy in the elderly: A cross-sectional study. *Int J Geriatr Psychiatry*. 2008; 23(7): 685–692.

History

▶ 51-Year-old paraplegic male presents with acute renal failure and sepsis (Figs. 107.1–107.4)

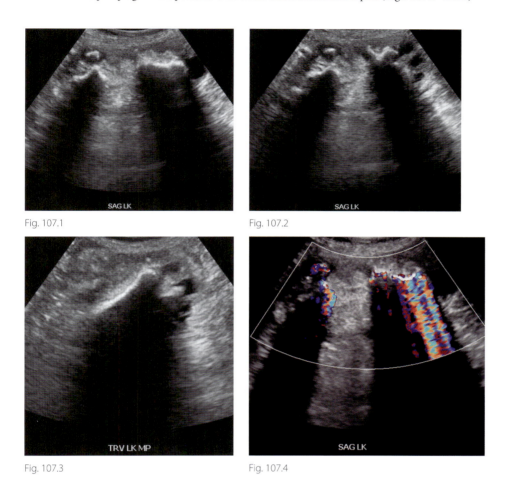

Fig. 107.1

Fig. 107.2

Fig. 107.3

Fig. 107.4

Case 107 Staghorn Calculus

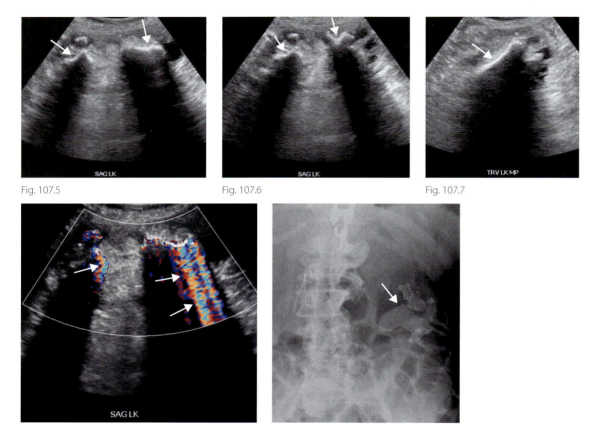

Fig. 107.5

Fig. 107.6

Fig. 107.7

Fig. 107.8

Fig. 107.9

Imaging Findings

► Brightly echogenic material (arrows in Figs. 107.5–107.7) with sharp distal shadowing fills the collecting system of the left kidney. Note scalloped margins (arrows in Figs. 107.5 and 107.6) conforming to the end of the calyces and long straight segment (arrow in Fig. 107.7) along the infundibula. The renal cortex is thin and echogenic. No hydronephrosis or fluid collections noted
► There is extensive twinkle artifact (arrows in Fig. 107.8) on color Doppler imaging
► Frontal abdominal radiograph demonstrates a large left staghorn calculus (arrow in Fig. 107.9). Note inferior vena cava filter and spinal rods

Differential Diagnosis

► Hyperparathyroidism and multiple renal calculi
► Air in urinary collecting system
► Emphysematous pyelonephritis
► Xanthogranulomatous pyelonephritis (XGP)

Teaching Points

► Renal calculi: increased incidence in older Caucasian males
  ▪ Predisposing conditions: dehydration, urinary tract stasis, hyperuricemia, hyperparathyroidism, hypercalciuria
  ▪ No cause identified in most patients
► A staghorn calculus is defined as a large, branching (antler-shaped) calculus filling the renal pelvis and extending into all or some of the calyces
  ▪ Composed of struvite (magnesium ammonium phosphate) ± calcium carbonite apatite
  ▪ Associated with urea splitting bacteria (*Proteus* >> *Pseudomonas, Morganella*, and *Klebsiella*)
  ▪ 3:1 female-to-male ratio
  ▪ Risk factors: previous urinary tract infection, nephrolithiasis (can act as nidus), obstruction, catheters, neurogenic bladder (diabetes, multiple sclerosis, spinal cord injury), urinary diversion

- Also called "infection stone" because bacteria are commonly present within the stone matrix causing the stone itself to be infected. Such bacteria are resistant to antibiotic therapy and are a source of recurrent infection
  - If not removed, will result in obstruction with risk of superinfection ± sepsis and destruction of the renal parenchyma
  - Predisposes to development of XGP
- ▶ Presentation: fever, hematuria, flank pain, sepsis
  - May be asymptomatic
- ▶ US findings
  - Echogenic mass filling much of the collecting system
  - Long straight margins along the infundibula and renal pelvis with scalloped or cuplike margins at end of calyces
  - Dense, sharp distal shadowing
  - Twinkle artifact on color Doppler US
- ▶ Hyperparathyroidism: can result in multiple, bilateral echogenic renal calculi with distal shadowing secondary to hypercalcemia
  - Calculi are typically smaller, separate, and do not conform to the shape of the collecting system
- ▶ Air in the urinary collecting system can occur secondary to infection (emphysematous pyelitis), reflux of air from the bladder following instrumentation, fistula with bowel, or trauma
  - Echogenic material filling the collecting system and conforming to shape
  - Dirty rather than sharp shadowing
  - Mobile
- ▶ Emphysematous pyelonephritis: echogenic foci with dirty shadowing consistent with air bubbles in the setting of a urinary tract infection
  - Air in renal parenchyma rather than collecting system
  - Not mobile
  - Patients acutely ill
- ▶ XGP: rare, chronic inflammatory process secondary to obstruction and infection of the collecting system with replacement of renal parenchyma by multiple cystic masses consisting of lipid-laden foamy macrophages (xanthoma cells), granulomas, and necrotic tissue
  - 80% have obstructing calculus, usually a staghorn calculus
  - Likely secondary to incomplete immune response to subacute bacterial infection
    - Most common organisms: *Proteus mirabilis* and *Escherichia coli*
  - Kidney eventually becomes nonfunctional
  - Inflammation can extend outside of kidney into perinephric fat, psoas muscle, adjacent organs, or subcutaneous tissues, better seen on CT
  - Most common in women, 40–60 years old, and diabetics
  - Clinical presentation
    - Abdominal or flank pain, fever, mass, weight loss, urinary tract infection, fistulas to the bowel or other organs, sinus tracts to skin surface
  - US findings
    - Enlarged kidney
    - Obstructing shadowing calculus in renal pelvis, often staghorn
    - Dilated collecting system, usually containing debris
    - Parenchyma replaced by multiple hypoechoic masses in varying stages of liquefaction, thinned residual parenchyma
    - Perinephric fluid collection or inflammatory tissue

26-Year-old woman 33 weeks pregnant presents with left flank pain. Note central echogenic, shadowing staghorn calculus (arrows in Figs. 107.10 and 107.11; long arrow in Fig. 107.12) in left kidney.

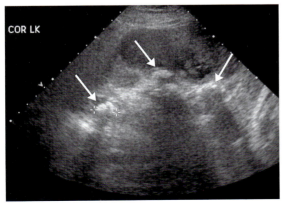

Fig. 107.10

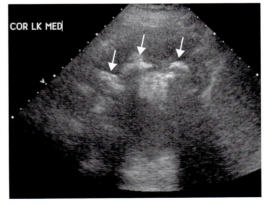

Fig. 107.11

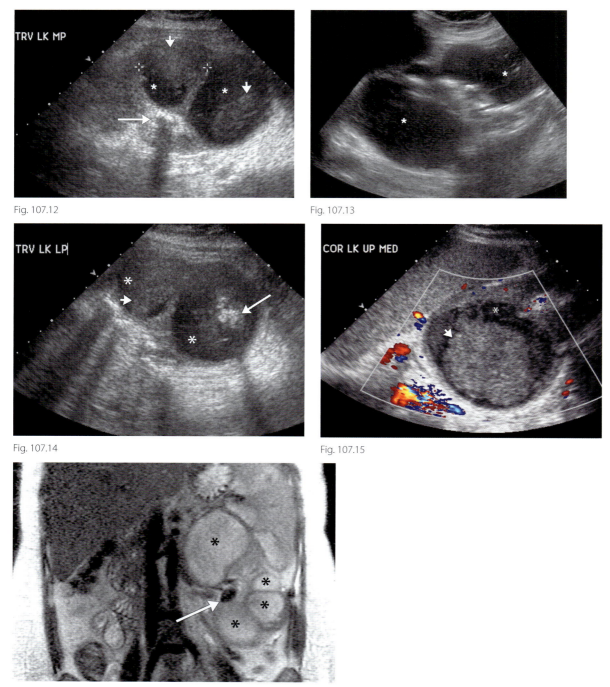

Fig. 107.12

Fig. 107.13

Fig. 107.14

Fig. 107.15

Fig. 107.16

► The peripheral renal cortex is largely replaced by multiple cystic masses (asterisks in Figs. 107.12–107.15), demonstrating increased through-transmission and a variable pattern of internal echoes with some appearing mass-like but avascular (short arrows in Figs. 107.12, 107.14, and 107.15) and other areas demonstrating punctate echogenic shadowing foci (long arrow in Fig. 107.14)

► Coronal T_2-weighted MRI image confirms replacement of left renal parenchyma by multiple cystic masses (asterisks in Fig. 107.16) with central low-signal (black) calculus (arrow)

► At surgery, the patient was found to have XGP
  ■ US mimics of XGP
    • Renal abscess: avascular, complex cystic renal mass, usually solitary, may have central calculus obstructing the collecting system, patients usually critically ill
    • Cystic renal cell carcinoma: complex cystic mass could appear similar to focal XGP but should show some central Doppler flow in solid component and no association with staghorn calculus

Management

▶ Staghorn calculus

  ▪ Complete removal necessary because residual fragments may regrow and harbor bacteria resulting in recurrent infection

▶ XGP

  ▪ Process irreversible, and nephrectomy treatment of choice

  ▪ Partial nephrectomy for localized XGP

Further Reading

1. Craig WD, Wagner BJ, Travis MD. Pyelonephritis: Radiologic–pathologic review. *RadioGraphics*. 2008; 28: 255–277.

2. Preminger GM, Assimos DG, Lingeman JE, et al. AUA guideline on management of staghorn calculi: Diagnosis and treatment recommendations. *J Urol*. 2005: 173: 1991–2000.

3. Kim JC. US and CT findings of xanthogranulomatous pyelonephritis. *Clin Imaging*. 2001; 25(2): 118–121.

Case 108

History

▶ 41-Year-old female referred for evaluation of left renal lesion seen on outside imaging study (Figs. 108.1–108.4)

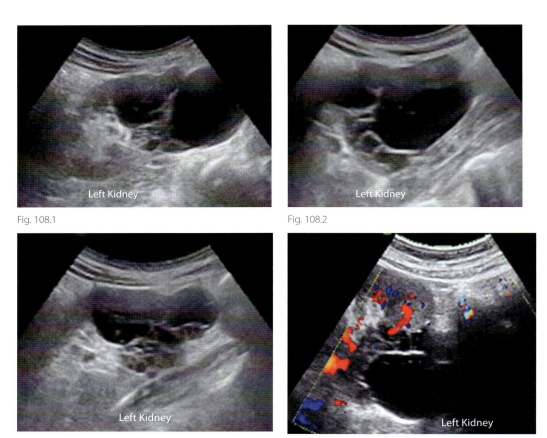

Fig. 108.1

Fig. 108.2

Fig. 108.3

Fig. 108.4

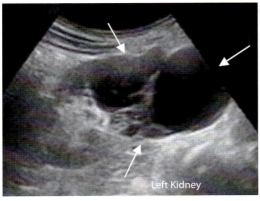

Fig. 108.5

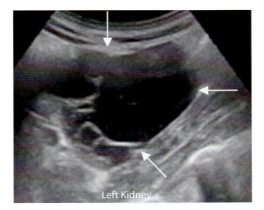

Fig. 108.6

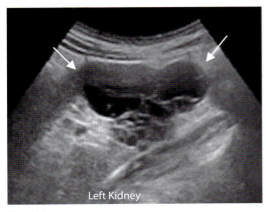

Fig. 108.7

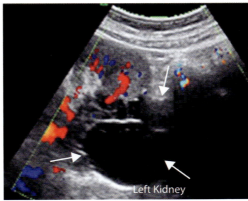

Fig. 108.8

Imaging Findings

► Multilocular cystic mass (arrows in Figs. 108.5–108.8) in the lower pole of the left kidney with numerous septations
► The locules vary in size with no communication between the cystic areas
► No solid component, although the septations appear more confluent superiorly
► No internal flow noted on color Doppler (Fig. 108.8)

Differential Diagnosis

► Localized cystic renal disease
► Cystic renal cell carcinoma
► Multicystic dysplastic kidney (MCDK)
► Mixed epithelial and stromal tumor (MEST)

Teaching Points

► Cystic nephroma (CN): rare, nonhereditary benign mixed mesenchymal and epithelial neoplasm
► Histology
   ▪ Multiple simple cysts and fibrous septa; no solid areas
   ▪ May be part of a spectrum of stromal epithelial lesions including MEST
   ▪ Some authors consider CN and MEST as variations of the same pathology
   ▪ Pathologic classification of renal neoplasms is currently under revision
► Incidence
   ▪ Children: males < 4 years of age
   ▪ Adults: most common in premenopausal women aged 40–60 years
      • Five times more common in females than males

- ► Presentation
  - ▪ Children: painless abdominal/flank mass
  - ▪ Adults: abdominal/flank pain, hematuria, or incidental finding
- ► US findings
  - ▪ Well-defined, relatively large (7–9 cm) cystic renal mass with numerous anechoic cysts of varying sizes
  - ▪ Often has a thick fibrous capsule
  - ▪ Cysts may herniate into renal pelvis or proximal ureter
  - ▪ Thin echogenic septations
  - ▪ ± Calcifications
  - ▪ Rarely, small cysts or confluent septations may mimic solid component
- ► Localized cystic renal disease
  - ▪ Rare, unlikely to progress
  - ▪ Collection of simple cysts of varying size separated by normal or atrophied renal parenchyma (most easily detected on CT or MR)
  - ▪ Unilateral
  - ▪ Not encapsulated
- ► Cystic renal cell carcinoma
  - ▪ May have a similar appearance, but typically has a solid component, thick, vascular septations, or mural calcification
- ► MCDK
  - ▪ Nonhereditary developmental disorder
  - ▪ Multiple noncommunicating cysts (often smaller than cysts in CN) replace the renal parenchyma
  - ▪ In adults, the kidney may completely regress or become quite small; persistent cysts may calcify
  - ▪ Usually involves entire kidney, but may be focal
    - • If focal, may have a similar appearance to CN
  - ▪ Associated with contralateral vesicoureteral reflux in up to 40% of cases
- ► MEST
  - ▪ Recently described benign mixed mesenchymal and epithelial tumor
  - ▪ Controversial as to whether this is a variation of CN or if the two entities are part of a spectrum of the same disease
  - ▪ Differs from CN histologically in that the lesion contains solid components, including tubules and stroma in addition to the cysts and fibrous septations
  - ▪ Perimenopausal women: 11 times more common in females, average age of 56 years
  - ▪ Associated with exogenous estrogen use and oral contraceptives
  - ▪ Best differentiated from CN on imaging by depiction of solid elements, enhancing mural nodules or septations, mural calcifications
    - • Significant overlap in appearance with cystic renal cell carcinomas

Management

- ► Difficult to confidently differentiate CN, MEST, and localized cystic renal disease from cystic renal cell carcinoma; hence, surgical excision often recommended
  - ▪ Contrast-enhanced CT or MR: identification of enhancing solid component increases concern for malignancy
  - ▪ Partial nephrectomy if benign diagnosis considered most likely
  - ▪ Local recurrence may occur

Further Reading

1. Silver IM, Boag AH, Soboleski DA. Best cases from the AFIP: Multilocular cystic renal tumor: Cystic nephroma. *RadioGraphics.* 2008; 28(4): 1221–1226.
2. Hopkins JK, Giles HW Jr, Wyatt-Ashmead J, et al. Best cases from the AFIP: Cystic nephroma. *RadioGraphics.* 2004; 24(2): 589–593.
3. Wood CG, Stromberg LJ, Harmath CB, et al. CT and MR imaging for evaluation of cystic renal lesions and diseases. *RadioGraphics.* 2015; 35: 125–141.
4. Srigley JR, Delahunt B, Eble JN, et al. The International Society of Urological Pathology (ISUP) Vancouver Classification of Renal Neoplasia. *Am J Surg Pathol.* 2013; 37: 1469–1489.

Case 109

History

▸ 71-Year-old diabetic male with rising creatinine (Figs. 109.1–109.4)

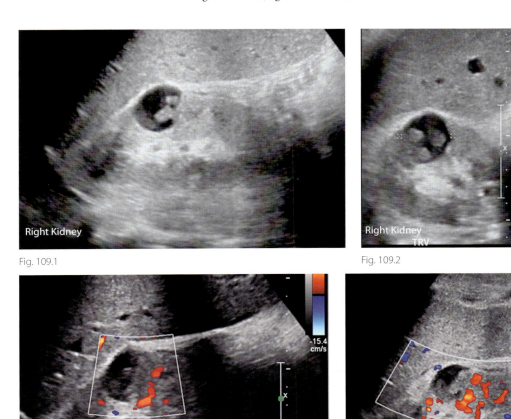

Fig. 109.1

Fig. 109.2

Fig. 109.3

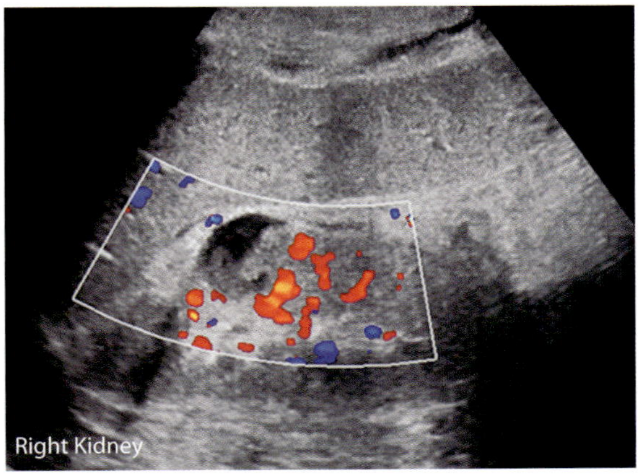

Fig. 109.4

Case 109 Complex (Hemorrhagic) Renal Cyst

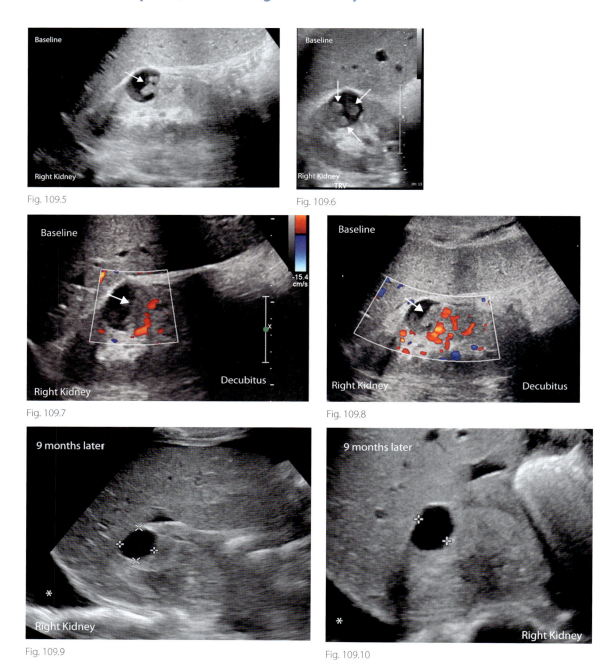

Fig. 109.5

Fig. 109.6

Fig. 109.7

Fig. 109.8

Fig. 109.9

Fig. 109.10

Imaging Findings

▶ Baseline grayscale images reveal several round, nodular components of moderate echogenicity (arrows in Figs. 109.5 and 109.6) within a right renal cyst (calipers in Fig. 109.6). Two of these appear mural based

▶ Color Doppler images obtained with the patient in the decubitus position demonstrate layering of the echogenic material (arrows in Figs. 109.7 and 109.8) and no detectable internal vascularity

▶ On follow-up examination obtained 9 months later, the right renal cyst appears completely anechoic (calipers in Figs. 109.9 and 109.10), most consistent with resolution of hemorrhage. Incidentally noted is a right pleural effusion (asterisks in Figs. 109.9 and 109.10)

Differential Diagnosis

► Cystic renal cell carcinoma (RCC)
► Renal abscess

Teaching Points

► Hemorrhage into renal cysts occurs either spontaneously or secondary to trauma
  ▪ Patients may present with abrupt and severe pain
  ▪ Many patients are asymptomatic
  ▪ Occurs in males more often than females
► US findings of hemorrhagic cysts
  ▪ Variable internal echogenicity depending on time course: anechoic, low-level echoes, occasionally echogenic
    • Diffuse internal echoes or focal clot
    • May have a reticular pattern similar to a hemorrhagic ovarian cyst

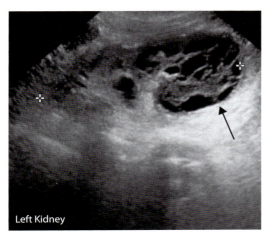

Fig. 109.11

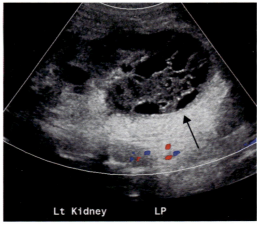

Fig. 109.12

This 54-Year-old female presented with acute flank pain. There is a complex cyst (arrows in Figs. 109.11 and 109.12) at the lower pole of the left kidney (calipers in Fig. 109.11) with a reticular pattern of fibrin stranding, confluent areas of homogeneous clot, and cystic spaces. Note increased through-transmission (increased brightness) deep to the cystic lesion. On color Doppler imaging (Fig. 109.12), no internal vascularity was noted. Hemorrhage within the cyst was confirmed on MR (not shown).
    • Clot may appear nodular
    • Layering of internal echoes with the patient in the decubitus position suggests that these echoes represent hemorrhage, debris, or pus rather than a solid tumor nodule
    • However, because hemorrhage into a cystic renal cell carcinoma could obscure visualization of the solid component, follow-up is recommended
    • A hemorrhagic cyst with diffuse, homogeneous internal echoes may mimic a solid lesion on grayscale imaging
  ▪ No internal vascularity
  ▪ Thin, regular wall
  ▪ Increased through-transmission
► Renal abscess
  ▪ Patients may present with flank pain, fever, and leukocytosis
  ▪ US findings
    • Round, cystic structure with internal echoes (diffuse, nodular—especially fungal balls—or layering)
    • Surrounding hyperemia
    • Thick or irregular wall
► Cystic RCC
  ▪ Complex cystic structure with solid vascular component

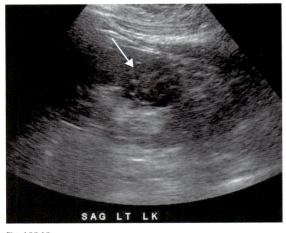

Fig. 109.13

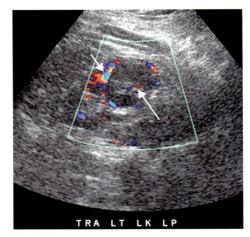

Fig. 109.14

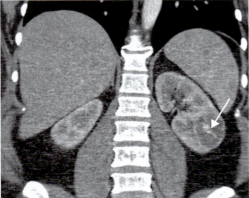

Fig. 109.15

This patient presented with acute kidney injury. Incidentally noted is a complex cyst at the lower pole of the left kidney with low-level internal echoes and septations (arrow in Fig. 109.13). The wall is vascular (short arrow in Fig. 109.14), and there is a small amount of internal vascularity (long arrow in Fig. 109.14). Coronal contrast-enhanced CT scan demonstrates enhancement of the septations (arrow in Fig. 109.15). Histology revealed a cystic papillary RCC.

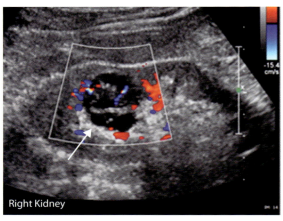

Fig. 109.16

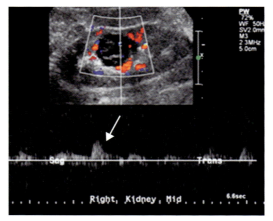

Fig. 109.17

Note complex right renal cyst (arrow in Fig. 109.16) with thick irregular, vascular septations on color Doppler image in a 67-year-old male. Arterial blood flow (arrow in Fig. 109.17). was detected on spectral Doppler within the septations These findings are strongly suspicious for a cystic RCC, which was proven at surgery.

Management

▶ Although the Bosniak classification of complex renal cysts on CT has never been proven to definitively correlate with the US appearance of complex renal cysts, it is often used as a general guideline for management

▶ Renal cysts are classified on CT according to the Bosniak classification as follows

- Type I: simple round cysts with water attenuation coefficient and imperceptible wall
- Type II: minimally complicated cysts—few thin (< 1 mm) septa, thin calcification, nonenhancing high-attenuation (proteinaceous or hemorrhagic fluid), < 3 cm, well marginated
- Type II F: probably benign (~25% malignant); more septations, thickened or enhancing septations or wall, thick calcification, hyperdense on CT without enhancement
- Type III: indeterminate (~54% malignant)—thick or multiple septations, mural nodules, hyperdense on CT
- Type IV: inevitably malignant—solid enhancing components

▶ Renal cysts with thick septations, calcifications, questionable solid or nodular components, or internal vascularity are further evaluated with contrast-enhanced CT or MR to search for solid components

- Contrast-enhanced US can also be used to evaluate for solid components, although it is not approved by the U.S. Food and Drug Administration for this use in the United States
- The presence of solid component suggests cystic RCC

▶ Renal cysts with few, thin septations, thin mural calcifications, and low-level internal echoes may be followed with US at 6-month intervals to ensure stability

Further Reading

1. Jamis-Dow CA, Choyke PL, Jennings SB, et al. Small (≤ 3 cm) renal masses: Detection with CT versus US and pathologic correlation. *Radiology.* 1996; 198: 785–788.
2. Israel GM, Bosniak MA. How I do it: Evaluating renal masses. *Radiology.* 2005; 236: 441–450.

Case 110

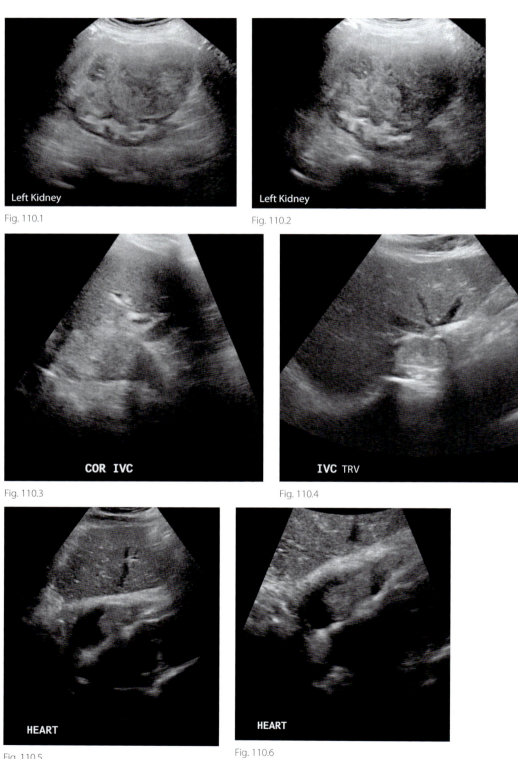

Fig. 110.1

Fig. 110.2

Fig. 110.3

Fig. 110.4

Fig. 110.5

Fig. 110.6

Case 110 Renal Cell Carcinoma With Tumor Thrombus Extending Into the Inferior Vena Cava and Right Atrium

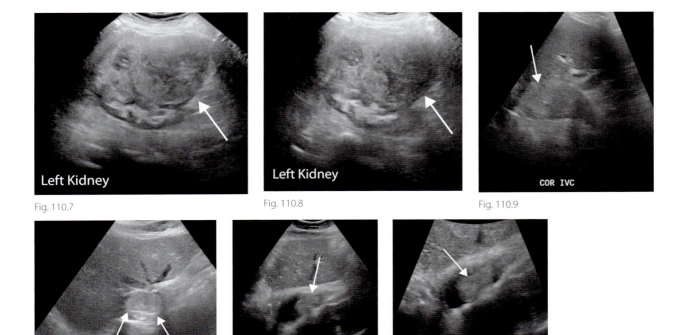

Fig. 110.7

Fig. 110.8

Fig. 110.9

Fig. 110.10

Fig. 110.11

Fig. 110.12

Imaging Findings

▶ Large heterogeneous predominantly echogenic exophytic mass (arrows in Figs. 110.7 and 110.8) arising from the lateral aspect of the left kidney

▶ Note relatively homogeneous echogenic tumor thrombus (arrows in Figs. 110.9 and 110.10) extending into and expanding the inferior vena cava (IVC) on coronal (Fig. 110.9) and transverse (Fig. 110.10) images. The left renal vein could not be visualized due to body habitus

▶ Tumor thrombus extends above the diaphragm into the right atrium (arrows in Figs. 110.11 and 110.12)

Differential Diagnosis

▶ Oncocytoma
▶ Angiomyolipoma (AML)
▶ Renal lymphoma
▶ Adrenocortical carcinoma

Teaching Points

▶ Renal cell carcinomas (RCCs) are malignant tumors derived from the renal tubular epithelium and account for approximately 90% of primary malignant adult renal neoplasms

▶ Presentation
  ▪ Sixth and seventh decades
  ▪ Male predilection of 2:1
  ▪ Asymptomatic, hematuria, flank pain, palpable mass, weight loss, anorexia, fatigue, and paraneoplastic syndromes such as fever, polycythemia, hypercalcemia, hypokalemia, and hypertension

▶ Risk factors
  ▪ Cigarette smoking, long-term dialysis, obesity, history of prior RCC, and genetic predisposition
  ▪ Increased incidence in patients with Von Hippel–Lindau syndrome and tuberous sclerosis

- ► US findings
  - ▪ Usually a solid renal mass, either homogeneous or heterogeneous, with variable echogenicity
  - ▪ Approximately 10% of small RCCs (< 3 cm) are echogenic, mimicking the US appearance of an AML
  - ▪ Cystic components, calcification, and hemorrhage may be observed
  - ▪ Internal vascularity
  - ▪ Invasion of renal vein/IVC is less commonly seen nowadays due to earlier detection of small RCCs as incidental finding on cross-sectional imaging
  - ▪ Synchronous tumors (1% bilateral, 10% multifocal)
- ► Imaging features of a solid renal mass will not reliably differentiate RCC from oncocytoma, lymphoma, or metastasis, although invasion of the renal vein or IVC would only be expected with an RCC
- ► Oncocytomas: benign renal adenomas composed of oncocytes—large epithelial cells with abundant granular eosinophilic cytoplasm containing numerous mitochondria
  - ▪ Peak incidence is at age 55 years
  - ▪ Male-to-female ratio of 2:1
  - ▪ Most patients are asymptomatic and present with an incidentally discovered mass on a CT, MR, or US of the abdomen
  - ▪ US findings are nonspecific
    - • Solid, homogeneous cortical renal mass with smooth, sharp margin that may be indistinguishable on US from a small (< 3 cm) RCC
    - • However, extremely unlikely to be as large as the renal mass illustrated previously
    - • Spoke-wheel pattern of radiating central vessels, although this pattern may occasionally be seen in RCCs as well
    - • Stellate central scar usually not visible on US and not a specific finding for oncocytoma on CT or MR because central necrosis in RCCs may have a similar appearance

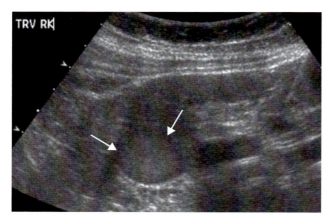

Fig. 110.13

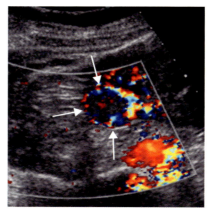

Fig. 110.14

55-Year-old male with acute kidney injury (Figs. 110.13 and 110.14). Note sharply marginated homogeneous slightly echogenic solid renal mass (arrows in Fig. 110.13) demonstrating internal vascularity on color Doppler with vessels radiating centrally (spoke-wheel pattern) (arrows in Fig. 110.14) in this patient with a surgically proven oncocytoma. By imaging features alone, this mass is indistinguishable from a RCC.

- ► Lymphoma: can present as a hypoechoic solid renal mass, but more often multiple hypoechoic masses of varying size
- ► Metastases: often multiple solid renal masses, variable echogenicity
- ► AML: Echogenic renal mass with posterior attenuation due to fat content
  - ▪ If large or hemorrhagic, may appear heterogeneous
  - ▪ No renal vein invasion
- ► Adrenocortical carcinoma: large heterogeneous suprarenal solid mass
  - ▪ Could compress and displace the kidney, but superior to kidney rather than a lateral mass as in this case
  - ▪ Absence of "claw sign" of renal parenchyma that often partially surrounds an exophytic RCC
  - ▪ Large tumors often invade renal vein and IVC with similar US appearance to RCC

Management

- ► Imaging cannot distinguish oncocytoma from a small RCC (< 3 cm)
- ► Hence, surgical resection generally recommended for solitary solid renal masses that do not show macroscopic fat on MR or CT
- ► However, advances in immunohistology may allow differentiation of benign from malignant renal lesions
  - ▪ Thus, biopsy increasingly performed in young, elderly, or sick patients with contraindications to surgery, especially with small solid renal lesions, because RCCs < 3 cm in diameter are unlikely to metastasize

- If oncocytoma considered likely histologically, renal sparing surgery or surveillance imaging can be considered
- CT and MRI used for staging RCCs
- Patients with RCCs should be evaluated for vascular invasion and synchronous tumors
  - Intraluminal tumor thrombus should be resected in operative candidates
  - Extent of vascular invasion determines surgical approach but does not affect prognosis
- Surgical excision is the gold standard treatment for nonmetastatic RCCs
- Partial nephrectomy or cryo/radiofrequency ablation are options for exophytic or small peripheral RCCs without vascular invasion or metastases

Acknowledgment

Figure 110.14 reprinted with permission from Pellerito JS and Polak JF. *Introduction to Vascular Sonography*, p. 528. Copyright Elsevier, 2012.

Further Reading

1. Ng CS, Wood CG, Silverman PM, et al. Renal cell carcinoma: Diagnosis, staging, and surveillance. *Am J Roentgenol.* 2008; 191: 1220–1232.
2. Sheth S, Scatarige JC, Horton KM, et al. Current concepts in the diagnosis and management of renal cell carcinoma: Role of multidetector CT and three-dimensional CT. *RadioGraphics.* 2001; 21(Suppl 1): S237–S254.
3. Kim HL, Zisman A, Han KR, et al. Prognostic significance of venous thrombus in renal cell carcinoma: Are renal vein and inferior vena cava involvement different? *J Urol.* 2004; 171: 588–591.
4. Lou L, Teng J, Lin X, et al. Ultrasonographic features of renal oncocytoma with histopathologic correlation. *J Clin Ultrasound.* 2014; 42(3): 129–133.

Case 111

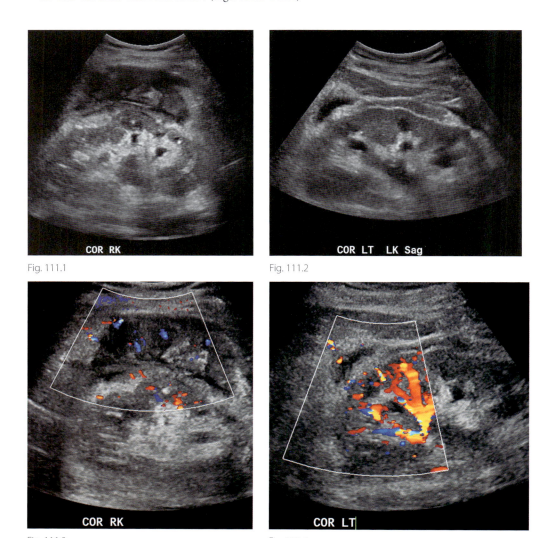

Fig. 111.1

Fig. 111.2

Fig. 111.3

Fig. 111.4

Case 111 Diffuse Large B-Cell Lymphoma Involving the Perinephric Space

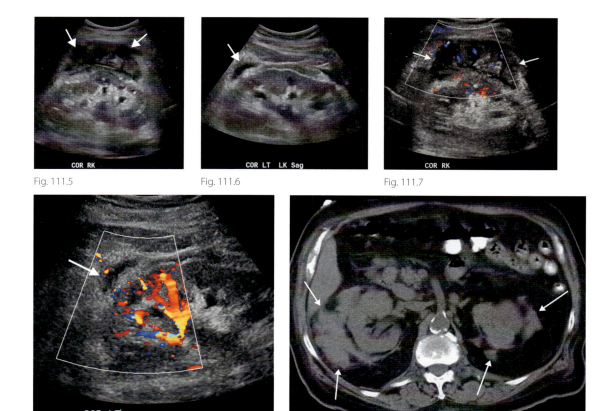

Fig. 111.5

Fig. 111.6

Fig. 111.7

Fig. 111.8

Fig. 111.9

Imaging Findings

▶ Bilateral vascular hypoechoic perinephric masses (arrows in Figs. 111.5–111.8), larger on the right
▶ Mild left hydronephrosis
▶ The renal cortex is thin and echogenic bilaterally
▶ Non contrast-enhanced CT scan confirms bilateral perinephric soft tissue masses (arrows in Fig. 111.9)

Differential Diagnosis

▶ Perinephric hematoma
▶ Perinephric abscess

Teaching Points

▶ Renal involvement with lymphoma is most commonly seen with widespread non-Hodgkin lymphoma and can be secondary to hematogenous spread or direct invasion
  ▪ Most often bilateral
▶ Autopsy data suggest renal involvement is present in approximately one-third of cases, although imaging findings are only detected in < 10% of patients
▶ Clinical presentation
  ▪ Most patients are asymptomatic
  ▪ Rarely, patients may present with flank pain, hematuria, constitutional symptoms, or acute renal failure
▶ Multiple US imaging patterns
  ▪ The kidneys may appear completely normal if the nodules are too small to visualize by US or if there is diffuse infiltration. Hence, a normal renal US appearance does not exclude the possibility of involvement of the kidneys by lymphoma
  ▪ Multiple homogeneous hypoechoic solid renal masses (Figs. 111.10 and 111.11): most common US pattern, usually bilateral, vascularity variable, indistinguishable from chloromas

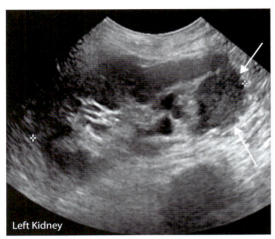

Fig. 111.10

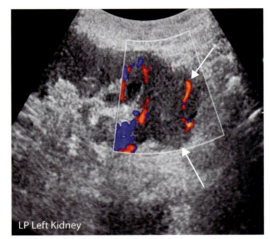

Fig. 111.11

Vascular mass (arrows in Figs. 111.10 and 111.11) isoechoic to the renal cortex at the lower pole of the left kidney (calipers in Fig. 111.10) in a second patient with large B-cell lymphoma. This patient had multiple bilateral cortical renal masses, although only one is shown.

- Solitary renal mass (rare)
- Masses do not typically invade the renal vein
- Diffuse infiltration resulting in an enlarged hypoechoic kidney that maintains its reniform shape but with disruption of the normal US architecture due to loss of corticomedullary differentiation and infiltration of the echogenic renal sinus
- Direct invasion from retroperitoneal lymphadenopathy, often at the renal hilum, which may lead to hydronephrosis and encase the blood vessels
- Perinephric soft tissue mass, as in the initial case, usually hypoechoic and vascular; often crescentic in shape (Figs. 111.5–115.8), which may appear to engulf the kidney
- Due to the homogeneous histology, these masses may be extremely hypoechoic, even anechoic, and therefore mimic renal cysts or perinephric fluid (Fig. 111.12), although there is usually no significant acoustic enhancement or increased through-transmission posterior to the mass

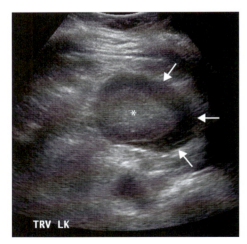

Fig. 111.12

Hypoechoic, nearly anechoic, soft tissue perinephric mass (arrows in Fig. 111.12) surrounding the lower pole of the kidney (asterisk) mimicking perinephric fluid in a third patient with renal lymphoma

- ▶ More heterogeneous appearance, including calcifications, may develop following treatment
- ▶ Perinephric hematoma
  - Heterogeneous perinephric mass, variable echogenicity
  - Avascular on color Doppler imaging

- ▶ Perinephric abscess
  - ▪ Heterogeneous perinephric mass, variable echogenicity
  - ▪ Peripheral but no internal vascularity
  - ▪ Unlikely to be bilateral
- ▶ Chloroma (granulocytic sarcoma)
  - ▪ Rare, extramedullary solid neoplasm of myeloid precursor cells encountered in the setting of hematological malignancies such as acute myelogenous leukemia (AML)
  - ▪ Skin, soft tissues, bone, and lymph nodes are the most commonly involved organs
  - ▪ May be diagnosed at presentation, during relapse, or may signify an impending blast crisis in patients with chronic myelogenous leukemia
  - ▪ Variable clinical presentation ranging from asymptomatic to mass effect
  - ▪ Nonspecific imaging findings, manifesting as either solid soft tissue masses (arrows in Figs. 111.13–111.15) or a diffuse infiltrative process
  - ▪ Imaging with fluorodeoxyglucose positron emission tomography (FDG-PET) demonstrates radiotracer uptake (Fig. 111.16)
  - ▪ Biopsy is often needed for final diagnosis
  - ▪ Differentiation from lymphoma, metastases, or multifocal renal cell carcinoma, which can all present as multiple hypoechoic solid renal masses, may be difficult, although a clinical history of AML with new renal masses should raise the possibility of chloroma

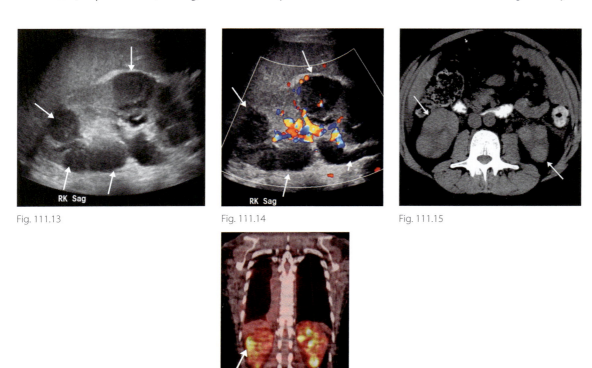

Fig. 111.13   Fig. 111.14   Fig. 111.15

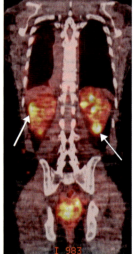

Fig. 111.16

54-Year-old female with renal failure and history of AML. There are bilateral hypoechoic minimally vascular renal masses (arrows in Fig. 111.13 and long arrows in Fig. 111.14). Note dilatation of proximal ureter (short arrow in Fig. 111.14). Axial non-contrast CT demonstrates multiple hyperattenuating renal masses (arrows in Fig. 111.15). Coronal fused image from a whole-body ^{18}F-FDG-PET CT demonstrates multifocal radiotracer uptake within the renal masses (arrows in Fig. 111.16).

Management

▶ Percutaneous core biopsy with flow cytometry is usually indicated if the imaging pattern suggests the presence of renal lymphoma

▶ Patients are treated with chemotherapy

Further Reading

1. Sheth S, Ali S, Fishman E. Imaging of renal lymphoma: Patterns of disease with pathologic correlation. *RadioGraphics*. 2006; 26: 1151–1168.
2. Paydas S, Zorludemir S, Ergin M. Granulocytic sarcoma: 32 cases and review of the literature. *Leukemia Lymphoma*. 2006; 47: 2527–2541.
3. Fritz J, Vogel W, Bares R, et al. Radiologic spectrum of extramedullary relapse of myelogenous leukemia in adults. *Am J Roentgenol*. 2007; 189: 209–218.

History

▶ 45-Year-old woman with fever and severe left flank pain (Figs. 112.1–112.4)

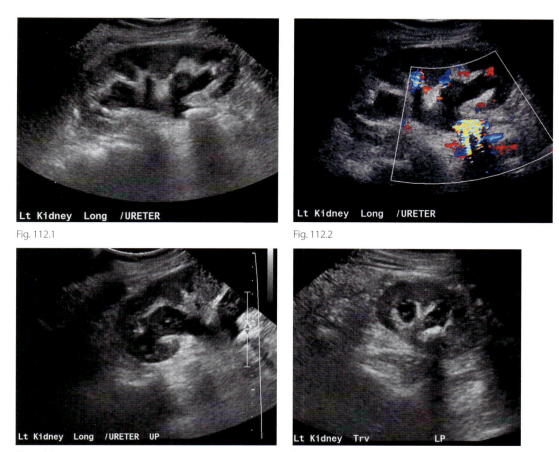

Fig. 112.1

Fig. 112.2

Fig. 112.3

Fig. 112.4

Case 112 Pyonephrosis

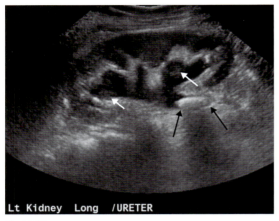

Fig. 112.5

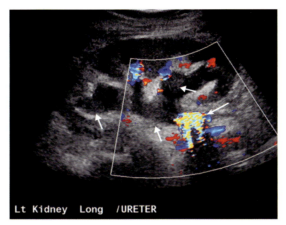

Fig. 112.6

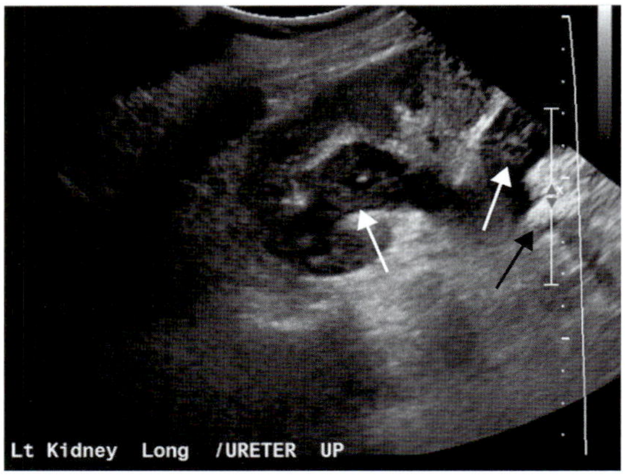

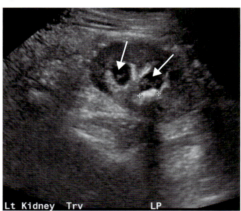

Fig. 112.7

Fig. 112.8

Imaging Findings

► Grayscale images of the left kidney demonstrate moderate hydronephrosis containing low-level echogenic material (white arrows in Figs. 112.5–112.8) as well as an obstructing brightly echogenic shadowing calculus (black arrows in Figs. 112.5 and 112.7) at the ureteropelvic junction (UPJ)

► Color Doppler sagittal image (Fig. 112.6) demonstrating twinkle artifact (black arrow with white rim) from the stone

► Transverse grayscale image (Figs. 112.8) demonstrates a second echogenic shadowing calculus (calipers)

Differential Diagnosis

► Hydronephrosis
► Artifact
► Blood clot or hemorrhage in renal collecting system
► Fungal balls in collecting system
► Urothelial carcinoma

Teaching Points

► Pyonephrosis: infected urine in an obstructed collecting system or "pus under pressure"
  ▪ Associated with pyelonephritis
  ▪ In young adults, UPJ obstruction and calculi are the most common causes of pyonephrosis
  ▪ In elderly patients, malignant ureteral obstruction is typically the predisposing factor
► Medical emergency: can lead to rapid destruction of renal parenchyma, bacteremia, and sepsis
► Presentation: fever, flank pain, pyuria
  ▪ Occasionally patients can be asymptomatic

- ► US is the imaging modality of choice for the diagnosis of pyonephrosis
- ► US findings
  - ▪ Dilatation of the pelvicaliceal system
  - ▪ Echogenic, mobile, avascular debris within collecting system (most reliable sign)

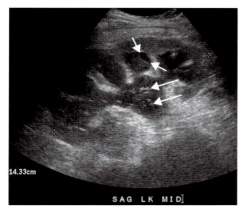

Fig. 112.9

55-Year-old male presenting with fever and flank pain. Sagittal grayscale image demonstrates moderate hydronephrosis. Low-level echoes are noted throughout the dilated collecting system that layer in one of the mid pole calyces (short arrows in Fig. 112.9). In addition, scattered punctate echogenic foci are noted, most prominent in the renal pelvis (long arrows in Fig. 112.9). Findings are nonspecific but can be seen with pyonephrosis, hemorrhage, or even debris.

- ▪ Layering or masslike collection of echoes less likely to be artifactual (Fig. 112.10)

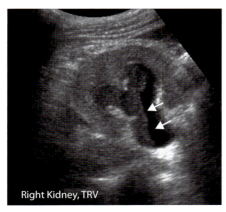

Fig. 112.10

This 48-year-old woman presented with right upper quadrant pain and fever. Note hypoechoic layering material in the dilated intrarenal collecting system (arrows in Fig. 112.10) on this transverse grayscale image of the right kidney consistent with layering purulent material given the clinical presentation.

- ► On CT, it is difficult to differentiate simple hydronephrosis from pyonephrosis
  - ▪ Indirect signs such as fluid–fluid levels, uroendothelial thickening, and renal parenchymal or perinephric inflammatory changes may point to the diagnosis
- ► Uncomplicated hydronephrosis
  - ▪ Urine in the collecting system is normally anechoic
- ► Artifact (false-positive diagnosis of pyonephrosis)
  - ▪ Low-level echoes mimicking pyonephrosis may be noted in obese patients due to poor penetration and attenuation of the US beam
  - ▪ Increasing the grayscale gain may create artifactual echoes within the collecting system
  - ▪ Layering or movement of echogenic material with change in patient position is helpful in differentiating artifactual from real echoes
- ► Blood clot or hemorrhage in collecting system
  - ▪ Echogenic material that may obstruct and dilate the collecting system
  - ▪ May mimic US appearance of pyonephrosis

- Associated with trauma (including renal biopsy), anticoagulation, renal mass
  - May be spontaneous
- Afebrile
► Fungal balls in the collecting system
  - Echogenic, nonshadowing, mobile, avascular soft tissue masses in the collecting system
  - May cause obstruction and hydronephrosis
► Urothelial carcinoma
  - Focal mass in collecting system that may cause obstruction
  - May be vascular
  - Associated with hematuria
  - Afebrile

Management

► Adjust gain and focal zone, maximize resolution (highest possible transducer frequency), and assess for mobility to ensure that intraluminal echoes are real and not artifactual
► Decompression of the renal collecting system with a percutaneous nephrostomy tube or urological retrograde nephroureterostomy tube placement
► Antibiotics

Further Reading

1. Demertzis J, Menias CO. State of the art: Imaging of renal infections. *Emerg Radiol*. 2007; 14: 13–22.
2. Vourganti S, Agarwal PK, Bodner DR, et al. Ultrasonographic evaluation of renal infections. *Radiol Clin North Am*. 2006; 44: 763–775.

History

▶ 29-Year-old pregnant female with left flank pain (Figs. 113.1–113.4)

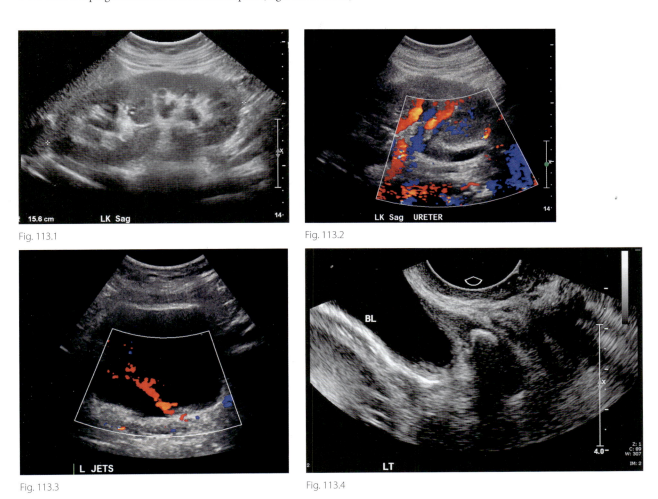

Fig. 113.1

Fig. 113.2

Fig. 113.3

Fig. 113.4

Case 113 Ureterovesical Junction Calculus

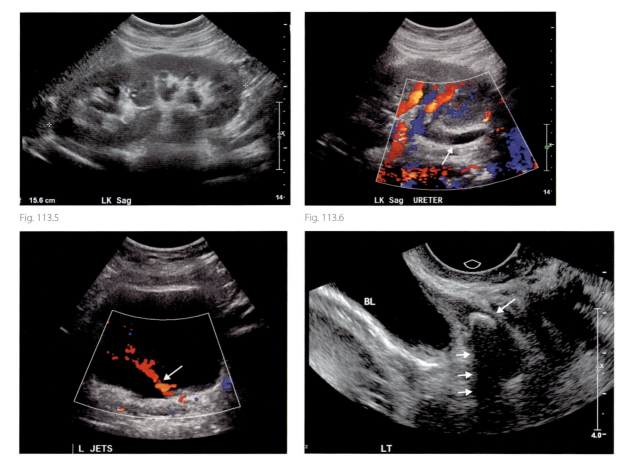

Fig. 113.5

Fig. 113.6

Fig. 113.7

Fig. 113.8

Imaging Findings

► Mild left hydronephrosis (Fig. 113.5) with dilated ureter (arrow in Fig. 113.6) and no stone seen on transabdominal images at ureterovesical junction (UVJ) ((Fig. 113.7)
► Color Doppler image of the bladder (Fig. 113.7) reveals a left ureteral jet (arrow)
► Transvaginal image demonstrating dilated distal left ureter and echogenic calculus (long arrow in (Fig. 113.8) near UVJ with posterior shadowing (short arrows). BL (bladder)
► The presence of the ureteral jet on color Doppler imaging (arrow in Fig. 113.7) indicates that the stone is not completely obstructing the distal ureter

Differential Diagnosis

► Physiologic hydronephrosis of pregnancy
► Ureteral or bladder urothelial carcinoma

Teaching Points

► Renal colic occurs in approximately 12% of the population in the United States
  ▪ Three times more common in men
► Risk factors
  ▪ Low fluid intake
  ▪ High animal fat diet

- Stasis: congenital UPJ obstruction, ureteroceles, tubular ectasia, polycystic kidney disease, calyceal diverticulum, horseshoe kidneys, cross-fused renal ectopia
- Crohn's disease
- Chemotherapy
▶ Symptomatic renal calculi occur in 1/1500 pregnancies
  - Incidence similar to that of nonpregnant female population
  - More common in second or third trimester
  - If stones do not pass, preterm labor, intractable pain, or urosepsis may occur
▶ Non-contrast CT is the gold standard for diagnosis of ureteral calculi in the general population, but it should be avoided during pregnancy due to risk of fetal exposure to ionizing radiation
▶ Hence, US is the imaging modality of choice for suspected renal colic in pregnancy, although US has limited sensitivity for the detection of calculi < 5 mm in diameter
▶ US findings
  - Dilatation of intrarenal collecting system
  - ± Dilatation of ureter
  - Echogenic calculus with posterior shadowing; depends on size, not composition; calculi are easiest to visualize on US when they are lodged at the UPJ and proximal ureter or at the UVJ and distal ureter, especially during pregnancy; it is very difficult to detect calculi in the mid ureter on US
  - Distal twinkle color Doppler artifact
  - Absence of ureteral jet on color Doppler suggests complete obstruction
▶ Transvaginal US evaluation of the distal ureters and UVJ is an important adjunct to transabdominal US due to better resolution with the higher frequency transvaginal probe
  - Note that in this case the stone in the distal ureter near the UVJ was only seen on transvaginal images and was not seen on the transabdominal US

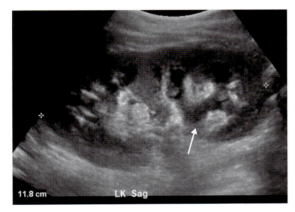

Fig. 113.9

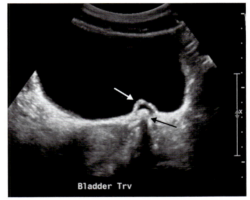

Fig. 113.10

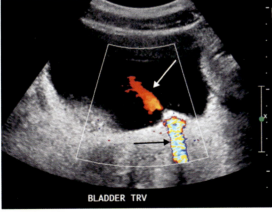

Fig. 113.11

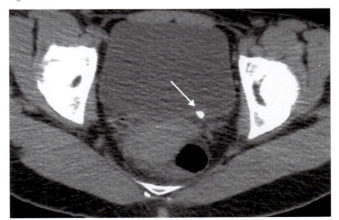

Fig. 113.12

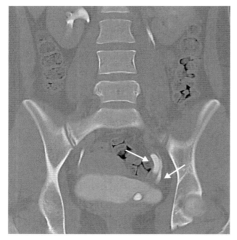

Fig. 113.13

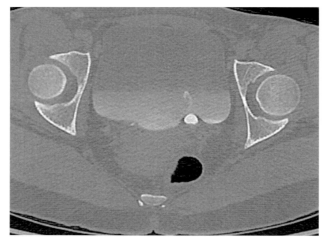

Fig. 113.14

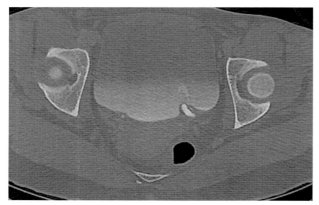

Fig. 113.15

This 24-year-old woman presented with left-sided flank pain. Imaging findings included the following:

▶ Note there is only dilatation of the collecting system of the lower pole of the left kidney (arrow in Fig. 113.9). The collecting system in the upper pole of the left kidney is not dilated

▶ Transabdominal views of the bladder (Fig. 113.10) reveal a small left ureterocele with a thin echogenic wall (white arrow) containing an echogenic calculus (black arrow) with posterior shadowing. Note that there is a small amount of anechoic fluid (urine) surrounding the calculus

▶ Color Doppler image (Fig. 113.11) demonstrates a left ureteral jet (white arrow) indicating that the stone is not completely obstructing the distal ureter. Note color mosaic or twinkle artifact (black arrow) posterior to the stone

▶ Axial non-contrast CT scan (Fig. 113.12) demonstrates the stone at the left UVJ (arrow)

▶ Following the administration of intravenous contrast, two distal left ureters (arrows in Fig. 113.13) can be seen on the coronal reformatted CT scan

▶ Axial contrast-enhanced CT images (Figs. 113.14 and 113.15) demonstrating two separate jets of contrast indicating that the two ureters insert into the bladder very close to each other and that neither is completely obstructed by the stone

▶ In patients with a duplicated collecting system, the Weigert–Meyer rule predicts that the upper pole moiety ureter will insert medially and inferiorly to the lower pole moiety ureter, which has a normal orthotopic insertion into the bladder. Reflux is more common into the lower pole ureter, whereas ureteroceles and obstruction occur more commonly at the ectopic insertion of the upper pole ureter. However, in this case, it was the lower pole moiety ureter that ended in a ureterocele

▶ Physiologic dilatation of the collecting system during pregnancy
　▪ Right-sided in 80–90% of cases, may be bilateral

▶ Urothelial carcinoma
　▪ May cause unilateral hydronephrosis due to tumor obstructing the ureter or UVJ
　▪ Tumor is typically hypoechoic and would not shadow
　▪ Blood flow is variably present on Doppler examination
　▪ Uncommon in this age group

Management

► MR urography or reduced-dose CT may also play a role in centers with experience using these technologies

► 70–80% of pregnant patients with ureteral calculi can be treated conservatively with analgesia, hydration, and antibiotics in the setting of infection

► If conservative therapy fails, ureteral stent placement, ureteroscopy, or percutaneous nephrostomy may be required

Further Reading

1. Isen K, Hatipoglu NK, Dedeoglu S, et al. Experience with the diagnosis and management of symptomatic ureteric stones during pregnancy. *Urology*. 2012; 79: 508–512.
2. Moesbergen TC, de Ryke RJ, Dunbar S, et al. Distal ureteral calculi: US follow-up. *Radiology*. 2011; 260: 575–580.

Case 114

History

► 47-Year-old male with gross hematuria (Figs. 114.1–114.4)

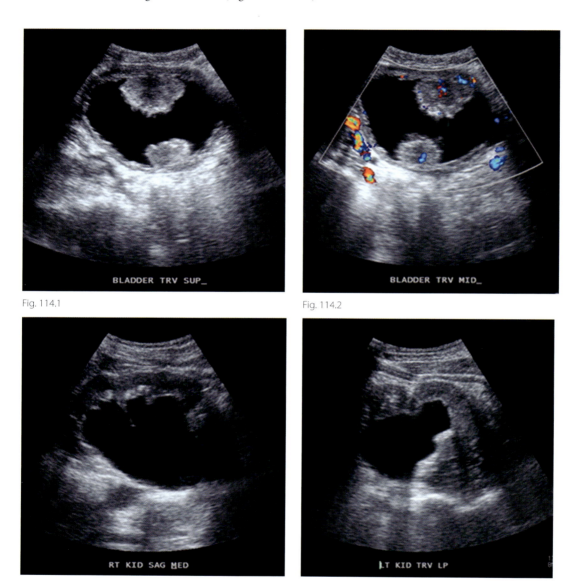

Fig. 114.1

Fig. 114.2

Fig. 114.3

Fig. 114.4

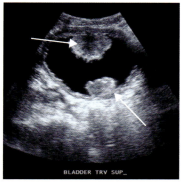
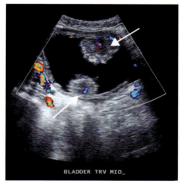
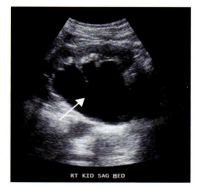

Fig. 114.5   Fig. 114.6   Fig. 114.7

Imaging Findings

▶ Two round, heterogeneous echogenic vascular masses arising from the dependent and nondependent bladder wall, respectively (arrows in Fig. 114.5). The bladder wall is diffusely thickened

▶ Minimal internal vascularity is present on color Doppler US (arrows in Fig. 114.6)

▶ Moderate to severe hydronephrosis (arrow in Fig. 114.7) is noted in both kidneys secondary to obstruction of the collecting system at the level of ureterovesicular junction. Only right kidney is shown here

Differential Diagnosis

▶ Bladder metastasis or direct invasion by adjacent tumor
  ▪ Prostate or cervical cancer, most commonly
▶ Clot, debris, fungus ball
▶ Benign bladder masses
  ▪ Leiomyoma, paraganglioma, lipoma, papilloma, cystitis cystica, neurofibroma
▶ Inflammatory fibrous pseudotumor

Teaching Points

▶ More than 70,000 new cases of bladder cancer are diagnosed yearly
▶ Classic presentation: painless hematuria, dysuria, urgency, increased frequency or pelvic pain
▶ 3:1 male-to-female ratio
▶ Most frequent histologic type is transitional cell carcinoma, often located at trigone or along lateral and posterior bladder wall, followed by squamous cell and adenocarcinoma
▶ Bladder masses may be incidentally found during sonographic evaluation of the kidneys or bladder for other indications
▶ Contrast-enhanced CT and/or MRI better demonstrate extent of involvement
▶ CT image through the bladder confirms the two large bladder masses (arrows in Fig. 114.8). Note thickening of the bladder wall and dystrophic calcifications in addition to clot and debris

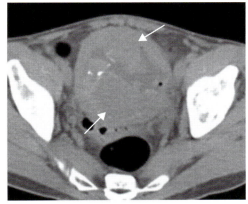

Fig. 114.8

- Important to distinguish between solid mass and hemorrhage/clot, particularly in setting of hematuria
  - Imaging should be performed with the bladder well distended
- Internal vascularity suggests neoplasm
- Clot/debris/fungus balls: typically dependent and often mobile, although can be adherent to bladder wall. No internal vascularity should be present (arrows in Fig 114.9 and Fig. 114.110)
  - Often associated with hemorrhagic cystitis and hydroureteronephrosis, likely secondary to bladder outlet or ureterovescicle obstruction by blood products (Fig. 114.11)

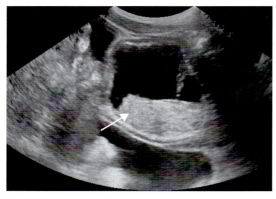

Fig. 114.9

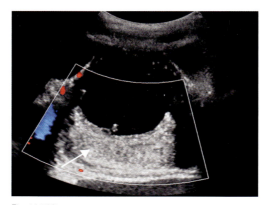

Fig. 114.10

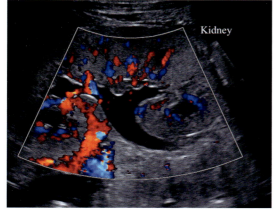

Fig. 114.11

- Bladder metastases: rare, occur with melanoma, gastric, lung, and breast cancer. Have a nonspecific solid US appearance
- Benign bladder masses have a nonspecific US appearance, usually presenting as solid nodules with or without vascularity
- Inflammatory fibrous pseudotumor is a rare benign proliferative lesion of the submucosa with a nonspecific radiologic appearance

Management

- Contrast-enhanced CT or MRI to delineate the presence of enhancing tissue and extent of disease (i.e., circumferential infiltration and extension through bladder wall)
- Cystoscopy with tissue biopsy for diagnosis and local staging
  - Some lesions can be resected transurethrally
- Clinical staging with combination of cystoscopy/biopsy findings and contrast-enhanced CT/MR imaging to evaluate for distant disease or synchronous lesions (i.e., ureter, renal pelvis)

Further Reading

1. Wong-You-Cheong JJ, Woodward PJ, Manning MA, et al. Inflammatory and nonneoplastic bladder masses: Radiologic–pathologic correlation. *RadioGraphics*. 2006; 26: 1847–1868.
2. Wong-You-Cheong JJ, Woodward PJ, Manning MA, et al. Neoplasms of the urinary bladder: Radiologic–pathologic correlation. *RadioGraphics*. 2006; 26: 553–580.

History

► 54-Year-old male with elevated transaminase and nausea (Figs. 115.1–115.4)

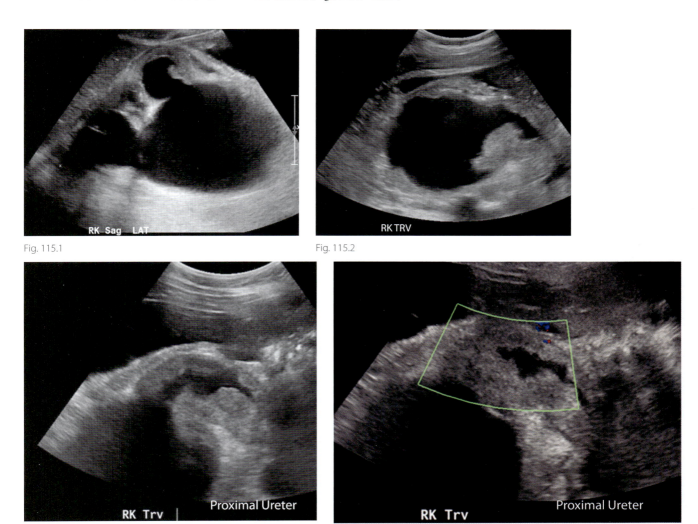

Fig. 115.1

Fig. 115.2

Fig. 115.3

Fig. 115.4

Case 115 Urothelial Carcinoma of the Ureter

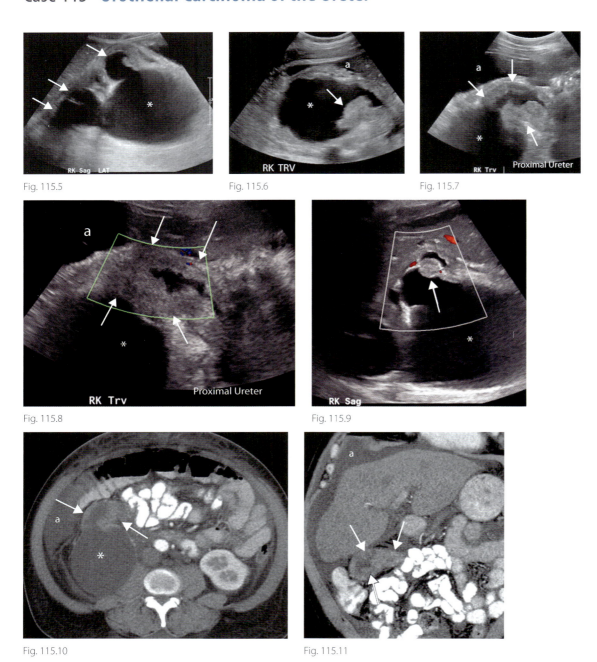

Fig. 115.5

Fig. 115.6

Fig. 115.7

Fig. 115.8

Fig. 115.9

Fig. 115.10

Fig. 115.11

Imaging Findings

▶ Severe right hydronephrosis with massive dilatation of the renal pelvis (asterisks in Figs. 115.5–115.9) and calyces (arrows in Fig. 115.5) consistent with right ureteropelvic junction (UPJ) obstruction

▶ Nodular soft tissue mass causing circumferential thickening of the wall of the proximal right ureter (arrows in Figs. 115.7 and 115.8) extending into the renal pelvis (arrow in Fig. 115.6)

▶ A very small amount of flow is noted on color Doppler imaging (Fig. 115.8)

▶ Note small amount of ascites ("a" in Figs. 115.6–115.8)

▶ Synchronous smaller, round avascular tumor (arrow in Fig. 115.9)

▶ Axial (Fig. 115.10) and coronal (Fig. 115.11) contrast-enhanced CT scans confirm findings: severe UPJ obstruction (asterisk in Fig. 115.10) due to infiltrating soft tissue mass in the proximal right ureter (arrows in Figs. 115.10 and 115.11). Ascites (a in Figs. 115.10 and 115.11)

Differential Diagnosis

► Lymphoma
► Renal tuberculosis
► Blood clot, pus, or fungal ball in the collecting system

Teaching Points

► Urothelial carcinomas, previously termed transitional cell carcinoma, are malignant tumors derived from the urothelium
  ▪ Can arise throughout the collecting system, including the calyces, renal pelvis, ureter, or bladder
  ▪ Often multifocal
  ▪ Account for approximately 5% of genitourinary tumors
  ▪ Incidence is increasing
► Presentation
  ▪ Elderly, peak incidence seventh decade
  ▪ Male predilection of 3:1
  ▪ Hematuria, dull or colicky flank pain, asymptomatic
► Clinical course
  ▪ Usual pattern of tumor spread is by local invasion or to regional lymph nodes
  ▪ Bone (especially spine) most common site for distant metastases
  ▪ Vascular (renal vein/inferior vena cava) invasion uncommon
  ▪ Synchronous or metachronous tumors common (bladder ~40% within 5 years and upper urinary tract ~12% within 28 months)
► Risk factors
  ▪ Cigarette smoking
  ▪ Exposure to cyclophosphamide, chemical and petrochemical toxins, aniline dye, coal, tar
  ▪ Urinary stasis (congenital structural anomalies)
  ▪ Chronic urinary tract infections
  ▪ Chronic analgesic abuse
  ▪ Balkan nephropathy
► US findings
  ▪ Most too small to be detected on US
  ▪ Intraluminal polypoid soft tissue mass ± dilatation of proximal collecting system
  ▪ Thickening of urothelium
  ▪ Calcifications in 2–7%
► Lymphoma: usually hypoechoic, rarely involves ureter
► Chronic tuberculosis: decreased renal size, scarring, strictures, focal caliectasis, parenchymal and collecting system calcifications
► Blood clot, pus or fungal ball: intraluminal mass of variable echogenicity
  ▪ Mobile
  ▪ Avascular
  ▪ No significant mural thickening
  ▪ Blood clot: often has an onion-like striated pattern on US, high attenuation on non-contrast CT, hematuria
  ▪ Pus or fungal ball: signs of infection, pyuria ± bacteriuria, diffuse and more uniform mural thickening, not as extensive or thick as in this case

Management

► Urine cytology and brushings to confirm diagnosis, occasionally percutaneous fine needle aspiration
► Cystoscopy, contrast-enhanced CT, and MRI for tumor staging and identification of vascular invasion and synchronous tumors
► Prognosis related to stage and age
  ▪ Five-year survival approximately 57% for upper tract tumors
► Treatment
  ▪ Endoscopic laser removal for low-risk tumors
  ▪ More extensive surgery for larger, invasive, more aggressive tumors
  ▪ Topical and systemic chemotherapy
► Cystoscopy with urine cytology every 3–6 months for at least 3 years if high-grade tumor; otherwise yearly to search for metachronous lesions

Further Reading

1. Leder RA, Dunnick NR. Transitional cell carcinoma of the pelvicalices and ureter. *Am J Roentgenol.* 1990; 155: 713–722.
2. Browne RF, Meehan CP, Colville J, et al. Transitional cell carcinoma of the upper urinary tract: Spectrum of imaging findings. *RadioGraphics.* 2005; 25: 1609–1627.
3. Wong-You- Cheong JJ, Wagner BJ, Davis CJJr. Transitional cell carcinoma of the urinary tract: Radiologic–pathologic correlation. *RadioGraphics.* 1998; 18: 123–142.
4. Fritz GA, Schoellnast H, Deutschmann HA, et al. Multiphasic multidetector-row CT (MDCT) in detection and staging of transitional cell carcinomas of the upper urinary tract. *Eur Radiol.* 2006; 16: 1244–1252.

History

▶ 86-Year-old female with urinary tract infection (Figs. 116.1–116.3)

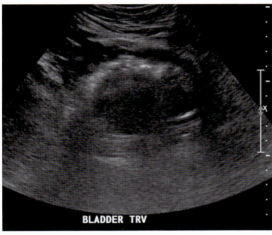

Fig. 116.1

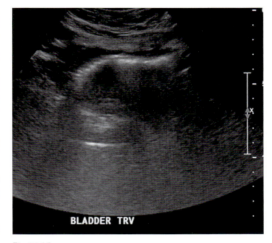

Fig. 116.2

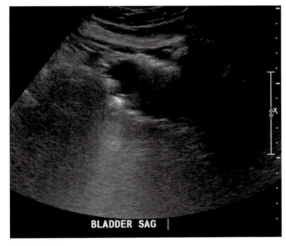

Fig. 116.3

Case 116 Emphysematous Cystitis

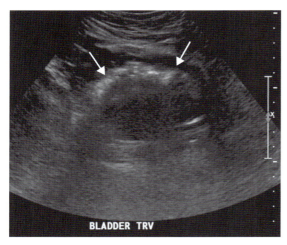

Fig. 116.4

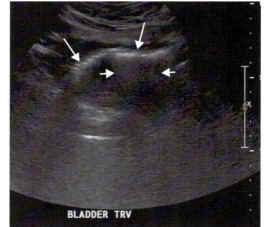

Fig. 116.5

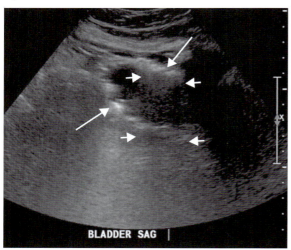

Fig. 116.6

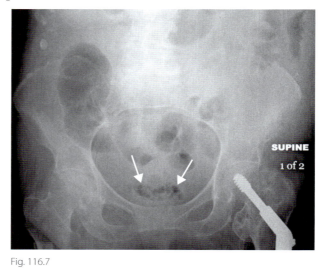

Fig. 116.7

Fig. 116.8

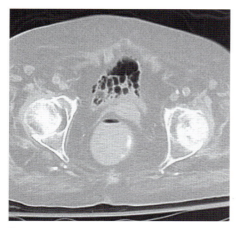

Fig. 116.9

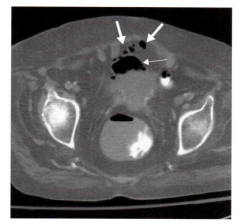

Fig. 116.10

Imaging Findings

▶ Linear markedly echogenic reflectors (arrows in Fig. 116.4 and long arrows in Figs. 116.5 and 116.6) with dirty shadowing (short arrows in Figs. 116.5 and 116.6) in both the nondependent and the dependent wall of the bladder

▶ Radiograph (Fig. 116.7) and axial non contrast-enhanced CT image (Fig. 116.8) confirm finding of air within the bladder wall (arrows in Figs. 116.7 and 116.8)

▶ Note the bubbly appearance of the air on lung windows (Fig. 116.9) from the CT scan consistent with air located in the bladder wall at the base of the bladder. Air in the bladder lumen would be confluent rather than in multiple locules

▶ More cephalad axial CT image demonstrates air in the surrounding soft tissues anterior to the bladder (thick arrows in Fig. 116.10) in the prevesical space as well as air in the lumen of the bladder (thin arrow in Fig. 116.10)

Differential Diagnosis

▶ Recent instrumentation

▶ Bladder fistula to either bowel or vagina secondary to carcinoma, Crohn's disease, or diverticulitis

▶ Bladder wall calcification (tuberculosis or schistosomiasis)

Teaching Points

▶ Emphysematous cystitis is characterized by gas within the bladder wall and/or lumen
  ▪ Caused by gas-forming organisms: most commonly *Escherichia coli* >> *Klebsiella pneumoniae, Enterobacter aerogenes,* and *Clostridium perfringens*
  ▪ Uroepithelium will become ulcerated, necrotic, and may slough
  ▪ Patients are extremely ill
  ▪ Overall mortality rate approximately 7%

▶ Risk factors: diabetes mellitus and urinary stasis (often neurogenic bladder)

▶ More common in women

▶ US findings
  ▪ Echogenic foci with ring-down artifact or dirty shadowing in bladder wall or lumen
  ▪ Intraluminal air will be nondependent and mobile
  ▪ Bladder wall may be thickened and echogenic

▶ Other causes of pneumaturia include recent instrumentation or urinary tract fistula to bowel or vagina

▶ Pneumaturia can be distinguished from emphysematous cystitis because the former results in air found only in the bladder lumen, which on US will appear as mobile echogenic confluent foci with dirty shadowing located nondependently in the bladder lumen
  ▪ Patients with emphysematous cystitis will demonstrate nonmobile foci of air within both the dependent and the nondependent portions of the bladder wall, and in addition may develop intraluminal air

▶ Bladder wall calcification rarely may develop in the setting of chronic infection such as tuberculosis or schistosomiasis
  ▪ Echogenic mural foci with clean sharp shadowing will be observed rather than dirty shadowing
  ▪ The bladder wall is often thickened, and the bladder may become small in capacity
  ▪ Patients with chronic schistosomiasis have an increased incidence of bladder calculi and squamous cell carcinoma

Management

▶ Treatment: nonsurgical management with bladder drainage, antibiotics, and correction of hyperglycemia

Further Reading

1. Grayson DE, Abbott RM, Levy AD, et al. Emphysematous infections of the abdomen and pelvis: A pictorial review. *RadioGraphics*. 2002; 22(3): 543–561.
2. Thomas AA, Lane BR, Thomas AZ, et al. Emphysematous cystitis: A review of 135 cases. *BJU Int*. 2007; 100(1): 17–20.

Section V   Small Parts

History

▶ 46-Year-old male with testicular pain (Figs. 117.1 and 117.2)

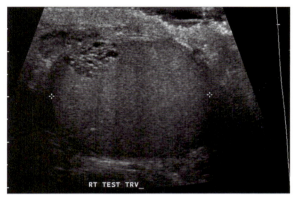

Fig. 117.1

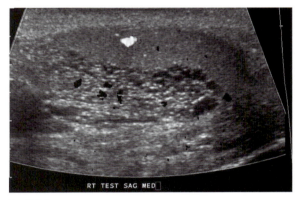

Fig. 117.2

Case 117 Dilated Rete Testis

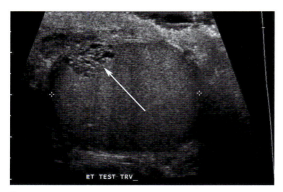

Fig. 117.3

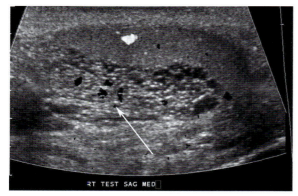

Fig. 117.4

Imaging Findings

▶ Multiple serpiginous anechoic tubular structures (arrow in Fig. 117.3) along the expected course of the mediastinum testis
▶ Notably, this abnormality appears focal and masslike on the transverse images, but in the sagittal plane is linear and tubular (arrow Fig. 117.4)

Differential Diagnosis

▶ Cystic testicular neoplasm
▶ Testicular abscess
▶ Intratesticular cysts
▶ Tunica albuginea cysts
▶ Intratesticular varicocele

Teaching Points

▶ Associated with epdidymal obstruction (spermatoceles or epididymal cysts) or secondary to trauma or inflammation. Most common in older men
▶ Usually bilateral and often asymmetric
▶ Tubular cystic structures along the length of the echogenic mediastinum testis
▶ Elongated shape, but can appear focal and masslike if only viewed in a single plane
▶ No internal vascularity
▶ Cystic testicular tumors
  ▪ Usually nonseminomatous germ cell tumors, especially teratomas. Complex US appearance with cystic or necrotic areas within a vascularized soft tissue component
▶ Testicular abscess
  ▪ Complex fluid-filled mass, which needs to be distinguished from tumors on the basis of clinical symptoms

- Intratesticular cyst
  - Incidental finding, also likely to be found along the mediastinum testis. Similar to tubular ectasia, intratesticular cysts will be anechoic and simple in appearance, discrete, and focal, whereas tubular ectasia will elongate along the course of the mediastinum
- Tunica albuginea cysts
  - Simple-appearing, small cysts along the margins of the testicle
- Intratesticular varicocele
  - Multiple tubular vessels within the testicle, which enlarge with Valsalva maneuver and, unlike tubular ectasia of the rete testis, demonstrate internal color-flow vascularity unless thrombosed

Management

- Tubular ectasia of the rete testis is an incidental finding with no clinical significance
- It is important to recognize this entity as a benign finding and not to confuse it with true pathology

Further Reading

1. Dogra VS, Gottlieb RH, Rubens DJ, et al. Benign intratesticular cystic lesions: US features. *RadioGraphics*. 2001; 21(Suppl 1): S273–S281.
2. Tartar MV, Trambert MA, Balsara ZN, et al. Tubular ectasia of the testicle: Sonographic and MR imaging appearance. *Am J Roentgenol*. 1993; 160: 539–542.

Case 118

▶ 40-Year-old male with chronic scrotal pain (Figs. 118.1–118.3)

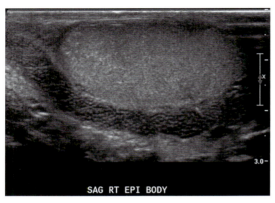

Fig. 118.1

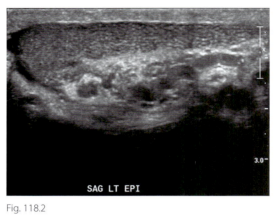

Fig. 118.2

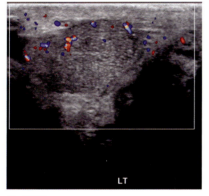

Fig. 118.3

Case 118 Tubular Ectasia of the Epididymis (Post-Vasectomy Change)

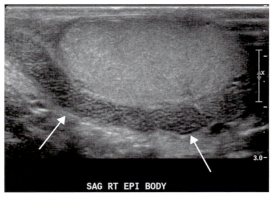

Fig. 118.4

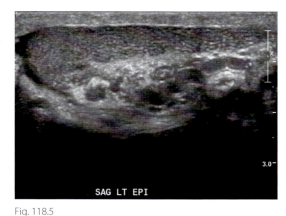

Fig. 118.5

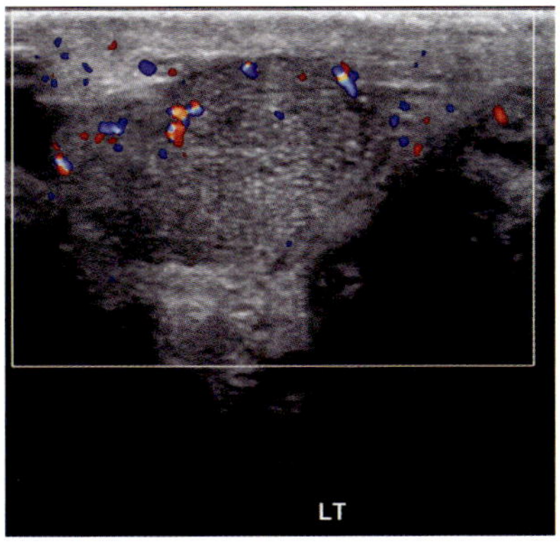

Fig. 118.6

Imaging Findings

▶ Both epididymi are enlarged and hypoechoic with a diffusely speckled appearance (Right, arrows Fig. 118.4; Left, Fig. 118.5)
▶ Peripheral vascularity without appreciable increased flow (Fig. 118.6)

Differential Diagnosis

▶ Normal epididymis
▶ Epididymitis
▶ Tuberculous epididymitis
▶ Tubular ectasia of the rete testis

Teaching Points

▶ Chronic testicular pain of unclear etiology is reported in one-third of patients following vasectomy
▶ Tubular ectasia of the epididymis is caused by engorgement of the epididymis from outflow obstruction
  ▪ Seen only with the more commonly employed closed-ended vasectomy technique
▶ US findings
  ▪ Diffusely enlarged pleural
  ▪ Hypoechoic
  ▪ Bilateral
  ▪ Speckled appearance secondary to parallel wavy echogenic lines that appear as echogenic dots in cross section
    • The linear speckled reflectors represent interfaces between engorged epididymal tubules and their walls
  ▪ Usually hypovascular
  ▪ Spermatic granuloma (echogenic foci with posterior shadowing)
  ▪ Spermatoceles (cysts in epididymis)
  ▪ Testes normal

- Normal epididymis: hypoechoic, homogeneous
  - Not as thick or speckled
- Epididymitis: enlarged, hypoechoic, increased vascularity
  - Not speckled, rarely bilateral
- Tuberculous epididymitis: thick, irregular, calcified, evidence of tuberculosis elsewhere, may spread to testis
- Tubular ectasia of the rete testis: similar speckled appearance along mediastinum of the testis
  - Does not involve epididymis

Management

- No treatment necessary other than analgesics for symptomatic relief

Further Reading

1. Ishigami K, Abu-Yousef MM, El-Zein Y. Tubular ectasia of the epididymis: A sign of postvasectomy status. *J Clin Ultrasound*. 2005; 33: 447–451.
2. Reddy NM, Gerscovich EO, Jain KA, et al. Vasectomy-related changes on sonographic examination of the scrotum. *J Clin Ultrasound*. 2004; 32: 394–398.

History

▶ 74-Year-old male with right testicular pain (Figs. 119.1–119.3)

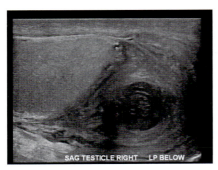

Fig. 119.1

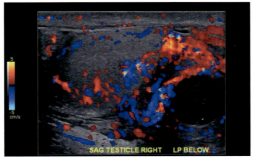

Fig. 119.2

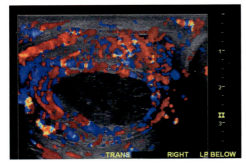

Fig. 119.3

Case 119 Epididymo-orchitis with Epididymal Abscess

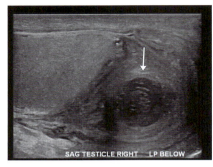

Fig. 119.4

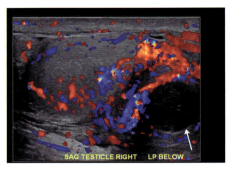

Fig. 119.5

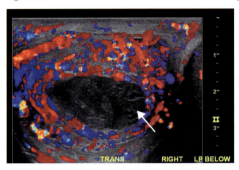

Fig. 119.6

Imaging Findings

▶ The tail of the right epididymis is enlarged and heterogeneous, although primarily hypoechoic (Fig 119.4)
▶ Marked hyperemia of epididymis as well as the adjacent testicular parenchyma (Figs. 119.5 and 119.6)
▶ Note sharply marginated, nearly anechoic, and completely avascular area (arrows in Figs. 119.4–119.6) demonstrating increased through-transmission indicative of complex fluid collection in tail of right epididymis

Differential Diagnosis

▶ Epididymo-orchitis (without abscess)
▶ Adenomatoid tumor
▶ Epididymal cystadenoma
▶ Testicular torsion

Teaching Points

▶ Epididymitis: common cause of acute scrotal pain
  ▪ Urethral discharge or pyuria may be present
▶ Most often secondary to retrograde bacterial infection
  ▪ *Neisseria gonorrhoeae* and *Chlamydia trachomatis* in men < 35 years old
  ▪ *Escherichia coli* in young children and men > 35 years old
▶ Imaging features
  ▪ Enlarged, heterogeneous, hypoechoic (secondary to edema) epididymis
  ▪ Usually begins in the tail of the epididymis
  ▪ Increased vascularity on color Doppler—may be observed even in absence of grayscale abnormalities
  ▪ Hydrocele often present
▶ May be complicated by epididymal abscess formation or orchitis
▶ Epididymal abscess: focal avascular complex fluid collection within the inflamed epididymis
  ▪ Echogenicity of abscess may be variable
▶ Orchitis: increased vascularity ± heterogeneity of the adjacent testicular parenchyma
  ▪ May progress to testicular abscess or infarction

- Both the clinical presentation (absence of signs of infection) and the radiological appearance should allow for definitive differentiation from other epididymal masses and testicular torsion
- Adenomatoid tumor: typically presents as a painless palpable extratesticular mass
  - Solid lesion with internal vascularity
  - Surrounding epididymis will be normal
- Epididymal cystadenoma: rare, associated with Von Hippel–Lindau syndrome
  - Variable US appearance: cystic mass ± small papillary projections, solid with small cystic areas, completely solid
  - More common in head of epididymis
  - May be associated with dilatation of the rete testis
- Testicular torsion: presents with acute scrotal pain that may mimic epididymitis
  - Doppler US findings diagnostic: no blood flow to testis and no increased flow to epididymis

Management

- Antibiotic therapy for epididymitis and epididymo-orchitis
- Percutaneous or surgical drainage of abscesses may be required if antibiotic therapy fails

Further Reading

1. Avery LL, Scheinfeld MH. Imaging of penile and scrotal emergencies. *RadioGraphics*. 2013; 33: 721–740.

Case 120

History

- 14-Year-old male with history of sudden-onset severe left scrotal pain that began 3 hours prior to presentation while playing lacrosse (Figs. 120.1–120.3)

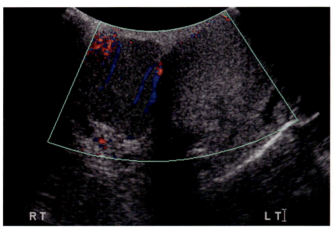

Fig. 120.1

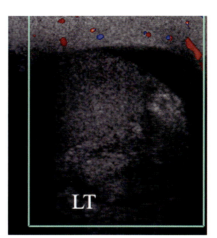

Fig. 120.2

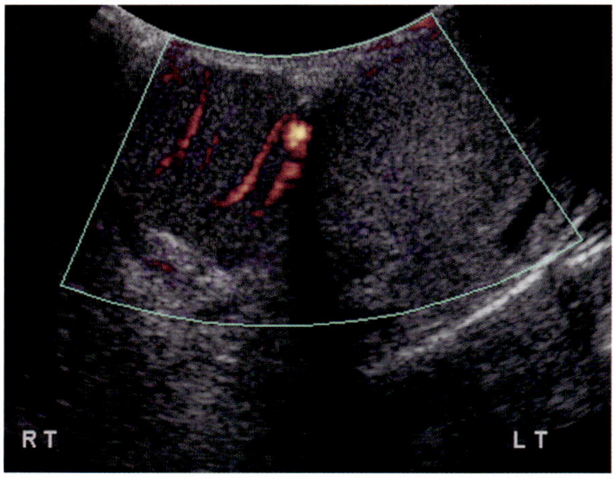

Fig. 120.3

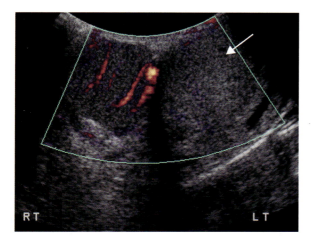

Fig. 120.4

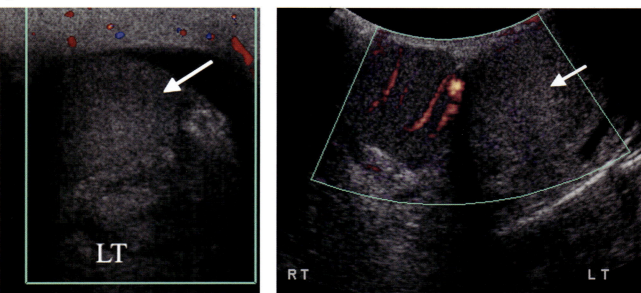

Fig. 120.5   Fig. 120.6

Imaging Findings

► Heterogeneous echotexture in the left testis, which is enlarged (arrows in Figs. 120.4 and 120.5)
► Small reactive hydrocele
► Flow in the normal right testicle with absent flow in the left testicle on color and power Doppler images (arrow in Figs. 120.5 and 120.6)

Differential Diagnosis

► Torsion/detorsion
► Epididymo-orchitis
► Torsion of testicular appendage
► Testicular tumor

Teaching Points

► Urologic emergency: irreversible damage can be seen after 4 hours of ischemia
► Predisposition by anatomical variants—for example, bell clapper deformity in which the testes lack normal attachment to the tunica vaginalis and hang freely

- ▶ Supravaginal torsion (torsion occurring above the tunica vaginalis) more common in infants. Intravaginal torsion much more common overall
- ▶ Sonography is imaging modality of choice. Findings include the following
  - ■ Decreased or absent central parenchymal flow
  - ■ Heterogeneous and hypoechoic echogenicity of the testis, which suggests testicular infarction
  - ■ Enlarged testis and epididymis
  - ■ Spiral twist of the spermatic cord causing a whirlpool pattern
  - ■ Hydrocele
  - ■ Edema of the scrotal wall
- ▶ In torsion/detorsion, grayscale and color Doppler appearances may be normal or even hyperemic
- ▶ In early torsion and partial torsion, grayscale and color Doppler appearances may be normal or minimally decreased
- ▶ Absent testicular vascular flow is sine qua non of testicular torsion: the other differential diagnoses would demonstrate some degree of flow to the testicle
- ▶ In epididymo-orchitis or testicular tumor, the vascular flow is likely to be increased diffusely or focally in the presence of an intratesticular mass

Management

- ▶ Acute presentation: rapid intervention with surgical detorsion and orchipexy to prevent testicular infarction
- ▶ Bilateral orchipexy should be performed, given the higher risk of subsequent torsion on the contralateral side because the bell clapper deformity is typically bilateral
- ▶ If the testicle is no longer viable, orchiectomy or partial orchiectomy is performed

Further Reading

1. Bhatt S, Dogra VS. Role of US in testicular and scrotal trauma. *RadioGraphics*. 2008; 28(6): 1617–1629.
2. Dogra VS, Rubens DJ, Gottlieb RH, et al. Torsion and beyond: New twists in spectral Doppler evaluation of the scrotum. *J Ultrasound Med*. 2004; 23(8): 1077–1085.

History

► 24-Year-old soccer player presents with scrotal pain following trauma (Figs. 121.1–121.4)

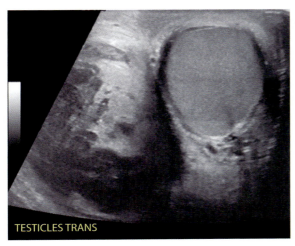

TESTICLES TRANS

Fig. 121.1

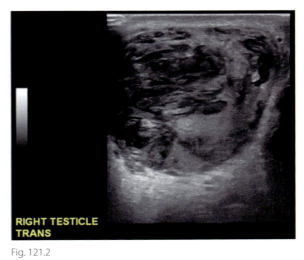

RIGHT TESTICLE TRANS

Fig. 121.2

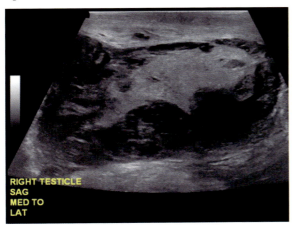

RIGHT TESTICLE SAG MED TO LAT

Fig. 121.3

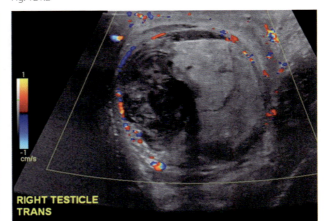

RIGHT TESTICLE TRANS

Fig. 121.4

Case 121 Testicular Rupture

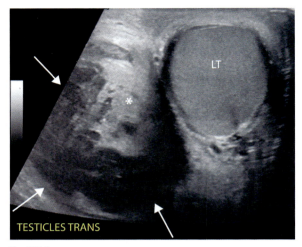

Fig. 121.5

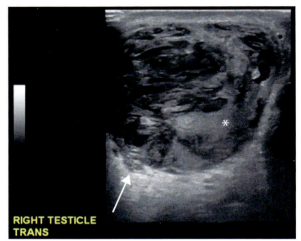

Fig. 121.6

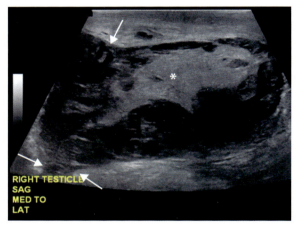

Fig. 121.7

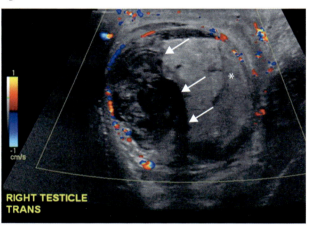

Fig. 121.8

Imaging Findings

▶ Enlarged right testis with irregular hypoechoic area (arrows in Figs. 121.5 and 121.8) that is avascular on color Doppler (Fig. 121.8) and sharply demarcated from the residual normal testicular parenchyma (asterisks in Figs. 121.5–121.8) consistent with intratesticular hematoma

▶ Irregularity of the testicular contour with focal bulging (arrows in Figs. 121.6 and 121.7) indicates disruption of the tunica albuginea with extrusion of testicular contents into the scrotal sac consistent with testicular rupture

▶ Normal left testis (LT in Fig. 121.5)

Differential Diagnosis

▶ Testicular fracture without capsular rupture
▶ Intratesticular hematoma
▶ Underlying testicular malignancy
▶ Testicular torsion

Teaching Points

▶ Testicular rupture most commonly presents with acute pain following blunt trauma (sports injuries, biking or motor vehicle accidents)
▶ US findings of intratesticular hematoma
  ▪ Focal avascular heterogeneous parenchymal area, variable echogenicity but usually hypoechoic and sharply demarcated from residual normal parenchyma, may be multifocal

- ▶ US findings of testicular rupture
  - ▪ Discontinuity of echogenic tunica albuginea (TA) or poorly defined irregular, disrupted testicular contour with extrusion of testicular contents into the scrotal sac
  - ▪ Hematocele and scrotal wall thickening common
- ▶ Testicular fracture: linear hypoechoic area traversing testicular parenchyma
  - ▪ TA intact and testicular contour smooth if rupture has not occurred
- ▶ Testicular malignancy: focal parenchymal mass, may mimic hematoma although more likely to be vascular
  - ▪ May present with pain and intratesticular hemorrhage following trauma
  - ▪ Therefore, follow-up US to exclude an underlying mass should be performed in all patients with intratesticular hematomas that are conservatively managed
- ▶ Testicular torsion: may present with pain following trauma
  - ▪ Enlarged diffusely heterogeneous, hypoechoic testis with smooth contour
  - ▪ TA intact
  - ▪ Entire testis avascular

Management

- ▶ Conservative management of testicular trauma if the TA is intact
- ▶ If the TA is disrupted, emergent surgery mandatory to prevent ischemic necrosis, atrophy, abscess formation, and loss of spermatogenesis
- ▶ US not 100% accurate for diagnosing testicular rupture
  - ▪ Surgical exploration recommended if no blood flow to testis or if US findings equivocal with high clinical suspicion for rupture

Further Reading

1. Fournier GR, Laing FC, McAninch JW. Scrotal ultrasonography in the management of testicular trauma. *Urol Clin North Am*. 1989; 16: 377–385.
2. Deurdulian C, Mittelstaedt CA, Chong WH, et al. US of acute scrotal trauma: Optimal technique, imaging findings, and management. *RadioGraphics*. 2007; 27: 357–369.

Case 122

History

▶ 20-Year-old male presents with a rapidly enlarging right testis (Figs. 122.1–122.3)

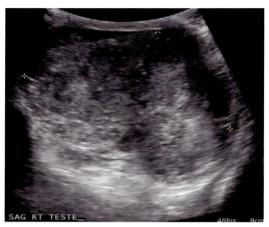

Fig. 122.1

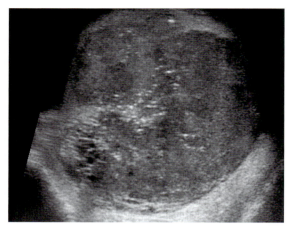

Fig. 122.2

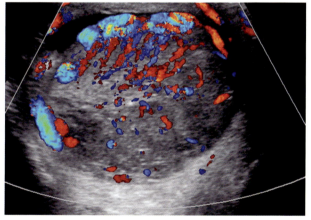

Fig. 122.3

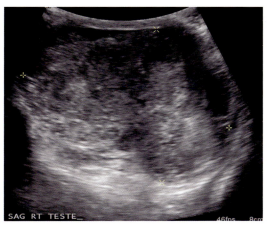

Fig. 122.4

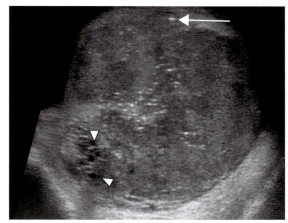

Fig. 122.5

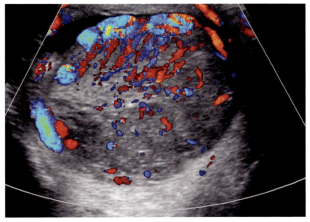

Fig. 122.6

Imaging Findings

▶ Markedly enlarged right testis
▶ Large heterogeneous mass involving the right testis with hypoechoic as well as echogenic areas (Fig. 122.4)
▶ Cystic areas are present within the mass (arrowheads in Fig. 122.5)
▶ Distortion of the testicular contour, raising suspicion that the tumor is invading the tunica albuginea (arrow in Fig. 122.5)
▶ Marked increased vascularity within the mass on color Doppler US (Fig. 122.6)

Differential Diagnosis

▶ Seminoma
▶ Lymphoma/Leukemia
▶ Metastases

Teaching Points

▶ Mixed germ cell tumors are the most common nonseminomatous germ cell tumors of the testis. They occur in younger patients compared to patients in which seminomas occur, < 35 years of age, and are generally more aggressive than pure seminomas. On US, they tend to appear more heterogeneous than seminomas and may contain cystic areas as well as coarse calcifications
▶ Nonseminomatous germ cell tumors also include embryonal cell carcinoma, yolk sac tumors, choriocarcinomas, and teratomas
▶ Seminomas: most common germ cell tumor of the testis. They most commonly present in the fourth and fifth decades of life. Patients with undescended testes have an increased risk of developing a seminoma. On US, pure seminomas present as homogeneous hypoechoic intratesticular masses with increased vascularity

- Non-Hodgkin lymphoma: most common secondary testicular tumor, usually affecting men older than 50 years of age. Testicular lymphoma is bilateral in approximately 38% of cases and is usually associated with systemic lymphoma but can be the presenting sign in 10% of patients. Patients present with testicular enlargement, and US will demonstrate bilateral or multiple hypoechoic masses, often quite large with increased vascularity
- Leukemic infiltrate: usually associated with acute leukemia, during remission because the testicle is a sanctuary site for leukemic cells. It is more common in children, and the sonographic appearance is similar to lymphoma
- Metastatic disease: from other primary tumors is rare, most commonly from prostate and lung primary cancers

Management

- Serum tumor markers
- Staging CT, MRI, and/or PET scan
- Radical orchiectomy followed by chemo- or radiation therapy if appropriate

Further Reading

1. Horstman WG, Melson GL, Middleton WD, et al. Testicular tumors: Findings with color Doppler US. *Radiology*. 1992; 185: 733–737.

History

► 26-Year-old male with a palpable testicular mass (Figs. 123.1 and 123.2)

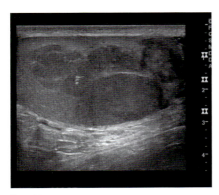

Fig. 123.1

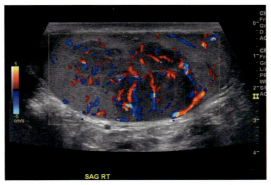

Fig. 123.2

Case 123 Testicular Seminoma

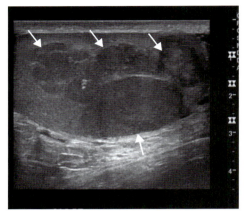

Fig. 123.3

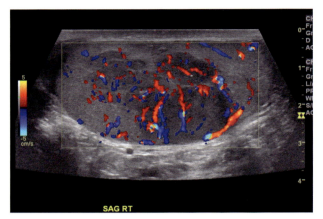

Fig. 123.4

Imaging Findings

► Multiple heterogeneous, predominately hypoechoic intratesticular masses (arrows in Fig. 123.3)
► Masses demonstrate increased vascularity on Color Doppler US (Fig. 123.4)

Differential Diagnosis

► Mixed germ cell tumor
► Non-germ cell tumor
► Metastases
► Lymphoma
► Focal orchitis
► Hematoma

Teaching Points

► Seminoma: most common subtype of testicular germ cell tumor
► Peak incidence: fourth and fifth decades
► Risk factors: prior testicular tumor, cryptorchidism, positive family history
► Metastasis: most common via lymphatic spread, typically to the retroperitoneal lymph nodes
  ▪ Hematogenous spread to distant organs can occur late in the disease
► Presentation: painless testicular lump; occasionally pain following scrotal trauma
► US is the initial imaging test of choice
  ▪ Most common US appearance: homogeneous hypoechoic, well-marginated, vascular mass ± lobular border
  ▪ Multifocal nodules, bilateral tumors, heterogeneity, cystic areas, or calcifications less common
  ▪ Irregularity of the tunica suggests capsular invasion
► Mixed germ cell tumors (combination of seminoma, choriocarcinoma, embryonal cell carcinoma, teratoma, and yolk sac tumors): second most common type of testicular neoplasm
  ▪ Occur in younger individuals
  ▪ Typically heterogeneous in appearance, more likely to have cystic areas and calcifications
  ▪ Overlap in appearance with pure seminoma
► Non-germ cell tumors: solid, vascular masses, variable echogenicity
  ▪ Not distinguishable from germ cell tumors by US criteria alone
► Lymphoma and metastases: more common in older patients (> 60 years old)
  ▪ Typically multiple, bilateral hypoechoic masses
  ▪ Lymphoma often very vascular
► Focal orchitis: hypoechoic, vascular area, may have an irregular border or skin thickening
  ▪ Painful, often concurrent epididymitis
  ▪ Follow-up US will demonstrate resolution post antibiotic therapy
► Hematoma: variable echogenicity, no internal vascularity, often more irregular, linear or angular margins

Management

▶ Evaluate for retroperitoneal lymphadenopathy, especially near the renal hila

▶ CT for staging

▶ Treatment: orchiectomy plus radiation therapy; adjuvant chemotherapy for advanced disease

▶ Prognosis is good with overall cure rate of 90%

▶ Yearly US to search for contralateral testicular neoplasm, particularly if history of cryptorchidism or infertility

Further Reading

1. Woodward PJ, Sohaey R, O'Donoghue MJ, et al. From the archives of the AFIP: Tumors and tumor-like lesions of the testis: Radiologic–pathologic correlation. *RadioGraphics*. 2002; 22: 189–216.

2. Krohmer SJ, McNulty NJ, Schned AR. Testicular seminoma with lymph node metastases. *RadioGraphics*. 2009; 29: 2177–2183.

Case 124

▶ 24-Year-old male presents for management of a testicular abnormality detected incidentally on a scrotal sonogram performed for scrotal pain (Figs. 124.1 and 124.2)

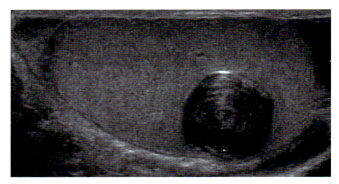

Fig. 124.1

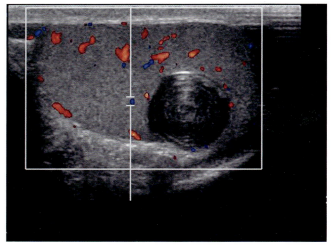

Fig. 124.2

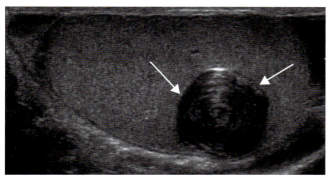

Fig. 124.3

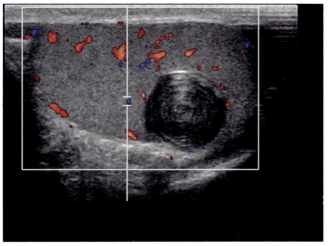

Fig. 124.4

Imaging Findings

▶ Well-circumscribed peripheral intratesticular mass (arrows in Fig. 124.3)
▶ Whorled internal appearance with echogenic layers like an onion skin (Figs. 124.3 and 124.4)
▶ Lack of internal vascularity

Differential Diagnosis

▶ Testicular cyst
▶ Germ cell neoplasm
▶ Cystic dilatation of the rete testis
▶ Tunica albuginea cyst

Teaching Points

▶ Epidermoid cysts are benign, well-circumscribed lesions of germ cell origin and account for approximately 1% of testicular tumors
▶ Approximately one-third are discovered incidentally on physical exam
▶ They occur at any age, most commonly during the second to fourth decades
▶ Pathologically, epidermoid cysts have a fibrous wall lined with keratinizing squamous epithelium and contain cheesy white keratin
▶ Sonographic appearances include the characteristic internal whorled pattern or "onion skin" appearance, peripheral calcifications, or a hypoechoic mass with central calcifications. Lesions may be solitary or bilateral
▶ A very important feature is the lack of internal vascularity that differentiates these lesions from malignant germ cell tumors such as seminomas or teratomas

► Other benign avascular intratesticular lesions include intratesticular cysts, which are anechoic with enhanced through-transmission, and cystic dilatation of the rete testis, which appears as a cluster of cystic lesions in the region of the rete testis. Tunica albuginea cysts are easily recognized by their cystic nature and characteristic localization within the tunica

Management

► If obtained, serum tumor markers should be negative
► Testicular-sparing local excision (enucleation) for histologic confirmation and differentiation from premalignant teratomas

Further Reading

1. Manning MA, Woodward P. Testicular epidermoid cysts: Sonographic features with clinicopathologic correlation. *J Ultrasound Med*. 2010; 29(5): 831–837.
2. Shah KH, Maxted WC, Duhn B. Epidermoid cysts of the testis: A report of three cases and an analysis of 141 cases from the world literature. *Cancer*. 1981; 47: 577–582.

History

▶ 40-Year-old male with nontender left scrotal mass (Figs. 125.1 and 125.2)

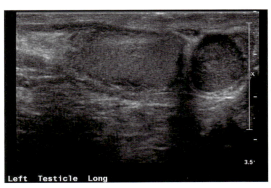

Fig. 125.1

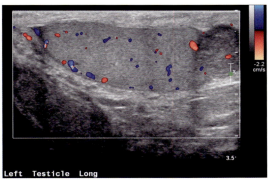

Fig. 125.2

Case 125   Adenomatoid Tumor of the Epididymis

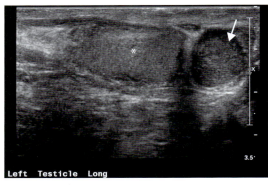

Fig. 125.3

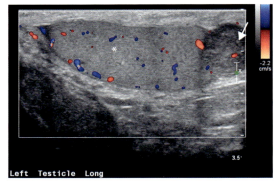

Fig. 125.4

Imaging Findings

► Well-circumscribed hypoechoic mass (white arrows in Figs. 125.3 and 125.4) arising from the tail of the left epididymis. The mass is separate from the left testis (asterisks in Figs. 125.3 and 125.4)
► Color Doppler US image (Fig. 125.4) demonstrates decreased vascularity within the mass (white arrow) compared to the left testis

Differential Diagnosis

► Other benign extratesticular tumors: fibroma, hemangioma, lipoma, leiomyoma, neurofibroma, sperm granuloma, fibrous pseudotumor, adrenal rests
► Malignant extratesticular tumors: liposarcoma, rhabdomyosarcoma, lymphoma, metastasis
► Polyorchidism
► Chronic epididymitis

Teaching Points

► Adenomatoid tumor is the most common intrascrotal extratesticular neoplasm in adults
  ▪ Most frequently located in the tail of the epididymis
  ▪ Rarely arises from the tunica of the testis or the spermatic cord
  ▪ Unilateral, solitary
  ▪ < 5 cm
► Presentation: incidental finding or palpable painless mass in men ≥20 years old
► US findings: nonspecific
  ▪ Solid, well-circumscribed mass of variable echogenicity—usually isoechoic or hypoechoic compared with testis
► Role of US in evaluating a scrotal mass in an adult is largely to differentiate extratesticular masses (usually benign) from intratesticular masses (high likelihood of malignancy)
  ▪ However, in children, extratesticular solid masses may be malignant
  ▪ US usually unable to definitely characterize extratesticular solid masses
► Risk factors for malignancy in extratesticular scrotal masses: large size, heterogeneity, areas of necrosis, infiltrative or ill-defined margins, increased vascularity, or extratesticular neoplasms presenting in children
  ▪ Malignant epididymal lesions are extremely rare
► Lipomas and liposarcomas: usually arise from the scrotal wall or spermatic cord, isoechoic to subcutaneous fat with linear echogenic striations
  ▪ Liposarcomas larger, more vascular, infiltrative margin
► Leiomyomas, fibromas, fibrous pseudotumors: hypoechoic, posterior attenuation or shadowing, may contain focal echogenic areas of calcification
► Polyorchidism: similar in shape and echogenicity to normal testis, but may be smaller
► Chronic epididymitis: enlarged, vascular, heterogeneous epididymis, ± calcifications, central fluid collections due to necrosis or abscess, history of epididymitis or pain

Management

► Confirmation of diagnosis with intraoperative frozen section followed by excision

Further Reading

1. Akbar SA, Sayyed TA, Jafri SZH, et al. Multimodality imaging of paratesticular neoplasms and their mimics. *RadioGraphics*. 2003; 23: 1461–1476.
2. Smart JA, Jackson EK, Redman SL, et al. Ultrasound findings of masses of the paratesticular space. *Clin Radiol*. 2008; 63: 929–938.

Case 126

History

▶ 50-Year-old male presents with a palpable penile mass (Figs. 126.1–126.3)

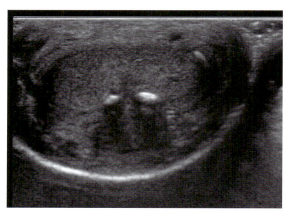

Fig. 126.1

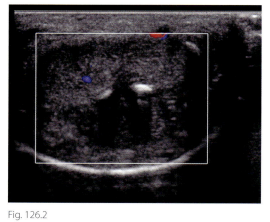

Fig. 126.2

Fig. 126.3

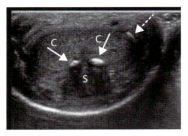
Fig. 126.4

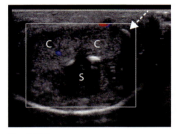
Fig. 126.5

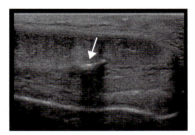
Fig. 126.6

Imaging Findings

▶ Transverse grayscale (Fig. 126.4), color Doppler (Fig. 126.5), and longitudinal grayscale (Fig. 126.6) images of the distal penis show echogenic linear foci with posterior acoustic shadowing (straight arrows) within the tunica albuginea between the corpora cavernosa (C) and corpus spongiosum (S)
▶ Linear echogenic focus with shadowing in the tunica albuginea overlying the dorsolateral aspect of the left corpus cavernosum (dashed arrows in Figs. 126.4 and 126.5)
▶ No soft tissue mass or abnormal vascularity

Differential Diagnosis

▶ Foreign body
▶ Penile implant
▶ Vascular calcifications

Teaching Points

▶ Chronic disorder characterized by plaques/scarring in the fibrous sheaths covering the corpora cavernosa and tunica albuginea, usually involves the dorsal and distal aspect of the penis
  ▪ Typically presents between the ages of 40 and 60 years
  ▪ Associated with other fibrotic conditions, such as Dupuytren's contracture
▶ Presentation: penile pain; palpable nodule; induration; curvature, deformity, or shortening of the penis during erection; sexual dysfunction
▶ US initial imaging modality of choice: enables detection, localization, and characterization (fibrous vs. calcified) of plaques, even if nonpalpable
  ▪ Also used to monitor medical therapy
▶ US findings
  ▪ Calcified plaques: linear, echogenic, posterior acoustic shadowing, likely stable
  ▪ Fibrous plaques: focal thickening of tunica albuginea
  ▪ Hypoechoic halo around a noncalcified plaque may indicate active disease
▶ Penile radiography performed with mammography equipment: more sensitive than US for detecting calcified plaques, but will not detect fibrous plaques
▶ MRI: as sensitive as US, useful in detecting noncalcified plaques at the penile base
  ▪ Plaques: low signal intensity on T1- and T2-weighted images
  ▪ Gadolinium enhancement suggests active inflammation
▶ Foreign body: echogenic ± shadowing, history of trauma, unlikely to be in classic location
▶ Penile implant: larger echogenic structure with shadowing, placed in corpus cavernosum
▶ Vascular calcifications: often two parallel echogenic lines, flow in lumen on color Doppler

Management

▶ Initial medical therapy with oral pentoxifylline
▶ Intralesional injections of verapamil or interferon α-2b
▶ Surgery (plaque excision with grafting) if sexual function limited

Further Reading
1. Prando D. New sonographic aspects of Peyronie disease. *J Ultrasound Med.* 2009; 28: 217–232.
2. Kalokairinou K, Konstantinidis C, Domazou M, et al. US imaging in Peyronie's disease. *J Clin Imaging Sci.* 2012; 2: 63.

Case 127

History

► 54-Year-old male with left lower extremity pain and swelling (Figs. 127.1–127.4)

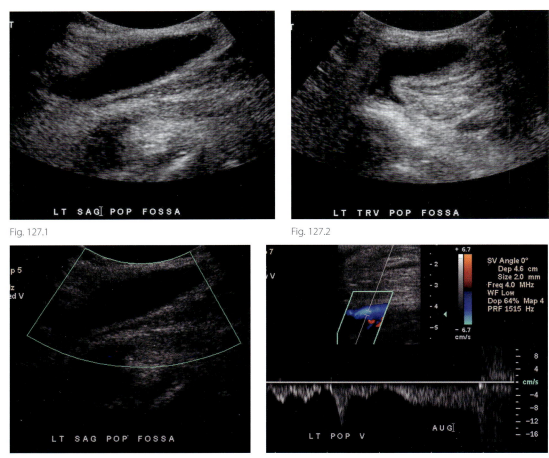

Fig. 127.1

Fig. 127.2

Fig. 127.3

Fig. 127.4

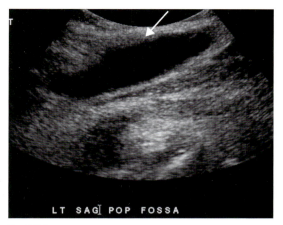

Fig. 127.5

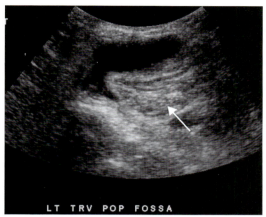

Fig. 127.6

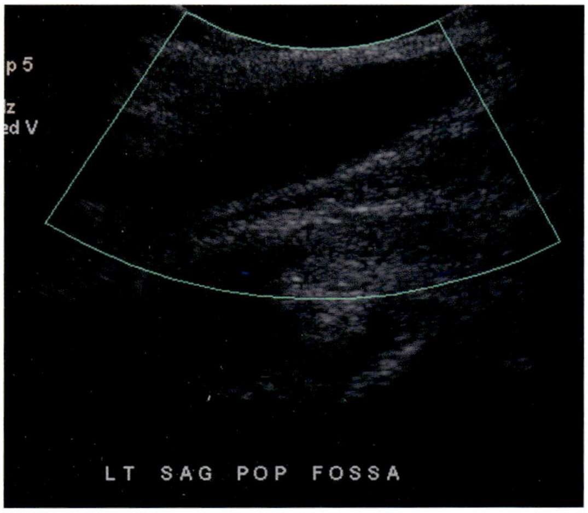

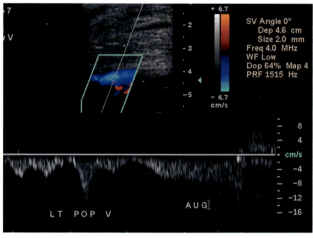

Fig. 127.7

Fig. 127.8

Imaging Findings

▶ Large popliteal cyst on sagittal US (arrow in Fig. 127.5)
▶ Cyst wraps around the medial head of the gastrocnemius muscle (arrow in Fig. 127.6) and connects to the knee joint on transverse view
▶ No internal vascularity
▶ Normal flow in the popliteal vein (Fig. 127.8)

Differential Diagnosis

▶ Knee joint effusion
▶ Prepatellar bursitis
▶ Popliteal artery aneurysm
▶ Cystic neoplasm

Teaching Points

▶ Baker cyst is caused by abnormal distension of the gastrocnemius–semimembranosus bursa, communicating with the knee joint
▶ May be asymptomatic or associated with knee pain, posterior knee tightness, or present as a palpable popliteal fossa mass
▶ Often associated with internal knee joint conditions that increase intra-articular pressure and lead to overproduction of synovial fluid, such as rheumatoid arthritis or meniscal tear
▶ Large or ruptured Baker cysts can dissect along the posteromedial calf muscles anterior to the gastrocnemius muscle, clinically mimicking deep venous thrombosis or thrombophlebitis

- US appearance
  - Fluid-filled collection medially in the popliteal fossa between the medial head of the gastrocnemius muscle and the semimembranosus tendon, best seen on transverse views
    - Internal echoes due to debris and fibrin strands if inflamed or infected
    - May contain calcified loose bodies resulting from osteochondromatosis
    - May appear more solid in rheumatoid arthritis due to synovial hypertrophy and pannus formation, ± increased vascularity
- Knee joint effusion
  - Commonly in the suprapatellar bursa between anterior lower femur and quadriceps tendon
  - Associated with traumatic, inflammatory, or degenerative knee conditions
- Prepatellar bursitis
  - In people who spent much time kneeling, such as house maids, nuns, carpet layers, and coal miners
  - Located in the anterior portion of the knee between the patella and skin
- Popliteal artery aneurysm
  - Pulsatile popliteal fossa mass
  - Vascular on color Doppler US with arterial flow
- Cystic neoplasm
  - Suspect if large cystic mass in non-inflamed knee with neurological symptoms

Management

- If asymptomatic, no treatment necessary
- Percutaneous aspiration with or without steroid injections if symptomatic
- Anti-inflammatory drugs to reduce inflammation and pain
- Arthroscopic surgery when associated with internal knee derangement
- MRI for confirmation in atypical cases

Further Reading

1. Ward EE, Jacobson JA, Fessell DP, et al. Sonographic detection of Baker's cysts: Comparison with MRI. *Am J Roentgenol.* 2001; 176: 373–380.

History

▶ 29-Year-old male with pain and swelling of the finger persisting for 1 month following trauma (Figs. 128.1–128.3)

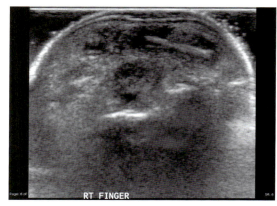

Fig. 128.1

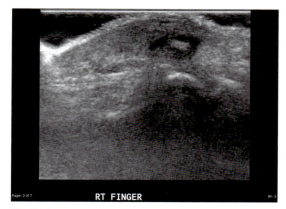

Fig. 128.2

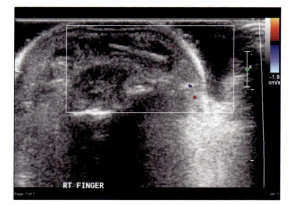

Fig. 128.3

Case 128 Foreign Body (Wood Splinter)

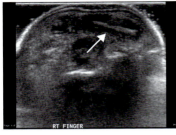
Fig. 128.4

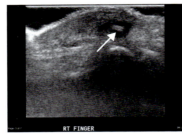
Fig. 128.5

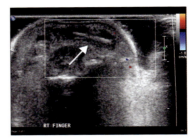
Fig. 128.6

Imaging Findings

▶ Linear echogenic structure (arrows in Figs. 128.4–128.6) without posterior shadowing in the volar subcutaneous soft tissues of the finger
▶ Note surrounding hypoechoic halo of tissue
▶ There is no increased vascularity on color Doppler image (Fig. 128.6)

Differential Diagnosis

▶ Embedded needle
▶ Subcutaneous air
▶ Abscess
▶ Subcutaneous fibroma

Teaching Points

▶ US is very sensitive for localizing radiolucent foreign bodies, such as wood or plastic, with a reported sensitivity of 95% in the hand and wrist
  ▪ Wooden splinters, thorns, and plastic are not typically identifiable on radiographs
  ▪ Glass, gravel, stones, and metal are typically radiopaque
  ▪ However, US may be helpful in identifying slivers of glass that are too small to be detected on radiographs
▶ A high-frequency linear array transducer provides optimal resolution
▶ US findings
  ▪ Echogenic reflector, conforming to shape of foreign body
  ▪ Echogenicity independent of composition
  ▪ Splinters, thorns, or plastic will not demonstrate posterior shadowing
  ▪ Hypoechoic rim of inflammatory granulomatous tissue and/or fibrosis
  ▪ ± Surrounding fluid collection
  ▪ May see surrounding hyperemia on color Doppler due to inflammation, but not always if the injury is long-standing
  ▪ Superinfection could result in a draining tract to the skin, increased vascularity, or surrounding punctate echogenic foci of air with dirty shadowing
▶ Metal or glass fragments: linear and echogenic
  ▪ Typically demonstrate posterior shadowing
  ▪ ± Twinkle artifact on color Doppler
▶ Subcutaneous air: possibly echogenic and linear
  ▪ More often irregular or punctate echogenic foci with dirty shadowing and twinkle artifact
▶ Abscess: fluid collection ± irregular, clumpy echogenic foci of air and increased peripheral vascularity
▶ Fibroma: hypoechoic well-circumscribed mass, variable vascularity, but no central linear echogenic reflector or history of antecedent trauma

Management

▶ Excision
▶ US localization of the foreign body for intraoperative or percutaneous removal

Further Reading

1. Boyse TD, Fessell DP, Jacobson JA, et al. US of soft-tissue foreign bodies and associated complications with surgical correlation. *RadioGraphics*. 2001; 21: 1251–1256.
2. Jacobson JA, Powell A, Craig JG, et al. Wooden foreign bodies in soft tissue: Detection at US. *Radiology*. 1998; 206: 45–48.

History

▶ 65-Year-old female with painful swelling on dorsum of the hand (Figs. 129.1 and 129.2)

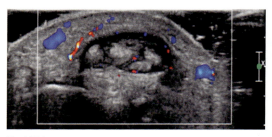

Fig. 129.1

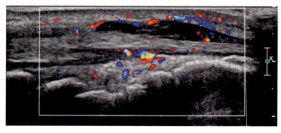

Fig. 129.2

Case 129 Tenosynovitis of the Extensor Tendons in the Fourth Compartment of the Dorsum of the Hand Secondary to Rheumatoid Arthritis

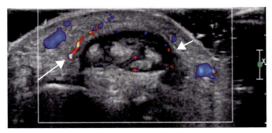

Fig. 129.3

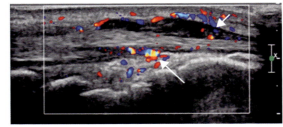

Fig. 129.4

Imaging Findings

► Fluid containing internal echoes and hypervascular thickened synovium (short arrows in Figs. 129.3 and 129.4) surround the extensor tendons in the fourth compartment of the dorsum of the hand
► Normal echogenicity and fibrillar pattern of tendons
► Hyperemia and edema of overlying subcutaneous fat (long arrows in Figs. 129.3 and 129.4)

Differential Diagnosis

► Tendinosis
► Complex fluid in radiocarpal joint recess

Teaching Points

► Tenosynovitis: inflammation of the synovial membrane covering a tendon with thickening and hyperemia of the synovium ± accumulation of fluid within the tendon sheath
► Risk factors: rheumatoid or other inflammatory arthritis, diabetes, repetitive trauma, gout, pseudogout, and infection (especially fungal)
► Presentation: pain, swelling, difficulty moving the joint
► US features
  ▪ Distension of tendon sheath with anechoic to hypoechoic complex fluid containing low-level internal echoes due to debris, hemorrhage, or infection
  ▪ Synovial thickening: vascular, variable echogenicity
  ▪ Fluid is compressible; hypertrophied synovium is not
  ▪ Color/power Doppler can help differentiate hypoechoic fluid from hyperemic synovium
  ▪ Underlying tendon usually is normal: echogenic, fibrillar pattern, hypovascular, intact
    • Unless associated tendinopathy or rupture
  ▪ Adjacent bony erosions (if related to inflammatory arthritis)
  ▪ Color Doppler may demonstrates hyperemia and edema in surrounding soft tissues
► Dynamic examination used to demonstrate integrity of tendon and/or restriction of tendon movement
► Tendinosis: tendon thickened, hypoechoic (diffuse or focal) with loss of fibrillar pattern, vascularity variable, no surrounding fluid or thickened synovium
► Complex joint effusion: adjacent to bone, not surrounding tendons, fluid complex or anechoic
  ▪ Most commonly associated with inflammatory arthritis, pseudogout, gout, trauma, and infection
  ▪ Tophi and urate crystal often echogenic

Management

► Assess for integrity of tendon, associated tendon pathology, and exclude infection
► Most patients respond to conservative therapy: rest, splinting, and anti-inflammatory medications
► Corticosteroid injections may relieve symptoms in up to 50% of patients
► Surgical decompression may be required if no response to conservative therapy
► Follow-up US to assess treatment response

Further Reading

1. Robinson P. Sonography of common tendon injuries. *Am J Roentgenol.* 2009; 193: 607–618.
2. McNally EG. Ultrasound of the small joints of the hands and feet: Current status. *Skeletal Radiol.* 2008; 37: 99–113.

Case 130

History

► 42-Year-old female with midline neck lump for several years (Figs. 130.1–130.3)

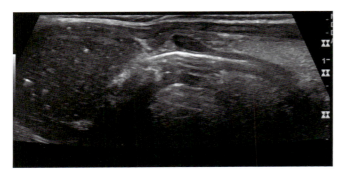

Fig. 130.1

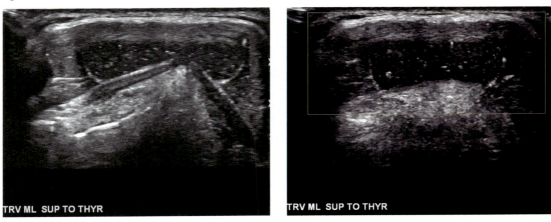

Fig. 130.2

Fig. 130.3

Case 130 Thyroglossal Duct Cyst

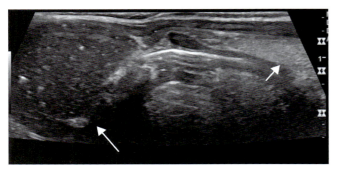

Fig. 130.4

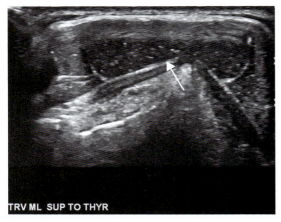

TRV ML SUP TO THYR

Fig. 130.5

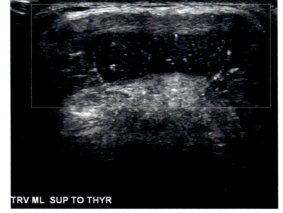

TRV ML SUP TO THYR

Fig. 130.6

Imaging Findings

▶ Complex midline cystic mass (long arrows in Figs. 130.4 and 130.5) with internal echoes and debris superior to the thyroid gland (short arrow in Fig. 130.4)
▶ Avascular on color Doppler US (CDUS) (Fig.130.6)
▶ US-guided aspiration biopsy performed for diagnosis

Differential Diagnosis

▶ Dermoid/epidermoid cyst
▶ Ectopic thyroid
▶ Pyramidal lobe
▶ Branchial cleft cyst
▶ Infected lymphatic malformation

Teaching Points

▶ Thyroglossal duct cyst (TGDC) most commonly presents as a palpable midline cystic mass, sometime parasagittal slightly to the left anywhere from the base of the tongue to the thyroid isthmus, although most are located at the level of the hyoid bone or infrahyoid
▶ Caused by persistence of the thyroglossal duct with secretory epithelium resulting in cyst or sinus formation
▶ Most are benign with 1% risk of malignancy, especially if calcified or containing soft tissue mass
▶ US appearance
  ▪ Simple midline cyst (> 50% of cases) above level of the thyroid gland
  ▪ Complex midline cystic mass containing internal echoes due to proteinaceous material or pseudocolloid, especially if infected
  ▪ Posterior acoustic enhancement despite internal debris
  ▪ No flow on CDUS

- ► Dermoid/epidermoid cyst
  - ■ May have similar US appearance to a TGDC
  - ■ Diagnosis based on histologic differentiation
- ► Ectopic thyroid
  - ■ Homogeneous soft tissue mass with thyroid echotexture signature
  - ■ Suprahyoid, often at base of the tongue
  - ■ Lack of posterior acoustic enhancement
  - ■ ^{99m}TC pertechnetate scan for confirmation
- ► Pyramidal lobe
  - ■ Congenital thyroid lesion
  - ■ Extending superiorly from thyroid isthmus
- ► Branchial cleft cyst
  - ■ Simple or complex cystic mass in the lateral neck due to failure of obliteration most commonly of the second branchial cleft
  - ■ Mostly suprahyoid in location
- ► Lymphatic malformation
  - ■ May involve parotid gland or infiltrate the submandibular space
  - ■ Mainly cystic/tubular spaces with or without septations
  - ■ Internal echoes if infected

Management

- ► US-guided aspiration in equivocal cases to establish diagnosis and exclude infection or malignant degeneration
- ► Surgical resection with the Sistrunk procedure, including removal of the duct at the base of the tongue, the cyst, and the medial part of the hyoid bone

Further Reading

1. Ahuja A, King AD, King W, et al. Thyroglossal duct cysts: Sonographic appearance in adults. *Am J Neuroradiol*. 1999; 20: 579–582.
2. Valentino M, Quiligotti C, Villa A, et al. Thyroglossal duct cysts: Two cases. *J. Ultrasound*. 2012; 15: 183–185.

Case 131

History

- 45-Year-old female with neck fullness (Figs. 131.1–131.4)

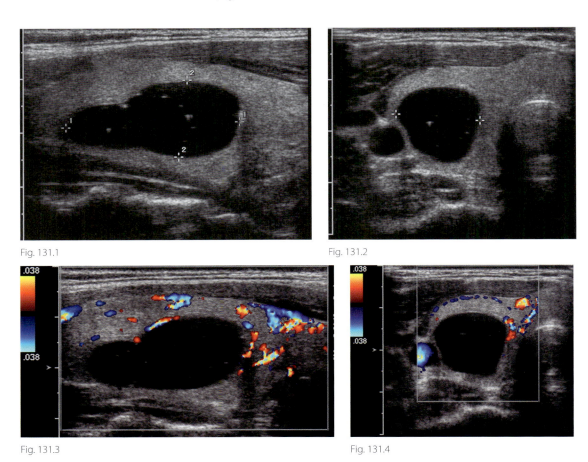

Fig. 131.1

Fig. 131.2

Fig. 131.3

Fig. 131.4

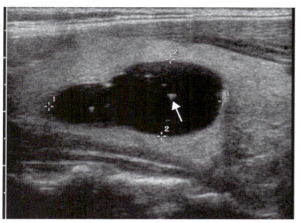

Fig. 131.5

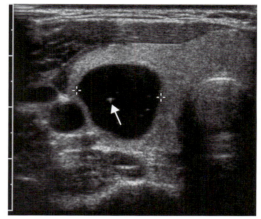

Fig. 131.6

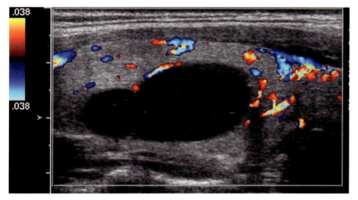

Fig. 131.7

Imaging Findings

▶ Cystic thyroid nodule with tiny echogenic foci with subtle "ring-down" or "comet tail" artifact (Figs. 131.5 and 131.6)
▶ No internal flow on color Doppler US (Fig. 131.7)

Differential Diagnosis

▶ Malignant nodule (papillary thyroid carcinoma) with cystic degeneration
▶ Solid indeterminate thyroid nodule with cystic degeneration
▶ Thyroid metastasis with cystic degeneration

Teaching Points

▶ Completely cystic (or predominantly cystic) thyroid nodules account for up to 28% of all thyroid nodules
▶ Cystic thyroid nodules can be composed of colloid, internal hemorrhage, and cellular debris, and they typically represent either hyperplastic or adenomatous nodules that have undergone cystic degeneration
▶ Cystic nodules are overwhelmingly benign, although the presence of a solid vascularized component and microcalcifications may herald the presence of malignancy, especially cystic papillary thyroid carcinoma
▶ Echogenic foci with "ring-down" or "comet tail" artifact within the cyst fluid represent inspissated colloid (arrows in Fig. 131.8)

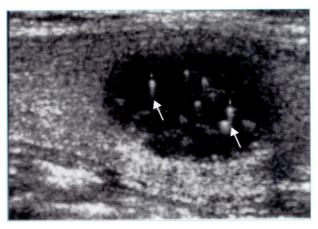

Fig. 131.8

▶ A "spongiform" nodule with multiple internal cystic spaces separated by innumerable avascular septations is an alternative appearance of a colloid nodule and is also associated with benignity

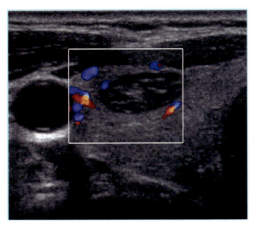

Fig. 131.9

▶ Spongiform nodule (Fig. 131.9) with no internal vascularity in another patient—also associated with benignity
▶ Intervention/treatment is not indicated unless a cystic thyroid nodule causes patient symptoms or pain
▶ Indeterminate thyroid nodules require fine needle aspiration biopsy (FNAB)
▶ Cystic metastases are extremely rare and suspected if the patient has an extrathyroidal primary tumor. FNAB is required for definitive diagnosis

Management

▶ A truly cystic nodule of the thyroid does not require any further intervention or treatment if the patient is asymptomatic
▶ If cystic nodules reach a large size and cause patient discomfort and pain, they can be treated with cyst aspiration and percutaneous ethanol injection
▶ Complex cystic lesion with solid components, especially if vascular, requires further investigation with FNAB for definite diagnosis

Further Reading

1. Bonavita JA, Mayo J, Babb J, et al. Pattern recognition of benign nodules at ultrasound of the thyroid: Which nodules can be left alone? *Am J Roentgenol.* 2009; 193: 207–213.
2. Frates MC, Benson CB, Charboneau JW, et al. Management of thyroid nodules detected at US: Society of Radiologists in Ultrasound consensus conference statement. *Radiology.* 2005; 237: 794–800.

History

▶ 24-Year-old female presents with tremor (Figs. 132.1–132.6)

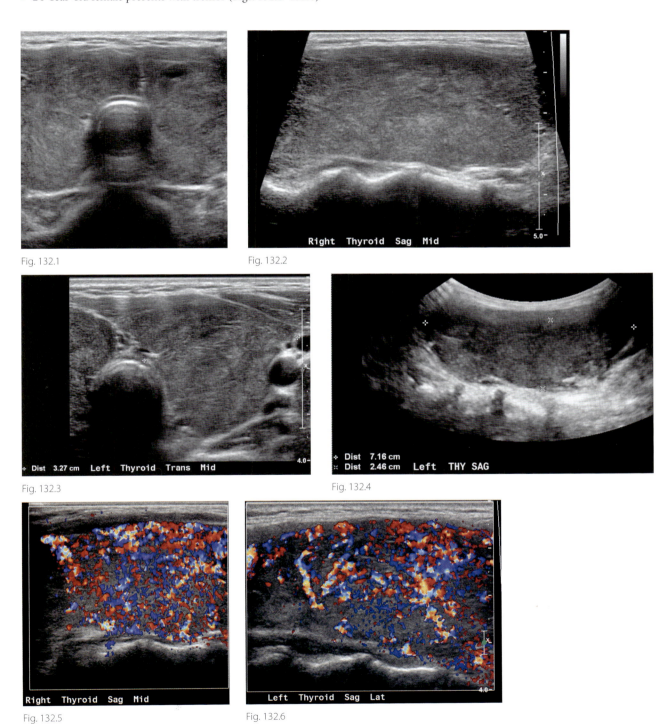

Fig. 132.1

Fig. 132.2
Right Thyroid Sag Mid
5.0

Fig. 132.3
Dist 3.27 cm Left Thyroid Trans Mid
4.0

Fig. 132.4
Dist 7.16 cm
Dist 2.46 cm Left THY SAG

Fig. 132.5
Right Thyroid Sag Mid

Fig. 132.6
Left Thyroid Sag Lat
4.0

Case 132 Graves Disease

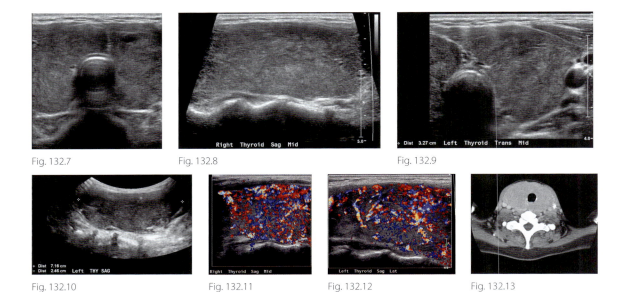

Fig. 132.7

Fig. 132.8

Fig. 132.9

Fig. 132.10

Fig. 132.11

Fig. 132.12

Fig. 132.13

Imaging Findings

▶ Heterogeneous, diffusely enlarged thyroid gland (Figs. 132.7–132.10). Note calipers measuring left lobe (Figs. 132.9 and 132.10)
▶ A lower frequency curved array transducer was required to obtain a longitudinal image of the entire left lobe (calipers in Fig. 132.10), which measures 7.2 × 2.5 × 3.3 cm
▶ Marked diffuse hyperemia of both lobes of the thyroid on color Doppler (Figs. 132.11 and 132.12)
▶ Contrast-enhanced CT scan demonstrating massive enlargement of the thyroid gland (Fig. 132.13) surrounding the trachea

Differential Diagnosis

▶ Hashimoto thyroiditis
▶ Subacute thyroiditis
▶ Multinodular goiter

Teaching Points

▶ Graves disease (diffuse toxic goiter)
  ▪ Autoimmune disorder caused by antibodies directed against the thyroid-stimulating hormone receptor (TSHR) with resultant secretion of excess thyroid hormone (T3 and T4)
  ▪ Most common cause of hyperthyroidism in the United States (60–80% of cases)
  ▪ 7–10 times more common in women
  ▪ Peak incidence: ages 20–50 years
  ▪ Etiology: possible genetic predisposition and/or viral or bacterial trigger
  ▪ Presentation: tachycardia/palpitations, nervousness, tremor, irritability, weight loss, excessive sweating, heat intolerance, exophthalmos, periorbital edema, pretibial myxedema, fatigue and weakness
▶ Diagnosis: Undetectable serum thyroid stimulating hormone (TSH) and elevated unbound T4
  ▪ Radionuclide imaging: extremely high uptake levels distinguish Graves disease (and toxic nodules) from other types of thyroiditis
▶ US findings: nonspecific
  ▪ Diffuse enlargement of thyroid gland
  ▪ Hypoechoic to isoechoic and homogeneous to slightly heterogeneous compared to normal thyroid tissue
  ▪ Marked increased vascularity of thyroid parenchyma in active stages on color Doppler, termed "thyroid inferno"
▶ Doppler characteristics have not been shown to correlate with laboratory or nuclear medicine assessment of thyroid function

- Hashimoto thyroiditis
  - Acutely the thyroid may be enlarged and relatively homogeneous; the patient may be euthyroid or slightly hyperthyroid
  - As the gland becomes infiltrated with lymphocytes and plasma cells, a heterogeneous pattern with numerous small hypoechoic areas 1–6 mm in size (termed micronodulation) will develop and patients become hypothyroid
  - Ultimately fibrosis occurs, and the gland becomes small and lobulated with echogenic septations. Vascularity is normal or decreased
- Subacute thyroiditis (de Quervain thyroiditis)
  - Acutely the thyroid may be enlarged and hypoechoic or develop focal areas of decreased echogenicity
  - Later the gland becomes indistinct and heterogeneous with normal or decreased vascularity
  - Hallmarks are pain on palpation and association with fever or viral syndrome
  - The patient may be transiently hyperthyroid
- Multinodular goiter
  - Enlarged, lobular thyroid containing numerous nodules of varying size
  - Echogenicity of the nodules varies from patient to patient, but nodules are usually similar in echotexture in a given individual
  - Patients are typically hypothyroid, unless there is an autonomous functioning adenoma

Management

- Beta-blockers can offer prompt relief of the adrenergic symptoms of hyperthyroidism
- Antithyroid drugs
- Radioactive iodine: common in the United States; used elsewhere if drug regimen does not result in remission
  - Graves ophthalmopathy develops or worsens following radioactive iodine in up to 15% of patients
  - Surgical decompression may be required
- Subtotal thyroidectomy: young, pregnant patients; severe disease

Further Reading

1. Tessler FN, Tublin ME. Thyroid sonography: Current applications and future directions. *Am J Roentgenol.* 1999; 173(2): 437–443.
2. Reid JR, Wheeler SF. Hyperthyroidism: Diagnosis and treatment. *Am Fam Physician.* 2005; 72(4): 623–630.

Case 133

History

▶ 20-Year-old female presents with hypothyroidism (Figs. 133.1–133.3)

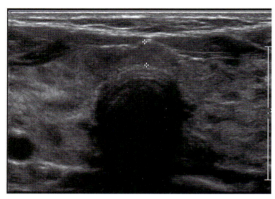

Fig. 133.1

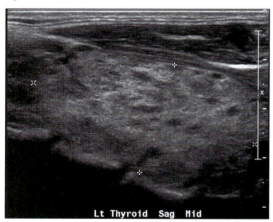

Fig. 133.2

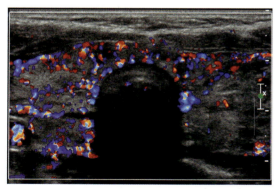

Fig. 133.3

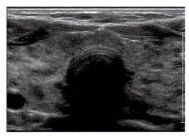

Fig. 133.4

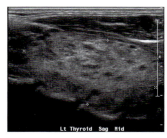

Fig. 133.5

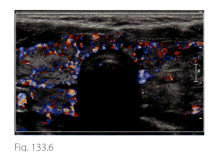

Fig. 133.6

Imaging Findings

▶ Diffusely heterogeneous thyroid parenchyma with numerous small subcentimeter (< 6 mm), hypoechoic, round foci (Figs. 133.4 and 133.5). This appearance is termed micronodulation. Thyroid isthmus (calipers in Fig. 133.4); Left lobe measured by calipers in Fig. 133.5
▶ Color Doppler imaging demonstrates moderately increased vascularity throughout the thyroid gland (Fig. 133.6)

Differential Diagnosis

▶ Graves disease
▶ Subacute granulomatous thyroiditis (de Quervain thyroiditis)

Teaching Points

▶ Hashimoto thyroiditis, or chronic autoimmune lymphocytic thyroiditis, is an autoimmune thyroid disease characterized by circulating antibodies to thyroid peroxidase, thyroglobulin, and/or thyroid-stimulating hormone receptors
▶ Histology: diffuse infiltration of thyroid gland with lymphocytes and plasma cells; secondary fibrotic reaction
▶ Most common cause of hypothyroidism in the United States
▶ Most patients present in the third to fifth decades
  ▪ Four- to sixfold increased incidence in females
  ▪ Overall incidence: 3.5/1000
▶ Signs and symptoms: fatigue, weight gain, dry skin, cold intolerance, hair loss, puffy face, periorbital edema, painless enlargement of the thyroid
  ▪ Many patients asymptomatic
▶ US findings depend on time course
  ▪ Acute
    • Enlarged, hypoechoic gland with heterogeneous, coarse echotexture
    • Micronodulation: innumerable, small (< 1–6 mm) hypoechoic nodules representing focal infiltration or aggregates of lymphocytes and plasma cells; this pattern is reported to have a positive predictive value of 95%
    • Often hypervascular on color Doppler, but vascularity variable
  ▪ Intermediate or subacute
    • Gland becomes normal in size
    • Hypoechoic areas become larger and more confluent, termed "giraffe pattern" (see Figs. 133.7 and 133.8)

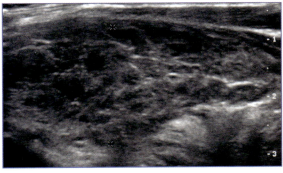

Fig. 133.7

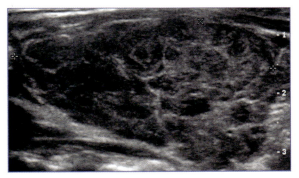

Fig. 133.8

43-Year-old woman with a 2-year history of fatigue and mild hypothyroidism. The numerous hypoechoic areas throughout the thyroid parenchyma are larger and more confluent than what is characteristic of the micronodulation pattern of acute Hashimoto thyroiditis illustrated in Figs. 133.4 and 133.5. This is termed the "giraffe pattern." These areas are separated by linear echogenic septations, some of which extend to the surface of the gland. The margin of the gland is slightly nodular.

- Chronic
  - Gland decreases in size and vascularity
  - Hypoechoic areas become larger and more confluent
  - Echogenic fibrous septations
  - Nodular contour due to retraction from the fibrous septations

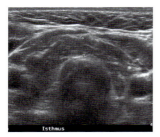 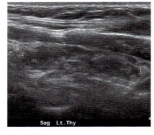 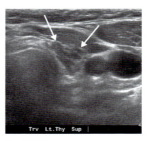

Fig. 133.9   Fig. 133.10   Fig. 133.11

A 54-year-old woman with a 20-year history of Hashimoto thyroiditis presents for yearly follow-up to exclude focal lesions. The thyroid gland (calipers in Figs. 133.9 and 133.10; arrows in Fig. 133.11) is hypoechoic and markedly decreased in size, with a lobular contour due to retraction from numerous echogenic fibrous septations traversing the thyroid parenchyma. There are no focal nodules.

- Grave disease: autoimmune disease
  - Patients present with hyperthyroidism
  - Diffuse enlargement of the thyroid gland, which classically is homogeneous and hypoechoic with a smooth contour
  - Markedly increased vascularity, termed "thyroid inferno"
  - However, Doppler-detected vascularity does not correlate with thyroid function
- Subacute granulomatous thyroiditis (de Quervain thyroiditis): inflammatory condition, likely viral in origin, usually spontaneously remits
  - Patients typically present following a viral upper respiratory syndrome with fever, enlargement of the thyroid, and pain on palpation
  - Patients often transiently hyperthyroid but may become hypothyroid
  - Enlargement of the thyroid gland, often heterogeneous with indistinct, patchy hypoechoic areas due to edema, variable vascularity

Management

- Lifelong thyroid replacement therapy with levothyroxine
- Yearly surveillance with US due to increased incidence of papillary thyroid cancer and thyroid lymphoma
  - Hence, when fine needle aspiration is performed of a nodule in a patient with underlying Hashimoto thyroiditis, flow cytometry is generally recommended in addition to standard cytologic evaluation

Acknowledgment

Figures 133.9–133.11 courtesy of Dr. Lynwood Hammers, Hammers Healthcare, New Haven, Connecticut.

Further Reading

1. Yeh HC, Futterweit W, Gilbert P. Micronodulation: Ultrasonographic sign of Hashimoto thyroiditis. *J Ultrasound Med*. 1996; 15: 813–819.

History

▶ 35-Year-old male with palpable right thyroid nodule (Figs. 134.1–134.3)

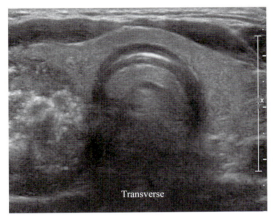

Fig. 134.1

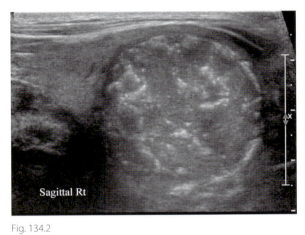

Fig. 134.2

Fig. 134.3

Case 134 Papillary Thyroid Cancer

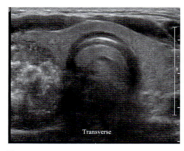

Fig. 134.4

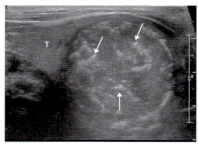

Fig. 134.5

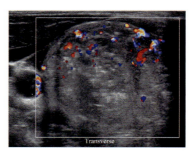

Fig. 134.6

Imaging Findings

► Large, solid nodule (Figs. 134.4–134.6) in the inferior pole of the right lobe of the thyroid with punctate echogenic, nonshadowing microcalcifications (arrows in Fig. 134.5); T, normal thyroid parenchyma
► Note increased internal vascularity on color Doppler image (Fig. 134.6)

Differential Diagnosis

► Hyperplastic or colloid nodule
► Follicular neoplasm
► Medullary thyroid cancer
► Anaplastic thyroid cancer
► Lymphoma
► Metastatic disease

Teaching Points

► Thyroid nodules are present in up to 50% of adults
  ▪ However, only 5–10% of thyroid nodules are malignant
► The reported incidence of thyroid cancer is increasing
  ▪ In part secondary to increased detection, including incidental findings on imaging studies such as carotid US or CT/MRI of the chest and neck
► Risks factors for thyroid cancer include the following
  ▪ Nodule found in male
  ▪ Childhood exposure to radiation
  ▪ Positive family history of thyroid cancer or multiple endocrine neoplasia type 2 (MEN2) syndrome
► Four main histologic types of thyroid cancer (CA): papillary (PTC) (80%), follicular (10%), medullary (5%), and anaplastic (< 5%)
  ▪ Papillary, follicular, and anaplastic tumors are epithelial-derived tumors
  ▪ Medullary CAs arise from the parafollicular cells (C cells), which secrete calcitonin
  ▪ PTC is most common and has the best prognosis, with a 20-year survival rate of approximately 90–95%
  ▪ Metastatic spread to cervical lymph nodes more common with PTC
  ▪ Hematogeneous spread more common with follicular thyroid CA
► Sonographic features of a thyroid nodule worrisome for papillary thyroid cancer include the following
  ▪ Calcification, especially nonshadowing microcalcifications (positive predictive value = 70%)
  ▪ Marked hypoechogenicity (more hypoechoic than strap muscles)
  ▪ Lobular, infiltrative, or invasive margins
  ▪ Nodules taller than wide
  ▪ Association with abnormal lymph nodes (microcalcifications, cystic areas, round, clustered, loss of echogenic central hilum, nodular cortex, increased or disorganized vascularity)
  ▪ Above US characteristics neither 100% sensitive nor specific
  ▪ The diffuse sclerosing variant of PTC is particularly common in children and may present with extensive involvement of an entire lobe with a speckled appearance due to the presence of innumerable tiny echogenic foci (see Figs. 134.7 and 134.8)

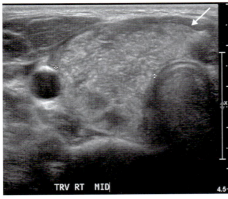

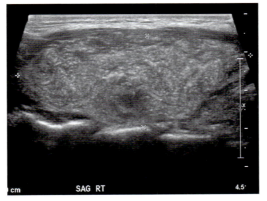

Fig. 134.7

Fig. 134.8

The entire right lobe of the thyroid (calipers in Figs. 134.7 and 134.8) is enlarged and diffusely infiltrated with tumor that extends into the isthmus (arrow in Fig. 134.7) in this 18-year-old female. Note speckled appearance due to the presence of numerous tiny echogenic, nonshadowing foci.

► Sonographic features that are likely to be benign include the following
  ▪ Cystic nodules, especially containing echogenic foci with ring-down or "comet tail" artifact (likely representing colloid)
  ▪ Spongiform (honeycomb) nodules
  ▪ Predominantly cystic nodules (solid component < 25% without vascularity or calcification)
► However, there is considerable overlap between benign and malignant US features
► Follicular neoplasm (Figs. 134.9 and 134.10)
  ▪ Homogeneous round solid nodule isoechoic or echogenic compared to thyroid parenchyma
  ▪ Thin peripheral hypoechoic halo
  ▪ Central linear hypoechoic areas, may have radiating linear pattern, possibly secondary to edema or hemorrhage
  ▪ Follicular neoplasms are considered surgical lesions because the diagnosis of follicular CA is based on the identification of capsular, vascular, and/or lymphatic invasion rather than cytologic characteristics
  ▪ Distant metastases more common than metastasis to cervical lymph nodes

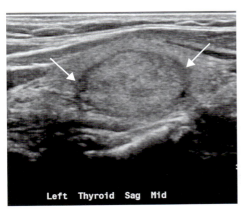

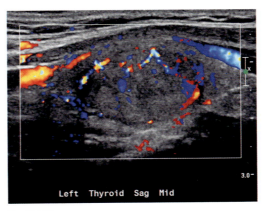

Fig. 134.9

Fig. 134.10

Echogenic vascular nodule with hypoechoic central areas in the left lobe of the thyroid in a 48-year-old female with a surgically proven follicular thyroid cancer. Note thin hypoechoic halo (arrows in Fig. 134.9), another common finding in follicular neoplasms. US characteristics, including whether the hypoechoic halo is thin or regular, cannot differentiate between benign and malignant follicular lesions.

► Medullary thyroid CA (Figs. 134.11 and 134.12): 10–20% associated with MEN2, more aggressive than PTC or follicular CAs, serum calcitonin used as serum marker
  ▪ Tumors tend to be larger with irregular infiltrating margins and often contain macrocalcifications
  ▪ Extracapsular invasion and lymph node metastases are common at presentation
  ▪ However, US findings are nonspecific and overlap with other types of thyroid cancer

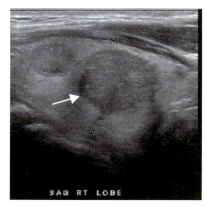

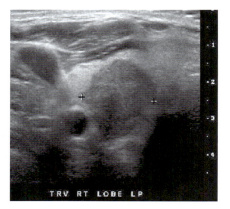

Fig. 134.11   Fig. 134.12

70-Year-old male with markedly elevated serum calcitonin level. Note 2-cm markedly hypoechoic nodule (arrow in Fig. 134.11 and calipers in Fig. 134.12) in the lower pole of the right lobe of the thyroid. The nodule is taller than wide on the transverse image (Fig. 134.12), with a lobular, infiltrating margin. These features are highly predictive of malignancy but could be seen with PTC as well as medullary thyroid CA.

▶ Anaplastic thyroid CA (Figs. 134.13–134.16): < 5% of all thyroid CAs, typically presents in older patients, extremely poor prognosis
  ▪ Large infiltrating tumors
  ▪ Variable echogenicity
  ▪ Vascular
  ▪ Extracapsular invasion and lymph node metastases common at presentation

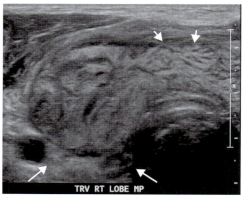

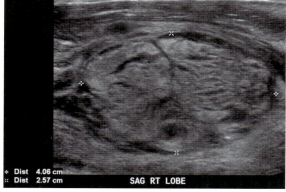

Fig. 134.13   Fig. 134.14

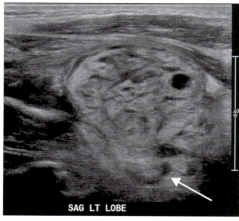

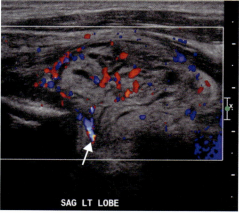

Fig. 134.15   Fig. 134.16

78-Year-old female presented with rapidly enlarging thyroid and cervical lymphadenopathy. Both the right and the left lobes of the thyroid as well as the isthmus (short arrows in Fig 134.13) are enlarged and infiltrated by tumor, which is vascular and heterogeneous but primarily echogenic with serpiginous to round anechoic areas. Almost no normal thyroid parenchyma is identified. Extracapsular invasion is noted (long arrows in Fig. 134.13 and arrows in Figs. 134.15 and 134.16) and was confirmed at surgery. The tumor is vascular on color Doppler (Fig. 134.16)

▶ Lymphoma (Figs. 134.17–134.19): more likely to be homogeneous, hypoechoic; less likely to have calcifications; increased incidence in patients with Hashimoto thyroiditis

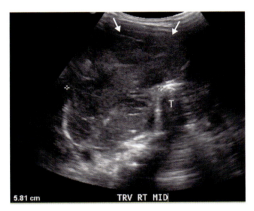

Fig. 134.17

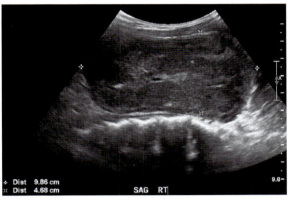

Fig. 134.18

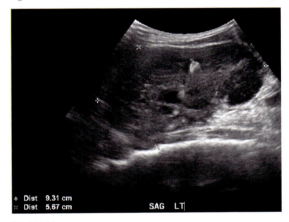

Fig. 134.19

52-Year-old male with a history of diffuse B-cell lymphoma. Note massively enlarged right lobe of the thyroid (calipers Figs. 134.17 and 134.18) extending into the isthmus (arrows in Fig. 134.17) overlying the trachea (T in Fig. 134.17). The left lobe of the thyroid (calipers in Fig. 134.19) appears similar and has several anechoic areas likely representing hemorrhage or necrosis.

▶ Metastases to thyroid: uncommon, variable echogenicity and vascularity, less likely to have calcifications

Management

▶ Diagnosis of PTC is made by fine needle aspiration
▶ Considerable controversy regarding which thyroid nodules should undergo aspiration
  ▪ Different organizations have published slightly different guidelines
▶ Total thyroidectomy with central lymph node dissection is recommended for most patients with PTC
  ▪ ^{131}Iodine commonly used as adjuvant radiotherapy
▶ US screening of the lateral neck to search for metastatic lymph nodes prior to surgery is increasingly performed because lateral neck dissection is recommended for patients with positive lymphadenopathy in levels 2–5.

Acknowledgment

Figures 134.7–134.12 and 134.17–134.19 courtesy of Dr. Lynwood Hammers, Hammers HealthCare, New Haven, Connecticut.

Further Reading

1. Bonavita JA, Mayo J, Babb J, et al. Pattern recognition of benign nodules at ultrasound of the thyroid: Which nodules can be left alone? *Am J Roentgenol.* 2009; 193: 207–213.

2. Moon WJ, Jung SL, Lee JH, et al. Benign and malignant thyroid nodules: US differentiation—Multicenter retrospective study. *Radiology.* 2008; 247: 762–770.

3. Smith-Bindman R, Lebda P, Feldstein VA, et al. Risk of thyroid cancer based on thyroid US imaging characteristics. *JAMA.* 2013; 173: 1788–1796.

4. Frates MC, Benson CB, Charboneau JW, et al. Management of thyroid nodules detected at US: Society of Radiologists in Ultrasound consensus conference statement. *Radiology.* 2005; 237: 794–800.

5. Haugen BR, Alexander EK, Bible KC, et al. 2015 American Thyroid Association Management Guidelines for Adult Patients with Thyroid Nodules and Differentiated Thyroid Cancer. *Thyroid.* 2016; 26: 1–133.

History

▶ 42-Year-old female presenting with a palpable right neck mass (Figs. 135.1–135.3)

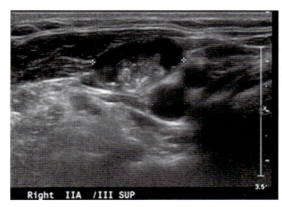

Fig. 135.1

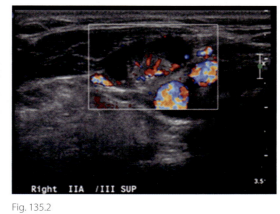

Fig. 135.2

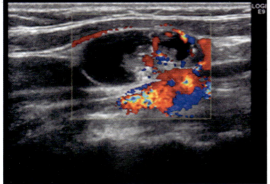

Fig. 135.3

Case 135 Lymph Node Metastasis From Papillary Thyroid Cancer

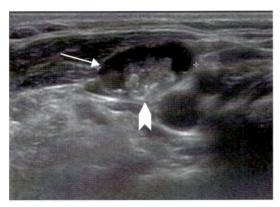

Fig. 135.4

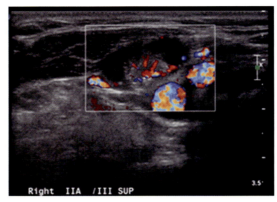

Fig. 135.5

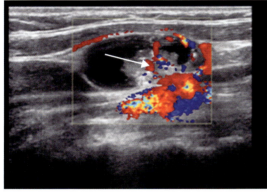

Fig. 135.6

Imaging Findings

► Enlarged and rounded right cervical lymph node level IIA/III with cystic changes (arrow in Fig. 135.4)
► Echogenic foci within the solid component represent microcalcifications (arrowhead in Fig. 135.4)
► No normal hilum or cortex
► Increased vascularity on color Doppler US (Fig. 135.5) with an irregular arborizing pattern in the nodular solid tissue (arrow in Fig. 135.6)

Differential Diagnosis

► Cystic metastasis from other head and neck malignancy, particularly squamous cell carcinoma
► Infectious lymphadenitis, including tuberculosis
► Sebaceous cyst/epidermoid cyst

Teaching Points

► Papillary thyroid carcinoma commonly metastasizes to cervical lymph nodes
► Following surgery, patients with papillary thyroid cancer are typically screened yearly for recurrence with stimulated serum thyroglobulin and US evaluation of the central and lateral neck compartments bilaterally for at least 5 years.
► Microcalcifications and cystic changes have a high specificity and positive predictive value for metastatic papillary thyroid cancer, although cystic changes can occasionally be seen in patients with metastatic lymph nodes from head and neck squamous cell cancers
► Microcalcifications and cystic degeneration of a right cervical lymph node on the axial images from a neck CT (arrow in Fig. 135.7) and corresponding neck US (arrow in Fig. 135.8)

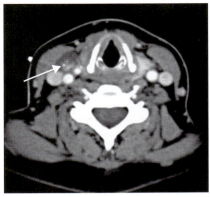

Fig. 135.7

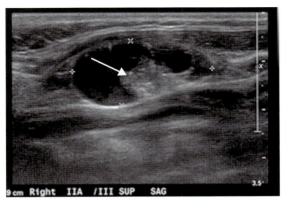

Fig. 135.8

► Other sonographic features commonly associated with nodal metastasis include the following
  ■ Round shape, loss of echogenic hilum, and irregular blood supply with loss of the central feeding vessel (arrows in Figs. 135.9 and 135.10)

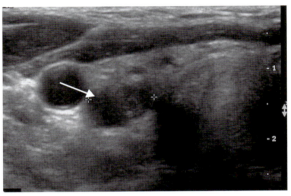

Fig. 135.9

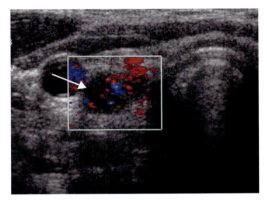

Fig. 135.10

  ■ Diffusely hypoechoic or echogenic lymph nodes with loss of the central echogenic hilum (arrow in Fig. 135.11); asymmetric, lobulated cortex; and diffuse hypervascularity (arrow in Fig. 135.12)

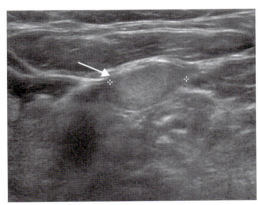

Fig. 135.11

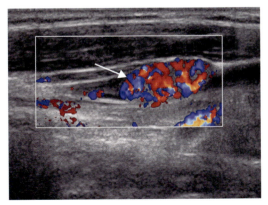

Fig. 135.12

  ■ Overlap with reactive lymph nodes does exist—when in doubt, recommend fine needle aspiration
► Infectious lymphadenitis: multiple enlarged hypoechoic lymph nodes but typically do not contain cystic areas or microcalcifications
► Sebaceous cyst would more likely demonstrate low-level internal echoes consistent with debris and is located in the epidermis

Management

▶ US is recommended for preoperative staging and nodal mapping

▶ Cervical lymph nodes are amenable to US fine needle aspiration

  ▪ Aspirate and send for thyroglobulin levels if node is cystic

▶ Abnormal lymph nodes from each compartment need to be sampled. The goal is to minimize the extent of surgery but to perform a full lymph node dissection in any compartment with positive cytology

▶ Determining the level of cervical node involvement is important for preoperative planning because level I, VI, and VII nodes require central neck dissection, whereas level II–V nodes require lateral neck dissection. Some surgeons now perform a central lymph node dissection in all patients

▶ In selected cases, especially after multiple neck surgeries for recurrence, alcohol ablation is performed by percutaneous injection into the abnormal lymph node

Further Reading

1. Ahuja AT, Ying M. Sonographic evaluation of cervical lymph nodes. *Am J Roentgenol*. 2005; 184: 1691–1699.
2. Sohn YM, Kwak JY, Kim EK, et al. Diagnostic approach for evaluation of lymph node metastasis from thyroid cancer using ultrasound and fine-needle aspiration biopsy. *Am J Roentgenol*. 2010; 194: 38–43.

History

► 45-Year-old female with flank pain and multiple renal calculi (Figs. 136.1–136.4)

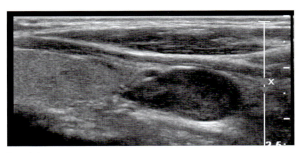

Fig. 136.1

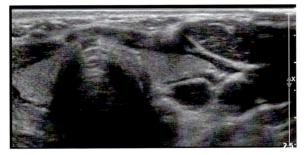

Fig. 136.2

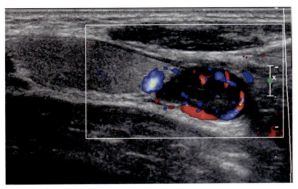

Fig. 136.3

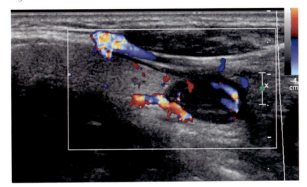

Fig. 136.4

Case 136 Parathyroid Adenoma, Primary Hyperparathyroidism

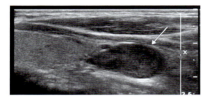

Fig. 136.5

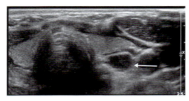

Fig. 136.6

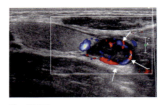

Fig. 136.7

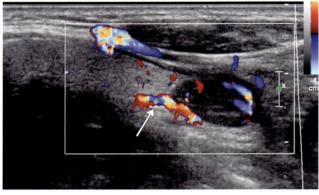

Fig. 136.8

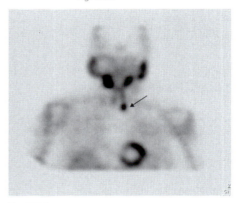

Fig. 136.9

Imaging Findings

▶ Hypoechoic oval, solid mass inferior and posterior to the lower pole of the left lobe of the thyroid (arrows in Fig. 136.5 and 136.6)
▶ Peripheral arc-like blood flow (arrows in Fig. 136.7) with a dominant polar feeding artery (arrow in Fig. 136.8)
▶ Delayed image from nuclear medicine parathyroid sestamibi scan demonstrates persistent uptake in the parathyroid adenoma (arrow in Fig. 136.9)

Differential Diagnosis

▶ Lymph node
▶ Parathyroid hyperplasia
▶ Parathyroid carcinoma
▶ Exophytic thyroid nodule

Teaching Points

▶ Four parathyroid glands are normally present: right and left upper (posterior to the superior/mid portion of the thyroid lobes) and right and left lower (posterior and inferior to the lower poles of the thyroid gland, usually within 2 cm)
▶ Ectopic parathyroid glands can be located anywhere from the submandibular gland to the superior mediastinum or in the thyroid gland itself
▶ 90% of cases of primary hyperparathyroidism (HPT) are due to a single adenoma
  ▪ Three times more common in females
  ▪ Multiple parathyroid adenomas (PTAs) may occur in older patients
  ▪ Parathyroid hyperplasia more common in patients with secondary HPT
▶ Presentation: hypercalcemia, elevated parathyroid hormone levels
  ▪ Majority asymptomatic
  ▪ Patients may present with nephrolithiasis, flank pain, bone and joint pain, abdominal pain, nausea and vomiting in severe cases
▶ Parathyroid adenoma—US findings
  ▪ Hypoechoic, homogeneous, ovoid, extrathyroidal solid mass
  ▪ Usually > 1.0 cm in size
  ▪ Rarely intrathyroidal
  ▪ Rarely complex cystic mass (1–4%)
    • Can aspirate and measure parathyroid hormone (PTH) from cystic fluid

- Vascular
  - Feeding polar artery or arc-like peripheral vascularity
- Increased flow to ipsilateral thyroid lobe
▶ Lymph nodes: classically reniform in shape with a hypoechoic cortex, echogenic central hilum, and central hilar artery and vein
▶ Parathyroid hyperplasia: homogeneous enlargement of multiple parathyroid glands that are usually smaller than adenomas
▶ Parathyroid carcinoma: rare, incidence approximately 1.25 cases/10 million people
- En bloc surgical excision is treatment of choice
- Five-year survival, 90%; 10-year survival, 50%
- Males = females
- Patients present with severe HPT as tumors secrete PTH
  - Serum calcium and PTH levels usually much higher (> 14 mg/dl) than in patients with HPT secondary to PTAs
  - Accounts for < 1% of all cases of HPT
  - Hypercalcemia treated with volume loading and calcium-wasting loop diuretic, but often difficult to control and results in significant morbidity
- May present with palpable mass (rare in patients with PTAs or parathyroid hyperplasia)
- US findings
  - No size threshold, but usually > 2 cm, rarely < 1.5 cm
  - Irregular, lobular shape
  - Heterogeneous echotexture, internal cystic components
  - Vascular: internal vascularity may be radial and irregular, no polar feeding vessel
  - Infiltration of surrounding soft tissues

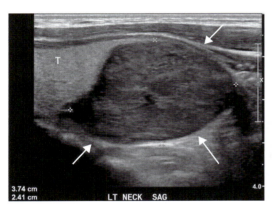

Fig. 136.10

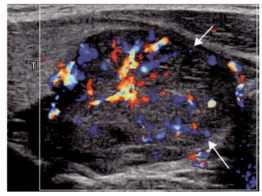

Fig. 136.11

Large (3.7 cm) heterogeneously hypoechoic, vascular solid mass (arrows in Figs. 136.10 and 136.11) inferior to the lower pole of the left lobe of the thyroid (T in Figs. 136.10 and 136.11)
▶ May be impossible by imaging alone to differentiate from large PTA
▶ Diagnosis often made at surgery when the parathyroid gland is found to be adherent to surrounding soft tissues secondary to local invasion
▶ Exophytic thyroid nodule: should see connection to thyroid gland, isoechoic to thyroid, less vascular than typical PTA

Management

▶ US considered imaging modality of choice for PTA localization in patients with hypercalcemia
▶ With accurate preoperative localization, minimally invasive surgery can be performed
▶ If imaging not classic, consider fine needle aspiration to measure PTH levels
▶ Four-dimensional CT or nuclear medicine sestimibi study next imaging modalities of choice to localize PTAs in patients with hypercalcemia and negative US

Further Reading

1. Reeder SB, Desser TS, Weigel RJ, et al. Sonography in primary hyperparathyroidism. *J Ultrasound Med.* 2002; 21: 539–552.
2. Mittendorf EA, McHenry CR. Parathyroid carcinoma. *J Surg Oncol.* 2005; 89(3): 136–142.
3. Busaidy NL, Jimenez C, Habra MA, et al. Parathyroid carcinoma: A 22-year experience. *Head Neck.* 2004; 26(8): 716–726.

Case 137

History

▶ 74-Year-old male with palpable right testicular mass (Figs. 137.1–137.4)

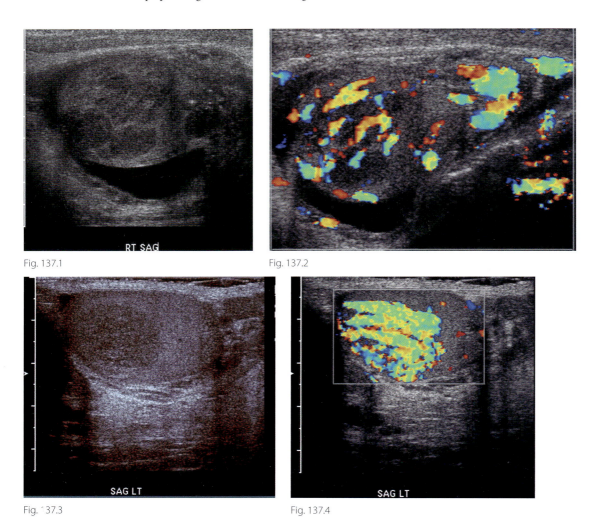

Fig. 137.1

Fig. 137.2

Fig. 137.3

Fig. 137.4

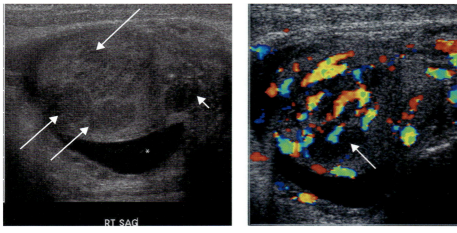

Fig. 137.5   Fig. 137.6

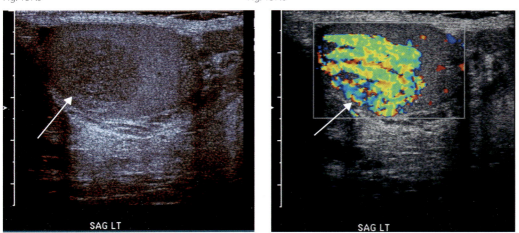

Fig. 137.7   Fig. 137.8

Imaging Findings

► Enlarged right testicle with multiple hypoechoic vascular masses, and diffuse infiltration of the testicle (long arrows in Figs. 137.5 and 137.6) and epididymal tail (short arrows in Figs. 137.5 and 137.6). Associated right hydrocele (asterisk in Fig. 135.5)
► Hypoechoic, mass in left testicle (arrow in Figs. 137.7 and 137.8) that was also hypervascular

Differential Diagnosis

► Leukemia
► Seminoma
► Metastases
► Testicular abscesses
► Sarcoidosis

Teaching Points

► Most common testicular tumor in men > 60 years old
► Accounts for 1–8% of all testicular tumors
► Most common secondary testicular neoplasm usually non-Hodgkin lymphoma, primary testicular lymphoma rare
► Most common bilateral testicular tumor, accounts for 50% of bilateral testicular neoplasms
► Presentation: painless testicular mass
  ▪ Often with lymph node involvement

461

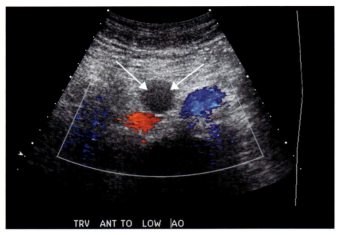

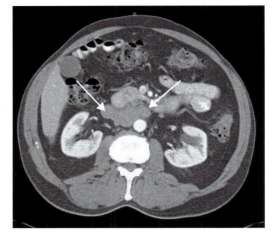

Fig. 137.9   Fig. 137.10

- ▪ Aortocaval lymphadenopathy on US and CT (arrows in Figs. 137.9 and 137.10)
- ▪ Extension into the epididymis and spermatic cord in up to one-half of cases (short arrow in Figs. 137.5 and 137.6)
- ► US appearance
  - ▪ Nonspecific, similar to seminoma
  - ▪ Commonly hypoechoic with focal masses or diffuse infiltration
  - ▪ Increased flow on color Doppler US, may mimic inflammatory process
  - ▪ Retroperitoneal lymphadenopathy
- ► Leukemia: second most common metastatic testicular neoplasm, often found in children during bone marrow remission because testicles provide a "sanctuary" for leukemic cells due to the blood–testis barrier; US appearance similar to lymphoma
- ► Seminoma: most common single cell tumor of testis, peak incidence fourth and fifth decades, most common tumor in undescended testes; US appearance similar to lymphoma, although less often multiple and bilateral
- ► Metastases: most frequently from prostate and lung, followed by melanoma, renal, colon, and stomach; variable US appearance— hypoechoic, echogenic or heterogeneous, typically bilateral, rare without evidence of other sites of metastases
- ► Testicular abscesses: rare, usually complication of epididymitis/orchitis with heterogeneous fluid-filled mass on US and clinical signs of inflammation with peripheral but not central vascularity
- ► Sarcoidosis: epididymal involvement > testicle; US: hypoechoic but often avascular

Management

- ► Chemotherapy if known history of lymphoma
- ► If no history of lymphoma, orchiectomy may be required for definitive diagnosis due to lack of specificity of US findings as was performed in this patient yielding large B-cell lymphoma

Further Reading

1. Lantz AG, Power N, Hutton B, et al. Malignant lymphoma of the testis: A study of 12 cases. *Can Urol Assoc J.* 2009; 3(5): 393–398.
2. Surti KM, Ralls PW: Sonographic appearance of plasmablastic lymphoma of the testes. *J Ultrasound Med.* 2008; 27: 965–967.

Case 138

History

► 36-Year-old male with history of enzyme deficiency diagnosed soon after birth (Figs. 138.1–138.4)

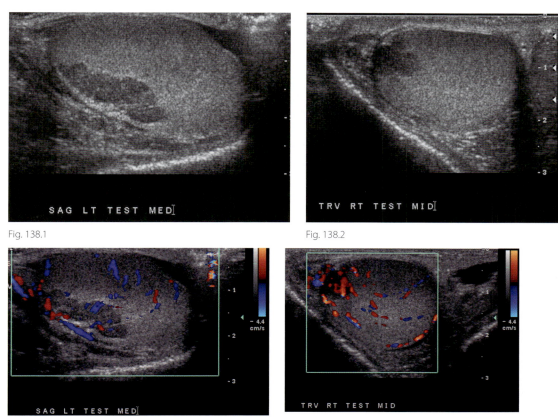

Fig. 138.1

Fig. 138.2

Fig. 138.3

Fig. 138.4

Case 138 Testicular Adrenal Rest Tumor-Like Masses in a Patient With Congenital Adrenal Hyperplasia

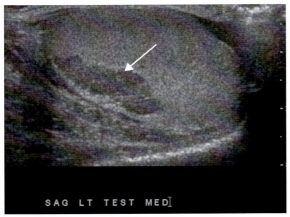

Fig. 138.5

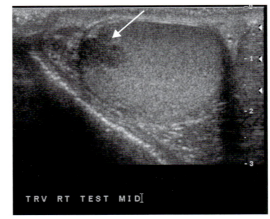

Fig. 138.6

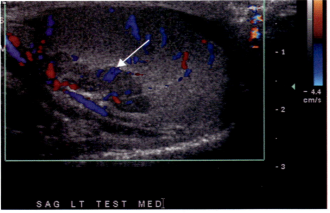

Fig. 138.7

Imaging Findings

► Hypoechoic, lobulated, well-circumscribed elongated masses in both testicles (arrows in Figs. 138.5 and 138.6)
► Increased flow on color Doppler US (CDUS) (arrow in Fig. 138.7)

Differential Diagnosis

► Germ cell tumors
► Lymphoma/leukemia
► Metastases
► Leydig cell hyperplasia
► Tubular ectasia of rete testis

Teaching Points

► Congenital adrenal hyperplasia (CAH)
  ▪ Autosomal recessive disorder due to adrenocortical enzyme (CYP 21) defect (21-hydroxylase deficiency) resulting in impaired production of cortisol and mostly aldosterone that may lead to Addisonian crisis with salt wasting and dehydration
► Increased pituitary adrenocorticoid hormone (ACTH) production leads to adrenal gland hyperplasia and overproduction of adrenal androgens, causing precocious puberty
► Testicular adrenal rests

- Benign corticotropin-dependent testicular lesions; often asymptomatic; however, also rare cause of a testicular mass/testicular enlargement
- Aberrant collection of adrenal cells entrapped within the developing gonad during fetal development (adrenal glands develop adjacent to gonads)
- Can lead to gonadal dysfunction and infertility; usually bilateral
► US findings
- Multiple, bilateral testicular masses, eccentrically located, typically adjacent to mediastinum testis
- Predominantly hypoechoic, rare heterogeneously echogenic with or without shadowing
- May be hyper-, hypo-, or normovascular on CDUS
► CT findings
- Prominent nodular bilateral adrenal glands on CT (arrows in Fig. 138.8)

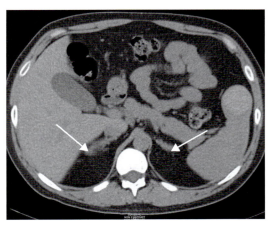

Fig. 138.8

- Germ cell tumors, lymphoma/leukemia, and metastases: may all present as hypoechoic or heterogeneous multiple, bilateral testicular lesions, but without the clinical and/or laboratory findings of CAH
- Testicular abscesses: usually sequela of epididymitis/orchitis, hypoechoic and indistinguishable by US from neoplasms; clinical history helpful
- Leydig cell hyperplasia: majority of testicular stromal tumors; may have similar clinical and US presentation, but not with CAH
- Tubular ectasia of rete testis: can be mistaken for testicular neoplasm; cystic lesions seen located near mediastinum testis. No flow on CDUS

Management

► Important to recognize as benign lesions to avoid unnecessary orchiectomy
► No further workup if patient has appropriate hormonal abnormality associated with CAH and shows appropriate US findings
► In equivocal cases, US-guided biopsy intraoperatively with testicle exposed
► Treatment with glucocorticoid replacement therapy can stabilize or cause regression of testicular lesions

Further Reading

1. Claahsen-van der Grinten HL, Otten BJ, Stikkelbroeck MML, et al. Testicular adrenal rest tumours in congenital adrenal hyperplasia. *Clin Endocrinol Metab.* 2009; 23(2): 209–220.
2. Nagamine WH, Mehta SV, Vade A. Testicular adrenal rest tumors in a patient with congenital adrenal hyperplasia. *J Ultrasound Med.* 2005; 24: 1717–1720.

Case 139

History

▶ 41-Year-old male with right testicular pain (Figs. 139.1–139.4)

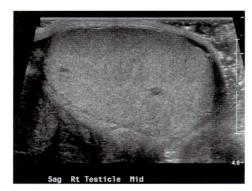

Fig. 139.1

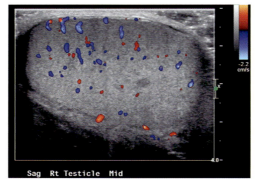

Fig. 139.2

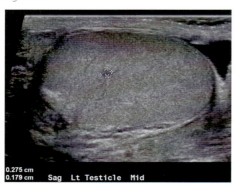

Fig. 139.3

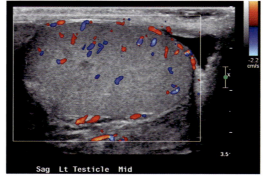

Fig. 139.4

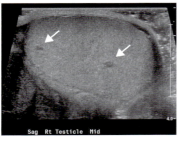

Fig. 139.5

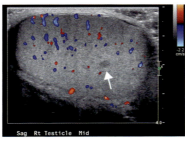

Fig. 139.6

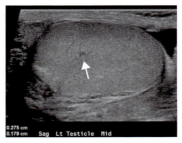

Fig. 139.7

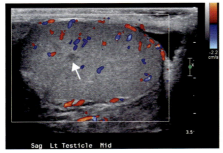

Fig. 139.8

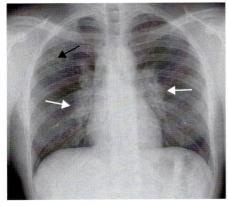

Fig. 139.9

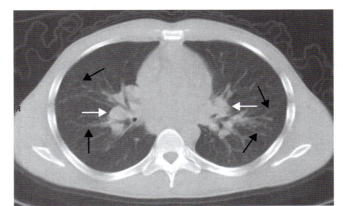

Fig. 139.10

Imaging Findings

▶ Several bilateral < 5mm hypoechoic foci in the testicular parenchyma (arrows in Figs. 139.5–139.8), which are not vascular on color Doppler imaging (Figs. 139.6 and 139.8)

▶ Note bilateral hilar lymphadenopathy (white arrows in Figs. 139.9 and 139.10) and pulmonary fibrosis (black arrows in Figs. 139.9 and 139.10) on chest radiograph and axial CT scan respectively consistent with known diagnosis of sarcoidosis

Differential Diagnosis

▶ Leukemia
▶ Lymphoma
▶ Metastases
▶ Testicular microabscesses
▶ Focal testicular infarcts

Teaching Points

▶ Idiopathic multisystemic disease characterized by the formation of noncaseating granulomas
  ▪ Most commonly presents in second through fourth decades
  ▪ 10–20 times more prevalent in African Americans than in Caucasians
  ▪ 10 times more common in women
▶ Male genitourinary involvement is rare (< 1% of patients with systemic sarcoid)
  ▪ Epididymis most commonly involved organ
  ▪ Testicular sarcoid usually associated with epididymal involvement, but isolated testicular sarcoid may occur
▶ Clinical manifestations of testicular sarcoidosis: painless testicular nodularity, diffuse mass, mild pain and swelling, recurrent epididymitis (if coexisting epididymal involvement); often asymptomatic
▶ US findings are nonspecific
  ▪ Multiple small bilateral hypoechoic lesions within the testicular parenchyma
  ▪ Epididymal lesions commonly associated
  ▪ Homogeneous infiltrative lesion involving the entire testis rare
  ▪ Echogenic lesions uncommon
▶ Testicular sarcoid should always be considered when an intratesticular lesion is seen in a patient with known sarcoidosis
  ▪ Other supportive findings: constitutional symptoms, chest imaging findings, and negative testicular tumor markers—human chorionic gonadotropin, α-fetoprotein, and lactate dehydrogenase
  ▪ In atypical cases, an open testicular biopsy or orchiectomy may be indicated
▶ On MRI, foci of testicular sarcoid are low signal on T2-weighted images and enhance following the administration of gadolinium
▶ Testicular lymphoma (non-Hodgkin), leukemia, and metastases (lung, prostate, renal, gastrointestinal, melanoma) may have a similar US appearance, presenting with multiple bilateral hypoechoic testicular masses
  ▪ In elderly men, metastases are more common than primary testicular tumors
  ▪ The testes are a "sanctuary" for lymphoma and leukemia because chemotherapy does not cross the blood–testicular barrier. Hence, disease can persist in the testes when the patient is in remission
  ▪ These etiologies are more likely to be vascular
▶ Microabscesses: multiple hypoechoic areas in the testes with peripheral vascularity, reactive hydrocele, ± skin thickening; may be bilateral
▶ Focal testicular infarcts: avascular hypoechoic areas in the testes often caused by vasculitis. Larger areas of infarction may be sequelae of torsion or incompletely treated epididymitis

Management

▶ Corticosteroids provide symptomatic relief and reduce the size of testicular lesions
▶ Methotrexate, azathioprine, and infliximab used to treat steroid-resistant systemic disease
▶ Epididymal sarcoid is associated with infertility; hence, serial semen analysis and sperm banking should be considered

Further Reading

1. Ghazle HH, Bhatt S. Testicular sarcoidosis: Sonographic findings. *J Diagn Med Sonogr*. 2011; 27: 126–130.
2. Woodward PJ, Sohaey R, O'Donoghue MJ, et al. From the archives of the AFIP: Tumors and tumor like lesions of the testis: Radiologic–pathologic correlation. *RadioGraphics*. 2002; 22: 189–216.
3. Rao PK, Sabanegh ES. Genitourinary sarcoidosis. *Rev Urol*. 2009; 11: 108–113.

History

▶ 59-Year-old male with acute left testicular swelling (Figs. 140.1–140.3)

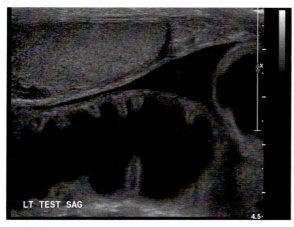

Fig. 140.1

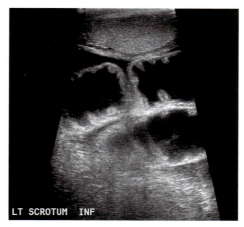

Fig. 140.2

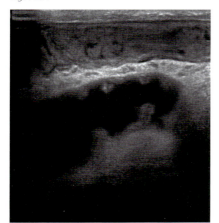

Fig. 140.3

Case 140 Scrotal Hernia

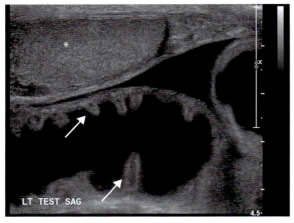

Fig. 140.4

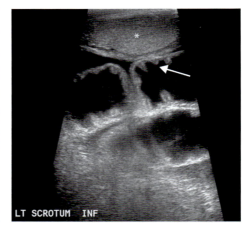

Fig. 140.5

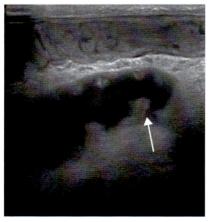

Fig. 140.6

Imaging Findings

► Large extratesticular mass due to large amount of small bowel herniating into left scrotal sac and filling both sides of the scrotal sac, compressing the left testicle (asterisk in Figs. 140.4 and 140.5). Notice valvulae conniventes (arrows in Figs. 140.4 and 140.5)
► Note free fluid within left scrotal sac and small bowel within the inguinal canal (arrow in Fig. 140.6)

Differential Diagnosis

► Femoral hernia
► Hydrocele
► Hematocele
► Pyocele

Teaching Points

► Protrusion of intra-abdominal cavity contents into the scrotal sac through the inguinal canal
► 25 times more common in men than women
► Two types: direct and indirect hernias defined by their relationship to the inferior epigastric vessels
  ▪ Direct: medial to inferior epigastric vessels; contents herniate through a weak area in the fascia transversalis; occurs in adults
  ▪ Indirect: lateral to inferior epigastric vessels due to embryonic failure of closure of the processes vaginalis after testis has passed through; occurs in adults and children
► Commonly presents as a paratesticular mass, usually diagnosed by physical exam
► Often contains bowel (small bowel or colon), omentum, and omental fat or fatty mass such as a lipoma
► Complications include obstruction, incarceration, and strangulation

► US findings
  ▪ Dilated bowel loops with or without peristalsis
  ▪ Echogenic mass, suggestive of fat
  ▪ Dilated bowel loops may be traced back to the inguinal canal
  ▪ Presence of flow on Doppler US may help to differentiate incarcerated/strangulated from viable bowel
  ▪ If these characteristic features are not present—difficult to differentiate scrotal hernia from other extratesticular multicystic masses such as hydroceles, hematoceles, or pyoceles
► CT Findings
  ▪ Enormous left inguinal hernia containing small bowel, fat, and mesenteric vessels on CT (arrows in Fig. 140.7 and 140.8). Mild dilatation and hypo-enhancement of small bowel wall, suggestive of vascular compromise (Figs. 140.7 and 140.8)

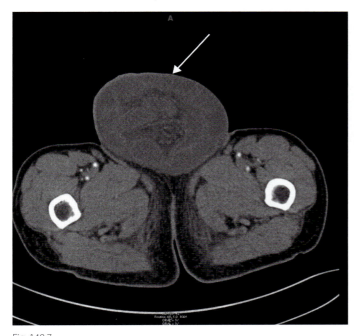

Fig. 140.7

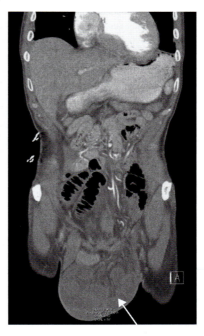

Fig. 140.8

  ▪ Femoral hernia: occurs below the inguinal ligament via the femoral canal and not via the inguinal canal. More common in women than in men due to wider bony structure of the female pelvis
  ▪ Hydrocele, hematocele, and pyocele: collections that accumulate between the visceral and tunical layers of the tunica vaginalis, usually confined to the anterolateral portion of the scrotum. Hydroceles contain simple fluid; hematoceles and pyoceles are complex fluid collections with or without septations and often due to trauma, post surgery, or infection

Management

► Surgical hernia repair (herniorraphy) if large and symptomatic to avoid obstruction, incarceration, and strangulation
► Watchful waiting without surgery if the hernia is small and only minimally symptomatic due to risk of post herniorraphy pain syndrome

Further Reading
1. Stavros AT, Rapp C. Dynamic ultrasound of hernias of the groin and anterior abdominal wall. *Ultrasound Q.* 2010; 26(3): 135–169.
2. Rapp C: Ultrasound of abdominal wall hernias. *J Diagn Med Sonogr.* 1999; 15: 231–235.

Case 141

► 35-Year-old male with fever and left-sided scrotal pain and swelling (Figs. 141.1–141.3)

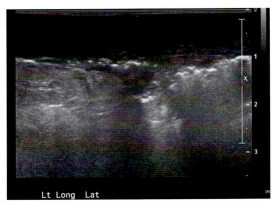

Fig. 141.1

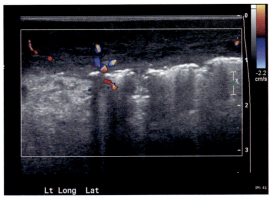

Fig. 141.2

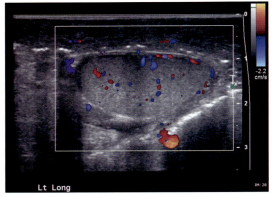

Fig. 141.3

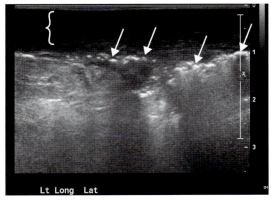

Fig. 141.4

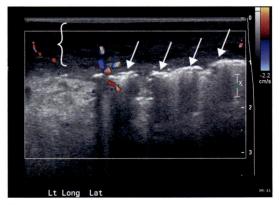

Fig. 141.5

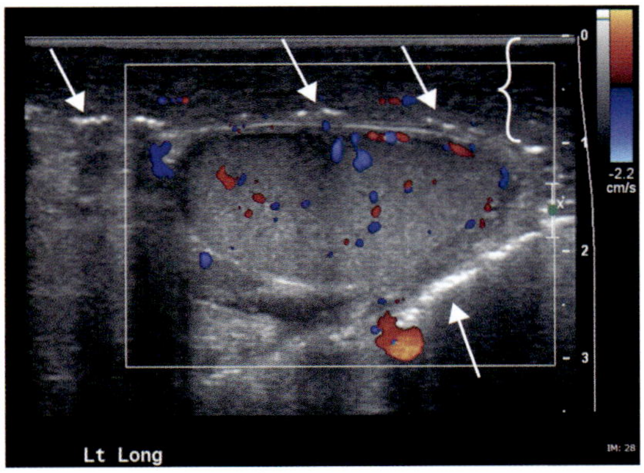

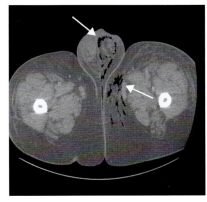

Fig. 141.6

Fig. 141.7

Imaging Findings

▶ Note extensive skin thickening and edema (brackets in Figs. 141.4–141.6) of the left scrotal wall with slightly increased vascularity on color Doppler imaging (Figs. 141.5 and 141.6)

▶ Multiple hyperechoic foci with dirty posterior acoustic shadowing (arrows in Figs. 141.4–141.6) are present in the scrotal wall consistent with air in the soft tissues

▶ The left testis is homogenous in echotexture with normal vascularity (Fig. 141.6)

▶ Axial CT scan confirms the presence of foci of gas within the scrotal skin, perineum, and subcutaneous tissue of the medial upper left thigh (arrows in Fig. 141.7), which is pathognomonic of Fournier gangrene

Differential Diagnosis

▶ Scrotal cellulitis
▶ Incarcerated scrotal hernia

Teaching Points

▶ Fournier gangrene is a rapidly progressive necrotizing fascitis involving the genital, perineal, and perianal regions
- Strong predilection for diabetic patients
- Progression of gangrene is often fulminant
- Surgical emergency with a potentially high mortality rate
- Classically a polymicrobial mixed aerobic and anaerobic infection
- Most common in elderly males, aged 60–70 years, but occasionally reported in young men, women, and children
- Most series report a 10:1 male-to-female ratio

▶ Clinical manifestations: scrotal swelling/hyperemia, pain, pruritus, fever, crepitus on palpation

▶ Risk factors: diabetes, alcohol abuse, malnutrition, immunosuppression, trauma

- ▶ Plain radiograph findings
  - ▪ Multiple lucencies in soft tissues overlying scrotum and perineum representing air in soft tissues
- ▶ US findings
  - ▪ Thickened, edematous scrotal wall (or labia) containing echogenic foci demonstrating "dirty" posterior acoustic shadowing secondary to reverberation artifact, diagnostic of gas within the scrotal wall
  - ▪ Increased vascularity of scrotal wall may be noted
  - ▪ Testis and epididymis typically normal in size, vascularity, and echotexture
  - ▪ Air and edema may be noted in soft tissue of perineum or upper, medial thigh
- ▶ CT has greater sensitivity for detecting subcutaneous air as well as accuracy in determining disease extent compared to physical exam or US and helps in planning surgical treatment
- ▶ Scrotal cellulitis: thick, edematous vascular scrotal wall without evidence of air. Often associated reactive hydrocele, pyocele, or scrotal/epididymal/testicular fluid collection representing abscess. May be associated with underlying epididymitis or orchitis
  - ▪ On transverse US views, tiny echogenic foci in the edematous, thickened scrotal wall may be confused with air in patients with severe cellulitis. However, these should be easily recognized on sagittal images as echogenic septations of connective tissue outlined by fluid within the scrotal wall. In addition, dirty posterior shadowing or ring-down artifact will not be present
- ▶ Incarcerated scrotal hernia: gas will be located in the obstructed bowel lumen separate from the scrotal wall and testicles

Management

- ▶ Intravenous broad-spectrum antibiotics with immediate and complete debridement of the necrotic tissue is the treatment of choice

Further Reading

1. Levenson RB, Singh AK, Novelline RA. Fournier gangrene: Role of imaging. *RadioGraphics*. 2008; 28: 519–528.
2. Avery LL, Scheinfeld MH. Imaging of penile and scrotal emergencies. *RadioGraphics*. 2013; 33(3): 721–740.

History

▶ 68-Year-old female with left-sided chest pain following a motor vehicle accident (Figs. 142.1 and 142.2)

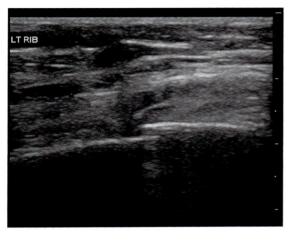

Fig. 142.1

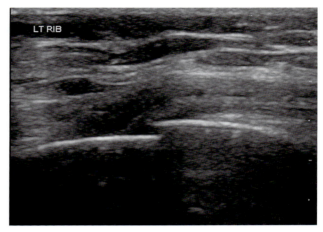

Fig. 142.2

Case 142 Rib Fracture Secondary to Trauma

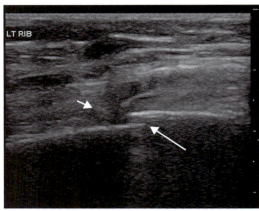
Fig. 142.3

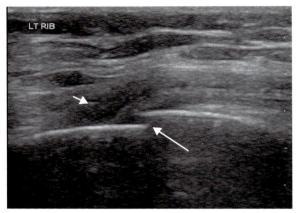
Fig. 142.4

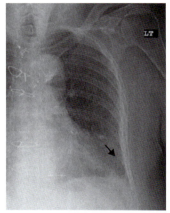
Fig. 142.5

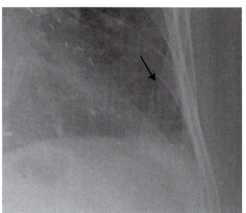
Fig. 142.6

Imaging Findings

▶ Step off of echogenic bony cortex in a left rib with elevation and overlapping of one of the fragments (long arrows in Figs. 142.3 and 142.4). Adjacent small anechoic area anteriorly elevating the fascial planes is consistent with hematoma (short arrows in Figs. 142.3 and 142.4)
▶ Minimally displaced rib fracture is confirmed on chest radiograph and magnified view of the ribs (arrows in Figs. 142.5 and 142.6)

Differential Diagnosis

▶ Pathologic rib fracture
▶ Expansile rib lesion
▶ Normal pleural line

Teaching Points

▶ Presentation: chest wall pain post trauma
▶ Look for complications of rib fractures, such as local hematoma, pneumothorax, and hemothorax
  ▪ Pneumothorax may be diagnosed on US by the absence of the sliding lung sign and absence of the normal comet tail artifact extending from the pleural line
▶ The presence of multiple rib fractures increases risk for more serious internal injury
▶ US reported to be more sensitive than radiography in detecting rib fractures
  ▪ Particularly difficult to detect nondisplaced fractures on radiographs
  ▪ Can perform a focused US exam and image precisely at the point of maximum pain and tenderness
  ▪ Especially useful in children because it avoids use of ionizing radiation

- ▶ US findings
  - ▪ Sharp disruption of echogenic bony cortex
  - ▪ ± Overriding fragment, displacement, or angulation
  - ▪ Adjacent avascular anechoic to hypoechoic hematoma
- ▶ Healing fracture: visualization of callus formation around fracture which will appear hypoechoic on US, often with focal areas of calcification (irregular clump-like or punctate areas of increased echogenicity with posterior shadowing), bony surface will become irregular, fracture margin less sharp and more rounded
  - ▪ Usually after 2 months no fracture line visible, but cortical bump/thickening remains
- ▶ Pathologic rib fracture: consider if rib fracture occurs with minimal or no trauma
  - ▪ Lung, kidney, hepatocellular carcinoma, and bowel all common primary sites to metastasize to ribs
  - ▪ Wider area of cortical disruption without such sharp margins as seen with traumatic fracture
  - ▪ Less likely to see overriding fragments; more likely to see areas where echogenic bony cortex appears to be absent or multiple fragments
  - ▪ Associated soft tissue mass demonstrating internal blood flow on color Doppler
  - ▪ ± Areas of calcification within the mass
  - ▪ May be difficult to differentiate from healing fracture with callus formation, but usually larger, more easily detectable soft tissue mass
- ▶ Expansile rib lesion: metastasis or bone neoplasm
  - ▪ Expansile soft tissue mass, may be vascular
  - ▪ May erode bony cortex or present as pathologic fracture

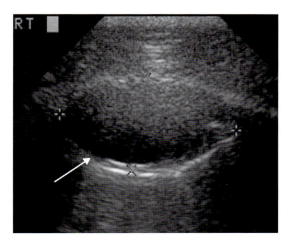

Fig. 142.7

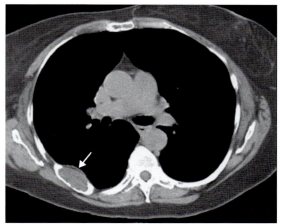

Fig. 142.8

This 60-year-old male presented with right-sided back pain. Note expansile hypoechoic rib lesion on US (cursors in Fig. 142.7) with loss of integrity of the bony cortex, which is poorly visualized anteriorly and appears disrupted posteriorly (arrow in Fig. 142.7). Correlative CT confirms the presence of the expansile soft tissue mass (arrow in Fig. 142.8) in a patient with a plasmacytoma. Nonvisualization of the bony cortex could be due to erosion or pathologic fracture.

- ▶ Normal US appearance of pleural margin: thin echogenic line with comet tail artifact extending from the visceral pleura that will slide under the parietal pleural with respiration; would not have a break or be displaced as in this case

Management

- ▶ Isolated rib fractures, without associated injuries, may be managed on an outpatient basis with analgesia and reduced activity
- ▶ Evaluate to exclude pneumothorax or hemothorax, which may require chest tube placement
- ▶ US can guide targeted administration of therapeutic intercostal analgesia

Acknowledgment

Figures 142.1–142.6 courtesy Dr. William D. Middleton, Mallinckrodt Institute of Radiology, Washington University School of Medicine, St. Louis, Missouri.

Further Reading

1. Griffith JF, Rainer TH, Ching ASC, et al. Sonography compared with radiography in revealing acute rib fracture. *Am J Roentgenol*. 1999; 173: 1603–1609.
2. Paik SH, Chung MJ, Park JS, et al. High-resolution sonography of the rib: Can fracture and metastasis be differentiated? *Am J Roentgenol*. 2005; 184: 969–974.

Case 143

History

▶ 48-Year-old swimmer presents with right shoulder pain (Figs. 143.1 and 143.2)

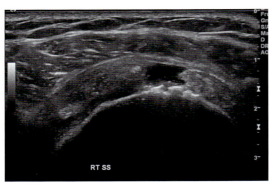

Fig. 143.1

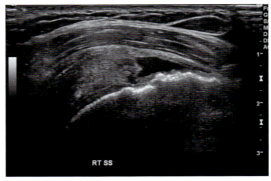

Fig. 143.2

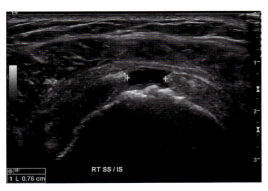

Fig. 143.3

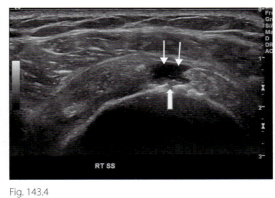

Fig. 143.4

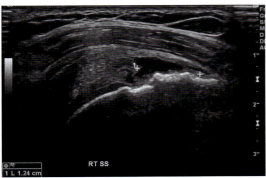

Fig. 143.5

Imaging Findings

► Full-thickness defect in the supraspinatus (SS) tendon that is filled with anechoic fluid (thin arrows in Fig. 143.4) and measured (cursors) in the short axis (Fig. 143.3) and long axis (Fig. 143.5) extending from the bursal surface to the articular surface
► Note torn edges of the retracted SS tendon and irregularity of the bony cortex (thick arrow in Fig. 143.4)

Differential Diagnosis

► Partial-thickness rotator cuff tear
► Anisotropy artifact
► Tendinopathy

Teaching Points

► The rotator cuff is composed of four tendons: the supraspinatus, infraspinatus, subscapularis, and teres minor tendons
  ▪ 95% of rotator cuff tears involve the supraspinatus tendon
  ▪ May extend posteriorly to involve infraspinatus tendon or, less often, anteriorly to involve the biceps and subscapularis tendons
► Etiology: chronic or repetitive microtrauma, subacromial impingement, tendon degeneration
► Presentation: shoulder pain and weakness with abduction
► Normal rotator cuff—US findings
  ▪ Homogeneous, echogenic, fibrillar echopattern
  ▪ Uniform in thickness (except where it tapers down at the insertion)
  ▪ Noncompressible with convex outer contour

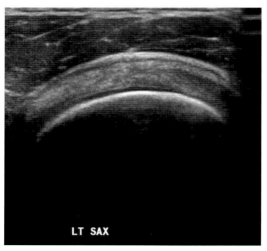
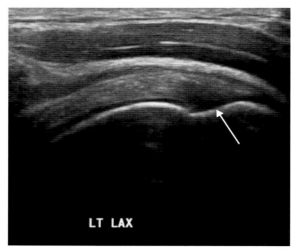

Fig. 143.6   Fig. 143.7

Short-axis (Fig. 143.6) and long-axis (Fig. 143.7) views of normal SS tendon with even thickness, homogeneous echogenicity, and fibrillar echopattern. Hypoechoic area at insertion of SS tendon (arrow in Fig. 143.7) is due to anisotropy and disappeared when the US beam was moved perpendicular to tendon.

▶ Full-thickness tear—US findings
  ▪ Anechoic or hypoechoic tendon gap filled with fluid or hypertrophied synovium extending from articular to bursal surface ± tendon retraction, uncovered humoral head (large tear)
  ▪ Concavity or "sagging" of the echogenic peribursal fat into the tendon gap, more apparent with compression
  ▪ Cortical irregularity of humeral head (older patients)
  ▪ Fluid in subdeltoid bursa

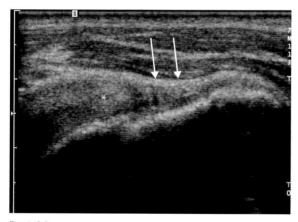

Fig. 143.8

Long-axis view from another patient with a complete rotator cuff tear (Fig. 143.8). Note retracted tendon (asterisk), loss of the normal superior convexity of the tendon with "sagging" of the echogenic peribursal fat into the tendon gap (arrows), and heterogeneous isoechoic material, likely synovial hypertrophy, in tendon gap.

▶ Partial tear—US findings
  ▪ Well-defined hypo, or anechoic area disrupting echogenic fibrillar pattern of tendon; remains constant on all angles
  ▪ Normal superficial convexity maintained
  ▪ May extend to articular or, less often, bursal surface
  ▪ Termed intrasubstance or interstitial tear if it does not reach surface
  ▪ Tendon thinning and volume loss
▶ Anisotropy artifact: scanning in an orientation such that the US beam is not perpendicular to the tendon fibers can create an artifactual hypoechoic area, usually involving the deep surface and relatively poorly marginated; will change with different orientations of the transducer
▶ Tedinopathy: tendon thickening, decreased echogenicity, heterogeneity without discrete defect

Management

► In expert hands, US and MRI have comparable accuracy for diagnosis of rotator cuff tear

► For partial tears, the arthroscopic approach is dependent on whether the tear reaches the articular or bursal surface

Acknowledgment

Figures 143.1–143.5 and 143.8 courtesy Dr. William D. Middleton, Mallinckrodt Institute of Radiology, Washington University School of Medicine in St. Louis, St. Louis, Missouri.

Further Reading

1. Teefey SA, Rubin DA, Middleton WD, et al. Detection and quantification of rotator cuff tears: Comparison of ultrasonographic, magnetic resonance imaging, and arthroscopic findings in seventy-one consecutive cases. *J Bone Joint Surg Am*. 2004; 86-A(4): 708–716.
2. Moosikasuwan JB, Miller TT, Burke BJ. Rotator cuff tears: Clinical, radiographic, and US findings. *RadioGraphics*. 2005; 25: 1591–1607.
3. Nazarian LN, Jacobson JA, Benson CB, et al. Imaging algorithms for evaluating suspected rotator cuff disease: Society of Radiologists in Ultrasound consensus conference statement. *Radiology*. 2013; 267: 589–595.

Case 144

▶ 43-Year-old male with acute ankle pain after stepping off a curb (Figs. 144.1–144.6)

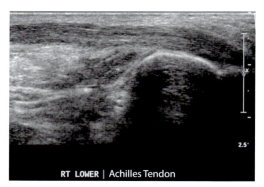

Fig. 144.1

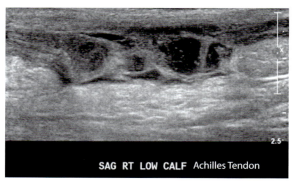

Fig. 144.2

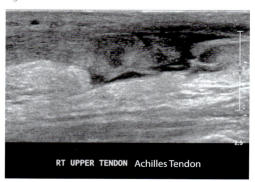

Fig. 144.3

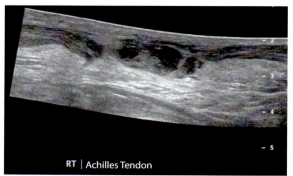

Fig. 144.4

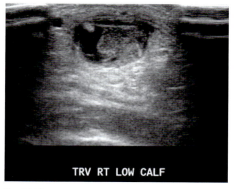

Fig. 144.5

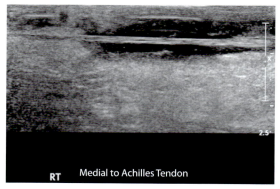

Fig. 144.6

482

Case 144 Complete Rupture of Achilles Tendon

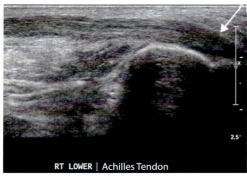

Fig. 144.7

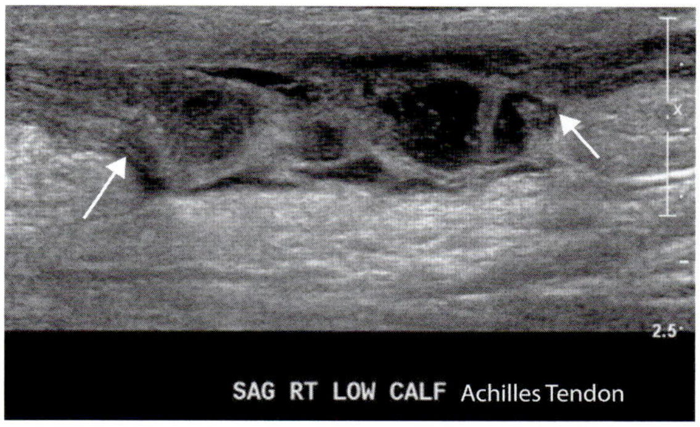

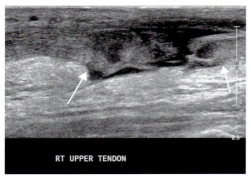

Fig. 144.8

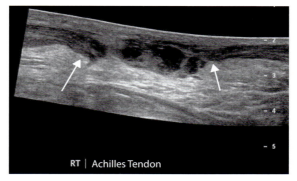

Fig. 144.9

Fig. 144.10

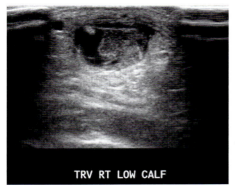

Fig. 144.11

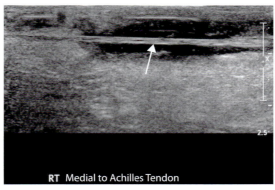

Fig. 144.12

Imaging Findings

- The distal Achilles tendon (AT) is slightly hypoechoic due to anisotropy, but the normal fibrillar pattern of the tendon is preserved and it inserts normally onto the calcaneus (arrow in Fig. 144.7)
- Sagittal (Figs. 144.8 and 144.9) and panoramic (Fig. 144.10) views of the upper AT demonstrate a full-thickness tear approximately 2–4 cm above the calcaneal insertion. The gap between the torn edges (arrows) is filled with heterogeneous material and fluid, also noted on transverse view (Fig. 144.11)
- The smaller plantaris tendon is intact medially (arrow in Fig. 144.12)

Differential Diagnosis

- Partial tear
- Tendinosis

Teaching Points

▶ Presentation: sudden-onset pain, relative weakness in plantar flexion
- Most common in middle-aged men
- Frequently occurs playing basketball or stepping off a curb

▶ Tear typically occurs 2 or 3 cm above calcaneal insertion, a relatively hypovascular area

▶ US findings of complete AT tear
- Complete disruption of tendon fibers
- Retraction of tendon, either tapered or balled up
- Refractive shadowing at torn edge; can use to localize edge of torn tendon so as to accurately measure length of tendon gap
- Gap may fill in with fluid, hemorrhage, or adjacent echogenic fat

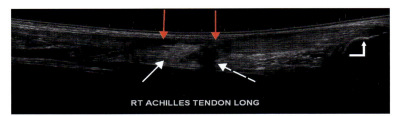

Fig. 144.13

Panoramic sagittal view of a second patient with full-thickness AT tear with retraction of the proximal tendon stump and herniation of echogenic fat (solid white arrow in Fig. 144.13) into the gap between the torn ends of the AT (red arrows). Linear refractive shadowing (dashed white arrow) denotes torn edge of distal tendon. Normal attachment of the distal AT to the calcaneus (angled arrow).

▶ Dynamic imaging with US will demonstrate independent movement of the tendon stumps and increased retraction with a full-thickness tear

▶ Report distance from calcaneal insertion and myotendinous junction plus length of tendon gap in neutral position, flexion, and extension

▶ Pitfall: mistaking medial plantaris tendon (Fig. 144.12) for residual intact AT fibers (i.e., partial tear)
- Plantaris tendon may remain intact when AT is completely ruptured
- Follow plantaris tendon back to its normal course between the gastrocnemius and soleus muscles

▶ Partial tear: hypoechoic or anechoic area/cleft that partially disrupts tendon fibers and fibrillar echopattern, may be well-defined, associated with tendinosis

▶ Tendinosis: focal or diffuse fusiform swelling of tendon, hypoechoic, fibers intact, increased flow on power Doppler represents neovascularity (not inflammation) and correlates with symptoms

Management

▶ Immobilization
▶ Surgical repair

Acknowledgment

Figure 144.13 courtesy Dr. William D. Middleton, Mallinckrodt Institute of Radiology, Washington University School of Medicine in St. Louis, St. Louis, Missouri.

Further Reading

1. Hartgerink P, Fessell DP, Jacobson JA, et al. Full- versus partial-thickness Achilles tendon tears: Sonographic accuracy and characterization in 26 cases with surgical correlation. *Radiology*. 2001; 220: 406–412.
2. Alfredson H, Masci L, Ohberg L. Partial mid-portion Achilles tendon ruptures: New sonographic findings helpful for diagnosis. *Br J Sports Med*. 2011; 45: 429–432.

History

▶ 62-Year-old female with 2 weeks of left calf tenderness and swelling (Figs. 145.1 and 145.2)

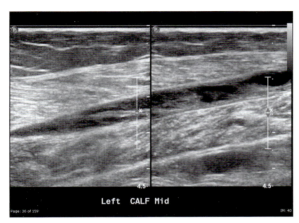

Fig. 145.1

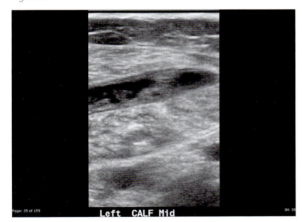

Fig. 145.2

Case 145 Plantaris Tendon Rupture

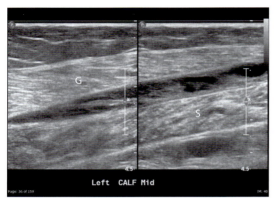

Fig. 145.3

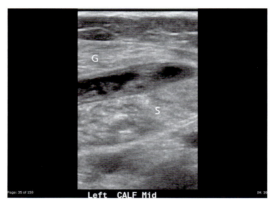

Fig. 145.4

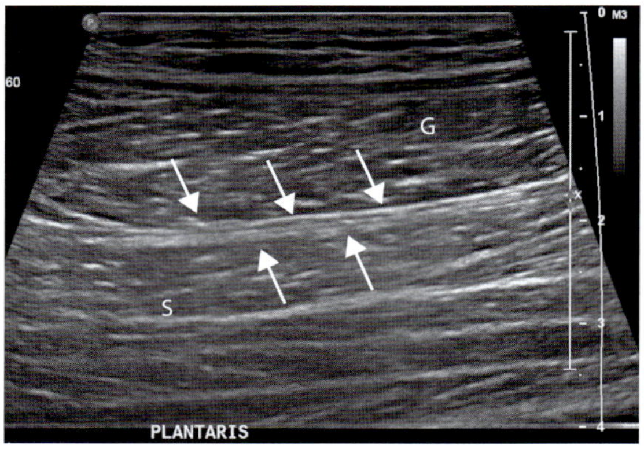

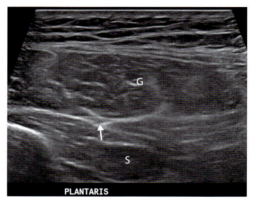

Fig. 145.5

Fig. 145.6

Imaging Findings

▶ Linear collection of fluid and echogenic material separating the more superficial gastrocnemius muscle (G in Figs. 145.3 and 145.4) from the deeper soleus muscle (S in Figs. 145.3 and 145.4) in the expected location of the plantaris tendon
▶ For comparison, note echogenic fibrillar appearance of normal plantaris tendon (arrows in Figs. 145.5 and 145.6) coursing between the gastrocnemius (G in Figs. 145.5 and 145.6) and soleus muscles (S in Figs. 145.5 and 145.6)

Differential Diagnosis

▶ Gastrocnemius muscle tear
▶ Soleus muscle tear
▶ Dissecting/ruptured Baker cyst

Teaching Points

▶ The plantaris tendon lies between the medial gastrocnemius muscle and the soleus muscle
▶ Approximately 10% of people lack one or both plantaris muscles and tendons
▶ Tears of the plantaris muscle most commonly occur at the myotendinous junction following running or jumping
  ▪ Sometimes referred to as " 'tennis leg"
  ▪ Often associated with tears of the gastrocnemius and soleus muscles or ACL, but may occur in isolation as in this case
▶ Clinical presentation
  ▪ "Stepped off the curb and felt a pop," rushed the net playing tennis
  ▪ Acute medial calf pain or stinging, calf swelling
  ▪ Pain worsens with dorsiflexion
  ▪ Can mimic deep venous thrombosis or muscle tear/sprain

- ► US findings
  - ▪ The normal plantaris tendon is a long thin echogenic structure with a fibrillar echotexture coursing between the bellies of the gastrocnemius and soleus muscles
  - ▪ Following a complete tear, the plantaris muscle retracts proximally; fluid and/or hematoma fills the tract of the torn tendon creating a linear tubular heterogeneous fluid collection between the gastrocnemius muscle anteriorly and the soleus muscle posteriorly
- ► Gastrocnemius or soleus muscle tears: hypoechoic heterogeneous material will disrupt the normal pennate sonographic architecture of the muscle
  - ▪ In this case, the abnormality is located at the interface between the two muscles
- ► Dissected or ruptured Baker cyst: tear-shaped heterogeneous fluid collection often superficial to the gastrocnemius muscle

Management

- ► Management is conservative
- ► Active stretching exercises should be avoided because stretching can exacerbate the tear

Further Reading

1. Leekam RN, Agur AM, McKee NH. Using sonography to diagnose injury of plantaris muscles and tendons. *Am J Roentgenol*. 1999; 172: 185–189.

Case 146

History

► 51-Year-old female with sudden onset of right calf pain (Figs. 146.1–146.4)

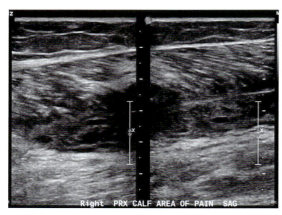

Fig. 146.1

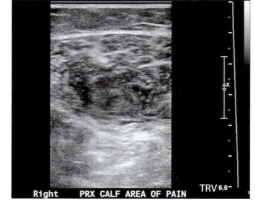

Fig. 146.2

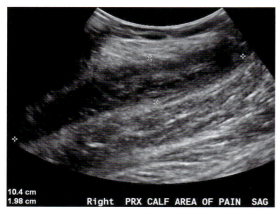

Fig. 146.3

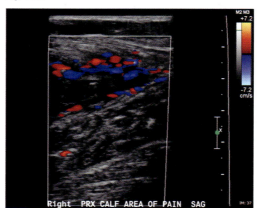

Fig. 146.4

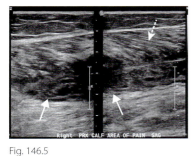

Fig. 146.5

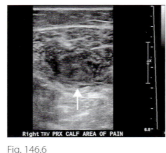

Fig. 146.6

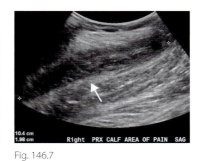

Fig. 146.7

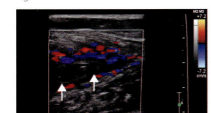

Fig. 146.8

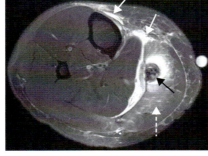

Fig. 146.9

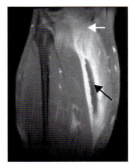

Fig. 146.10

Imaging Findings

▶ Heterogeneous hypoechoic area (white solid arrows in 146.5, arrow in Fig. 146.6, and calipers in Fig. 146.7) focally disrupting the normal pennate echopattern of the gastrocnemius muscle (dashed arrow in Fig. 146.5)

▶ The thin echogenic plantaris tendon (arrow in Fig. 146.7) between the gastrocnemius muscle anteriorly and soleus muscle posteriorly is intact

▶ The abnormal hypoechoic area is avascular (arrows in Fig. 146.8) on color Doppler imaging with peripheral hyperemia

▶ Axial T2-weighted with fat saturation MRI image (Fig. 146.9) and coronal contrast-enhanced T1-weighted MRI with fat saturation image (Fig. 146.10) demonstrate an ill-defined high signal intensity region due to edema (dashed arrow in Fig. 146.9) and increased enhancement (white arrow in Fig. 146.10) within the medial belly of the gastrocnemius muscle, extending to its origin. Note intramuscular nonenhancing collection, hypointense on both T2- and T1-weighted sequences (black arrows in Figs. 146.9 and 146.10 respectively), consistent with hematoma at the myofascial junction where tears commonly occur. On the T2-weighted image, high signal intensity fluid is observed to track along the fascial planes (solid white arrows in Fig. 146.9)

▶ Findings consistent with myofascial junction injury of the medial gastrocnemius muscle with associated hematoma and edema in the muscle belly

Differential Diagnosis

▶ Plantaris tendon tear
▶ Ruptured Baker cyst
▶ Intramuscular neoplasm

Teaching Points

▶ Muscle tears most often occur at the myofascial or myotendinous junctions
▶ Rupture of the myofascial junction of the medial head of gastrocnemius, known as "tennis leg," typically occurs in middle-aged individuals who present with sudden mid-calf pain, often with a snapping sensation
  ▪ Mechanism: simultaneous passive stretching and active contraction of the gastrocnemius muscle as occurs during active plantar flexion of the foot during simultaneous knee extension
▶ US findings
  ▪ Disruption of the pennate/fishbone echotexture of the muscle—echogenicity variable depending on time course
  ▪ Tears can be partial or complete
  ▪ Most common location is the medial head of the gastrocnemius muscle

- Special attention should be paid to the most anteromedial portion of the medial head of the gastrocnemius muscle to detect small tears
- Avascular with peripheral hyperemia on color Doppler
- Often associated with a fluid collection between the medial head of the gastrocnemius and the soleus muscles ± hemorrhage (as seen on MRI in this patient)
► MR imaging findings
- Feathery pattern of edema at the myofascial junction
- Intramuscular hematoma
- Perifascial fluid collections
- Retraction of the muscle and tendon if complete rupture
► Plantaris tendon rupture: similar clinical presentation, fluid collection between gastrocnemius and soleus muscles that retain their normal pennate echotexture, echogenic tendon that is normally present between these two muscles will be absent
- Comparison to contralateral side may be helpful
► Ruptured Baker cyst: similar clinical presentation, complex fluid collection in upper calf, often dissects anterior to the gastrocnemius muscle
► Intramuscular neoplasm: focal intramuscular mass of variable echogenicity, usually hypoechoic, expect internal vascularity without associated fluid collection
- Sarcomas and metastases (lung and melanoma) most common

Management

► Conservative management with ice packs, limb elevation, nonsteroidal anti-inflammatory drugs, avoidance of activity until pain-free
► Fasciotomy if complicated by development of compartment syndrome

Further Reading

1. Kwak HS, Lee KB, Han YM. Ruptures of the medial head of the gastrocnemius ("tennis leg"): Clinical outcome and compression effect. *Clin Imaging*. 2006; 30(1): 48–53.
2. Bianchi S, Martinoli C, Abdelwahab IF, et al. Sonographic evaluation of tears of the gastrocnemius medial head ("tennis leg"). *J Ultrasound Med*. 1998; 17: 157–162.

History

▶ 36-Year-old male with history of HIV, left lower extremity swelling, pain, and enlarging left popliteal mass (Figs. 147.1–147.4)

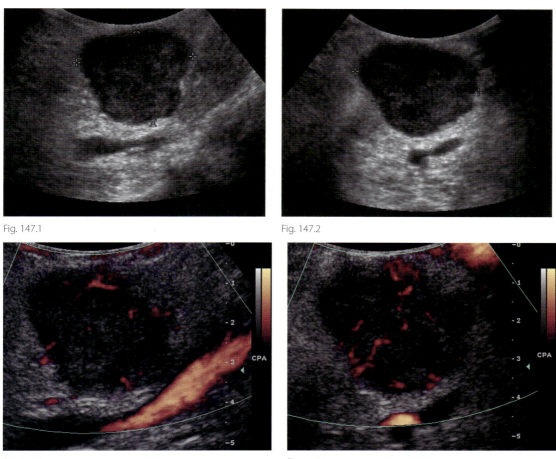

Fig. 147.1

Fig. 147.2

Fig. 147.3

Fig. 147.4

Case 147   Soft Tissue Mass (Metastatic Melanoma)

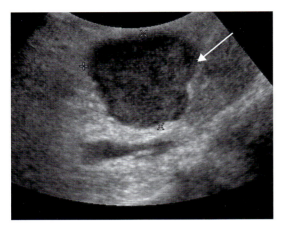

Fig. 147.5

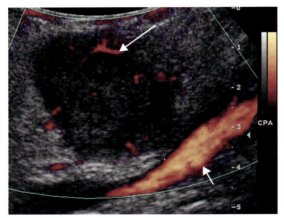

Fig. 147.6

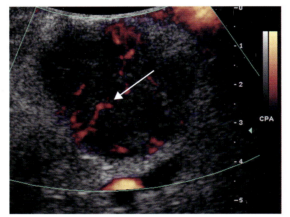

Fig. 147.7

Imaging Findings

▶ Solid, hypoechoic lobulated well-defined mass in the left popliteal fossa on sagittal (arrow in Fig. 147.5)
▶ Internal flow demonstrated on power Doppler US (arrows in Figs. 147.5 and 147.6) with patent popliteal vein (short arrow in Fig. 147.6)

Differential Diagnosis

▶ Baker cyst
▶ Popliteal artery aneurysm
▶ Lipoma
▶ Hematoma
▶ Sarcoma
▶ Lymphoma

Teaching Points

▶ Popliteal soft tissue mass
   ▪ Most caused by Baker cyst
   ▪ May also result from trauma, primary neoplasm such as sarcoma, or metastatic lesion from a variety of primary tumors
   ▪ If metastatic, most common primary: lung, melanoma, kidney, gastrointestinal tract, breast, and bladder
▶ US findings
   ▪ Variable
   ▪ Echogenicity can range from hypoechoic to isoechoic to echogenic with or without shadowing, depending on underlying primary
   ▪ Often vascular on color Doppler US

- Tumor vascularity correlates with areas of angiogenesis
  - Homogeneous or heterogeneous: areas of cystic necrosis and dystrophic calcification can be seen
- Melanoma: most serious form of skin cancer, which can spread quickly to any other part of the body. The rate of melanoma has increased dramatically in the past 30 years due to sun exposure. Highest rate in elderly (age > 80 years); however, not uncommon in young adults (age < 30 years). Usually history of prior melanoma
- Heterogeneous enhancing mass in popliteal fossa on MRI (arrow in Fig. 147.8)
- Intense metabolic activity in left popliteal fossa mass on fluorodeoxyglucose (FDG) positron emission tomography (PET)/CT scan (arrow in Fig. 147.9)

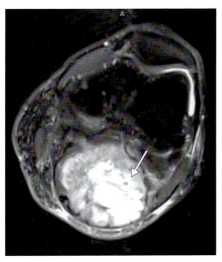 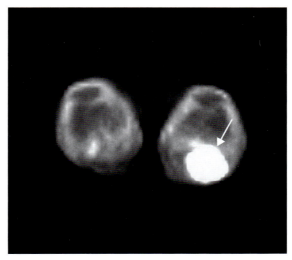

Fig. 147.8   Fig. 147.9

- Baker cyst: caused by abnormal distension of the gastrocnemius–semimembranosus bursa, communicating with the knee joint. More cystic and no internal vascularity. May contain debris if hemorrhagic or infected
- Popliteal artery (PA) aneurysm: pulsatile popliteal fossa mass with focal fusiform or saccular enlargement of PA. Arterial flow on Doppler US. May be partially or completely thrombosed
- Lipoma: mobile, well-defined soft tissue mass. Echogenicity ranges from hyperechoic to isoechoic and hypoechoic. May show internal echogenic septations. Little to no flow on Doppler US
- Hematoma: more echogenic in acute phase and no internal vascularity. Usually history of trauma and/or anticoagulation
- Sarcoma and lymphoma: similar US, MRI, and PET/CT appearance. Tissue sampling needed for definitive diagnosis

Management

- Further imaging with contrast-enhanced CT and/or MRI to determine extent of disease
- FDG PET/CT to assess for metabolic activity and other sites of involvement
- Percutaneous biopsy for definite diagnosis with appropriate immunohistochemistry
- Further treatment depending on underlying cause; surgical resection, chemotherapy, radiation, or immunotherapy

Further Reading

1. Toprak H, Erkan K, Serter A, et al. Ultrasound and Doppler US in the evaluation of superficial soft tissue lesions. *J Clin Imaging Sci*. 2014; 4: 12.
2. American Cancer Society. *Cancer Facts and Figures 2014*. Atlanta, GA: American Cancer Society; 2014: 20–21.
3. Abed R, Grimer RJ, Tillman RM, et al. Soft tissue metastases: Their presentation and origin. *J Bone Joint Surg Br*. 2009; 91(8): 1083–1085.

Section VI　Vascular

History

► 45-Year-old male with history of colon cancer presents with right leg swelling (Figs. 148.1 and 148.2)

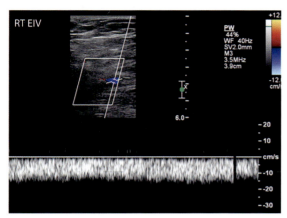

Fig. 148.1

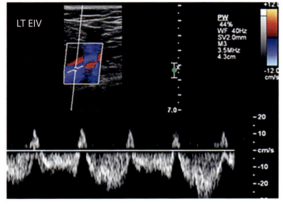

Fig. 148.2

Case 148   Abnormal Flat, Monophasic Spectral Doppler Waveform in Right External Iliac Vein

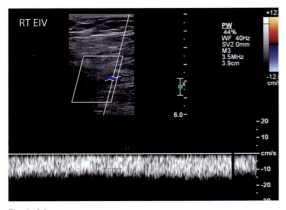

Fig. 148.3

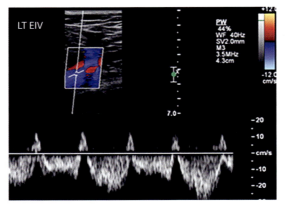

Fig. 148.4

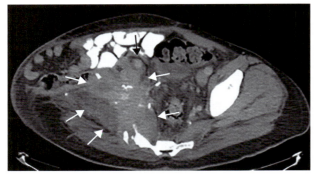

Fig. 148.5

Imaging Findings

► Flat, monophasic spectral Doppler waveform in the right external iliac vein (EIV) without respiratory variation (Fig. 148.3)
► Normal pulsatile spectral Doppler waveform with respiratory variation and transmitted cardiac pulsatility in the left EIV (Fig. 148.4)
► Contrast-enhanced CT scan demonstrates compression of the cephalad right EIV underneath the right external iliac artery (black arrow in Fig. 148.5) by a large destructive bony metastasis to the right acetabulum (white arrows in Fig. 148.5)

Differential Diagnosis

► Right common iliac vein (CIV) or cephalad EIV thrombosis
► May–Thurner syndrome
► Deep inspiration
► Inferior vena cava (IVC) thrombosis

Teaching Points

► Normal spectral Doppler waveforms in the EIV or common femoral vein (CFV) demonstrate respiratory phasicity with decreased velocity during inspiration or following the Valsalva maneuver. Transmitted cardiac pulsatility may be observed
  ▪ Waveforms should be symmetric right to left
  ▪ Even when a unilateral venous Doppler ultrasound examination of the lower extremities is performed, a spectral Doppler waveform in the contralateral EIV and/or CFV should be evaluated for comparison
► A unilateral flat or monophasic spectral Doppler waveform in the EIV or CFV indicates cephalad obstruction to flow that could be caused by the following
  ▪ Ipsilateral pelvic vein (CIV or cephalad EIV) thrombus
  ▪ External compression of ipsilateral pelvic veins by retroperitoneal or pelvic mass, renal transplant, May–Thurner syndrome
  ▪ Contralateral EIV or CFV spectral Doppler waveforms will demonstrate normal respiratory variation and/or cardiac pulsatility

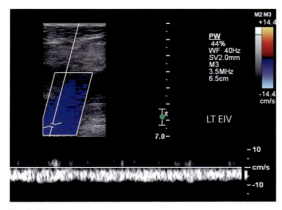

Fig. 148.6

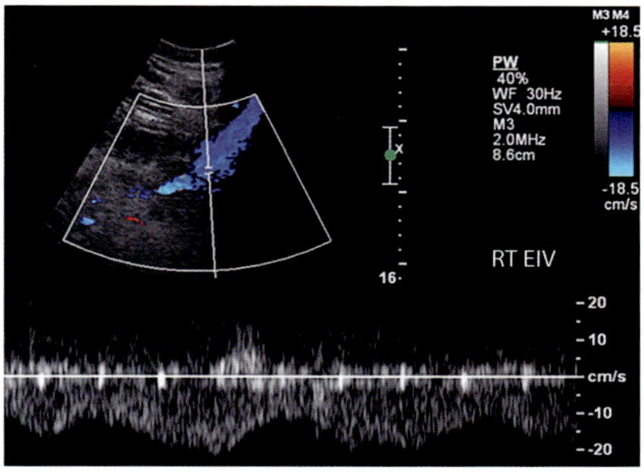

Fig. 148.7

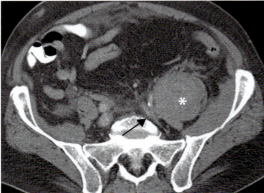

Fig. 148.8

58-Year-old male presents with left groin and pelvic pain following cardiac catheterization. Note flat monophasic spectral Doppler waveform in the left EIV (Fig. 148.6) due to compression of the left CIV (arrow in Fig. 148.8) by a retroperitoneal hematoma (asterisk in Fig. 148.8). The spectral Doppler waveform in the right EIV has normal respiratory variation (Fig. 148.7).

▶ Bilateral monophasic spectral Doppler waveforms in the EIVs and/or CFVs indicate cephalad obstruction to flow that could be caused by the following
  ▪ IVC or bilateral pelvic vein thrombus
  ▪ Extrinsic compression of IVC or bilateral iliac veins
  ▪ Obesity
  ▪ Ascites
  ▪ Advanced pregnancy
▶ In obese or pregnant patients, obtaining a spectral Doppler waveform during the Valsalva maneuver or while imaging in the lateral decubitus position is useful to prevent false-positive diagnosis of a flat EIV waveform
  ▪ The Valsalva maneuver will accentuate normal respiratory variation
  ▪ The decubitus position will prevent compression of the EIVs by overlying adipose tissue or the gravid uterus
▶ Cephalad right EIV or CIV occlusive deep venous thrombosis (DVT) would also result in a flat spectral Doppler waveform in the lower right EIV, indistinguishable from the findings presented in the first case
▶ May–Thurner syndrome or iliac vein compression syndrome
  ▪ Compression of the left CIV by the right common iliac artery
  ▪ Results in venous stasis and pooling of blood predisposing to development of DVT in the left lower extremity
  ▪ Will cause a flat monophasic spectral Doppler waveform in the left EIV and CFV
  ▪ Rarely, the right CIV may be compressed by the right common iliac artery, resulting in a flat right EIV/CFV spectral Doppler waveform
▶ Prolonged deep inspiration or excessive compression with the transducer can also cause flat spectral Doppler waveforms in the EIV and CFV
▶ IVC thrombosis or external compression would cause bilateral monophasic spectral Doppler waveforms in the EIVs and CFVs

Management

▶ If monophasic spectral Doppler waveforms are obtained in the EIV or CFV, search for retroperitoneal/pelvic mass or cephalad DVT in pelvic veins or IVC

▶ May–Thurner syndrome or external compression: venous stent

▶ Pelvic DVT: anticoagulation, thrombolysis for massive iliofemoral thrombosis, IVC filter if anticoagulation contraindicated

Further Reading

1. Bach AM, Hann LE. When the common femoral vein is revealed as flattened on spectral Doppler sonography: Is it a reliable sign for diagnosis of proximal venous obstruction? *Am J Roentgenol.* 1997; 168(3): 733–736.

History

▶ 64-Year-old male presents with bilateral leg swelling (Figs. 149.1 and 149.2)

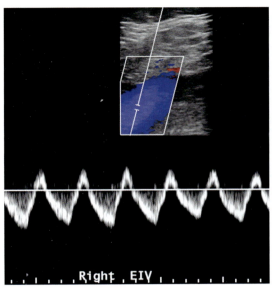

Fig. 149.1

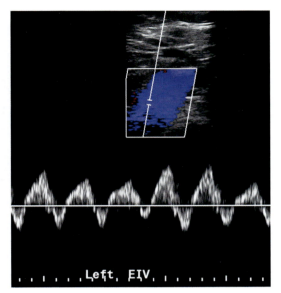

Fig. 149.2

Case 149 Abnormal Pulsatile or "Sawtooth" Waveforms in the Bilateral External Iliac Veins Due to Tricuspid Regurgitation

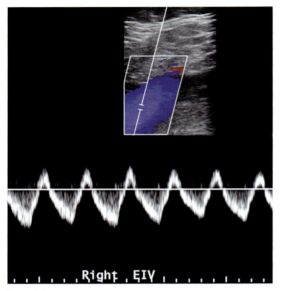

Fig. 149.3

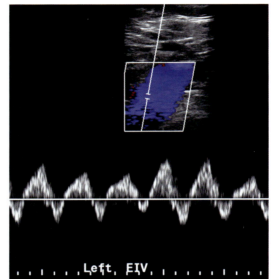

Fig. 149.4

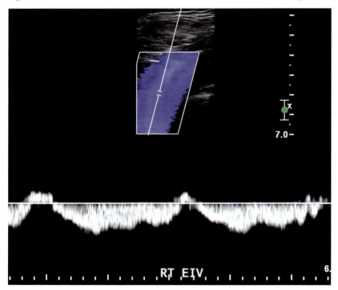

Fig. 149.5

Imaging Findings

▶ Jagged or "sawtooth" pulsatile spectral Doppler waveforms in the bilateral external iliac veins (EIVs) (Figs. 149.3 and 149.4) with flow above and below the baseline due to transmission of increased cardiac pulsatility in a patient with elevated right atrial pressure. The patient had moderate tricuspid regurgitation (TR) on cardiac echo

▶ Normal venous spectral Doppler waveform (Fig. 149.5) from a different patient. The normal spectral Doppler waveform in the EIV is nonpulsatile but phasic with decreased forward flow (i.e., reduced flow velocity) during inspiration because increased intra-abdominal pressure during inspiration will result in decreased venous return toward the heart

Differential Diagnosis

▶ Right heart failure
▶ Pulmonary hypertension

Teaching Points

► US is the imaging modality of choice for the diagnosis of deep venous thrombosis (DVT)
► The most common clinical presentation of DVT is leg pain and swelling, but these findings are nonspecific
  ▪ 70% of patients referred for evaluation of leg pain and swelling will have a cause other than DVT
  ▪ Patients presenting with bilateral leg swelling without risk factors for DVT, such as a history of malignancy or trauma, are much more likely to have cardiac disease rather than DVT as a cause of their symptoms
    • The likelihood of such patients harboring DVT is ≤ 5%
► TR occurs in < 1% of the population
► Etiology of TR
  ▪ Right ventriculomegaly
  ▪ Endocarditis
  ▪ Rheumatic heart disease
  ▪ Carcinoid
  ▪ Postinfarction
  ▪ Congenital abnormalities (e.g., Ebstein anomaly)
  ▪ Idiopathic
► Clinical presentation of TR
  ▪ Typically asymptomatic
  ▪ Bilateral leg swelling, hepatomegaly, jugular venous distension, pansystolic heart murmur
  ▪ May be associated with pulmonary hypertension
► US findings of TR
  ▪ Increased pulsatility or "sawtooth" spectral Doppler waveform in EIVs with flow above and below the baseline
  ▪ Similar waveform may be found in the hepatic or renal veins and inferior vena cava (IVC)
  ▪ Distension of the EIVs, hepatic veins, and IVC
  ▪ Pulsatile portal venous flow
► Pulmonary hypertension and right heart failure may cause a similar spectral Doppler waveform pattern in the bilateral EIVs

Management

► Diagnosis confirmed on cardiac echography
► Treatment options for primary TR include valvuloplasty and valvular repair
► Symptomatic relief for leg swelling with compression stockings, elevation

Further Reading

1. Sheiman RG, Weintrub JL, McArdle CR. Bilateral lower extremity US in the patient with bilateral symptoms of deep venous thrombosis: Assessment of need. *Radiology*. 1995; 196: 379–381.
2. Abu-Yousef MM, Kakis ME, Mufid M. Pulsatile venous Doppler flow in lower limbs: Highly indicative of elevated right atrium pressure. *Am J Roentgenol*. 1996; 167: 977–980.

Case 150

▶ 66-Year-old female with history of bilateral deep venous thrombosis and pulmonary embolism status post inferior vena cava filter placement presents with 3 days of right leg swelling. Images of the right common femoral and femoral veins were obtained (Figs. 150.1–150.4).

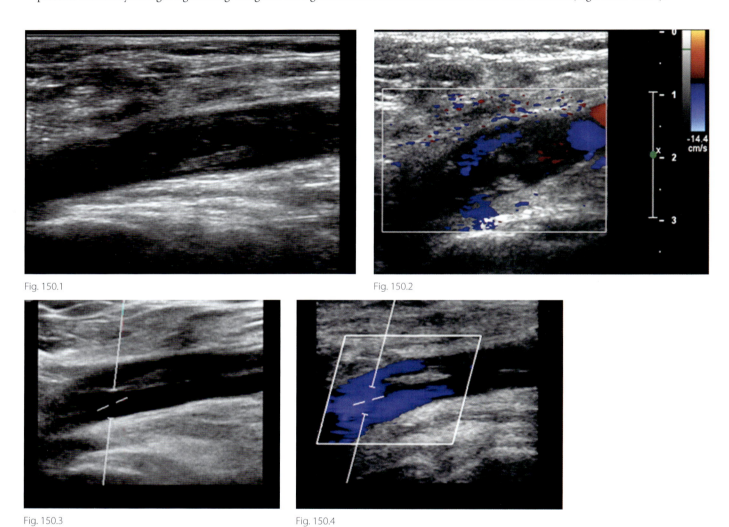

Fig. 150.1

Fig. 150.2

Fig. 150.3

Fig. 150.4

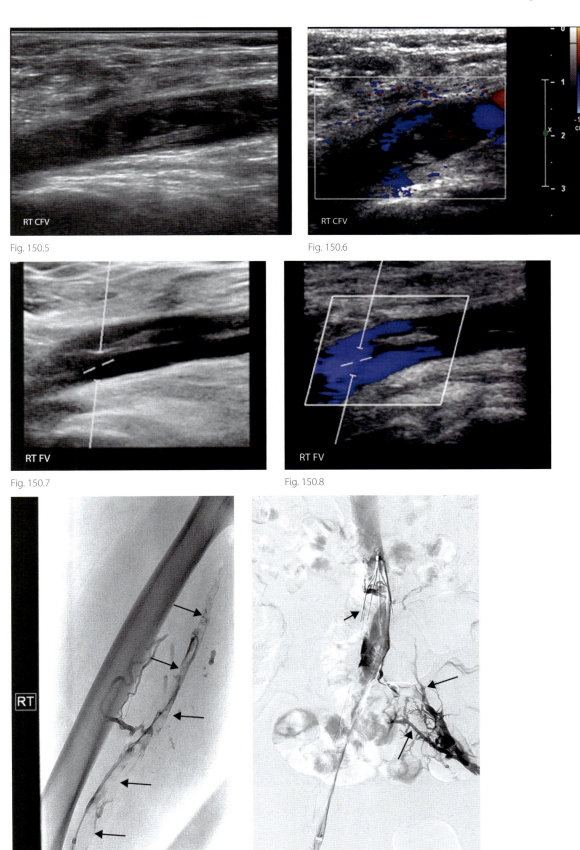

Fig. 150.5

Fig. 150.6

Fig. 150.7

Fig. 150.8

Fig. 150.9

Fig. 150.10

Imaging Findings

▶ Heterogeneous material expands and nearly fills the right common femoral vein on grayscale (Fig. 150.5) and color Doppler images (Fig. 150.6). Echogenic areas are more likely to represent chronic deep venous thrombosis (DVT), whereas the more homogeneous hypoechoic material is more likely to be acute thrombus in this patient with a history of prior bilateral DVT and inferior vena cava (IVC) filter placement

▶ Grayscale (Fig. 150.7) and color Doppler (Fig. 150.8) images of the femoral vein demonstrate linear echogenic intraluminal strands consistent with synechiae from prior episode of DVT

▶ Venogram (Figs. 150.9 and 150.10) demonstrating near occlusive DVT (arrows in Fig. 150.9) extending from the right popliteal vein through the iliac vein and into the previously placed IVC filter (short arrow in Fig. 150.10). Absence of significant collaterals is suggestive of an acute DVT component. The left lower extremity deep venous circulation is completely thrombosed with extensive pelvic collaterals (long arrows in Fig. 150.10)

Differential Diagnosis

▶ Extensive acute DVT

Teaching Points

▶ Most DVT originates in the calf veins
▶ Doppler US is the imaging modality of choice to assess for lower extremity DVT
  ▪ CT or MR venography useful if iliac or IVC extension is suspected and cannot be visualized with Doppler US
  ▪ Catheter venography is usually performed only when intervention is contemplated
▶ Risk factors: stasis, hypercoagulable states, endothelial injury
  ▪ Prior episode of DVT major risk factor for recurrent DVT
  ▪ Recurrence rate approximately 25%
▶ US findings of DVT
  ▪ Noncompressible venous segment (negative predictive value > 99.5%)
  ▪ Absent color flow if occlusive; color void if nonocclusive
  ▪ A flat spectral Doppler waveform without respiratory variation suggests more central obstruction to flow (either from external compression or intraluminal thrombus)
    • Unilateral: ipsilateral external iliac and/or common iliac veins
    • Bilateral: IVC or bilateral common/external iliac veins
  ▪ Lack of augmentation
▶ Sometimes difficult to differentiate acute from chronic or residual DVT on US
  ▪ Acute thrombus: expands vein, "floating thrombus", slightly compressible, usually more hypoechoic
  ▪ Chronic/residual thrombus: small vein (smaller than adjacent artery), linear echogenic thin fibrin stranding, thicker echogenic synechiae, mural calcification, wall thickening, adherent or calcified thrombus
  ▪ Collateral channels may develop within 2 weeks
  ▪ Significant overlap in US findings
  ▪ Most accurate means of differentiating recurrent acute DVT from chronic or residual DVT is documentation of DVT in a new location, correlation with new focal symptoms, or observation of progression on short-interval follow-up

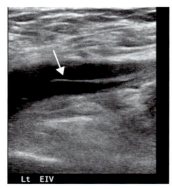

Fig. 150.11

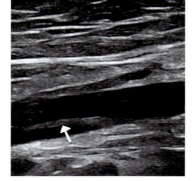

Fig. 150.12

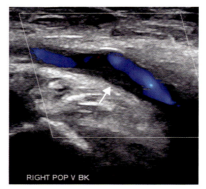

Fig. 150.13

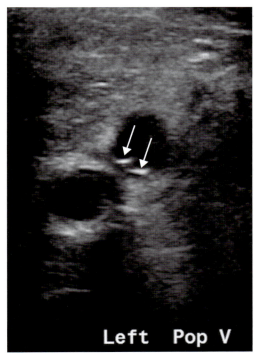
Fig. 150.14

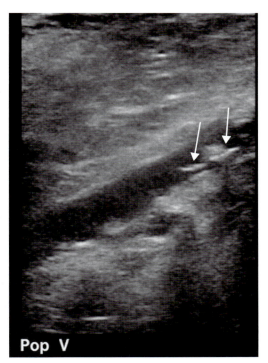
Fig. 150.15

► Findings suggesting chronic DVT
  ▪ Thin echogenic linear fibrin strand (arrow in Fig. 150.11)
  ▪ Thicker, less echogenic linear synechiae or scar (arrow in Fig. 150.12)
  ▪ Adherent hypoechoic smooth-surfaced nonocclusive thrombus (arrow in Fig. 150.13) is outlined by blue on color Doppler image and makes an obtuse angle with the vein wall in a patient on anticoagulation for DVT without recurrent symptoms
  ▪ Calcified mural scarring (arrows in Fig. 150.14) and/or calcified residual thrombus (arrows in Fig. 150.15)

Management

► Uncomplicated DVT: systemic anticoagulation for 3–6 months
► DVT with contraindication to anticoagulation, or development and/or progression of DVT while on therapeutic anticoagulation: IVC filter placement
► Transcatheter interventions (thrombolysis, angioplasty, stenting) indicated when there is extensive DVT, such as involvement of the iliac veins and IVC, or if there is development of phlegmasia cerulea dolens (loss of venous outflow that impedes arterial inflow, causing ischemia and gangrene), which is a medical emergency
► Follow-up Doppler US after completion of anticoagulation therapy is recommended in high-risk patients to establish baseline mapping of residual DVT. This will help distinguish chronic from acute on chronic DVT in patients presenting with recurrent symptoms

Further Reading

1. Useche J, Fernandez de Castro A, Galvis G, et al. Use of US in the evaluation of patients with symptoms of deep venous thrombosis of the lower extremities. *RadioGraphics*. 2008; 28: 1785–1797.
2. Atri M, Herba MJ, Reinhold C, et-al. Accuracy of sonography in the evaluation of calf deep vein thrombosis in both postoperative surveillance and symptomatic patients. *Am J Roentgenol*. 1996; 166: 1361–1367.
3. Hamper UM, DeJong MR, Scoutt LM. Ultrasound evaluation of the lower extremity veins. *Radiol Clin North Am*. 2007; 45: 525–547.

Case 151

History

▶ 62-Year-old male presents with a transient ischemic attack (Figs. 151.1–151.4)

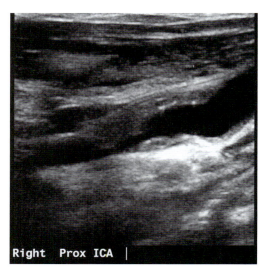

Fig. 151.1

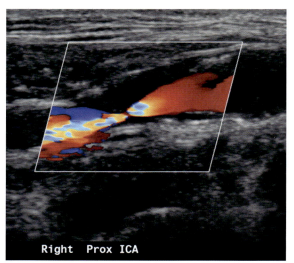

Fig. 151.2

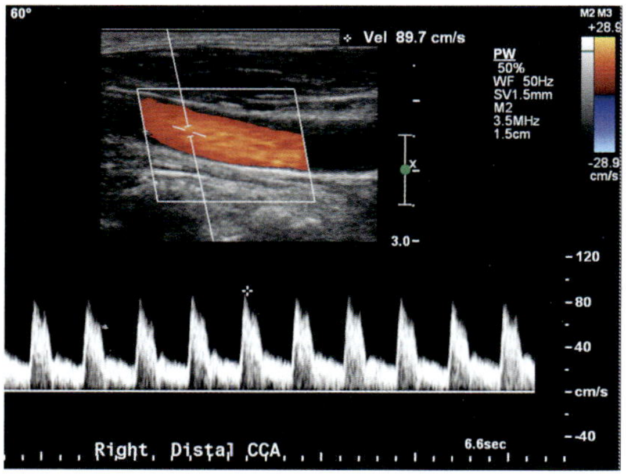

Fig. 151.3

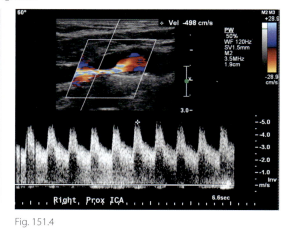

Fig. 151.4

Case 151 ≥ 70% Stenosis of the Right Internal Carotid Artery

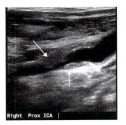
Fig. 151.5

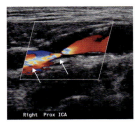
Fig. 151.6

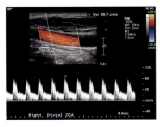
Fig. 151.7

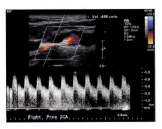
Fig. 151.8

Imaging Findings

► Heterogeneous predominantly hypoechoic plaque (arrows in Fig. 151.5) significantly narrows the residual lumen at the origin of the right internal carotid artery (ICA)

► Note color aliasing on color Doppler image (arrows in Fig. 151.6) at the site of the stenosis as well as distal to the stenosis indicating increased peak systolic velocity (PSV)

► Spectral Doppler waveforms in the distal right common carotid artery (CCA) (Fig. 151.7) and proximal right ICA (Fig. 151.8) demonstrate a markedly elevated PSV of 498 cm/s in the right ICA with turbulence and spectral broadening and a peak systolic velocity ratio (PSVR) between the ICA and CCA of 5.5

Differential Diagnosis

► 50–69% ICA stenosis
► Near occlusion of ICA

Teaching Points

► Duplex Doppler US is considered the noninvasive screening modality of choice to evaluate for an ICA stenosis
► ICA stenoses are generally stratified as follows
  ▪ Normal (no stenosis)
  ▪ < 50%
  ▪ 50–69%
  ▪ ≥ 70% but less than near occlusion
  ▪ Near occlusion
  ▪ Total occlusion
► The Society of Radiologists in Ultrasound (SRU) recommends using the following criteria for diagnosis of a ≥ 70% ICA stenosis but less than near occlusion
  ▪ PSV > 230 cm/s plus visible plaque and luminal narrowing
  ▪ ICA/CCA PSVR > 4
  ▪ ICA end diastolic velocity > 100 cm/s
► The Doppler waveform should be obtained with an angle of ≤ 60° and ≥ 45°
► PSV is generally considered the primary spectral Doppler criterion for grading an ICA stenosis
  ▪ However, if the PSV in the CCA is > 100 cm/s or < 60 cm/s, or if there is a contralateral high-grade stenosis or occlusion, the PSVR is likely a better criterion
► Although the SRU criteria are widely used, a relatively wide range of PSV and PSVR numbers have been reported to be highly accurate for the diagnosis of high-grade ICA stenosis (≥ 70–80%)
  ▪ Threshold numbers may be chosen to maximize sensitivity (lower numbers) or specificity (higher numbers)
  ▪ Whatever chart or threshold numbers are used in a given laboratory, spectral Doppler criteria should be concordant with grayscale and color Doppler imaging findings
  ▪ If no explanation can be found for a significant discordance between the Doppler criteria and the grayscale or color Doppler findings, correlative imaging should be considered
► SRU criteria for diagnosis of a moderate ICA stenosis (50–69%)
  ▪ PSV between 125 and 230 cm/s
  ▪ ICA/CCA PSV ratio between 2.0 and 4.0

- ► SRU criteria for diagnosis of a nearly occlusive ICA stenosis
  - ■ PSV often decreases (< 230 cm/s)
  - ■ Diastolic velocity may remain elevated
  - ■ Large amount of plaque and significant luminal narrowing on grayscale and color Doppler imaging
  - ■ High-resistance proximal waveform
  - ■ Distal tardus parvus waveform
- ► High-output states such as hypertension or thyrotoxicosis may cause increased PSV throughout the extracranial carotid arteries bilaterally in the absence of an underlying stenosis
- ► Vessel tortuosity or a contralateral high-grade stenosis or occlusion may cause unilateral increased PSV in the carotid arteries without an underlying stenosis

Management

- ► Numerous prospective multicenter trials have demonstrated that both carotid endarterectomy and carotid stent placement reduce the rate of ipsilateral ischemic events in symptomatic patients with ≥ 70% ICA stenosis
- ► Intervention provides some, but less significant, benefit in both symptomatic and asymptomatic patients with 50–69% ICA stenosis
- ► Recent data suggest that current state-of-the-art medical management may be better for moderate ICA stenosis

Further Reading

1. Grant EG, Benson CB, Moneta GL, et al. Carotid artery stenosis: Grayscale and Doppler US diagnosis—Society of Radiologists in Ultrasound consensus conference. *Radiology*. 2003; 229: 340–346.
2. Lanzino G, Rabinstein AA, Brown RD Jr, et al. Treatment of carotid artery stenosis: Medical therapy, surgery or stenting? *Mayo Clin Proc*. 2009; 84: 362–368.

History

▶ 77-Year-old male with right internal carotid artery (RICA) stent placement 12 months prior for a 90% RICA stenosis now presents for surveillance (Figs. 152.1–152.3). Known left internal carotid artery occlusion. History of cervical radiation therapy for squamous cell oropharyngeal cancer.

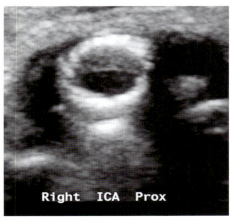

Fig. 152.1

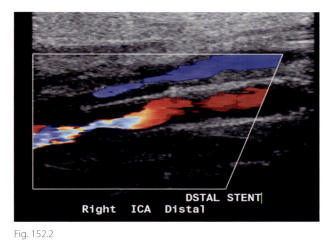

Fig. 152.2

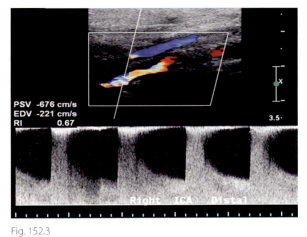

Fig. 152.3

Case 152 Right Internal Carotid Artery In-Stent Restenosis

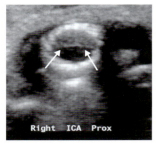

Fig. 152.4

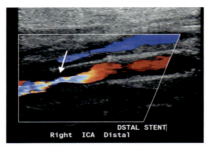

Fig. 152.5

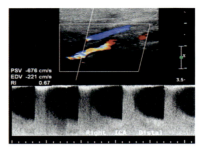

Fig. 152.6

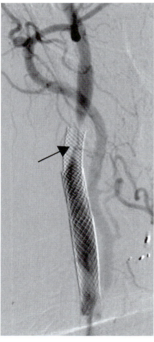

Fig. 152.7

Imaging Findings

► Transverse grayscale image demonstrating internal echoes (arrows in Fig. 152.4) within the distal aspect of the RICA stent consistent with neointimal hyperplasia
► On Color Doppler image, note narrowing of the distal lumen of the stent with focal color aliasing (arrow in Fig. 152.5) consistent with a high-grade stenosis
► Spectral Doppler US (Fig. 152.6) demonstrates spectral broadening as well as markedly elevated peak systolic velocity (PSV) of 676 cm/s with an end diastolic velocity of 221 cm/s within the distal stent
► PSV in the mid stent was 95 cm/s (not shown), giving a PSV ratio of approximately 7:1
► Digital subtraction angiogram confirms high-grade in-stent restenosis (arrow in Fig. 152.7), which was subsequently treated with angioplasty and deployment of an additional 6-mm drug-eluting stent (not shown)

Differential Diagnosis

► < 70% in-stent restenosis
► Stent thrombosis
► Stent fracture

Teaching Points

▶ Carotid endarterectomy (CEA) and carotid artery stenting (CAS) are the most commonly employed methods of treating carotid artery stenosis

▶ CAS has currently gained acceptance as a safe alternative to CEA, particularly in patients at high surgical risk, although guidelines for referral to CEA versus CAS remain in evolution as experience and technology develop
  ▪ Risk of periprocedural myocardial infarction and cranial nerve damage higher for CEA
  ▪ Risk of periprocedural stroke higher for CAS
  ▪ Most recommend CEA: heavily calcified or very hypoechoic plaque (increased risk of embolization), tortuous vessel, long lesion, if the patient cannot receive antiplatelet agents, and in patients older than age 75 years (although this last criterion is controversial)
  ▪ Most recommend CAS: high medical comorbidity, restenosis post CEA, "hostile" neck (status post surgery or radiation therapy), common carotid artery lesions, lesions inaccessible to surgeon

▶ The CREST (Carotid Revascularization Endarterectomy versus Stenting Trial) trial reported similar rates of restenosis for CAS and CEA after 2 years of follow-up
  ▪ 2–22%, depending on the study (average < 9%)

▶ Doppler US has an important role as the most widely used noninvasive method of following patients post CAS

▶ However, conventional Doppler US criteria are less accurate in patients who have undergone CAS because PSV within the stent is typically higher than in nonstented arteries, likely due to a combination of factors
  ▪ Decreased compliance of vessel wall from the stiff metallic stent
  ▪ Residual wasting of a stent that does not fully expand
  ▪ External compression of the stent by residual plaque
  ▪ Increased flow to the ICA if the stent is configured to reduce flow though the external carotid artery
  ▪ Velocities in the range of 125–200 cm/s (and even greater) are fairly common even in widely patent stents

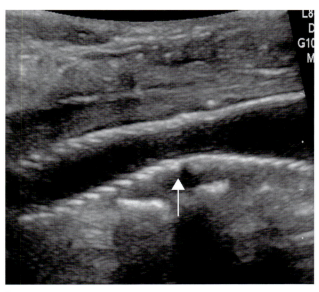

Fig. 152.8

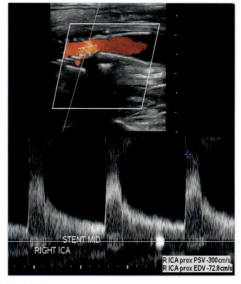

Fig. 152.9

Note residual wasting of the RICA stent (arrow in Fig. 152.8) with increased PSV of 300 cm/s (Fig. 152.9). However, there is no intraluminal echogenic material to suggest neointimal hyperplasia or plaque, and the increased PSV is likely related to the postprocedural configuration of the stent rather than in-stent restenosis.

▶ Published Doppler criteria for grading in-stent restenosis are quite variable, in part due to small study size, variations in stent composition, type and length of stents, as well as variation in protocols at different institutions in the reported studies
  ▪ All authors agree that PSV and PSV ratio criteria are considerably higher for a given degree of in-stent restenosis compared to the native carotid arteries
  ▪ Hence, grayscale and color Doppler appearance as well as change over time assume greater importance

▶ A meta-analysis by Pizzolato et al. (see Further Reading) concluded that a PSV of 300–350 cm/s could be used as a relatively good and sensitive predictor of high-grade in-stent restenosis

- ► CT angiogram and MR angiogram are complementary imaging modalities that are primarily used as a problem-solving test in difficult or complex cases following CAS
- ► < 70% in-stent restenosis

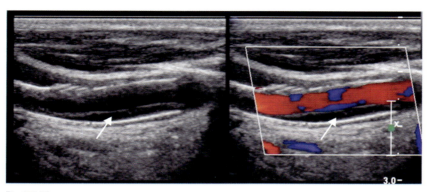

Fig. 152.10

Split-screen image demonstrating low-level internal echoes posteriorly (arrows in Fig. 152.10) within the stent lumen on grayscale (left) and color Doppler (right) images. However, there is no significant narrowing of the residual lumen or color Doppler aliasing to suggest increased velocity. Findings are consistent with a < 50% stenosis. Six-month interval follow-up should be considered to ensure stability and lack of progression.

- ► Stent thrombosis
  - ▪ Unusual complication
  - ▪ Complete absence of flow on color and spectral Doppler
  - ▪ Intraluminal echogenic material

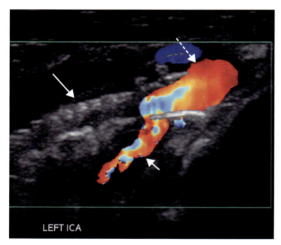

Fig. 152.11

Color Doppler image reveals no detectable flow in the left ICA stent above the carotid bifurcation (long arrow in Fig. 152.11). The lumen is filled with low-level echoes consistent with thrombus. Left external carotid artery (short arrow) and common carotid artery (dashed arrow) are patent.

- ► Stent fracture
  - ▪ Extremely rare complication
  - ▪ May be asymptomatic or present with pain ± trauma
  - ▪ Assess for discontinuity or irregularity of echogenic stent components
  - ▪ May result in significant narrowing of residual lumen and increased PSV

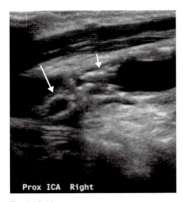

Fig. 152.12

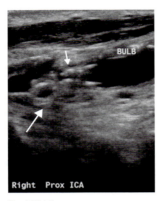

Fig. 152.13

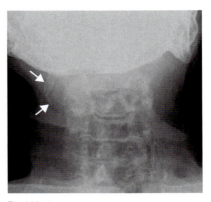

Fig. 152.14

On these longitudinal grayscale images (Figs. 152.12 and 152.13), the lower aspect of the right ICA stent (short arrows) appears compressed and funneled, but it is oriented parallel to the vessel lumen, as expected. However, the upper portion of the stent (long arrows) appears to be oriented perpendicular to the vessel lumen in the transverse plane, appearing in cross section. In addition, the upper fragment of the stent appears to be separated from the lower portion of the stent. X-ray of the neck confirms fracture of the stent with acute angulation of the separate components (arrows in Fig. 152.14).

Management

▶ Due to the risk of in-stent restenosis, most clinicians recommend following patients after stent placement with Doppler US at 1 month, 6 months, and then yearly, although protocols vary at different institutions
  ▪ Intervention in the asymptomatic patient generally not recommended until stenosis ≥ 75–80%
  ▪ Patients with lesser degrees of stenosis followed at shorter intervals, usually every 6 months
▶ Digital subtraction angiography with balloon angioplasty and/or stenting is used to confirm the diagnosis and treat in-stent restenosis

Further Reading

1. Pizzolato R, Hirsch JA, Romero JM. Imaging challenges of carotid artery in-stent restenosis. *J NeuroIntervent Surg.* 2014; 6: 32–41.
2. Lal BK. Recurrent carotid stenosis after CEA and CAS: Diagnosis and management. *Semin Vasc Surg.* 2007; 20: 259–266.

Case 153

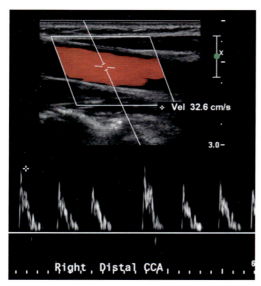

Fig. 153.1

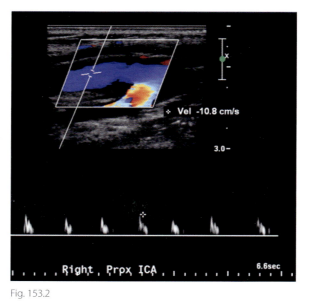

Fig. 153.2

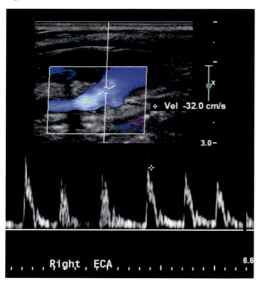

Fig. 153.3

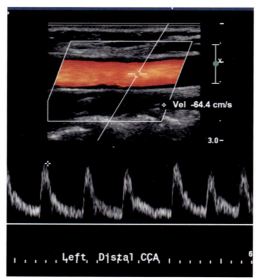

Fig. 153.4

Case 153 High-Resistance Waveforms in the Right Common and Proximal Internal Carotid Arteries Secondary to Occlusion of the Right Distal Internal Carotid Artery

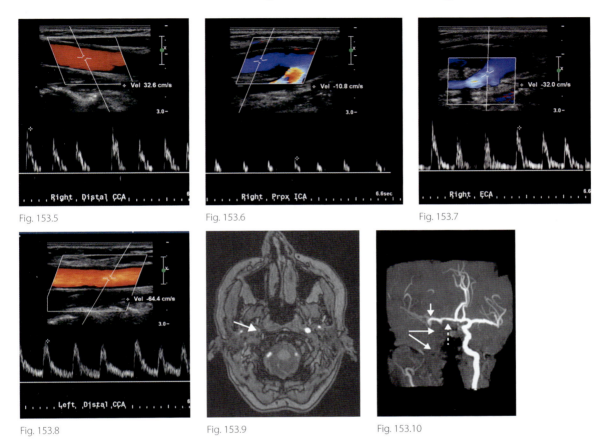

Fig. 153.5

Fig. 153.6

Fig. 153.7

Fig. 153.8

Fig. 153.9

Fig. 153.10

Imaging Findings

► Low peak systolic velocity (PSV) with complete absence of diastolic flow in the right common carotid artery (CCA) and proximal internal carotid artery (ICA) (Figs. 153.5 and 153.6, respectively) are consistent with a distal occlusion or high-grade stenosis. Findings are more pronounced in the right ICA where there is almost no flow. This waveform has been called a "knocking" or "staccato" waveform pattern

► The proximal ICA is widely patent; thus, the obstruction to flow must be distal to this point

► Increased diastolic flow in the right external carotid artery (ECA) (Fig. 153.7) compared to the ipsilateral ICA (Fig. 153.6) and contralateral ECA (not shown) is termed "internalization" of the ECA waveform and reflects compensatory, collateral flow due to distal occlusion in the ipsilateral ICA territory

► Left CCA spectral Doppler waveform (Fig. 153.8) demonstrates normal PSV and diastolic flow

► Time-of-flight MR angiogram (MRA) image (Fig. 153.9) and coronal three-dimensional maximum intensity projection reconstruction (Fig. 153.10) demonstrate occlusion of the distal cervical and intracranial right ICA (arrow in Fig. 153.9 and long solid arrows in Fig. 153.10) with retrograde filling of the right middle cerebral artery (MCA) (short arrow in Fig. 153.10) through the patent anterior communicating artery and A1 segment of the anterior cerebral artery (dashed arrow in Fig. 153.10)

Differential Diagnosis

► Ipsilateral MCA occlusion
► Ipsilateral distal ICA dissection
► Increased intracranial pressure
► Bilateral distal ICA or MCA occlusions
► Brain death
► Aortic regurgitation

Teaching Points

▶ Distal ICA and MCA occlusions or high-grade stenoses can be due to atherosclerosis, acute thrombosis, or dissection
▶ Normal spectral Doppler waveforms of the CCAs and ICAs
  ▪ Sharp systolic upstroke
  ▪ PSV: 60–100 cm/s
  ▪ Moderate amount of continuous forward diastolic flow
▶ US findings of distal CCA, ICA, or MCA occlusion or high-grade stenosis
  ▪ Reversed, absent, or substantially decreased diastolic flow in the proximal carotid segments
  ▪ Decreased PSV
  ▪ Systolic upstroke remains sharp
  ▪ Termed "high-resistance" waveform pattern
  ▪ More pronounced closer to the obstruction, eventually becoming a tiny blip of forward systolic flow (Fig. 153.6), termed the "knocking" or "staccato" waveform pattern
  ▪ Increased diastolic flow in the ipsilateral ECA, termed "internalization" of the ECA waveform, may be observed if the ECA provides collateral blood flow to the intracranial ICA/MCA circulation via periorbital or ophthalmic branches
  ▪ Increased PSV may be noted in the contralateral CCA and ICA due to compensatory flow
  ▪ If the occlusion/stenosis in the ICA is long-standing and the ECA supplies significant collateral flow to the distal ICA intracranial territory, decreased diastolic flow in the ipsilateral CCA may not be observed
▶ Ipsilateral MCA occlusion or high-grade stenosis
  ▪ Identical CCA and proximal ICA high-resistance waveforms with patent proximal ICA
▶ ICA dissection
  ▪ Most common in young patients who present with trauma or headache
  ▪ Typically originates at skull base extending toward carotid bulb
  ▪ Intramural hematoma more common than patent true and false lumens
  ▪ Identical US findings
    • Proximal high-resistance waveforms with decreased, absent, or reverse diastolic flow and low PSV
    • Widely patent proximal ICA near bifurcation without evidence of atherosclerosis
    • If the dissection has extended to the bulb, the intramural hematoma will cause homogeneous hypoechoic thickening of the arterial wall resulting in a long-segment smooth, tapering stenosis or complete occlusion of the ICA

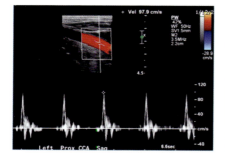
Fig. 153.11

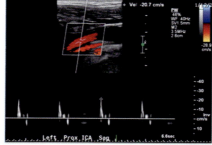
Fig. 153.12

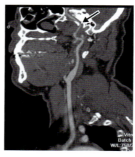
Fig. 153.13

Note high-resistance spectral Doppler waveforms more pronounced in the left ICA (Fig. 153.12) than the CCA (Fig. 153.11) in this 24-year-old female who presented with a severe headache. The proximal ICA is widely patent without evidence of plaque or atherosclerosis. Sagittal CT angiogram demonstrates smoothly tapered narrowing of the distal ICA (arrow in Fig. 153.13) at the skull base, most consistent with a spontaneous ICA dissection.

▶ Increased intracranial pressure, bilateral distal ICA/MCA occlusions, and brain death will result in bilateral CCA and proximal ICA high-resistance waveforms, more pronounced in ICAs
▶ Increased intracranial pressure
  ▪ Usually secondary to a mass lesion
  ▪ High-resistance waveforms more pronounced on the side of the mass lesion
▶ Bilateral ICA occlusions
  ▪ Increased flow in the bilateral ECAs and vertebral arteries, depending on intracranial collateral pathways

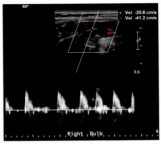

Fig. 153.14

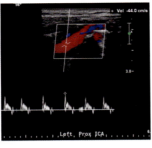

Fig. 153.15

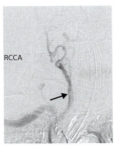

Fig. 153.16

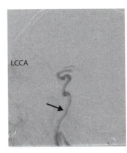

Fig. 153.17

Low-PSV, high-resistance spectral Doppler waveforms in the right carotid bulb (Fig. 153.14) and proximal left ICA (Fig. 153.15) in this 74-year-old female who presented with a massive stroke. There was no opacification of either the right or the left ICA on the subsequent angiogram. CCAs (arrows in Figs. 153.16 and 153.17)

► Brain death
  ▪ Extremely pronounced high-resistance waveforms in bilateral ICAs, often with reversed diastolic flow
  ▪ However, the diagnosis of brain death should not be made on US alone
► Aortic regurgitation
  ▪ Decreased, absent, or reversed diastolic flow in the bilateral proximal CCAs, reversed diastolic flow often pronounced and pan-diastolic
  ▪ PSV increased or normal
  ▪ Waveforms in the distal CCAs and ICAs should normalize, demonstrating normal diastolic flow
  ▪ Abnormal waveform usually only seen when aortic regurgitation is at least moderate to severe

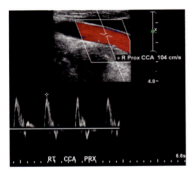

Fig. 153.18

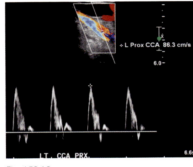

Fig. 153.19

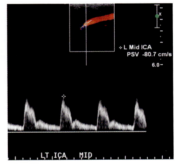

Fig. 153.20

No end diastolic flow is present in either the right (Fig. 153.18) or left (Fig. 153.19) CCAs in this patient with aortic regurgitation. However, PSV is not decreased, which differentiates this waveform pattern from the high-resistance waveform pattern previously described. In addition, the waveform is normal in the left (Fig. 153.20) and right (not shown) ICAs.

Management

► Observation of unilateral high-resistance waveforms with low PSV, more pronounced in the ICA than in the CCA, with a widely patent ICA, should prompt further evaluation with CT angiogram, MRA, or angiogram to assess for occlusion or high-grade stenosis of the distal ICA or MCA
► Bilateral high-resistance, low velocity waveforms in the CCAs and ICAs suggest bilateral or global pathology such as bilateral distal ICA occlusions, increased intracranial pressure, vasospasm, or brain death

Further Reading

1. Scoutt LM, Lin FL, Kliewer M. Waveform analysis of the carotid arteries. *Ultrasound Clin.* 2006; 1: 133–159.
2. Robbin ML, Lockhart ME. Carotid artery ultrasound interpretation using a pattern recognition approach. *Ultrasound Clin.* 2006; 1: 111–132.
3. Mattos MA, Hodgson KJ, Ramsey DE. Identifying total carotid occlusion with colour flow duplex scanning. *Eur J Vasc Surg.* 1992; 6: 204–210.
4. Kirsch JD, Wagner LR, James EM. Carotid artery occlusion: Positive predictive value of duplex sonography compared with arteriography. *J Vasc Surg.* 1994; 19: 642–649.

Case 154

History

- 67-Year-old female, preoperative evaluation (Figs. 154.1–154.6)

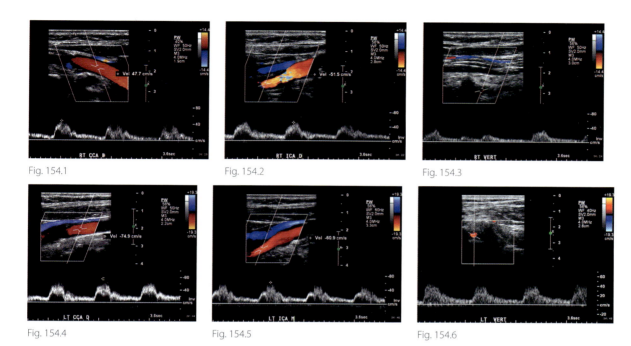

Fig. 154.1

Fig. 154.2

Fig. 154.3

Fig. 154.4

Fig. 154.5

Fig. 154.6

Case 154 Tardus Parvus Waveforms in the Carotid and Vertebral Arteries Secondary to Aortic Stenosis

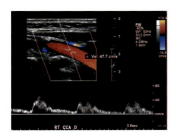

Fig. 154.7

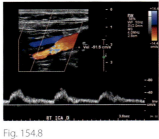

Fig. 154.8

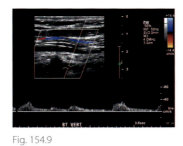

Fig. 154.9

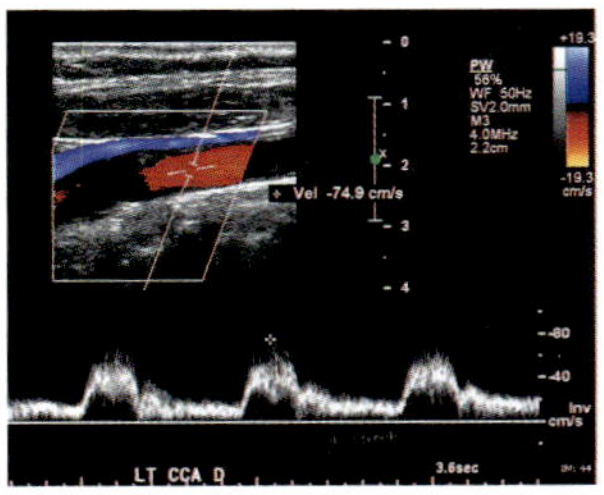

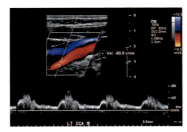

Fig. 154.10

Fig. 154.11

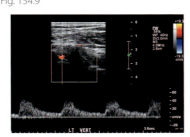

Fig. 154.12

Imaging Findings

- Spectral Doppler waveforms from the right and left common carotid, internal carotid, and vertebral arteries (Figs. 154.7–154.12) demonstrate delayed systolic acceleration with prolonged systolic upstroke, decreased peak systolic velocity, and rounding of the systolic peak in all vessels

Differential Diagnosis

- Innominate artery stenosis
- Stenosis of a common origin of the innominate and left common carotid arteries (Bovine arch)
- Coarctation of the aorta
- Decreased cardiac output

Teaching Points

- Aortic stenosis (AS) has become the most frequent cardiovascular problem after hypertension and coronary artery disease in Europe and North America
  - Affects approximately 2% of people older than age 65 years in developed countries
  - Most commonly presents as calcific AS in older patients (eighth and ninth decades)
    - More common in men than in women
  - Patients with calcified congenital bicuspid aortic valves commonly present slightly earlier
  - AS in younger patients is typically congenital in origin
  - AS secondary to rheumatic heart disease has become very rare in developed countries
- Most patients with mild to moderate disease are typically asymptomatic
- Clinical presentation of severe AS
  - Syncope and/or hypotension due to decreased cardiac output
  - Heart failure, shortness of breath especially at night or while lying down, swollen lower extremities
  - Chest pain/angina
  - Bruit
  - Endocarditis
- AS may be complicated by development of aortic regurgitation as the valve becomes deformed and incompetent

- ► Tardus parvus (TP) waveforms, characterized by slow systolic upstroke and a dampened rounded systolic peak with decreased peak systolic velocity (PSV), are often seen on spectral Doppler arterial waveforms distal to a high-grade stenosis
- ► Findings of AS on carotid Doppler US examination
  - ▪ Bilateral TP waveforms in the carotid and vertebral arteries
  - ▪ The TP appearance will be more pronounced the more distal to the aortic valve that the vessel is sampled—that is, more pronounced in the internal carotid artery in comparison to the common carotid artery (CCA)
  - ▪ Diffusely decreased PSV
  - ▪ Typically only seen with severe AS
- ► An innominate stenosis could result in TP waveforms in the right carotid and vertebral arteries, but not on the left
- ► A stenosis at the common origin of the right innominate and left CCA (bovine aortic arch) could result in TP waveforms in the bilateral carotid and right vertebral arteries, but not in the left vertebral artery
- ► Aortic coarctation most often results in a stenosis of the thoracic aorta distal to the origin of the left subclavian artery and, therefore, would not affect the carotid and vertebral artery waveforms
- ► Decreased cardiac output could result in diffusely decreased PSV (i.e., cause a parvus waveform) but would not be expected to slow the rate of systolic acceleration (i.e., not a tardus waveform)

Management

- ► Cardiac echo used to diagnose, grade, and follow patients with AS
- ► Urgent valve replacement is required in patients with symptomatic AS
- ► The management of asymptomatic patients with severe AS remains controversial
  - ▪ Sudden death is the major concern when asymptomatic patients are followed conservatively. However, the incidence is < 1% per year

Further Reading

1. Baumgartner H. Aortic stenosis: Medical and surgical management. *Heart*. 2005; 91(11): 1483–1488.
2. Rohren EM, Klewer MA, Carroll BA, et al. A spectrum of Doppler waveforms in the carotid and vertebral arteries. *Am J Roentgenol*. 2003; 181(6): 1695–1704.

History

► 57-Year-old female with heart failure, pre-cardiac transplant evaluation for carotid stenosis (Figs. 155.1–155.6)

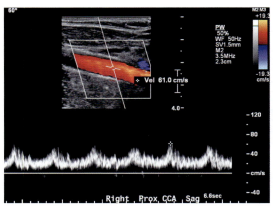

Fig. 155.1

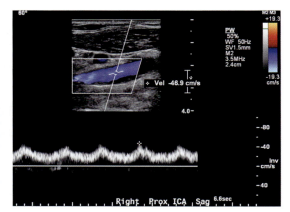

Fig. 155.2

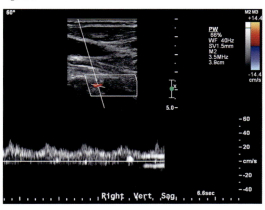

Fig. 155.3

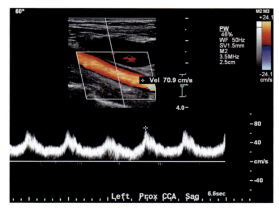

Fig. 155.4

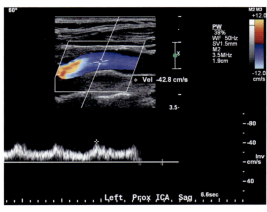

Fig. 155.5

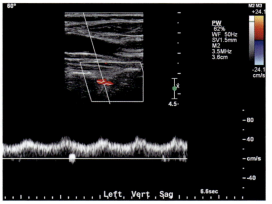

Fig. 155.6

Case 155 Abnormal Carotid Artery Waveforms Due to Left Ventricular Assist Device

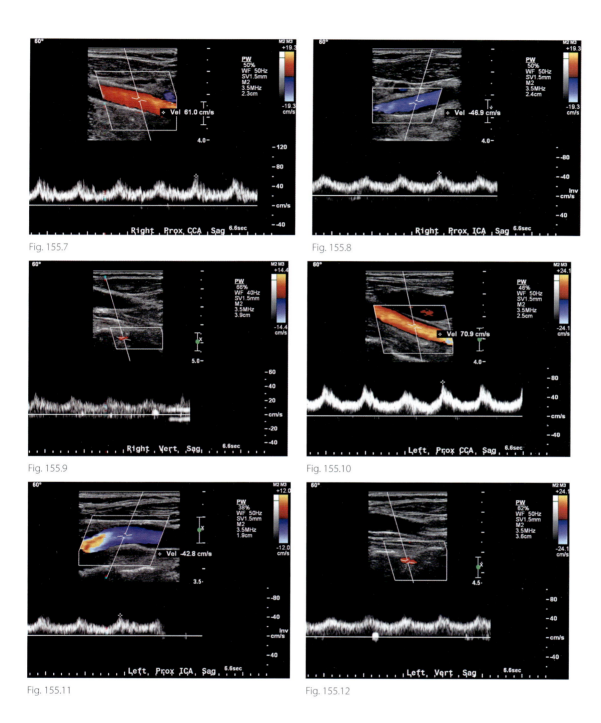

Fig. 155.7

Fig. 155.8

Fig. 155.9

Fig. 155.10

Fig. 155.11

Fig. 155.12

Imaging Findings

▶ Pronounced tardus parvus spectral Doppler waveforms characterized by delayed systolic upstroke (tardus), decreased peak systolic velocity (PSV) (parvus), and rounding of the systolic peaks involving the bilateral common carotid, internal carotid, and vertebral arteries (Figs. 155.7–155.12)

Differential Diagnosis

▶ Severe aortic stenosis
▶ Low cardiac output

Teaching Points

▶ Ventricular assist devices are surgically implanted mechanical devices that aid in pumping blood in patients with severe refractory cardiac failure
- May be placed in the left, right, or both ventricles
- Left ventricular assist devices (LVADs) are most common, but if pulmonary arterial resistance is high, right ventricular assistance may be necessary

▶ Used primarily in patients with heart failure refractory to medical management as a bridge to myocardial recovery (post myocardial infarction or cardiac surgery) or as a bridge to cardiac transplantation
- Occasionally placed as final treatment option for patients who are not cardiac transplant candidates

▶ LVADs act as a conduit, diverting blood from the apex of the left ventricle to the aorta through a mechanical pump placed in the left upper quadrant
- Current devices pump with continuous forward flow
- Patients will have no palpable or greatly diminished peripheral pulses following placement

▶ Complications
- Bleeding
- Infection
- Arrhythmia
- Organ failure
- Disseminated intravascular coagulopathy
- Peripheral arterial embolus (including stroke)

▶ Spectral Doppler findings on carotid US examination
- Monophasic, tardus parvus waveforms with delayed systolic upstroke, rounded and diminished systolic peak (PSV < 40 cm/s), and no flow below the baseline
- Less commonly, nonpulsatile flow pattern with no obvious systolic peak (waveform may appear venous)
- All major arterial branches from the aorta will have the same waveform—for example, the carotid, vertebral, subclavian, renal, and common femoral arteries

▶ Physiology
- Pumping of some blood by intrinsic residual myocardial reserve thought to account for blunted systolic peak
- Absence of a systolic peak likely to occur when the left ventricle is simply acting as passive conduit with all blood pumped by the device
- Continuous diastolic flow will be observed even in arteries with normally high-resistance circuits such as the common femoral and external carotid arteries due to forward pumping of blood throughout the cardiac cycle

▶ Aortic stenosis
- Severe aortic stenosis could cause similar pronounced tardus parvus arterial waveforms diffusely, including in the common carotid, internal carotid, and vertebral arteries bilaterally
- Could see similar waveforms in other aortic branches, although less commonly

▶ Low cardiac output states
- Could cause diffusely decreased PSV, including in the bilateral carotid and vertebral arteries, but without delay in systolic acceleration

Management

▶ Patients with LVADs maintained on anticoagulation due to risk of stroke
▶ PSV not a reliable criterion for grading ICA stenosis in such patients, and more reliance should be placed on grayscale and color Doppler findings as well as PSV ratio

Further Reading

1. Cervini P, Park SJ, Shah DK, et al. Carotid Doppler ultrasound findings in patients with left ventricular assist devices. Ultrasound Q. 2010; 26: 255–61.
2. Frazier OH, Myers TJ, Westaby S, et al. Clinical experience with an implantable, intracardiac, continuous flow circulatory support device: physiologic implications and their relationship to patient selection. Ann Thorac Surg. 2004; 77:133–142.

Case 156

History

▶ 55-Year-old male presents with chest pain and absent pulses (Figs. 156.1–156.5)

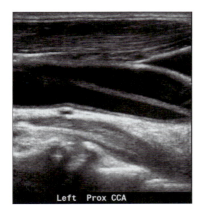

Fig. 156.1

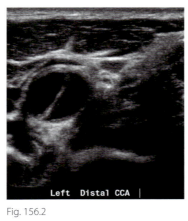

Fig. 156.2

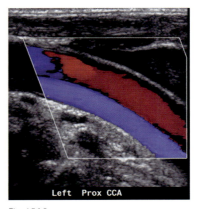

Fig. 156.3

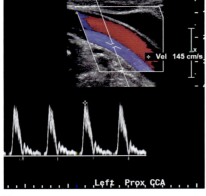

Fig. 156.4

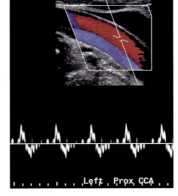

Fig. 156.5

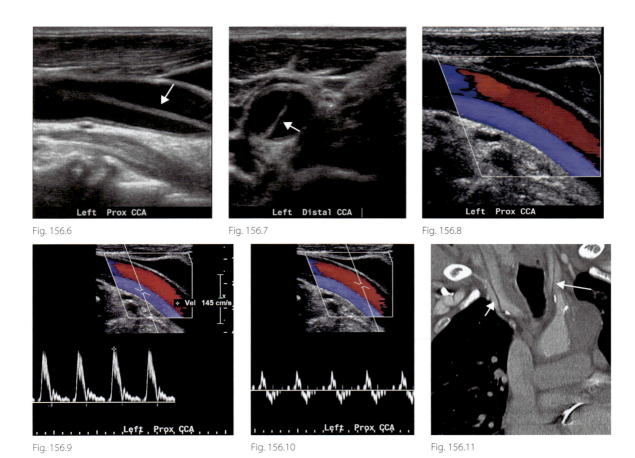

Fig. 156.6

Fig. 156.7

Fig. 156.8

Fig. 156.9

Fig. 156.10

Fig. 156.11

Imaging Findings

▶ Longitudinal (Fig. 156.6) and transverse (Fig. 156.7) grayscale US images of the left common carotid artery (CCA) demonstrate an echogenic linear intraluminal structure (arrows) consistent with dissection flap

▶ Longitudinal color Doppler image (Fig. 156.8) demonstrates that both the true and false lumens are patent with reversed flow in the false lumen

▶ Increased peak systolic velocity (PSV) of 145 cm/s (Fig. 156.9) in the true lumen (blue in Figs. 156.9 and 156.10) is likely due to compression by the false lumen (red in Figs. 156.9 and 156.10) that demonstrates a biphasic spectral Doppler waveform (Fig. 156.10)

▶ Coronal reconstructed CT (Fig. 156.11) demonstrates a dissection flap in the right innominate artery extending into the right CCA (short arrow) as well as a dissection flap in the left CCA (long arrow)

Differential Diagnosis

▶ Catheter in carotid artery
▶ Reverberation artifact

Teaching Points

▶ Etiology of CCA dissections
  ▪ Extension from dissection of the aortic arch
  ▪ Trauma
  ▪ Spontaneous
    • Implies weakness of the vessel wall such as underlying connective tissue disorder (Marfan or Ehlers–Danlos syndromes), arteritis, or cystic medial necrosis
▶ Pathophysiology

- Blood dissects into the arterial wall through an intimal tear that lifts the intima ± media off the adventitial layer
- Whether a patent false lumen develops versus mural hematoma depends on whether or not there is a re-entry point
▶ Presentation
  - Chest pain (from aortic dissection)
  - Neck or facial pain
  - Headache
  - Differential blood pressures in arms if innominate or subclavian artery involved
  - May be asymptomatic
▶ US findings
  - Echogenic linear intimal flap
    • Most often proximal
    • May be mobile
    • Thick or thin depending on whether the medial layer is included
  - False lumen may be patent or thrombosed
  - Patent false lumen may have a variable spectral Doppler waveform (high resistance with decreased diastolic flow, blunted or decreased PSV, reversed flow, bidirectional flow)
  - False lumen may compress true lumen, increasing PSV
  - Mural hematoma or thrombosed false lumen: thick hypoechoic homogeneous wall, may spiral around lumen, less common in CCA than internal carotid artery dissections
▶ Arterial catheter
  - Two (or three) parallel echogenic liness within vessel lumen
  - Would not create two discrete arterial lumens with different waveforms

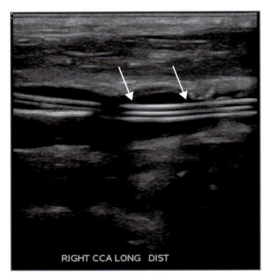

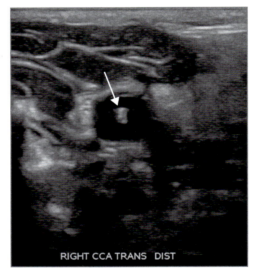

Fig. 156.12   Fig. 156.13

This 58-year-old female in the intensive care unit had a central venous catheter inadvertently placed into the right CCA. Note three parallel echogenic lines (arrows) within the vessel lumen on longitudinal (Fig. 156.12) and transverse views (Fig. 156.13).
▶ Reverberation artifact
  - Echogenic line or more often multiple lines parallel to vessel wall in near field
  - Would not be obliquely oriented or cause differential flow patterns

Management

▶ CCA dissections may be relatively stable and asymptomatic
  - 3–7% incidence of stroke
  - May not require intervention
▶ Assess the internal and external carotid arteries as well as the subclavian and innominate arteries with US to determine extent of dissection

► Further evaluation with MR angiography, CT angiography, or angiography to determine extent and/or aortic involvement often indicated

  ▪ Type A aortic dissections involving the ascending aorta require surgical or stent graft intervention

  ▪ Cardiac echo indicated to assess aortic valve for regurgitation and to exclude hemorrhagic pericardial effusion

Further Reading

1. Provenzale JM. Dissection of the internal carotid and vertebral arteries: Imaging Features. *Am J Roentgenol*. 1995; 165: 1099–1104.
2. Sturzenegger M, Mattle HP, Rivoir A, et al. Ultrasound findings in carotid artery dissection: Analysis of 43 patients. *Neurology*. 1995; 45: 691–698.

Case 157

History

▶ 51-Year-old male with vertigo (Figs. 157.1 and 157.2)

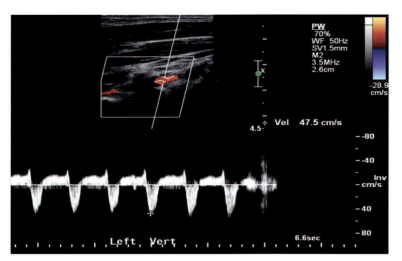

Fig. 157.1

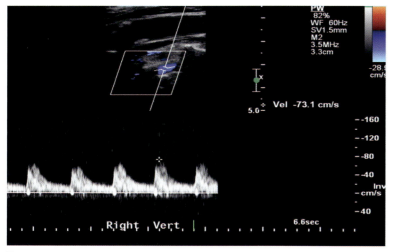

Fig. 157.2

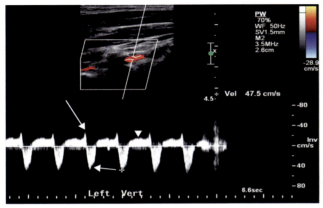

Fig. 157.3

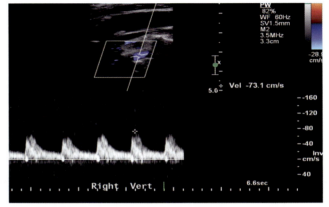

Fig. 157.4

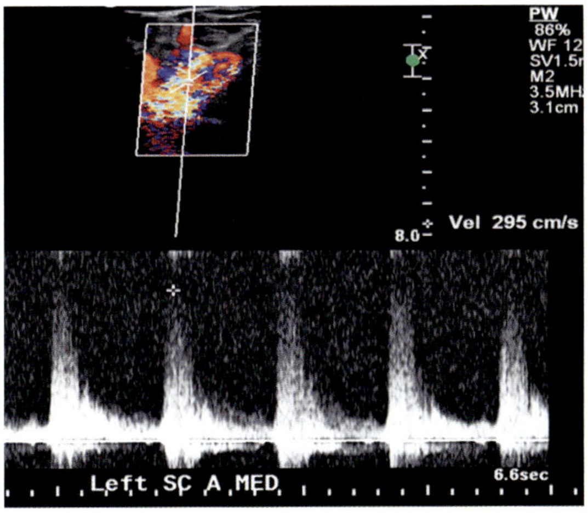

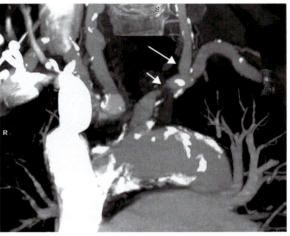

Fig. 157.5

Fig. 157.6

Imaging Findings

▶ Mid-systolic retraction (short arrow in Fig. 157.3) in left vertebral artery (VA) that extends below the baseline resulting in reversal of flow from mid to end systole. Flow is color coded red in the left VA, indicating that flow is reversed heading toward the transducer and away from the head

▶ Extremely thin/narrow initial systolic peak (long arrow in Fig. 157.3) with relatively low peak systolic velocity (PSV)

▶ Antegrade diastolic flow (arrowhead in Fig. 157.3)

▶ Normal right VA spectral Doppler waveform (Fig. 157.4) has a single systolic peak with normal PSV and sharp systolic upstroke. There is continuous forward flow throughout the cardiac cycle. Flow is color coded blue heading away from the transducer and toward the head (antegrade)

▶ PSV in the left subclavian artery (SCLA) is elevated at 295 cm/s (Fig. 157.5), consistent with a moderate to severe stenosis. Note focal color aliasing indicative of elevated PSV

▶ CT angiogram (Fig. 157.6) reveals severe stenosis (short arrow) in left SCLA proximal to the origin of the left VA (long arrow)

Differential Diagnosis

▶ Complete subclavian steal
▶ Vertebral artery dissection

Teaching Points

▶ Subclavian steal refers to reversal of flow in the VA due to occlusion or high-grade stenosis of the proximal SCLA or innominate artery proximal to the origin of the VA
- Blood flow to the arm is thus derived from the contralateral VA with blood flowing toward the head in the contralateral VA to the basilar artery, then down the ipsilateral VA to the SCLA and thence into the arm
- Rarely, collateral flow is supplied to the VA by the ipsilateral common carotid artery via the posterior communicating artery in the circle of Willis
- More common on the left

▶ Symptoms: lightheadedness, syncope, dizziness, ataxia, vertigo
- Worse when exercising arm
- May be asymptomatic and an incidental finding

▶ Complete subclavian steal: US findings
- Reversal of flow throughout entire cardiac cycle

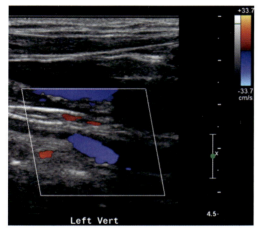

Fig. 157.7

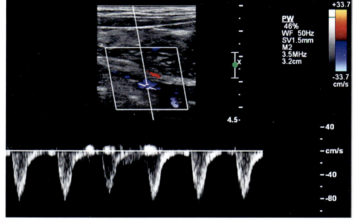

Fig. 157.8

In this patient with complete subclavian steal there is reversed flow throughout the entire cardiac cycle in the left VA; color coded blue (Fig. 157.7), which is the color below the baseline on the color Doppler scale and, therefore, heading away from the transducer/head toward the left SCLA. Flow is below the baseline with a "negative number" on the spectral Doppler image (Fig. 157.8) indicating reversed direction of flow.

▶ "Pre-steal" spectral Doppler waveform: US findings
- Transient flow reversal in mid systole with mid-systolic retraction
- Depth of mid-systolic retraction (above, to, or below baseline) loosely correlates with degree of SCLA stenosis
- Two systolic peaks
  - First is narrow with sharp upstroke
  - Second is rounder and wider
- Persistent forward diastolic flow
- Provocative maneuvers (exercising hand or inflating blood pressure cuff above systolic blood pressure, deflating, and resampling) may convert a pre-steal waveform to a complete steal or deepen the mid-systolic retraction

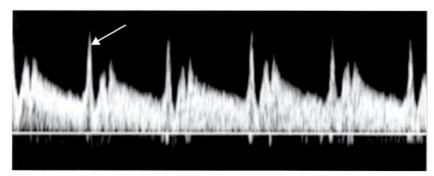

Fig. 157.9

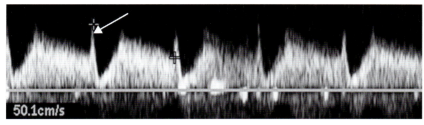

Fig. 157.10

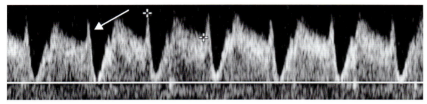

Fig. 157.11

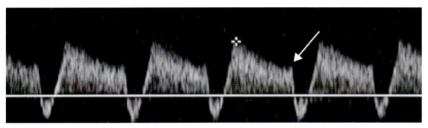

Fig. 157.12

Varying degrees of pre-steal waveforms in four different patients. Note sharp, pointed narrow early systolic peak (arrows in Figs. 157.9–157.12)) that is barely visible in Fig. 157.12, followed by varying depths of mid-systolic retraction: remaining above the baseline (Figs. 157.9 and 157.10), to the baseline (Fig. 157.11), and below the baseline (Fig. 157.12). The second systolic peak is rounded, wider, and blunter, and there is persistence of continuous forward diastolic flow in all waveforms. The depth of the mid-systolic retraction loosely correlates with the degree of subclavian artery stenosis.

► VA dissection
  ▪ May result in bidirectional flow, but reversed flow more likely in diastole
  ▪ No mid-systolic retraction

Management

► Pre-steal physiology rarely symptomatic and rarely requires intervention
► Many patients with complete flow reversal in the VA are completely asymptomatic
► Symptomatic patients
  ▪ Angioplasty with stenting
  ▪ Common carotid artery to distal subclavian artery surgical bypass

Further Reading

1. Kliewer MA, Hertzberg BS, Kim DH, et al. Vertebral artery Doppler waveform changes indicating subclavian steal physiology. *Am J Roentgenol.* 2000; 174(3): 815–819.
2. Horrow M, Stassi J. Sonography of the vertebral arteries: A window to disease of the proximal great vessels. *Am J Roentgenol.* 2001; 177: 53–59.

Case 158

History

▶ 63-Year-old male with back pain and pulsatile abdominal mass (Figs. 158.1–158.4)

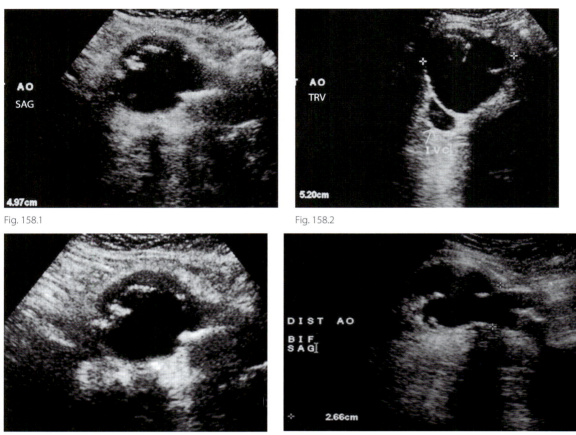

Fig. 158.1

Fig. 158.2

Fig. 158.3

Fig. 158.4

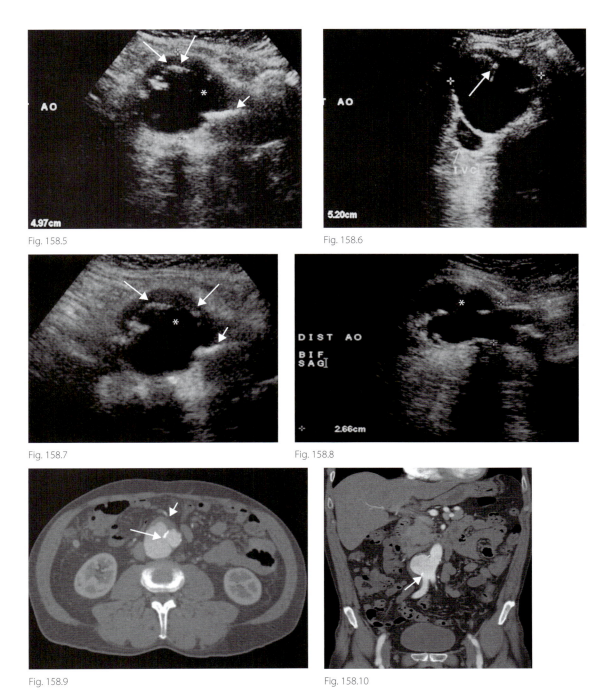

Fig. 158.5

Fig. 158.6

Fig. 158.7

Fig. 158.8

Fig. 158.9

Fig. 158.10

Imaging Findings

▶ 5.0 × 5.2-cm infrarenal saccular abdominal aortic aneurysm (AAA) (asterisks in Figs. 158.5, 158.7, and 158.8) arising from the anterior aortic wall and extending to the bifurcation (calipers in Fig. 158.8). Note peripheral crescent of intraluminal thrombus with echogenic surface (long arrows in Figs. 158.5–158.7). The wall of the aorta is focally echogenic with distal shadowing (short arrows in Figs. 158.5 and 158.7), consistent with mural calcification

- Axial (Fig. 158.9) and coronal (Fig. 158.10) contrast-enhanced CT scan confirms the US findings, including the saccular configuration, mural calcification (long arrows in Figs. 158.9 and 158.10), as well as mural thrombus (short arrow in Fig. 158.9)
- This patient presented with acute back pain and was emergently treated with endograft repair (EVAR)

Differential Diagnosis

- Pseudoaneurysm

Teaching Points

- Incidence of AAA highest in elderly, four times more common in men
  - Involves all three layers of aortic wall
  - Most are infrarenal and fusiform
  - Saccular: consider aortic dissection, trauma, infection, or vasculitis; greater risk of rupture
- Risk factors for AAA
  - Most are secondary to atherosclerosis
    - Smoking
    - Hypertension
    - Hypercholesterolemia
  - Family history (first-degree relative)
  - Connective tissue diseases
- Most patients are asymptomatic; a minority present with a pulsatile abdominal mass
- Patients with ruptured AAAs present with back or flank pain, ± hypotension
  - Risk of rupture related to size and growth rate
  - Risk of rupture higher and occurs at smaller AAA diameter in women
  - Mortality rate following rupture nearly 60%
- US screening has been proven to be cost-effective in reducing mortality from AAAs in men > 65 years old who have smoked or in women with family history of AAA
- US findings of AAAs
  - Measure from outer to outer wall on sagittal/coronal and transverse images
  - Diameter ≥ 3.0 cm or ≥ 1.5 times diameter of proximal aortic segment
  - ± Echogenic, calcified, or irregular wall
  - ± Intraluminal thrombus or plaque
  - Most AAAs are fusiform and infrarenal

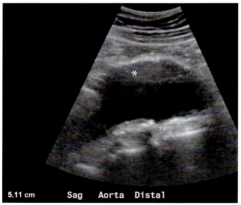

Fig. 158.11

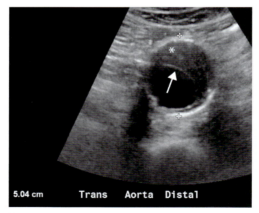

Fig. 158.12

This 58-year-old female presented with a pulsatile abdominal mass. Sagittal (Fig. 158.11) and transverse (Fig. 158.12) grayscale US images demonstrate a 5.1 × 5.0-cm fusiform AAA (calipers) as measured from outer wall to outer wall. In the sagittal plane, the aortic diameter should be measured perpendicular to the long axis of the lumen. Note small amount of mural thrombus or plaque (asterisks in Figs. 158.11 and 158.12) with an echogenic surface (arrow in Fig. 158.12). She was referred for EVAR.

- Saccular: focal, eccentric, ± disruption in wall; neck may be narrow or wide
- Relationship to origin of main renal arteries important for management: describe as suprarenal, juxtarenal, or infrarenal

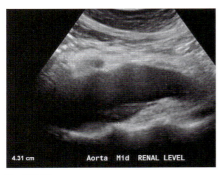

Fig. 158.13

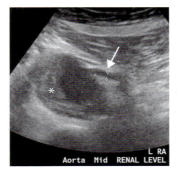

Fig. 158.14

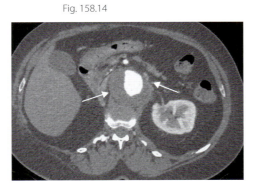

Fig. 158.15

Fig. 158.16

This 65-year-old male presented for screening for AAA and was found to have a suprarenal AAA. Sagittal grayscale US demonstrating a 4.3-cm AAA (calipers in Fig. 158.13) extending to the diaphragm. The AAA involves the origin of the left renal artery (arrows in Figs. 158.14 and 158.15), which is patent on color Doppler imaging (Fig. 158.15). Hence, the aneurysm is also juxtarenal. Note crescentic area of relatively echogenic mural-based thrombus within the AAA (asterisks in Figs. 158.14 and 158.15). Axial contrast-enhanced CT scan (Fig. 158.16) demonstrating the partially thrombosed AAA (arrows) that extends well above the superior pole of the left kidney.

▶ Pseudoaneurysm
  ▪ History of trauma, infection, or vasculitis
  ▪ Contained by zero, one, or two layers of the aortic wall
  ▪ Focal outpouching from aorta
  ▪ Neck may be wide or narrow
  ▪ "Yin-yang" color Doppler pattern within sac representing slowly swirling blood

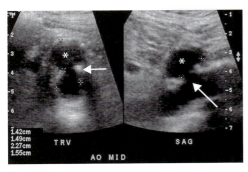

Fig. 158.17

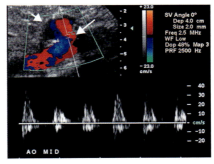

Fig. 158.18

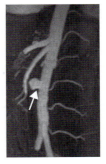

Fig. 158.19

85-Year-old male with a history of infectious aortitis after multiple complications from an anastomotic leak following surgery for a perforated cecal carcinoma. Partially thrombosed saccular AAA (asterisks in Fig. 158.17) arising from the anterior abdominal aortic wall with a wide neck (arrows in Fig. 158.17 and long arrow in Fig. 158.18). Note "yin-yang" (red/blue) color Doppler pattern in sac of pseudoaneurysm (PSA) with a small amount of intraluminal thrombus (short arrow on duplex color Doppler image, Fig. 158.18). Sagittal reconstructed MR angiogram demonstrates the wide-necked PSA (arrow in Fig. 158.19) arising from the anterior wall of the aorta.

Management

► Surveillance: asymptomatic AAAs < 5.0 cm
  ■ Timing controversial, shorter for AAAs close to 5 cm in diameter
► Intervention recommended for AAAs
  ■ > 5.0–5.5 cm in men
  ■ > 4.5–5.0 cm in women
  ■ Growth rate ≥ 1 cm per year
► CT has limited role in screening, but it is critical for treatment planning
► EVAR preferred over open surgical repair, depending on suitability of anatomy of AAA and aorta
  ■ Mortality for elective EVAR < 2% versus 3–5% for open repair
► Open repair for AAAs with unfavorable anatomy

Further Reading

1. American Institute of Ultrasound in Medicine. AIUM practice guideline for the performance of diagnostic and screening ultrasound examinations of the abdominal aorta in adults. *J Ultrasound Med.* 2011; 30: 121–126.
2. Shang EK, Nathan DP, Boonn WW, et al. A modern experience with saccular aortic aneurysms. *J Vasc Surg.* 2013; 57(1): 84–88.
3. LeFevre ML; U.S. Preventive Services Task Force. Screening for abdominal aortic aneurysm: U.S. Preventive Services Task Force recommendation statement. *Ann Intern Med.* 2014; 161(4): 281–290.

Case 159

History

► 67-Year-old female with a known abdominal aortic aneurysm presents with abdominal pain (Figs. 159.1–159.4)

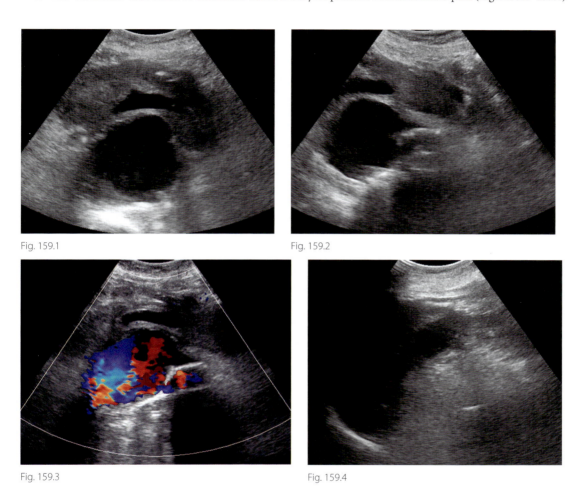

Fig. 159.1

Fig. 159.2

Fig. 159.3

Fig. 159.4

Case 159 Rupture of Abdominal Aortic Aneurysm

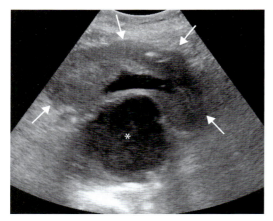

Fig. 159.5

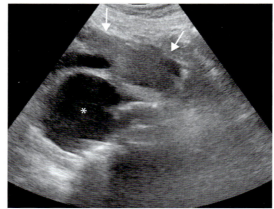

Fig. 159.6

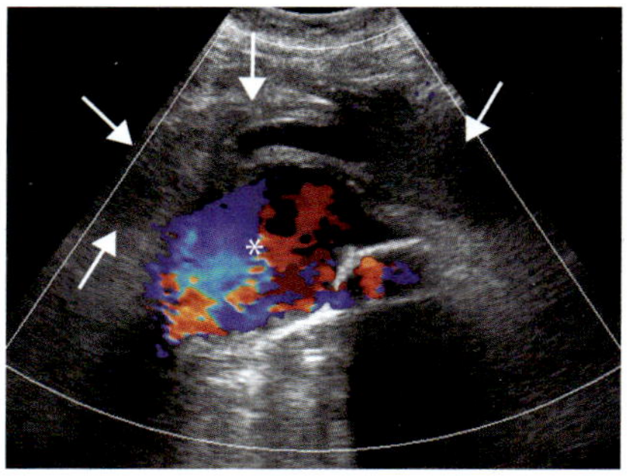

Fig. 159.7

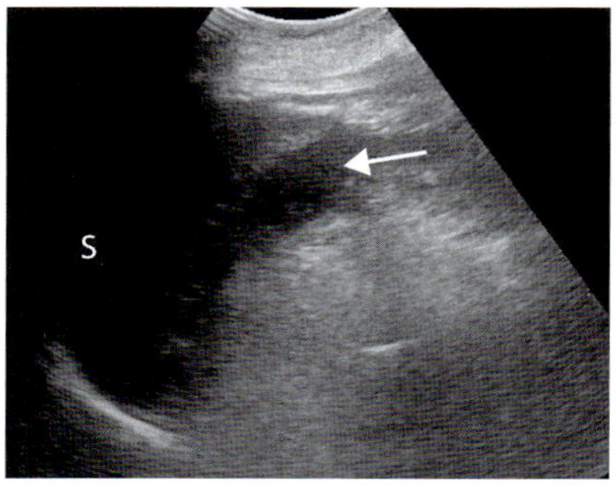

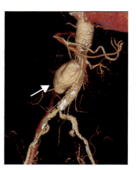

Fig. 159.8

Fig. 159.9

Imaging Findings

► Note abdominal aortic aneurysm (AAA) (asterisks in Figs. 159.5–159.7) measuring approximately 6 cm in diameter
► The AAA fills in with color on color Doppler (Fig. 159.7) without evidence of intraluminal thrombus
► A heterogeneous crescentic-shaped collection (arrows in Figs. 159.5–159.7) is noted anterior to the AAA, consistent with hematoma
► Note echogenic free fluid in the splenorenal fossa (arrow in Fig. 159.8), consistent with intraperitoneal hemorrhage. Spleen (S)
► Three-dimensional volume-rendered CT scan of the abdominal aorta done a few days prior to the US study demonstrates a saccular infrarenal aneurysm (arrow in Fig. 159.9)

Differential Diagnosis

► Aortic aneurysm without rupture, ascites
► Retroperitoneal fibrosis
► Lymphoma

Teaching Points

► An AAA is defined as dilatation of the abdominal aorta to ≥ 3 cm in diameter or > 1.5 times the diameter of the proximal segment
► Rupture of an AAA is the 10th leading cause of death in men older than age 55 years in the United States
► The U.S. Preventive Services Task Force recommends one-time US screening for AAA in men aged 65–75 years who have ever smoked and in women with a family history
► Risk of rupture is related to size and growth rate
  ▪ Intervention recommended for an AAA ≥ 5.0 to 5.5 cm in diameter in men
  ▪ Women have a lower incidence of AAA but a higher risk of rupture, rupture at smaller aortic diameter, and have a higher mortality rate. Hence, intervention recommended for an AAA ≥ 4.5 to 5.0 cm

- Presentation: classic triad of abdominal pain, hypotension, and pulsatile abdominal mass present in approximately 50% of patients
  - 80% have abdominal pain
- Early recognition is crucial: mortality rate increases to 75% if diagnosis is delayed, from 35% if rupture is promptly diagnosed
- Diagnostic US findings
  - Periaortic hematoma surrounding an AAA and echogenic intraperitoneal fluid
  - Echogenicity of periaortic hematoma is variable depending on time course
  - However, the presence of an AAA > 5 cm in a patient with abdominal/back pain and hypotension should raise concern for AAA rupture
- US highly sensitive for detecting AAAs (95–98%)
  - Much lower sensitivity for diagnosis of contained leak (4% reported in one study) or contained rupture because direct sonographic signs often absent
- False-positive diagnosis of AAA rupture may occur if intra-abdominal free fluid is present due to other causes, such as chronic ascites
- Retroperitoneal fibrosis or lymphoma
  - Periaortic hypoechoic material could be noted in both; much less likely to be heterogeneous or to contain anechoic areas
  - Lymphoma more likely to be mass-like and lobular; may lift aorta off spine, causing aorta to appear as if it is floating
  - Neither would be associated with AAA or free intraperitoneal fluid

Management

- If clinically stable, a CT scan may be indicated to delineate the anatomy and extent of bleeding
- Contrast-enhanced US (CEUS) (not yet approved by the U.S. Food and Drug Administration for noncardiac or nonhepatic indications) may allow rapid and noninvasive diagnosis
  - CEUS findings: delayed or prolonged aortic lumen opacification, focal non-enhancing mural region, contrast leakage into thrombus and around aneurysm, pooling of contrast dependently outside the aneurysm
- Emergent intervention with tube graft or endovascular stent graft

Further Reading

1. Catalano O, Lobianco R, Cusati B, et al. Contrast-enhanced sonography for diagnosis of ruptured abdominal aortic aneurysm. *Am J Roentgenol*. 2005; 184(2): 423–427.
2. Shuman WP, Hastrup W Jr, Kohler TR, et al. Suspected leaking abdominal aortic aneurysm: Use of sonography in the emergency room. *Radiology*. 1988; 168(1): 117–119.

Case 160

History

▶ 62-Year-old male presents for surveillance 1 year following endovascular abdominal aortic aneurysm repair (EVAR) (Figs. 160.1–160.4)

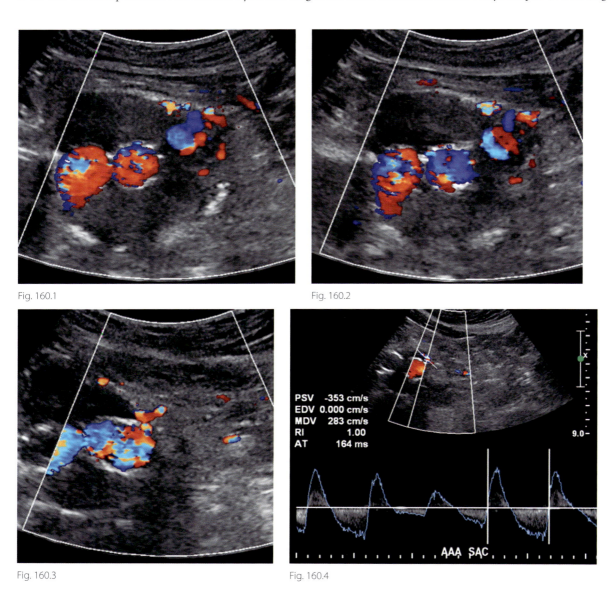

Fig. 160.1

Fig. 160.2

Fig. 160.3

Fig. 160.4

Case 160 Type II Endoleak From Inferior Mesenteric Artery

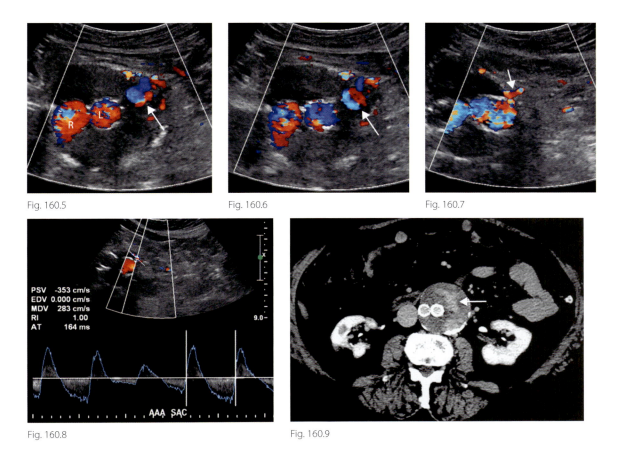

Fig. 160.5

Fig. 160.6

Fig. 160.7

Fig. 160.8

Fig. 160.9

Imaging Findings

▶ Transverse color Doppler images (Figs. 160.5–160.7) demonstrating patency of the right (R in Fig. 160.5) and left (L in Fig. 160.5) outflow limbs of the endograft within the calcified abdominal aortic aneurysm (AAA), which remained stable in size at 6.1 cm (measurement not shown)

▶ There is color Doppler flow within the sac of the AAA outside the endograft (arrows in Figs. 160.5 and 160.6) as well as a patent feeding vessel anterolaterally to the left (arrow in Fig. 160.7) consistent with a type II endoleak likely from the inferior mesenteric artery (IMA)

▶ Spectral Doppler waveform (Fig. 160.8) demonstrates a "to and fro" pattern, characteristic of a feeding vessel to an endoleak, similar to the waveform noted in the neck of a pseudoaneurysm

▶ Contrast-enhanced CT scan demonstrating contrast enhancement within the AAA outside the endograft consistent with contrast-enhanced flowing blood in a type II endoleak (arrow in Fig. 160.9)

Differential Diagnosis

▶ Motion artifact
▶ Type I endoleak
▶ Type III endoleak
▶ Type IV endoleak

Teaching Points

▶ Risk of rupture of an AAA related to size and growth rate
   ▪ Intervention recommended for AAAs 5 to 5.5 cm in maximal diameter or growth rate > 0.5 cm per 6 months
   ▪ Some intervene at 4.5–5 cm in females

- ▶ Short-term mortality and morbidity are lower for elective EVAR than for open repair
  - ▪ 3–5% mortality rate for open repair
  - ▪ < 2% mortality rate for EVAR
- ▶ Long-term mortality rates similar for EVAR and open repair
- ▶ Hence, EVAR is now the preferred method for elective treatment of AAAs, if anatomy is favorable
- ▶ However, more interventions required for patients s/p EVAR due to procedural complications
  - ▪ Endoleaks
    - • Most common complication, occurring in > 10% of patients
    - • Usually within the first 3 years
    - • Pose risk of AAA rupture, especially if large or AAA continues to increase in diameter
  - ▪ Graft migration
  - ▪ Structural failure
  - ▪ Continued growth of aneurysm
  - ▪ Thrombosis of graft
- ▶ Five types of endoleaks
  - ▪ Type I: incomplete seal between edge of endograft and aortic wall, top of graft (Ia) or bottom (Ib)
    - • Significant risk of rupture
    - • Revision recommended
  - ▪ Type II: retrograde flow into aneurysm sac through branch of the aorta
    - • Most common; most occur within first 30 days
    - • Relatively slow, low-pressure flow
    - • Approximately 50% spontaneously thrombose
    - • May be watched if small and no increase in AAA diameter
  - ▪ Type III: structural failure—break in graft, tear in fabric, separation of modules
    - • Less common with newer endografts
    - • Abdominal X-ray helpful for diagnosis
    - • Significant risk of rupture
    - • Revision required
  - ▪ Type IV: blood enters aneurysm sac due to graft porosity
    - • Occurs during the procedure
    - • Common, transient
    - • No treatment necessary because self-limited
  - ▪ Type V: AAA continues to enlarge post EVAR; however, no endoleak visualized on any imaging modality
    - • Uncommon
    - • Generally requires open repair
- ▶ US findings, type II endoleak
  - ▪ Color flow in AAA sac separate from graft lumen, usually in middle of AAA
    - • Anterior leak, usually from IMA or accessory renal artery
    - • Posterior leak, usually from lumbar artery
    - • Sometimes complex with more than one feeding vessel
  - ▪ Spectral tracing useful to differentiate true flow from color artifact
    - • Retrograde flow through branch vessel or "to and fro" flow pattern
  - ▪ Important to measure maximal diameter of AAA to ensure no interval growth
  - ▪ Blood flow into sac should not be traceable to the aortic lumen above or below the graft (type I endoleak) or to a break in the graft (type III endoleak)
- ▶ Motion artifact: less distinct area of color outside the endograft within the AAA, more speckled, less focal
- ▶ Mirror image artifact: focal color in the AAA similar in appearance to flow within the graft lumen, but posterior to the echogenic wall of the graft, and not lateral
- ▶ Type I endoleak
  - ▪ Risk factors
    - • Short neck (< 15 mm)
    - • Wide neck (> 32 mm)
    - • Calcification of thrombus at landing zone
    - • Angulation > 60°
    - • Dilated common iliac arteries
  - ▪ Color flow from the aortic lumen enters the AAA sac between the edge of the graft and the aortic wall

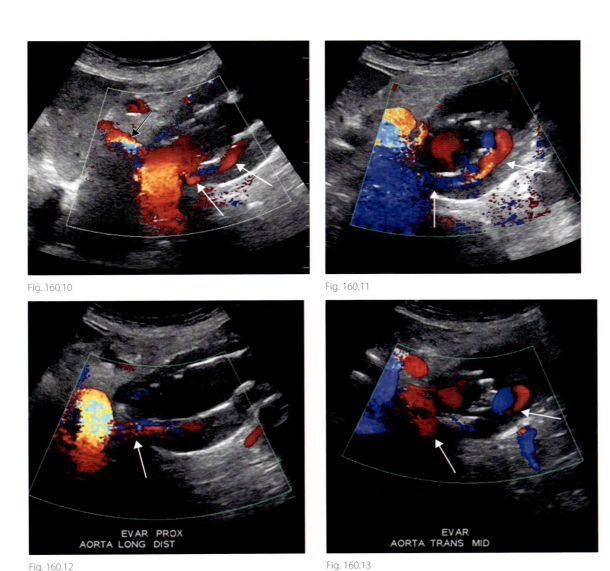

Fig. 160.10

Fig. 160.11

EVAR PROX
AORTA LONG DIST

Fig. 160.12

EVAR
AORTA TRANS MID

Fig. 160.13

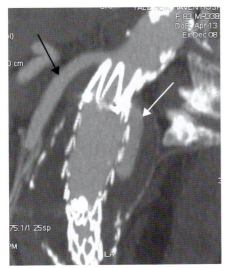

Fig. 160.14

66-Year-old male 6 months following EVAR with a fenestrated chimney graft extension and right renal artery stent. Color Doppler images demonstrate color flow between the top edge of the graft and the wall of the aorta (white arrows in Figs. 160.10–160.13) entering the aneurysm beyond the confines of the endograft consistent with a type Ia endoleak. Superior mesenteric artery (black arrows in Figs. 160.10 and 160.14).

Contrast-enhanced sagittal CT scan confirms endoleak (white arrow in Fig. 160.14) between the top edge of the covered portion of the graft and the aortic wall.

► Type III endoleak
- Color flow enters the AAA sac from a break in the wall of the endograft
- Usually in mid graft, may be difficult to differentiate from a type II endoleak
- Consider if color flow within aneurysm is immediately adjacent to wall of endograft or if the echogenic struts appear deformed or focally separated near leak

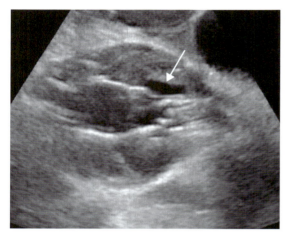

Fig. 160.15

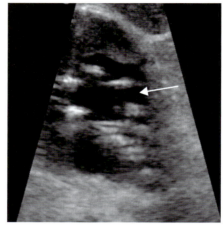

Fig. 160.16

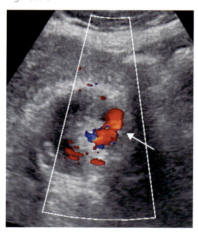

Fig. 160.17

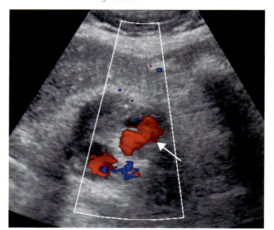

Fig. 160.18

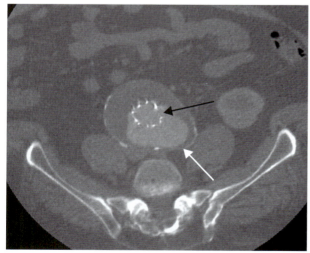

Fig. 160.19

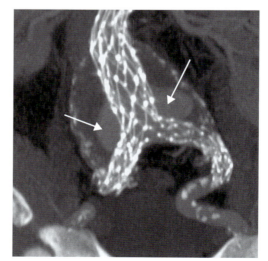

Fig. 160.20

52-Year-old male 3 years following EVAR. Grayscale images demonstrate anechoic area adjacent to the endograft (arrow in Fig. 160.15) and widening between the echogenic struts (arrow in Fig. 160.16). On color Doppler imaging, blood flow appears to exit directly from the graft into the aneurysm (arrows in Figs. 160.17 and 160.18), consistent with a type III endoleak at the bifurcation of the graft. Axial (Fig. 160.19) and coronal (Fig. 160.20) contrast-enhanced CT scans demonstrate an area of enhancement (white arrows in Figs. 160.19 and 160.20) immediately adjacent to the graft, consistent with a type III endoleak. Note break or widening between the struts (black arrow in Fig. 160.19).

► Type IV endoleak
  ▪ Only observed during placement, resolves spontaneously

Management

► Lifetime surveillance required following EVAR
  ▪ Protocols vary
  ▪ Contrast-enhanced (CE) CT or CEUS more sensitive than color Doppler US for endoleaks
  ▪ However, duplex Doppler US will detect most clinically significant endoleaks or increase in AAA diameter
  ▪ Due to risks of radiation exposure and intravenous contrast from serial CE CTs, most centers now rely on Doppler US for screening if initial CE CT is normal
  ▪ Measuring the maximal diameter of the AAA is extremely important
    • Any increase in diameter, especially > 5 mm, requires careful search for an endoleak that may require treatment
► Type II endoleaks
  ▪ Many spontaneously resolve
  ▪ If small, may be followed without intervention provided there is no increase in size of the aneurysm
  ▪ If large or AAA growing > 0.5 cm, intervention with embolization of inflow/outflow vessel(s)

Further Reading

1. Schmieder GC, Stout CL, Stokes GK, et al. Endoleak after endovascular aneurysm repair: Duplex ultrasound imaging is better than computed tomography at determining the need for intervention. *J Vasc Surg.* 2009; 50(5): 1012–1017.
2. Sato DT, Goff CD, Gregory RT, et al. Endoleak after aortic stent graft repair: Diagnosis by color duplex ultrasound scan versus computed tomography scan. *J Vasc Surg.* 1998; 28: 657–663.
3. Qadura M, Pervaiz P, Harlock JA, et al. Mortality and reintervention following elective abdominal aortic aneurysm repair. *J Vasc Surg.* 2013; 57: 1676–1683.
4. Schlosser FJV, Gusberg RJ, Dardik A, et al. Aneurysm rupture after EVAR: Can the ultimate failure be predicted? *Eur J Vasc Endovasc Surg.* 2009; 37: 15–22.

Case 161

History

► 43-Year-old male presents with flank and back pain (Figs. 161.1–161.6)

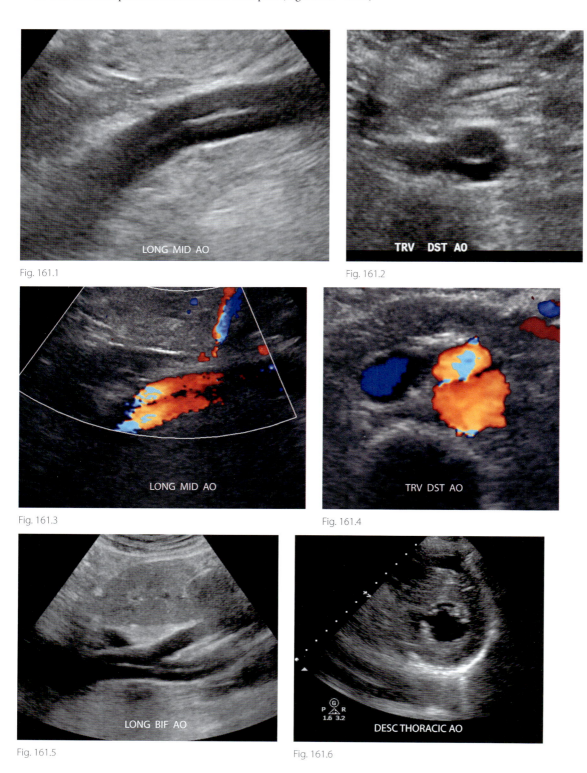

Fig. 161.1

Fig. 161.2

Fig. 161.3

Fig. 161.4

Fig. 161.5

Fig. 161.6

Case 161 Aortic Dissection Involving the Descending Thoracic Aorta, Abdominal Aorta, and Left Common Iliac Artery

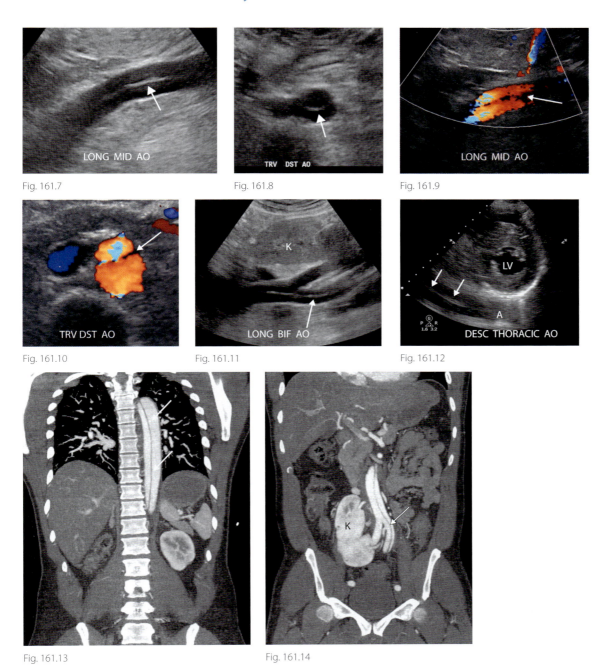

Fig. 161.7

Fig. 161.8

Fig. 161.9

Fig. 161.10

Fig. 161.11

Fig. 161.12

Fig. 161.13

Fig. 161.14

Imaging Findings

- ▶ Sagittal (Fig. 161.7) and transverse (Fig. 161.8) grayscale images of the abdominal aorta demonstrate a thin, echogenic dissection flap (arrows)
- ▶ Both true and false lumens are patent on color Doppler sagittal (Fig. 161.9) and transverse (Fig.161.10) images; dissection flap (arrows)
- ▶ The dissection flap (arrow in Fig. 161.11) extends into the left common iliac artery; right pelvic kidney (K)
- ▶ Cardiac echo (Fig. 161.12) demonstrates a thin, echogenic dissection flap (arrows) in the descending aorta (A); left ventricle (LV)
- ▶ Coronal reconstructed CT angiogram confirms dissection flap in the descending thoracic aorta (arrows in Fig. 161.13) extending into the abdominal aorta and left common iliac artery (arrow in Fig. 161.14). This was a type A aortic dissection reaching the level of the aortic valve (not shown). Right pelvic kidney (K)

Differential Diagnosis

► Reverberation artifact
► Calcified mural thrombus
► Arterial catheter

Teaching Points

► Dissection of the abdominal aorta usually occurs as an extension of a thoracic aortic dissection
  ■ Rarely isolated to abdominal aorta
  ■ Thrombosis of the false lumen can obstruct the distal aorta or branch vessels
  ■ Most common in men older than age 60 years
► Risk factors
  ■ Abdominal aortic aneurysm
  ■ Hypertension
  ■ Connective tissue disorders
  ■ Trauma
► Pathophysiology
  ■ Blood enters aortic wall through an intimal tear lifting intima ± media off adventitia
  ■ Whether or not a mural thrombus versus a patent false lumen develops depends on whether or not there is a re-entry point
► Presentation
  ■ Back, flank, or chest pain
  ■ Symptoms related to branch vessel compromise, such as mesenteric ischemia, hypertension, cold extremities, or claudication
► US findings
  ■ Echogenic intimal flap separating true and false lumens; may be difficult to see unless perpendicular to US beam
  ■ False lumen: larger and anterior to true lumen, but variable; may thrombose
  ■ Color Doppler: variable flow dynamics in the two lumens
  ■ Spectral Doppler: elevated peak systolic velocity in true lumen if compressed by false lumen, disorganized flow pattern in false lumen, more normal waveform in true lumen
  ■ Variable involvement of aortic branches
► Reverberation artifact
  ■ Echogenic line(s) parallel to anterior aortic wall, usually multiple and in near field, would not separate two lumens
► Mural thrombus
  ■ Calcified surface could appear linear and echogenic mimicking a dissection with thrombosed false lumen
  ■ Would not see blood flow on both sides
► Arterial catheter
  ■ Parallel echogenic lines separated by anechoic lumen, usually thicker
  ■ History of placement
  ■ Would not extend into branch vessels or create two lumens with differential flow patterns

Management

► Best evaluated with CT angiography
► Type A dissections (involving the aortic arch) require intervention
  ■ Risk of developing severe aortic regurgitation and/or pericardial tamponade
► Type B dissections usually managed conservatively unless associated with end organ ischemia or an abdominal aortic aneurysm ≥ 5 cm
  ■ Stenting of the true lumen or major branch vessels may be used to improve flow

Further Reading

1. Trimarchi S, Tsai T, Eagle KA, et al. Acute abdominal aortic dissection: Insight from the International Registry of Acute Abdominal Aortic Dissection (IRAD). *J Vasc Surg.* 2007; 46: 913–919.
2. Clevert DA, Rupp N, Reiser M, et al. Improved diagnosis of vascular dissection by ultrasound B-flow: A comparison with color-coded Doppler and power Doppler sonography. *Eur Radiol.* 2005; 15: 342–347.

History

▶ 87-Year-old male with acute-onset severe right leg pain (Figs. 162.1–162.4)

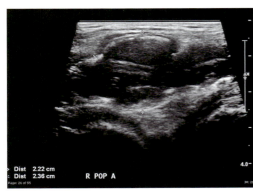

Fig. 162.1

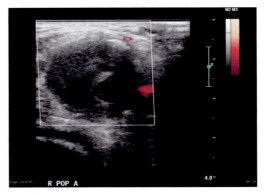

Fig. 162.2

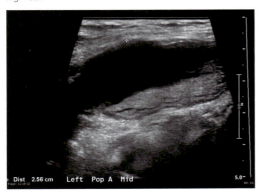

Fig. 162.3

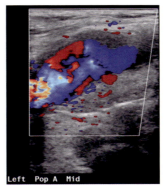

Fig. 162.4

Case 162 Thrombosed Right Popliteal Artery Aneurysm and Patent Left Popliteal Artery Aneurysm

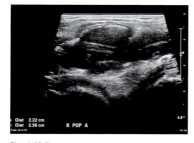

Fig. 162.5

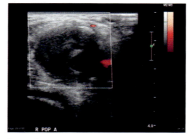

Fig. 162.6

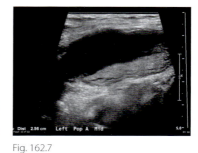

Fig. 162.7

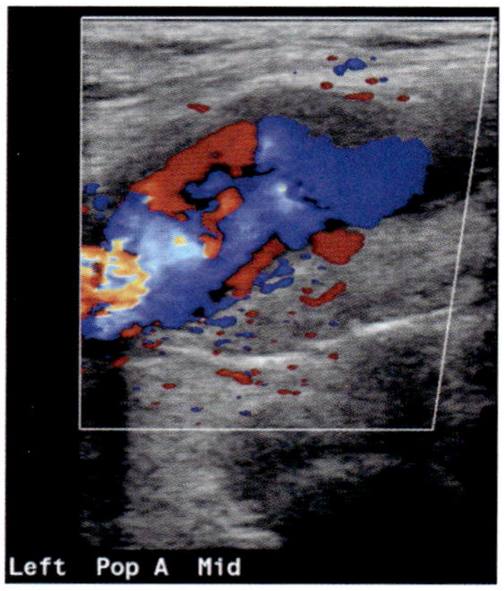

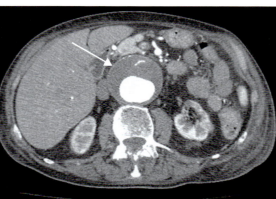

Fig. 162.8

Fig. 162.9

Imaging Findings

▶ Aneurysmal dilatation of the right popliteal artery (PA) (calipers in Fig. 162.5) measuring 2.2 cm in anteroposterior (AP) diameter with a heavily calcified arterial wall and hypoechoic mural thrombus

▶ The central lumen appears anechoic, but there is no flow on power Doppler (Fig. 162.6), consistent with acute complete thrombosis

▶ There is a patent left popliteal artery aneurysm (PAA) (Figs. 162.7 and 162.8) measuring 2.6 cm in AP dimension (calipers in Fig. 162.7) with echogenic mural thrombus

▶ Arterial phase contrast-enhanced CT scan demonstrates a large abdominal aortic aneurysm (AAA) (arrow in Fig. 162.9) with eccentric non-enhancing mural thrombus anteriorly

Differential Diagnosis

▶ Pseudoaneurysm
▶ Baker cyst
▶ Arterial dissection with thrombosed false lumen

Teaching Points

▶ The PA is the most common site of peripheral artery aneurysms and is considered aneurysmal if > 0.7 cm in AP diameter
  ▪ PAAs more common in older males
  ▪ 50–70% will have a contralateral PAA
  ▪ Associated with arterial aneurysms elsewhere
  ▪ All three layers of the vessel wall are involved in PAAs
▶ Causes of PAAs
  ▪ Atherosclerosis most common
  ▪ Connective tissue disease, especially Ehler–Danlos and Marfan syndromes
  ▪ Cystic adventitial disease: mucus-containing cysts within the wall of the PA
    • Can compress the lumen
    • Cysts usually identifiable on US as round anechoic spaces in vessel wall

- ▶ Clinical presentation
  - ▪ Asymptomatic
  - ▪ Palpable mass
  - ▪ Distal ischemia secondary to embolization or occlusion
  - ▪ Pain secondary to compression of adjacent nerve
  - ▪ Rupture is rare
- ▶ US findings
  - ▪ Fusiform or saccular dilatation of PA > 0.7 cm or 1.5 times the diameter of the proximal vessel segment
  - ▪ Evidence of atherosclerosis: calcified vessel wall, plaque, mural-based thrombus
  - ▪ Vessel lumen often narrowed or irregular secondary to intraluminal thrombus
- ▶ 30–40% of patients with PAAs will have an AAA
  - ▪ With bilateral PAAs, the incidence of AAA may be as high as 68%
- ▶ PA pseudoaneurysm
  - ▪ Contained by only one or two layers of the vessel wall or compacted surrounding connective tissue
  - ▪ History of high-impact injury, penetrating trauma, infection/sepsis
  - ▪ Rarely bilateral
  - ▪ More likely eccentric or saccular rather than fusiform
  - ▪ No association with AAA
- ▶ Baker cyst
  - ▪ Could mimic a PAA on physical exam, presenting as a palpable mass in the popliteal fossa
  - ▪ Often asymptomatic, but may present with calf pain secondary to rupture or inflammation/infection
  - ▪ Located superficial to the popliteal vessels between the gastrocnemius and semimembranosus tendons
  - ▪ Not vascular
- ▶ Arterial dissection
  - ▪ History of connective tissue disorder or trauma
  - ▪ Calcified echogenic intima displaced centrally separating true and false lumens rather than peripheral rim calcification of aneurysm
  - ▪ True and false lumen may both be patent; however, thrombosis of the false lumen may mimic mural-based thrombus in a PAA
  - ▪ Uncommon to be isolated to popliteal arteries or bilateral

Management

- ▶ US considered the modality of choice for diagnosis and follow-up of PAAs
- ▶ Check for associated AAA, especially if bilateral PAAs
  - ▪ Iliac artery aneurysms may also be found
- ▶ Thrombolytic therapy or bypass graft for acute occlusions
- ▶ Arterial bypass grafts for symptomatic patients (distal emboli) and if > 2 cm in diameter in asymptomatic patients

Further Reading

1. Wright LB, Matchett WJ, Cruz CP, et al. Popliteal artery disease: Diagnosis and treatment. *RadioGraphics*. 2004; 24: 467–479.

Case 163

History

► 62-Year-old male with nonhealing left foot ulcer (Fig. 163.1)

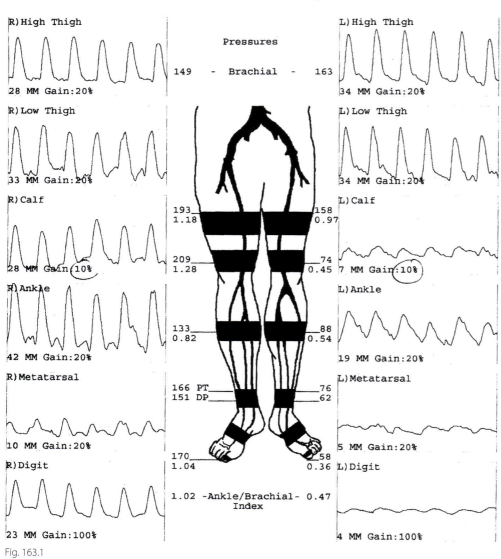

Fig. 163.1

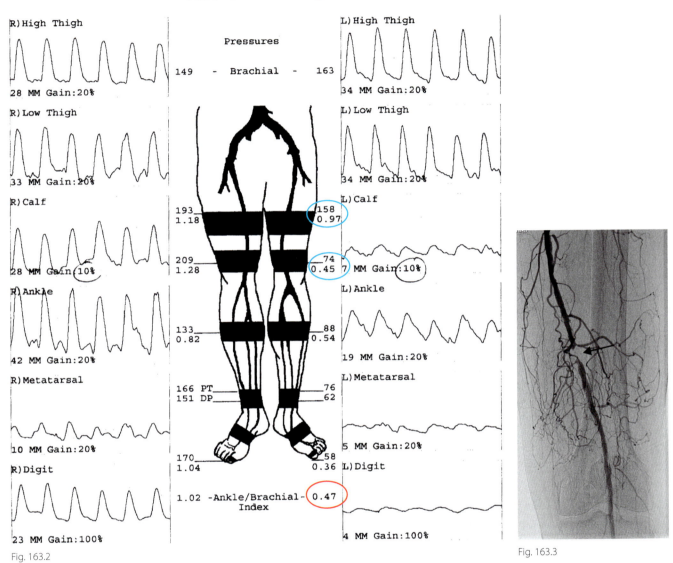

Fig. 163.2

Fig. 163.3

Imaging Findings

▶ 84 mm Hg pressure gradient between the upper (158 mm Hg) and lower thigh (74 mm Hg) (blue circles in Fig. 163.2) on the left without further significant decrease in pressure distally in the left calf or ankle

▶ The left ankle brachial index (ABI) is 0.47 (red circle in Fig. 163.2), consistent with moderate arterial insufficiency

▶ Pulse volume recordings (PVRs) demonstrate marked flattening of the waveform with loss of the dicrotic notch, delay in time to peak, and decreased amplitude in the left calf and below (Fig. 163.2) compared to the left lower thigh and right calf PVR waveforms

▶ Segmental pressures and PVR waveforms are normal on the right (Fig. 163.2)

▶ Digital subtraction angiogram demonstrating focal occlusion of the distal left superficial femoral artery (SFA) (arrow in Fig. 163.3) with distal reconstitution via collaterals. Note that even though there is complete occlusion of the SFA, there is only moderate arterial insufficiency due to the presence of abundant collateral supply

Differential Diagnosis

► High-grade stenosis versus occlusion of the distal left SFA

Teaching Points

► The ABI and PVR study is a noninvasive physiologic test that can be used to confirm diagnosis of peripheral arterial disease (PAD) in symptomatic individuals, provide prognostic data, and monitor treatment efficacy
► ABI: compares blood pressure (BP) in the brachial arteries with BP in the dorsalis pedis (DP) and posterior tibial (PT) arteries (cuff inflated at the ankle)
  ▪ The ABI is reported as the higher of the DP and PT pressures on a given side divided by the higher of the right and left brachial artery pressures
  ▪ ABI ≥ 0.90 is normal: virtually excludes arterial insufficiency
    • Musculoskeletal or neurologic conditions should therefore be considered a cause of lower extremity pain
  ▪ ABI < 0.90 but ≥ 0.60 indicates mild PAD; ABI < 0.60 and ≥ 0.40 indicates moderate PAD; ABI < 0.40 indicates severe PAD, possible critical limb ischemia
  ▪ Some authors believe that ABIs are not sufficiently accurate in differentiating between mild and moderate arterial insufficiency and favor describing an ABI < 0.90 but ≥ 0.40 as mild to moderate arterial insufficiency
  ▪ ABI ≥ 1.30 is indeterminate: indicates noncompressible vessels secondary to vessel wall calcification
    • Most commonly found in patients with diabetes or chronic renal disease
► Post exercise ABI: indicated in symptomatic patients with a normal resting ABI
  ▪ A decrease in the ABI of 0.15–0.20 following exercise is abnormal
► Serial ABI measurements: a decrease > 0.15 in isolation or > 0.10 associated with change in clinical status considered significant
► Toe brachial index (TBI): compares pressure in brachial artery to pressure in great toe
  ▪ Useful in diabetic patients because medial calcinosis rarely affects the digital arteries
  ▪ TBI < 0.70 is abnormal
► Segmental pressures and PVRs helpful in determining the level of arterial stenosis or occlusion
  ▪ Segmental pressures obtained using appropriately sized cuffs
  ▪ Four-cuff method (performed in this case): upper and lower thigh, upper calf, and ankle
  ▪ Three-cuff method: one measurement at the thigh level, upper calf, and ankle
  ▪ A pressure gradient > 20 mm Hg between different levels in the same limb or between the right and the left limb at the same level considered significant
► PVRs measure change in limb blood flow volume related to the temporal profile of the arterial pulse
  ▪ Normal PVR tracing: sharp systolic upstroke and dicrotic notch
  ▪ With increasing degree of stenosis, PVR waveforms distal to the stenosis become progressively abnormal: Initially there is loss of the dicrotic notch. With increasing stenosis, there is convex bowing of the downslope away from the baseline, the waveforms become progressively flatter, decrease in amplitude, and demonstrate a rounded peak and increased time to peak
► Limitations: unable to differentiate between occlusion and high-grade stenosis, short- versus long-segment disease, single versus multiple sites

Management

► Percutaneous intervention
  ▪ Short-segment stenosis: balloon angioplasty and/or stent placement
  ▪ Occlusion: primary stent placement
► Surgical intervention
  ▪ Arterial bypass grafts: more durable, require adequate outflow vessel

Further Reading

1. Wennberg PW. Approach to the patient with peripheral arterial disease. *Circulation*. 2013; 128(20): 2241–2250.
2. Rose SC. Noninvasive vascular laboratory for evaluation of peripheral arterial occlusive disease: Part II—Clinical applications: Chronic, usually atherosclerotic, lower extremity ischemia. *J Vasc Interv Radiol*. 2000; 11(10): 1257–1275.
3. McCann TE, Scoutt LM, Gunabushanam G. A practical approach to interpreting lower extremity noninvasive physiologic studies. *Radiol Clin North Am*. 2014; 52(6): 1343–1357.

History

▶ 77-Year-old male with right calf pain after walking two blocks, relieved by rest (Figs. 164.1–164.6)

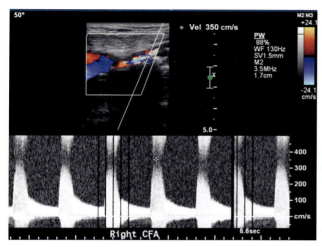

Fig. 164.1

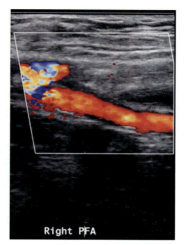

Fig. 164.2

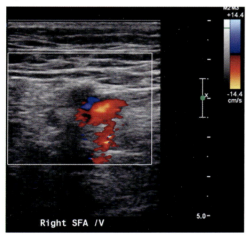

Fig. 164.3

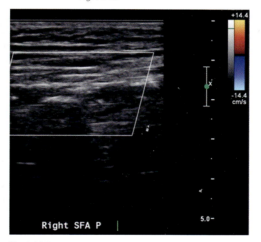

Fig. 164.4

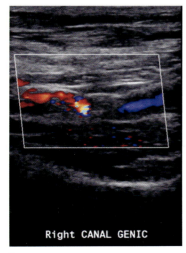

Fig. 164.5

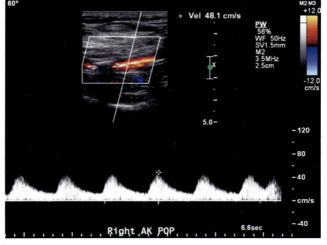

Fig. 164.6

Case 164 Right Common Femoral Artery Stenosis and Occlusion of Right Superficial Femoral Artery With Distal Reconstitution From Geniculate Collaterals

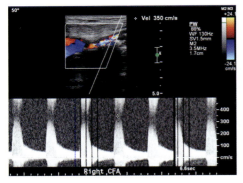

Fig. 164.7

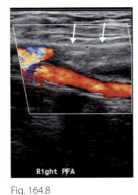

Fig. 164.8

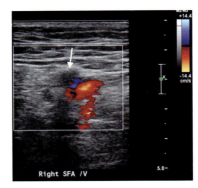

Fig. 164.9

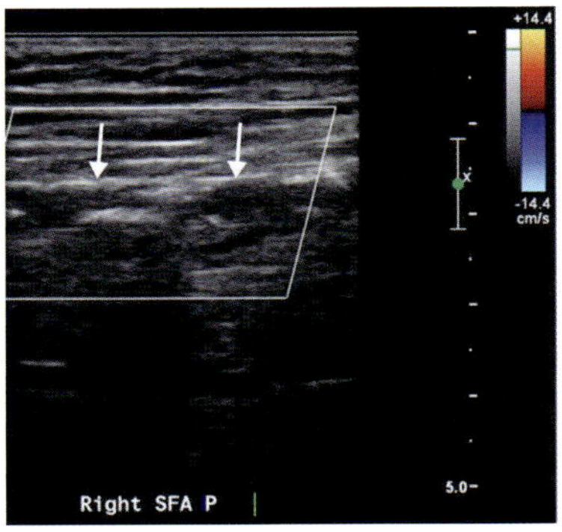

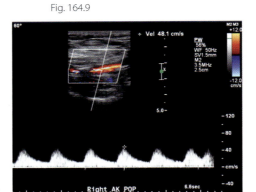

Fig. 164.10

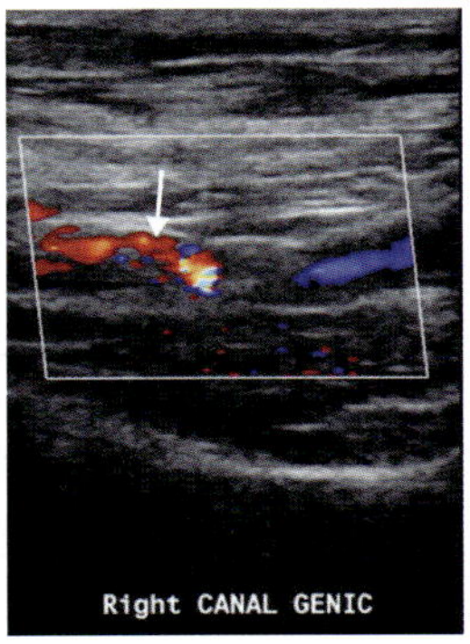

Fig. 164.11

Fig. 164.12

Image Findings

▶ Note aliasing, turbulence, fill in of spectral window, and increased peak systolic velocity (PSV) (350 cm/s), as well as narrowing of the lumen of the right common femoral artery (CFA) on duplex Doppler image (Fig. 164.7), consistent with a high-grade stenosis

▶ Sagittal (Figs. 164.8 and 164.10) and transverse (Fig. 164.9) color Doppler images reveal no flow in the superficial femoral artery (SFA) (arrows in Figs. 164.8–164.10), which is heavily calcified and filled with hypoechoic material consistent with plaque and/or thrombus

▶ The distal SFA (blue in Fig. 164.11) reconstitutes from a geniculate collateral (arrow in Fig. 164.11) that is tortuous, unaccompanied by a paired vein, and is not parallel to the expected course of the SFA

▶ Note tardus parvus waveform (delayed systolic acceleration and decreased PSV) with increased diastolic flow in the popliteal artery (Fig. 164.12)

Differential Diagnosis

▶ High-grade superficial femoral artery stenosis

Teaching Points

▶ Peripheral arterial disease is a major cause of disability in the United States, estimated to affect more than 8 million people
  ▪ Involves the lower extremities more commonly than the upper extremities
  ▪ Usually secondary to atherosclerotic plaque
  ▪ Can result in stenosis or occlusion, and involves single or multiple segments
  ▪ Typically presents a decade after myocardial ischemia
▶ Approximately 50% of patients are symptomatic
  ▪ Claudication: pain with exercise and relieved by rest
    • May progress to resting pain

- Arterial ulcerations
- Cold extremities
- Absent pedal pulses, cyanotic (blue) extremities, blanching of foot when elevated
► Risk factors
  - More common in men than in women
  - Smoking
  - Diabetes
  - Older age (> 65 years)
  - Elevated cholesterol levels
  - Hypertension
  - Obesity
  - History of coronary artery disease or stroke
► Workup
  - Screening with ankle–brachial indices and pulse volume recordings, ± Doppler US, which also can be used for confirmation
  - Treatment planning usually requires CT angiography, MR angiography, or digital subtraction arteriography
► At rest, the lower extremity arteries normally have a triphasic, high-resistance spectral Doppler waveform pattern with a sharp systolic upstroke, brief reversal of flow in early diastole, forward low-velocity flow in mid diastole, and absence of flow in late diastole

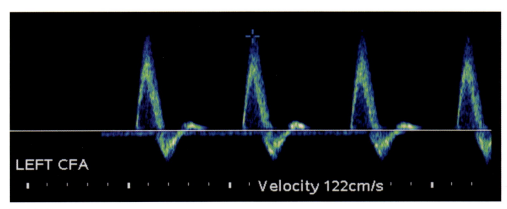

Fig. 164.13

Normal triphasic arterial spectral Doppler waveform of the left CFA in a 56-year-old male (Fig. 164.13)
► US findings of arterial occlusion
  - Echogenic plaque, vessel wall calcification, internal echoes obliterating the lumen
  - No fill in of arterial lumen on color or power Doppler
  - No spectral Doppler detectable flow in vessel lumen
  - Adjacent irregular collateral vessels without accompanying vein
  - May see monophasic high-resistance spectral Doppler waveform with sharp upstroke but decreased PSV in proximal arterial segment
  - Tardus parvus (TP) waveform in distal artery if reconstituted by collaterals
► Differentiating a stenosis from an occlusion on US
  - May not always be possible to differentiate a high-grade stenosis with minimal flow from a complete occlusion
  - Complete absence of flow on Doppler US is more suggestive of complete occlusion than a high-grade stenosis
  - However, low-velocity, low-volume flow in a nearly occlusive lesion may not be detectable by Doppler US, and heavily calcified shadowing atherosclerotic plaque may also limit Doppler detection of blood flow in a patent vessel
  - TP waveforms not expected distal to a mild stenosis and are indicative of a moderate to high-grade proximal stenosis or occlusion

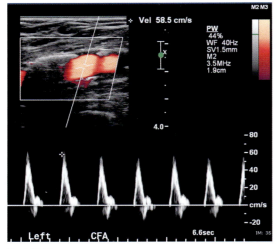

Fig. 164.14

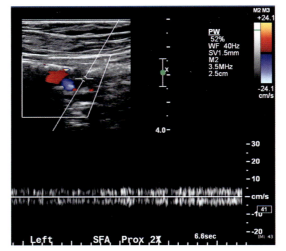

Fig. 164.15

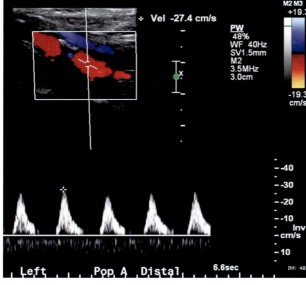

Fig. 164.16

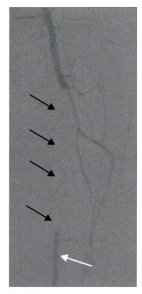

Fig. 164.17

59-Year-old male with left calf claudication. Spectral Doppler waveform (Fig. 164.14) in the left CFA has a normal triphasic pattern. Power Doppler demonstrates complete fill in of the lumen without evidence of stenosis. Spectral Doppler waveform obtained from the proximal left SFA (Fig. 164.15) shows no detectable flow. Symmetric artifact above and below the baseline mimicking a flat Doppler waveform is secondary to system noise and not true flow. The vessel wall is calcified, consistent with atherosclerosis. The popliteal artery waveform (Fig. 164.16) has a TP appearance with decreased PSV (27 cm/s compared to 59 cm/s in the CFA) and increased time to peak (delayed systolic acceleration). Carbon dioxide angiogram performed in this patient due to renal insufficiency shows a long-segment occlusion of the proximal left SFA (black arrows in Fig. 164.17) with reconstitution of the mid SFA (white arrow in Fig. 164.17) from a collateral artery arising from the profunda femoris artery.

► Maximizing Doppler detection of blood flow
  ▪ Power and spectral Doppler more sensitive than color Doppler
  ▪ Straight as opposed to angled color box
  ▪ Decrease scale or pulse repetition frequency
  ▪ Increase Doppler gain
  ▪ Increase color/write priority
  ▪ Decrease wall filter
► The TP spectral Doppler waveform is the sonographic analogue of the "pulsus tardus et parvus" sign on physical examination in patients with severe aortic stenosis, and it is characterized by delayed (tardus) and diminished (parvus) systolic upstroke and rounding of the systolic peak

- TP waveforms are typically observed distal to a moderate to high-grade stenosis or complete arterial occlusion with reconstitution of flow from collaterals
- The likelihood of a distal TP waveform increases with increasing grade of the proximal stenosis
► In in vitro experiments, TP waveforms were not observed in rigid, noncompliant distal vessel phantoms even with severe stenosis, resulting in a hypothesis that the TP waveform is related to a combination of stenosis severity, trans-stenotic pressure gradient, and post-stenotic vessel wall compliance
► The TP waveform is a useful indirect sign of a proximal stenosis in an arterial segment that may be difficult to directly image
  For example
  - Unilateral TP waveforms throughout the lower extremity from the level of the CFA to the arteries in the calf suggest the presence of a more proximal common or external iliac artery stenosis
  - Bilateral TP waveforms throughout the lower extremities suggest either bilateral common or external iliac artery stenoses or stenosis of the aorta (including aortic coarctation) or the aortic valve
  - TP waveforms distal to an arterial segment that cannot be directly imaged due to technical reasons (e.g., deep to heavily calcified arterial plaque or overlying bandages) suggest the presence of significant stenosis or occlusion
► Pitfalls in interpretation of TP waveforms include the following
  - TP waveforms indicate a proximal stenosis but are not specific for a given location
  - If the vessel wall is stiff due to calcification or atherosclerosis, development of the TP waveform may be blunted
    • Hence, a TP waveform is more likely to be seen distal to a stenosis in a younger patient without diabetes or long-standing hypertension
  - The TP appearance becomes more pronounced the farther from the stenosis that the vessel is sampled
  - Identification of TP waveforms is subjective, with considerable inter- and intraobserver variability
  - Acceleration time, the interval from end diastole to early systolic peak, and acceleration index, the slope of the same interval, provide a more objective method of evaluation
  - However, discriminatory cutoffs vary according to arterial segment

Management

► Observation, if collaterals are adequate and the patient is asymptomatic
► Angioplasty with stenting or arterial bypass graft, if the patient is symptomatic

Further Reading

1. Rooke TW, Hirsch AT, Misra S, et al. 2011 ACCF/AHA focused update of the guideline for the management of patients with peripheral artery disease (updating the 2005 guideline): A report of the American College of Cardiology Foundation/American Heart Association task force on practice guidelines. *Circulation.* 2011; 124: 2020–2045.
2. Norgren L, Hiatt WR, Dormandy JA, et al. Inter-society consensus for the management of peripheral arterial disease (TASC II). *J Vasc Surg.* 2007; 45(Suppl S): S5–S67.
3. Wennberg PW. Approach to the patient with peripheral arterial disease. *Circulation.* 2013; 128(20): 2241–2250.
4. Rose SC. Noninvasive vascular laboratory for evaluation of peripheral arterial occlusive disease: Part II—Clinical applications: Chronic, usually atherosclerotic, lower extremity ischemia. *J Vasc Interv Radiol.* 2000; 11(10): 1257–1275.

Case 165

History

▶ 67-Year-old male with right leg claudication (Figs. 165.1–165.4)

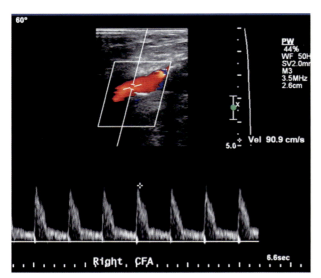

Fig. 165.1

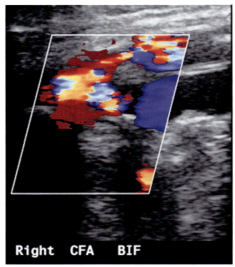

Fig. 165.2

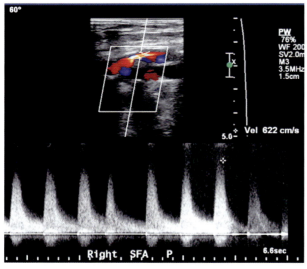

Fig. 165.3

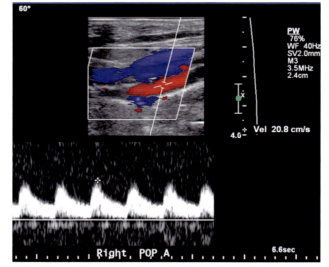

Fig. 165.4

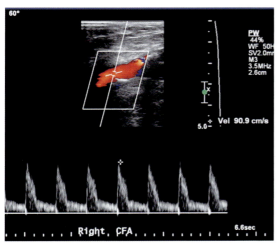

Fig. 165.5

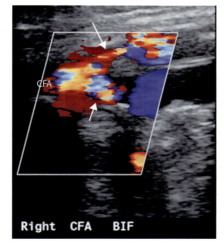

Fig. 165.6

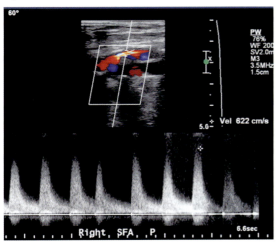

Fig. 165.7

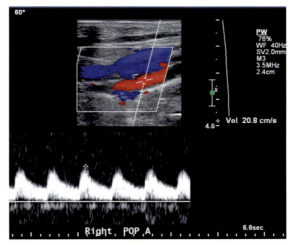

Fig. 165.8

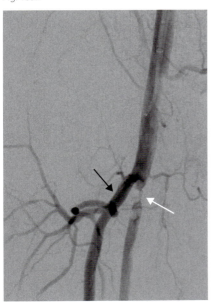

Fig. 165.9

Imaging Findings

▶ The right common femoral artery (CFA) is patent and normal in caliber with a sharp systolic upstroke, no evidence of turbulence (thin spectral envelop and no flow below the baseline), and normal peak systolic velocity (PSV) of 91 cm/s (Fig. 165.5). However, the presence of continuous forward diastolic flow, a low-resistance waveform pattern, is suggestive of distal disease and ischemia

▶ Color aliasing is present in the distal CFA, at the origin of the profunda femoris artery (PFA) (short arrow in Fig. 165.6), as well as at the origin of the superficial femoral artery (SFA), which is markedly narrowed (long arrow in Fig. 165.6)

▶ Markedly elevated PSV of 622 cm/s in the narrowed proximal SFA (Fig. 165.7), with spectral broadening and turbulent flow below the baseline consistent with a high-grade stenosis, > 70%. PSV ratio > 6:1

▶ Tardus parvus (TP) waveform in the popliteal artery (Fig. 165.8): low PSV, delayed systolic upstroke, and increased diastolic flow

▶ Angiogram demonstrating a severe stenosis at the origin of the SFA (white arrow in Fig. 165.9). Note prominence of the widely patent PFA (black arrow in Fig. 165.9), consistent with compensatory flow

Differential Diagnosis

▶ Focal dissection
▶ Cystic medial necrosis
▶ Thromboangitis obliterans (Buerger disease)

Teaching Points

▶ Peripheral arterial disease (PAD) is caused by a combination of endothelial dysfunction and inflammation with resultant plaque formation and is an independent risk factor for coronary artery and cerebrovascular disease
▶ Risk factors
  ▪ Smoking
  ▪ Hypertension
  ▪ Hyperlipidemia
  ▪ Obesity
  ▪ Diabetes mellitus
▶ Presentation
  ▪ 50% of patients are asymptomatic
  ▪ Intermittent claudication (muscle cramping with exercise that is relieved by rest)
  ▪ Increasing in severity to resting limb pain, ulceration, and gangrene
    • Pain worse at night or when extremity is elevated
  ▪ Paresthesia
  ▪ Decreased pedal pulses
  ▪ Blanching of skin with elevation of extremity, dependent rubor
▶ Spectral Doppler waveforms from normal lower extremity arteries at rest are triphasic with a sharp systolic upstroke, reversed flow in early diastole, and forward flow in mid to late diastole with no end diastolic flow
▶ Duplex Doppler US findings of lower extremity arterial stenosis
  ▪ Echogenic plaque, ± shadowing, ± heterogeneous
  ▪ Narrowing of the vessel lumen on grayscale and/or color and power Doppler
  ▪ Focal color aliasing
  ▪ Increased PSV at site of stenosis
    • 200–350 cm/s indicates moderate stenosis; > 350 cm/s indicates severe stenosis
    • Spectral broadening (loss of clear area under spectral tracing, also called fill in of spectral window)
    • Turbulence (flow below the baseline)
    • Loss of triphasic waveform
  ▪ PSV ratio (PSV at stenosis/PSV of proximal arterial segment)
    • > 2:1 consistent with a > 50% stenosis
    • > 4:1 consistent with > 75% stenosis
    • > 7:1 consistent with a > 90% stenosis
    • However, some authors prefer to simply state that a PSV ratio > 2:1 indicates a 50–99% stenosis without further differentiation of the degree of stenosis because intervention is based on symptoms
  ▪ Distal tardus parvus waveform usually signifies severe proximal stenosis or occlusion
▶ More precise determination of degree of stenosis is important following arterial bypass graft or stent placement because revision, reintervention, or close interval follow-up are generally warranted at > 70% stenosis
▶ Arterial dissection and cystic medial necrosis could both cause focal narrowing of the SFA with increased PSV but are not associated with echogenic shadowing plaque

- ► Cystic medial necrosis
  - Typically involves larger arteries (aorta and major branches)
  - Associated with Marfan and Ehlers–Danlos syndromes
  - May result in aneurysms and dissections
- ► Buerger disease
  - Recurrent acute and chronic inflammation resulting in severe stenosis or thrombosis of the small to medium-sized arteries and veins without significant atherosclerosis
  - Strongly associated with smoking, men younger than age 40 years

Management

- ► The ankle–brachial index with pulse volume recordings is the best screening test for PAD
- ► Duplex US or CT/MR angiography used to localize and grade stenosis
  - Conventional angiography usually done in the context of treatment
- ► Medical management versus revascularization with angioplasty, stent, or bypass graft depending on symptom severity, risk factors, and extent of disease
  - Revascularization for critical limb ischemia or lifestyle-limiting claudication
  - Decision regarding surgery versus interventional therapy depends on disease extent and quality of runoff arteries
  - In general, surgery has better long-term patency than endovascular intervention

Further Reading

1. Hiatt WR. Medical treatment of peripheral arterial disease and claudication. *N Engl J Med.* 2001; 344(21): 1608–1621.
2. Rooke TW, Hirsch AT, Misra S, et al. Management of patients with peripheral artery disease (compilation of 2005 and 2011 ACCF/AHA guideline recommendations): A report of the American College of Cardiology Foundation/American Heart Association Task Force on Practice Guidelines. *J Am Coll Cardiol.* 2013; 61(14): 1555–1570.

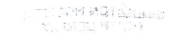

Case 166

History

► 82-Year-old asymptomatic male with left distal superficial femoral artery (SFA) to posterior tibial artery (PTA) bypass graft presents for surveillance 3 months following surgery (Figs. 166.1–166.3)

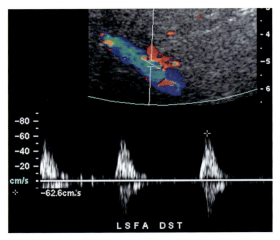

Fig. 166.1

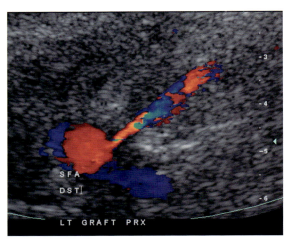

Fig. 166.2

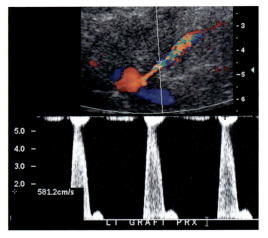

Fig. 166.3

Case 166 Stenosis of Arterial Bypass Graft

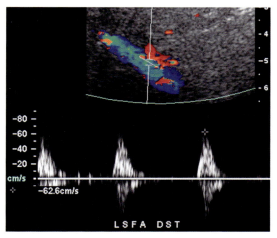

Fig. 166.4

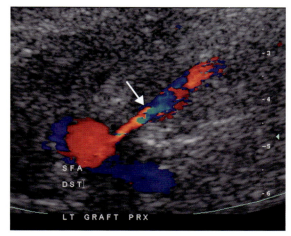

Fig. 166.5

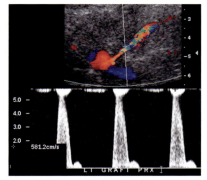

Fig. 166.6

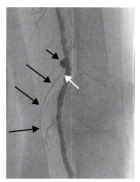

Fig. 166.7

Imaging Findings

▶ Peak systolic velocity (PSV) is 63 cm/s in the distal SFA just above the proximal anastomosis of the bypass graft (Fig. 166.4). The spectral Doppler waveform has a high-resistance monophasic pattern with no diastolic flow

▶ The distal SFA to PTA arterial bypass graft is narrowed at the proximal anastomosis. Note focal color aliasing (arrow in Fig. 166.5)

▶ PSV at the arterial anastomosis is markedly elevated at 581 cm/s, more than nine times the PSV in the native distal SFA, consistent with severe stenosis (Fig. 166.6). Note spectral broadening of the waveform, which is caused by turbulent flow

▶ Angiogram demonstrates a high-grade focal stenosis at the proximal anastomosis of the bypass graft (white arrow in Fig. 166.7). The distal graft is patent but markedly attenuated (long black arrows in Fig. 166.7). Dilated hood of graft (short black arrow in Fig. 166.7). The patient was successfully treated using balloon angioplasty (not shown)

Differential Diagnosis

▶ Mismatch of caliber of native artery and bypass graft

Teaching Points

▶ 20–30% of in situ or reversed vein arterial bypass grafts (ABGs) develop stenosis within the first year of surgery

▶ Causes of ABG failure include the following
  ▪ Immediate postoperative period: inadequate surgical technique or poor outflow arteries
  ▪ Early (first year): neointimal hyperplasia
  ▪ Late: progression of atherosclerosis

▶ The aim of surveillance is to detect and treat ABG stenosis prior to occlusion. Surveillance consists of interval history and physical examination, resting and post-exercise ankle–brachial indices (ABIs) with pulse volume recordings (PVRs), and Doppler US
  ▪ Baseline parameters are obtained in the immediate postoperative period
  ▪ Regular follow-up typically recommended every 3–6 months for at least 2 years

- Shorter interval follow-up, every 3 months, advised if a mild to moderate stenosis not yet requiring intervention is documented
► US findings of ABG stenosis
  - Narrowed graft on grayscale or color Doppler images
  - Increased PSV
    • Moderate stenosis (200–350 cm/s)
    • Severe stenosis (> 350 cm/s)
  - Increased PSV ratio (PSV at stenosis/PSV at prestenotic arterial segment)
    • Moderate stenosis (2.0–3.5)
    • Severe stenosis (> 3.5)
  - Increasing PSV on serial US examinations
  - PSV in graft < 45 cm/s, especially if PSV is globally decreased throughout the graft and associated with a focal area of increased PSV, but dependent on graft diameter because wider grafts have lower PSV
  - High-resistance monophasic waveforms throughout graft (especially if previously triphasic)
  - Tardus parvus spectral Doppler waveforms with blunted systolic upstroke, decreased PSV, and increased diastolic flow distal to the suspected area of stenosis
► Pitfalls in arterial Doppler US of ABGs
  - PSV is affected by the individual's cardiovascular status, inflow disease, outflow disease, tandem stenoses, and collateral channels
    • PSV ratios may be helpful in these cases: Estimated percentage stenosis approximately $100 \times (1 - 1/\text{PSV ratio})$
  - PSV > 200 cm/s or increased PSV ratio may be normal at the distal anastomosis due to graft to native artery size mismatch, especially in below-knee bypass grafts
  - Turbulent flow at anastomoses may be secondary to vessel tortuosity and not necessarily indicate underlying stenosis
  - High-resistance monophasic waveforms are not necessarily abnormal, especially in below-knee grafts

Management

► Treatment dependent on symptoms, ABIs/PVRs, and US findings; even if the stenosis is only moderate by US criteria, treatment may be indicated if symptoms and ABIs/PVRs are worsening
► Balloon angioplasty
► Stent placement or surgical revision may be considered in recurrent stenosis following angioplasty

Further Reading

1. Rooke TW, Hirsch AT, Misra S, et al. 2011 ACCF/AHA focused update of the guideline for the management of patients with peripheral artery disease (updating the 2005 guideline): A report of the American College of Cardiology Foundation/American Heart Association Task Force on Practice Guidelines. *Circulation.* 2011; 124: 2020–2045.
2. Norgren L, Hiatt WR, Dormandy JA, et al. Inter-society consensus for the management of peripheral arterial disease (TASC II). *J Vasc Surg.* 2007; 45(Suppl S): S5–S67.

History

▶ 62-Year-old male with groin pain following cardiac catheterization (Figs. 167.1–167.3)

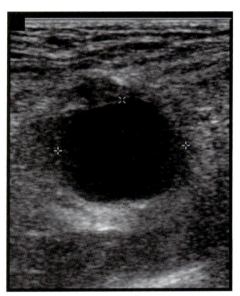

Fig. 167.1

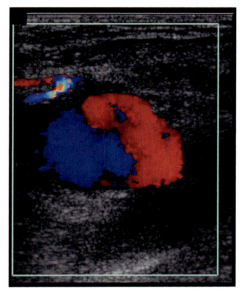

Fig. 167.2

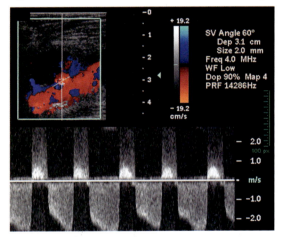

Fig. 167.3

Case 167 Pseudoaneurysm Arising From Right Common Femoral Artery

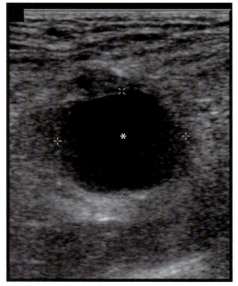

Fig. 167.4

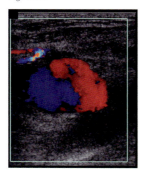

Fig. 167.5

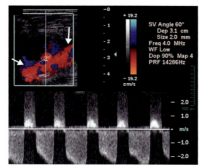

Fig. 167.6

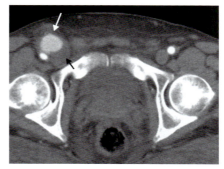

Fig. 167.7

Imaging Findings

▶ Anechoic cystic structure (asterisk and calipers in Fig. 167.4) anterior to the femoral vessels (not shown)

▶ "Yin-yang" appearance (red on one side and blue on the other) (Fig. 167.5) representative of swirling blood flow on color Doppler image; the classic color Doppler appearance of a pseudoaneurysm (PSA)

▶ "To-and-fro" blood flow on spectral Doppler waveform (Fig. 167.6) obtained in the neck of the PSA that arises from the right common femoral artery (CFA) (arrows in Fig. 167.6), with flow heading toward the PSA (above the baseline) in systole and reversal of flow (below the baseline) back toward the CFA during diastole

▶ Intravenous contrast partially fills an outpouching (white arrow in Fig. 167.7) arising from the right CFA on CT angiogram. Note crescentic area of lower attenuation within the PSA (black arrow in Fig. 167.7), consistent with partial thrombosis

Differential Diagnosis

▶ Hematoma

▶ Arteriovenous fistula (AVF)

Teaching Points

▶ PSAs post arterial catheterization result from focal disruption of the arterial wall with extravasation of blood that is contained in a sac by compressed perivascular soft tissues. Patency is maintained by persistent communication with the arterial lumen through a neck

  ▪ The neck can be long or short and either wide or narrow

- ► Risk factors post angiography
  - ▪ Anticoagulation
  - ▪ Obesity
  - ▪ Large sheath size
  - ▪ Poor technique (either at access or inadequate post intervention compression)
- ► Complications
  - ▪ Pain
  - ▪ Swelling
  - ▪ Compression of adjacent vessels or nerves due to mass effect
  - ▪ Rupture
  - ▪ Distal embolization
  - ▪ Local skin ischemia/necrosis
- ► US is the primary, and in most cases the only, modality necessary for diagnosis and treatment
- ► Important features to assess with US include the following
  - ▪ Size
  - ▪ Configuration (number of lobulations); may have tandem PSAs
  - ▪ Extent of mural thrombus
  - ▪ Length and diameter of neck
  - ▪ Status of underlying common femoral artery and vein

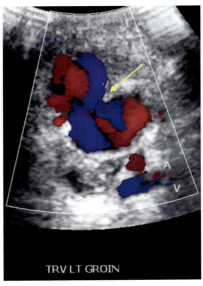

Fig. 167.8

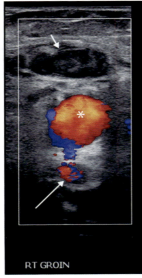

Fig. 167.9

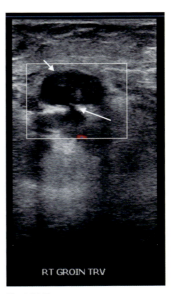

Fig. 167.10

Two different patients with bilobed PSAs post catheterization. Color Doppler image (Fig. 167.8) demonstrating a bilobed PSA above the left common femoral artery (CFA) (A in Fig. 167.8) and vein (V in Fig. 167.8). Each "lobe" has the classic "yin-yang" color flow appearance of blue/red. There is a wide neck between the two lobes of the PSA (arrow in Fig. 167.8). In a second patient, color Doppler image (Fig. 167.9) reveals a PSA (asterisk in Fig. 167.9) anterior to the right CFA (long arrow in Fig. 167.9). The neck connecting the patent component of the PSA to the CFA is linear and color coded blue. Anterior to the patent lobe of the PSA is an oval heterogeneous collection (short arrows in Figs. 167.9 and 167.10) that represents the more superficial lobe of the PSA, which is thrombosed. In Fig. 167.10, a short, narrow hypoechoic neck (long arrow) connects the thrombosed superficial lobe to the patent deep lobe. Only a small focus of color flow is seen in the patent lobe on this image due to the placement of the color box.

- ► US findings
  - ▪ Grayscale: anechoic or hypoechoic cystic structure near the artery, ± slowly swirling flow or intraluminal echoes consistent with thrombus formation
  - ▪ Color Doppler US: "yin-yang" pattern of swirling flow within the PSA sac; mural thrombus will appear as a color void
  - ▪ Spectral Doppler US of PSA neck: "to-and-fro" flow pattern—flow above the baseline heading toward the PSA sac in systole and flow below the baseline heading toward the artery in diastole

► PSAs may also occur following trauma, surgery, arterial instrumentation, and arterial dissection; in the setting of arteritis, fibromuscular dysplasia, and radiation therapy; and from erosion from malignancy or adjacent soft tissue infections. Mycotic PSAs can occur in the setting of bacteremia

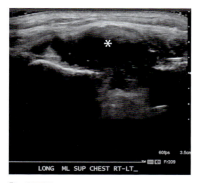

Fig. 167.11

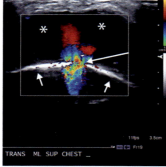

Fig. 167.12

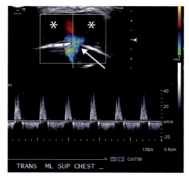

Fig. 167.13

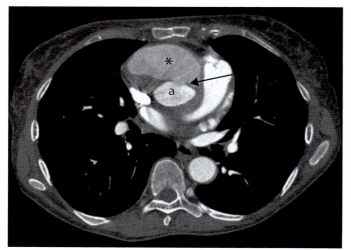

Fig. 167.14

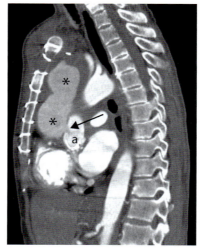

Fig. 167.15

This patient presented with chest pain following repair of an ascending aortic aneurysm. US images demonstrate an anechoic area (asterisks in Figs. 167.11–167.13) superficial to the echogenic wall of the ascending aorta (short arrows in Fig. 167.12). On color Doppler (Figs. 167.12 and 167.13), there is a jet of blood flowing from the ascending aorta into the anechoic region through a focal disruption in the echogenic aortic wall (long arrows in Figs. 167.12 and 167.13) diagnostic of a PSA. Color aliasing (yellow, orange, and turquoise color pixels in Figs. 167.12 and 167.13) indicates high-velocity flow in the neck of the PSA (long arrow in Fig. 167.12 and arrow in Fig. 167.13). Note "to-and-fro" flow above and below the baseline on the spectral Doppler tracing from the neck of the PSA (Fig. 167.13). Findings are confirmed on contrast-enhanced axial (Fig. 167.14) and sagittal (Fig. 167.15) CT scans of the chest. There is a large PSA (asterisks in Figs. 167.14 and 167.15) anterior to the ascending aorta ("a" in Figs. 167.14 and 167.15). Note that contrast density in the PSA is lower than in the aorta because it is diluted by non-contrast-enhanced blood that is slowly swirling within the PSA before re-entering the systemic circulation. Note focal disruption in the wall of the ascending aorta (arrows in Figs. 167.14 and 167.15).

► Hematoma: common following vascular access
  ▪ Heterogeneous hypoechoic perivascular mass or region
  ▪ Margins often indistinct and irregular, but may be well-defined
  ▪ No flow on Doppler US
  ▪ May not be able to differentiate between hematoma and completely thrombosed PSA
► AVF: less common following vascular access
  ▪ May appear as an anechoic, round structure with flow on color Doppler if the draining vein focally dilates
  ▪ Low-resistance spectral Doppler waveform in feeding artery and pulsatile high-velocity flow in draining vein
  ▪ No "yin-yang" color Doppler or "to-and-fro" spectral Doppler flow patterns
  ▪ Often shows perivascular soft tissue color bruit due to tissue vibration

Management

- ► PSAs < 2.5 cm in diameter without significant symptoms
  - Observation only: follow-up with weekly US for up to 1 month because the majority of these will spontaneously thrombose
  - Intraluminal thrombus within the PSA at the time of diagnosis increases the likelihood of spontaneous thrombosis
  - If coagulation factors are abnormal or if the patient is anticoagulated, spontaneous thrombosis less likely
- ► Larger PSAs and persistent or symptomatic small PSAs
  - US-guided thrombin injection of sac
  - Follow-up US in 24–48 hours recommended to confirm complete thrombosis
  - US-guided compression of PSA neck no longer preferred method of treatment due to comparatively greater patient discomfort and lower technical success rate
- ► US-guided injection of normal saline into the soft tissues surrounding the PSA neck to compress the neck and thereby cause thrombosis of the PSA is gaining in popularity
- ► Surgery or endovascular therapy with stent placement to exclude the PSA reserved for patients in whom percutaneous therapy has failed
- ► Surgery for infected PSAs and PSAs with significant mass effect (e.g., causing distal ischemia from femoral artery compression or neuropathy secondary to femoral nerve compression)

Further Reading

1. Ahmad F, Turner SA, Torrie P, et al. Iatrogenic femoral artery pseudoaneurysms—A review of current methods of diagnosis and treatment. *Clin Radiol*. 2008; 63(12): 1310–1316.
2. Morgan R, Belli AM. Current treatment methods for post catheterization pseudoaneurysms. *J Vasc Interv Radiol*. 2003; 14(6): 697–710.

Case 168

History

▶ 65-Year-old male status post cardiac catheterization with groin bruit (Figs. 168.1–168.3)

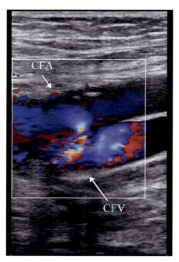

Fig. 168.1

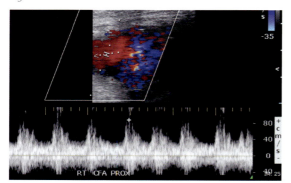

Fig. 168.2

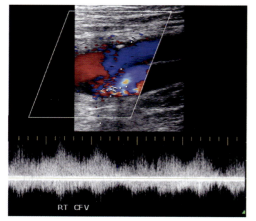

Fig. 168.3

Case 168 Arteriovenous Fistula Between Right Common Femoral Artery and Vein

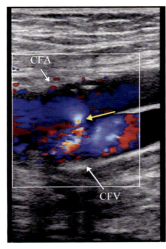

Fig. 168.4

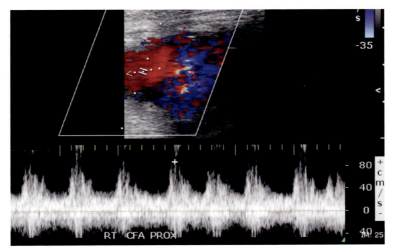

Fig. 168.5

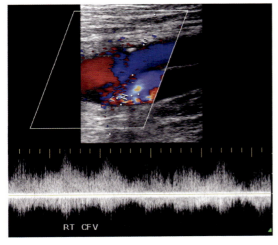

Fig. 168.6

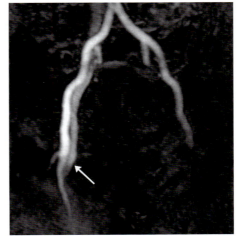

Fig. 168.7

Imaging Findings

► Note connection (yellow arrow in Fig. 168.4) between the right common femoral artery (CFA) and common femoral vein (CFV) indicative of a post-traumatic arteriovenous fistula (AVF)
► Aliasing or color mosaic at the site of the AVF is consistent with high-velocity flow
► There is a low-resistance spectral Doppler waveform with increased diastolic flow in the CFA (Fig. 168.5) above (cephalad to) the AVF; the spectral Doppler waveform in a normal CFA should have a high-resistance triphasic pattern
► The CFV above the AVF has a pulsatile, high-velocity turbulent waveform (Fig. 168.6)
► Note early venous filling of the right CFV, iliac veins, and inferior vena cava above the fistula on MR venogram (arrow in Fig. 168.7)

Differential Diagnosis

► Hematoma
► Pseudoaneurysm (PSA)

Teaching Points

► AVFs are abnormal communications between an artery and a vein bypassing the normal capillary bed
  ▪ Congenital or acquired
  ▪ In the groin, usually iatrogenic secondary to catheterization

- ► Presentation
  - ▪ Localized pain or swelling
  - ▪ Less commonly: bruit, lower extremity edema, distal ischemia, or right heart failure
- ► Physical findings
  - ▪ Machinery-like murmur or bruit
  - ▪ Hematoma
  - ▪ Pulsatile thrill
- ► US findings
  - ▪ Anechoic channel connecting artery and vein on grayscale imaging
  - ▪ High systolic and diastolic velocity (low-resistance spectral Doppler waveform) in the proximal artery with a normal triphasic waveform in the distal artery
  - ▪ Turbulent, pulsatile (arterialized) high-velocity flow in the draining vein above the AVF with a normal venous waveform below
  - ▪ Aliasing within the fistulous connection on color Doppler imaging
  - ▪ Color mosaic in the surrounding soft tissues due to soft tissue vibration artifact
- ► Soft tissue hematoma
  - ▪ Common finding post catheterization
  - ▪ Similar clinical presentation as AVF with localized pain and swelling
  - ▪ Echogenicity depends on time course: anechoic to echogenic, often heterogeneous
  - ▪ Sharply marginated to indistinct margins with blurring of soft tissue planes
  - ▪ Avascular
  - ▪ Spectral Doppler waveforms in adjacent artery and vein are usually normal; however, if compresses artery and vein, may see increased velocity and transmitted arterial pulsations to vein. Velocities usually not as high as in AVF
- ► PSA
  - ▪ More common than AVFs post catheterization
  - ▪ Similar clinical presentation
  - ▪ Sharply marginated anechoic rounded structures on grayscale, attached by a neck to the adjacent artery
  - ▪ "Yin-yang" pattern of swirling blood flow on color Doppler
  - ▪ "To-and-fro" spectral Doppler waveform within the neck (if thin), with flow above (during systole) and below (during diastole) the baseline

Management

- ► Small AVFs usually spontaneously resolve or thrombose
- ► Large or symptomatic AVFs require surgical or endovascular repair

Further Reading

1. Gonzalez SB, Busquets LC, Figueiras RG, et al. Imaging arteriovenous fistulas. *Am J Roentgenol.* 2009; 193: 1425–1433.
2. Glaser RL, McKellar D, Scher KS. Arteriovenous fistulas after cardiac catheterization. *Arch Surg* 1989; 124: 1313–1315.
3. Nasser TK, Mohler ER 3rd, Wilensky RL, et al. Peripheral vascular complications following coronary interventional procedures. *Clin Cardiol.* 1995; 18: 609–614.

Case 169

History

► 65-Year-old male with end-stage renal disease (ESRD) 2 months following surgical creation of a radiocephalic fistula referred for evaluation because the fistula is slow to mature (Figs. 169.1–169.4)

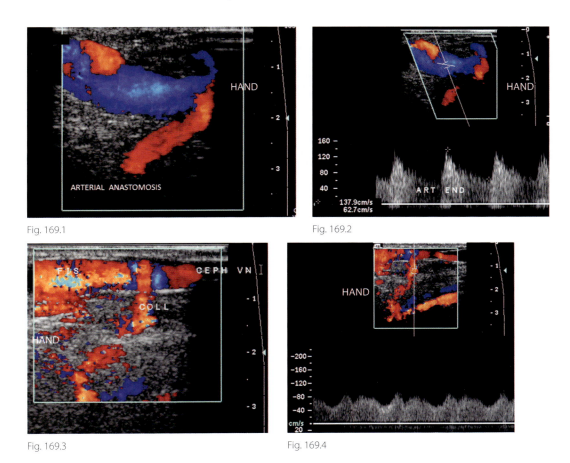

Fig. 169.1

Fig. 169.2

Fig. 169.3

Fig. 169.4

Case 169 Failure of Hemodialysis Access Fistula to Mature Secondary to Competing Collaterals

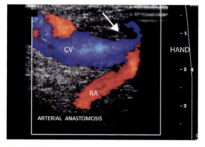

Fig. 169.5

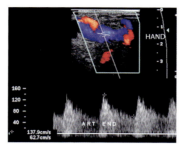

Fig. 169.6

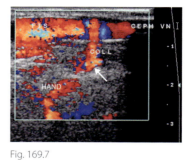

Fig. 169.7

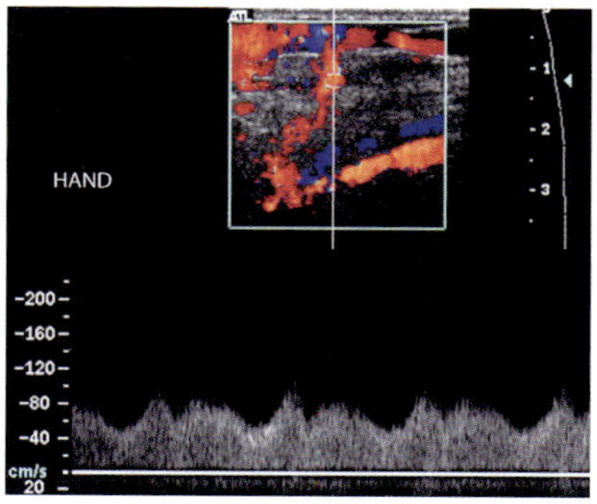

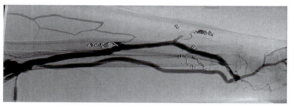

Fig. 169.8

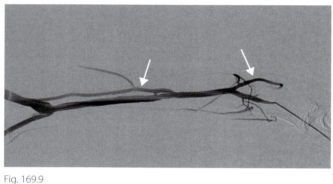

Fig. 169.9

Fig. 169.10

Imaging Findings

▶ Color Doppler image (Fig. 169.5) reveals a widely patent radial artery (RA) to cephalic vein (CV) anastomosis (arrow) but relatively diminutive cephalic venous outflow (CEPH VN in Fig. 169.7) with a large competing venous collateral (COLL, arrow in Fig. 169.7)
▶ Spectral Doppler tracing at the arterial anastomosis (Fig. 169.6) reveals a low-resistance waveform pattern with continuous forward diastolic flow but a relatively low velocity of 138 cm/s
▶ Note pulsatile venous Doppler waveform with high-velocity flow (80 cm/s) in the competing collateral channel (Fig. 169.8)
▶ A fistula venogram (Fig. 169.9) shows two large collaterals (arrows) arising from the outflow vein. These two collaterals as well as a few smaller collateral veins were coil embolized
▶ Follow-up fistulogram 1 month post embolization (Fig. 169.10) showed significantly improved forward flow through the fistula and increased outflow vein diameter

Differential Diagnosis

▶ Poor arterial inflow
▶ Stenosis at arterial anastomosis
▶ Venous outflow or central stenosis
▶ Competing venous collaterals
▶ Fistula too deep to be palpated

578

Teaching Points

► Hemodialysis is the primary, preferred bridge to renal transplantation
  ▪ Limited access sites are available: bilateral upper arms, bilateral forearms, and bilateral groins
  ▪ Each site lasts 2 or 3 years, on average
► Hemodialysis can be performed, in order of preference, via an arteriovenous fistula (AVF), arteriovenous graft (AVG), or central venous dialysis catheter
► AVFs are preferred because they last longer and have a substantially lower rate of complications, such as infection, pseudoaneurysm formation, and anastomotic stenosis
  ▪ However, AVFs may require 2 or 3 months to "mature" by developing adequate expansion of the outflow venous channel and increasing flow volume to accommodate repeated cannulation and dialysis
  ▪ More primary failures
► AVGs can be used for hemodialysis within 2 or 3 weeks of placement
  ▪ Although AVGs are less durable and have a much higher rate of infection, 60–80% of patients on dialysis in the United States use AVGs primarily because of the following
    • Late referral for dialysis
    • Clinical evaluation suggesting that the vessels in the arm are inadequate for creation of an AVF
► Central venous dialysis catheters often preferred by patients due to ease of placement, ease of use, and no impact on arms
  ▪ However, much higher incidence of infection
  ▪ Considered least desirable option by physicians
► "Fistula First" campaign introduced to increase the use of AVFs over AVGs
  ▪ Preoperative mapping with US recommended to find vessels considered adequate for fistula creation that are not apparent on physical examination
  ▪ Inflow artery: > 2 mm in diameter with a normal spectral Doppler waveform (high-resistance pattern with sharp systolic upstroke), adequate peak systolic velocity (PSV) that should be compared with contralateral side, no drop in PSV after fist clenching
  ▪ Outflow vein: > 2.5 mm without cephalad occlusion or calcification
  ▪ Begin with radial artery and cephalic vein in nondominant hand, next nondominant brachial artery and basilic/cephalic veins, then dominant forearm, lastly dominant upper arm
  ▪ Veins should be traced centrally to sternum to exclude central venous stenosis
  ▪ Map with patient sitting and arm dependent to distend veins
    • Can lightly apply tourniquet to dilate veins
    • Avoid mapping after dialysis when blood volume is reduced
► US findings suggesting that an AVF has matured adequately for hemodialysis
  ▪ Flow volume 500–600 ml/min
  ▪ Diameter ≥ 4–6 mm
  ▪ Depth < 5–6 mm
  ▪ Increased PSV and end diastolic velocity in native artery above fistula
  ▪ Increased PSV (200–400 cm/s) at anastomosis
  ▪ Velocity > 100 cm/s in fistula
► 20–50% of AVFs fail to mature
  ▪ Anatomic cause can be identified by US in 90%
  ▪ Approximately 78% salvage rate
► Risk factors
  ▪ Diabetes
  ▪ Female
  ▪ African American race
  ▪ Older age
  ▪ Obesity
  ▪ Vascular comorbidities
  ▪ Forearm >>> upper arm
► Causes of fistula failure
  ▪ Arterial inflow limitations: stenosis of proximal native artery or arterial anastomosis
  ▪ Venous outflow limitations: small vessel diameter, stenosis or occlusions, competing collateral branches
  ▪ Vessel too deep to be palpated by dialysis nurse or accessed even using US guidance
  ▪ Approximately 20% have more than one problem
  ▪ In approximately 10% of patients, no anatomic abnormality will be found
    • Possible poor cardiac output or inadequate arterial wall reactivity

- ▶ If an AVF does not appear to be maturing with lack of dilatation or poor palpable "thrill" over fistula, early evaluation with Doppler US or catheter angiography and subsequent intervention have been advocated to promote maturation
  - ▪ Many patients are referred directly for angiography without prior US because angiography is both diagnostic and therapeutic
- ▶ Competing draining venous collaterals or side branch steal
  - ▪ High-velocity flow through a side branch (or branches)
  - ▪ Significant reduction in diameter and velocity in the main venous outflow channel
  - ▪ More common in forearm
  - ▪ Usually occurs within 10 cm of arterial anastomosis
- ▶ Inflow arterial stenosis
  - ▪ Atherosclerosis or dissection of brachial or radial artery

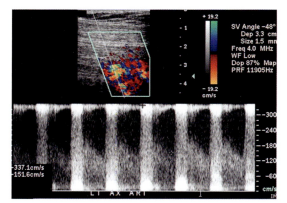

Fig. 169.11

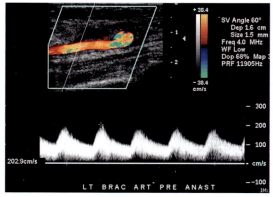

Fig. 169.12

This patient presented with absence of a palpable thrill over the arterial anastomosis of a brachial artery (BA) to basilic vein fistula created 1 month previously. Note increased PSV of 337 cm/s with spectral broadening in the axillary (AX) artery (Fig. 169.11) as well as a soft tissue color bruit due to tissue vibration from the high-velocity flow. The distal BA just proximal to the arterial anastomosis has a tardus parvus waveform pattern with a delayed systolic upstroke (Fig. 169.12) reflective of the proximal stenosis in the axillary artery. This was due to atherosclerotic plaque. Treatment with angioplasty improved flow in the BA, and the AVF subsequently matured adequately to support hemodialysis.

- ▶ Stenosis at arterial anastomosis

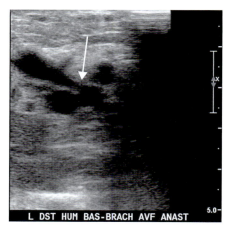

Fig. 169.13

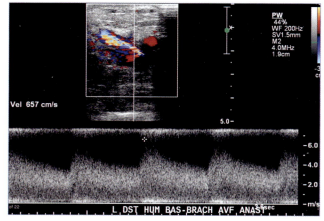

Fig. 169.14

Note narrowing at the arterial anastomosis (arrow in Fig. 169.13) and markedly increased PSV of 657 cm/s (Fig. 169.14) in this patient with low flow volume in a recently created BA to basilic vein fistula—findings consistent with a > 70% stenosis. This patient was effectively treated with angioplasty of the arterial anastomosis.

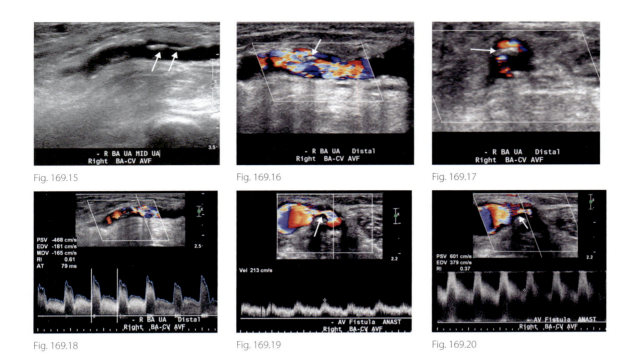

Fig. 169.15

Fig. 169.16

Fig. 169.17

Fig. 169.18

Fig. 169.19

Fig. 169.20

Note echogenic linear structure in mid BA (arrows in Figs. 169.15–169.17) consistent with a dissection flap in a patient with a brachial artery to cephalic vein AVF. PSV is increased from 119 cm/s in the proximal BA (not shown) to 468 cm/s at the level of the focal dissection (Fig. 169.18) with a PSV ratio of > 4:1, consistent with a > 70% stenosis. In addition, duplex Doppler images demonstrate narrowing (arrows in Figs. 169.19 and 169.20) just beyond the arterial anastomosis. Velocities increase from 213 cm/s (Fig. 169.19) at the anastomosis to 601 cm/s at the stenosis (Fig. 169.20) for a ratio of approximately 3:1. Findings are consistent with a high-grade post-anastomotic stenosis.

▶ Stenosis in outflow vein
- Scarring, fibrosis, vessel wall calcification (often from prior episodes of venous thrombosis)
- May occur in venous outflow of AVF (cephalic or basilic veins) or the more central veins (axillary and subclavian veins)
- History of prior central venous catheters increases risk

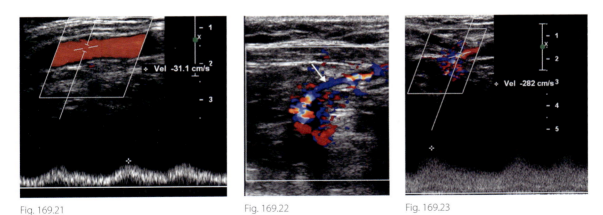

Fig. 169.21

Fig. 169.22

Fig. 169.23

This patient had extremely low volume flow through a recently created fistula. Peak velocity in the mid fistula is only 31 cm/s (Fig. 169.21). Color Doppler image (Fig. 169.22) demonstrates a long narrow segment of the basilic vein (arrow) where it joins the brachial vein in the upper arm with increased velocity of 282 cm/s (Fig. 169.23), consistent with a severe outflow stenosis. The patient was treated with angioplasty and stent placement.

▶ Complete occlusion/thrombosis of fistula

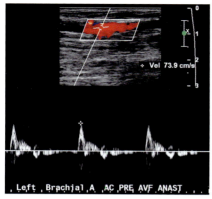

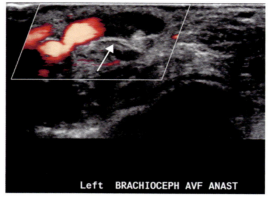

Fig. 169.24

Fig. 169.25

This patient presented 6 weeks following creation of a brachiocephalic AVF without a palpable thrill. There is a high-resistance waveform pattern with reversed early to mid-diastolic flow in the inflow brachial artery (Fig. 169.24). PSV is 74 cm/s. This is the normal waveform pattern and PSV of the native BA. However, after an AVF is created, the BA should develop a low-resistance waveform with increased PSV and continuous forward high-velocity diastolic flow due to the distal arteriovenous gradient. Further imaging with power Doppler (Fig. 169.25) reveals that the cephalic vein is completely occluded (arrow) just distal to the anastomosis.

► AVF too deep
  ▪ ≥ 4–6 mm
  ▪ More common in upper arm

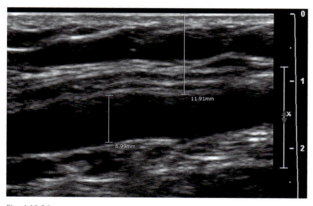

Fig. 169.26

The dialysis nurse was not able to palpate the upper arm fistula in this patient. Although the fistula was of adequate diameter (7 mm) and flow volumes were normal (800 ml/min; not shown), the fistula was too deep to be palpable at 12 mm (Fig. 169.26) below the skin surface and was treated with surgical superficialization (elevation).

Management

► Treatment options to promote maturation of an AV fistula depend on the underlying lesion
► Competing collateral draining veins
  ▪ Surgical ligation or percutaneous coil embolization to promote arterialization and dilatation of the main channel
► Inflow artery stenosis or arterial anastomotic stricture
  ▪ Angioplasty
  ▪ Stenting of inflow arterial stenosis may be performed
► Venous outflow stricture
  ▪ Angioplasty +/− stenting of the venous outflow: may require successive sessions in order to achieve desired diameter of at least 6 mm

- ▶ Vein too deep
  - ▪ Retunnel to superficialize and elevate
- ▶ Despite aggressive measures, current nonmaturation rate of hemodialysis AVFs is approximately 30%

Further Reading

1. Shamimi-Noori S, Resnick SA, Sato KT. Accessory draining vein embolization in the salvage of nonfunctioning arteriovenous fistulae. *J Vasc Interv Radiol.* 2013; 24(4): S38.
2. Falk A. Maintenance and salvage of arteriovenous fistulas. *J Vasc Interv Radiol.* 2006; 17(5): 807–813.

Case 170

History

▶ 74-Year-old male with a history of hypertension presents with back pain (Figs. 170.1–170.4)

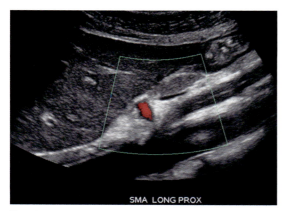

Fig. 170.1

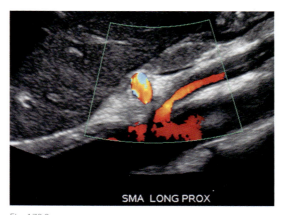

Fig. 170.2

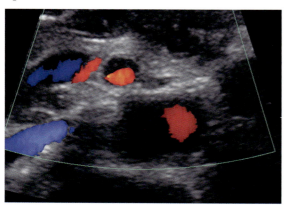

Fig. 170.3

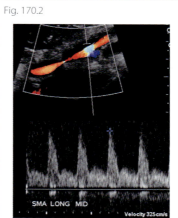

Fig. 170.4

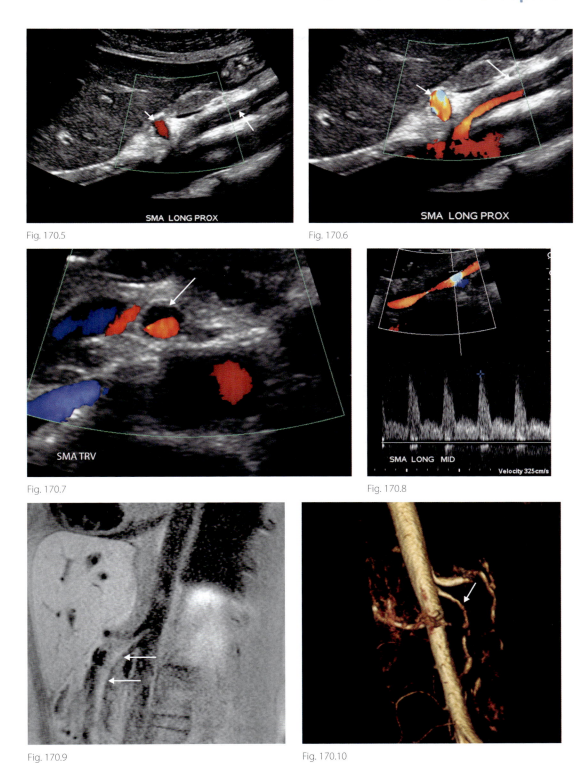

Fig. 170.5

Fig. 170.6

Fig. 170.7

Fig. 170.8

Fig. 170.9

Fig. 170.10

Imaging Findings

▶ Sagittal color Doppler image (Fig. 170.5) demonstrating linear echogenic intraluminal flap (long arrow) in superior mesenteric artery (SMA)

▶ The false lumen is thrombosed (long arrow in Fig. 170.6 and arrow in Fig. 170.7) with narrowing of the patent true lumen resulting in increased peak systolic velocity (PSV) of 325 cm/s (Fig. 170.8)

- The celiac artery (short arrows in Figs. 170.5 and 170.6) is incompletely visualized on these images but is widely patent without evidence of dissection
- Sagittal T1 black blood MR image of SMA (Fig. 170.9) demonstrates high signal intensity in the false lumen (arrows) consistent with thrombosis or intramural hematoma. Three-dimensional (3D) volume-rendered longitudinal image from MR angiogram (Fig. 170.10) confirms narrowing of the true lumen (arrow)

Differential Diagnosis

- Vasculitis
- Atherosclerosis

Teaching Points

- Spontaneous dissection of the SMA is rare
  - More common in males, aged 40–70 years
- Predisposing risk factors: fibromuscular dysplasia, connective tissue disorders, cystic medial necrosis, atherosclerosis, trauma
  - May occur secondary to extension from abdominal aortic dissection
- Presentation
  - Acute or chronic abdominal pain, sometimes worse after eating
  - Patients may be asymptomatic
- US findings
  - Echogenic intraluminal flap
    - Seen best on grayscale because color blooming artifact may obscure flap on color Doppler imaging
    - May not be apparent if false lumen is thrombosed

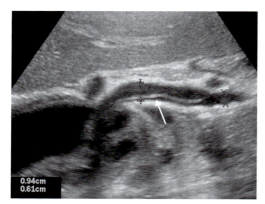

Fig. 170.11

Echogenic intraluminal flap (arrow in Fig. 170.11) in another patient with an SMA dissection extending from an abdominal aortic dissection. The SMA (calipers) is dilated, measuring up to 9 mm.

  - The false lumen may be patent and fill in with color or become thrombosed (similar appearance to intramural hematoma that develops when there is no exit point) with asymmetric hypoechoic thickening of vessel wall

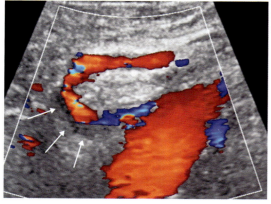

Fig. 170.12

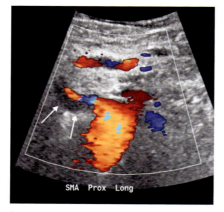

Fig. 170.13

Hypoechoic thrombosed false lumen (arrows in Figs. 170.12 and 170.13) compresses the true lumen, which is irregular and attenuated on color Doppler images from another patient, a 46-year-old male, with a spontaneous SMA dissection.

- True lumen often compressed by false lumen resulting in stenosis and elevated PSV
- SMA may be aneurysmally dilated
- Often begins 1–2 cm distal to origin, when not due to extension of aortic dissection
► Potential complications
- If true lumen significantly narrowed by thrombosed false lumen, bowel ischemia requiring bowel resection or revascularization may occur
- Separation of intima ± media from the adventitia layer results in weakening of the vessel wall, increasing the risk of pseudoaneurysm (PSA) formation

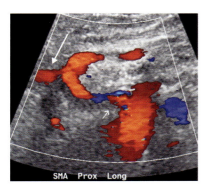 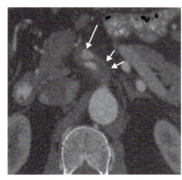 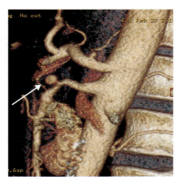

Fig. 170.14   Fig. 170.15   Fig. 170.16

Six-month follow-up US examination (Fig. 170.14) of same patient as shown in Figs. 170.12 and 170.13 reveals persistent narrowing of true lumen of SMA, thrombosis of the false lumen (hypoechoic mural thickening—short arrow in Fig. 170.14), and a focal outpouching (long arrow) that fills in with color consistent with interval development of a small patent PSA. Contrast-enhanced axial CT (Fig. 170.15) demonstrating thrombosed false lumen (short arrows) and patent PSA (long arrow). Volume-rendered sagittal 3D reconstruction from CT angiogram reveals the PSA as a focal outpouching (arrow in Fig. 170.16) arising from the SMA.

► Vasculitis: circumferential wall thickening
► Atherosclerosis: plaque or thrombus may have an echogenic surface, but unusual to be so homogeneous and involve such a long segment of SMA
- More often echogenic, calcified, and found at origin of SMA

Management

► Assess abdominal aorta and other major branches off abdominal aorta for dissection; screen for aneurysm and PSA
► Confirmation with CT or MR angiography if US equivocal
► Management controversial and symptom based
- Asymptomatic: surveillance ± anticoagulation and antihypertensive therapy
- Symptomatic: angioplasty (percutaneous transluminal angioplasty) with stent placement or surgical revascularization

Further Reading

1. Garrett HE. Options for treatment of spontaneous mesenteric artery dissection. *J Vasc Surg*. 2014; 59(5): 1433–1439.
2. Sheldon PJ, Esther JB, Sheldon EL, et al. Spontaneous dissection of the superior mesenteric artery. *Cardiovasc Intervent Radiol*. 2001; 24(5): 329–331.

Case 171

History

▶ 64-Year-old female with weight loss and chronic abdominal pain, made worse by eating (Figs. 171.1 and 171.2)

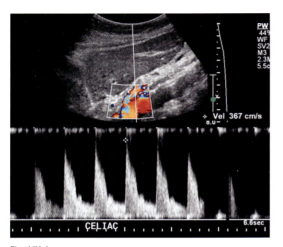

Fig. 171.1

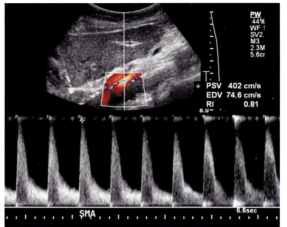

Fig. 171.2

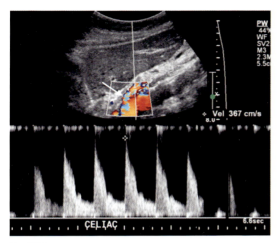

Fig. 171.3

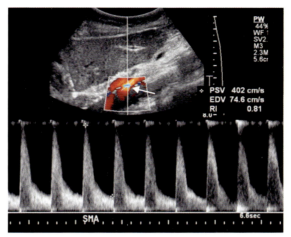

Fig. 171.4

Imaging Findings

▶ Color Doppler aliasing is present at the narrowed origins of the celiac artery (arrow in Fig. 171.3) and superior mesenteric artery (SMA) (arrow in Fig. 171.4)
▶ Spectral Doppler waveforms demonstrate increased peak systolic velocity (PSV) at the origins of the celiac artery at 367 cm/s and SMA at 402 cm/s, consistent with stenosis
▶ The wall of the abdominal aorta is irregular and calcified, consistent with atherosclerosis
▶ PSV in the abdominal aorta just cephalad to the origin of the celiac artery was 85 cm/s (not shown)

Differential Diagnosis

▶ Mesenteric dissection
▶ Vasculitis
▶ Normal postprandial exam
▶ Median arcuate ligament syndrome

Teaching Points

▶ Most common in females > 60 years of age
▶ Etiology
 ▪ Most cases due to atherosclerotic plaque at origins of the celiac artery (CA), SMA, or inferior mesenteric artery (IMA)
 ▪ Less common etiologies include vasculitis (especially fibromuscular dysplasia), dissection, radiation treatment, cocaine abuse, and tumor encasement
 ▪ Emboli may result in acute complete occlusion of the CA, SMA, and/or IMA
▶ Pathophysiology
 ▪ A robust collateral network normally exists between the mesenteric vessels (CA, SMA, and IMA) providing potentially redundant or backup blood flow to the gastrointestinal tract
 ▪ Thus, symptoms rarely occur if only one of the mesenteric vessels is chronically stenosed/occluded due to adequate collateral blood flow
 ▪ Development of symptoms due to decreased blood flow typically requires stenosis/occlusion of at least two of the mesenteric arteries
▶ Presentation
 ▪ Intestinal angina (postprandial abdominal pain)
 ▪ Weight loss
 ▪ Fear of food
 ▪ Anorexia
 ▪ Patients eat numerous small meals and still lose weight
▶ US findings
 ▪ Echogenic (± shadowing) atherosclerotic plaques in abdominal aorta and at the origin of mesenteric vessels
 ▪ Aliasing on color Doppler imaging

- Spectral Doppler criteria controversial: fasting PSV > 200 cm/s in the CA, > 275 cm/s in the SMA, and > 200 cm/s in the IMA have high sensitivity in predicting ≥ 70% stenosis
- The presence of tardus parvus waveforms in the distal mesenteric vessels increases specificity of elevated PSV at the origins
- Some authors advocate using other Doppler criteria: slightly higher PSVs, ratio of PSV in the mesenteric vessels to aortic PSV, or increase in end diastolic velocity (EDV)
- Change or lack of change in PSV or EDV following eating is no longer considered helpful because normal splanchnic blood flow demonstrates a wide range of responses to food intake

► Mesenteric arterial dissection
- Often extension of aortic dissection, but may occur spontaneously in absence of aortic dissection
- Thin echogenic intraluminal dissection flap
- Asymmetric thickening of the vessel wall due to mural hematoma or thrombosed false lumen
- Narrowing of lumen will result in color aliasing and increased PSV

► Mesenteric vasculitis
- Typically circumferential hypoechoic vessel wall thickening without evidence of atherosclerosis
- Narrowing of lumen will result in color aliasing and increased PSV

► Normal postprandial Doppler findings
- Variable increase in PSV and EDV, but unlikely to be > 200 cm/s in any vessel
- No narrowing of lumen or distal tardus parvus waveform

► Medial arcuate ligament syndrome
- Occurs in younger patients
- May cause postprandial epigastric pain
- Increased PSV and fishhook appearance of celiac artery during expiration or upright position
- PSV drops in inspiration
- SMA and IMA normal

Management

► US findings can be confirmed by CT or MRI angiography
► Treatment
- Surgery: endarterectomy or aortomesenteric arterial bypass graft
- Endovascular procedures: angioplasty and stent placement
- Patients not suitable for surgical or endovascular intervention treated medically with aspirin and/or warfarin; some may find short-term relief with nitrate therapy
► Follow-up post intervention
- Immediate baseline duplex Doppler US evaluation followed by serial exams every 6–12 months

Further Reading

1. Mitchell EL, Moneta GL. Mesenteric duplex scanning. *Perspect Vasc Surg Endovasc Ther*. 2006; 18(2): 175–183.
2. AbuRahma AF, Stone PA, Srivastava M, et al. Mesenteric/celiac duplex ultrasound interpretation criteria revisited. *J Vasc Surg*. 2012; 55(2): 428–436.

History

▶ 33-Year-old female with abdominal pain, worse after eating (Figs. 172.1–172.6)

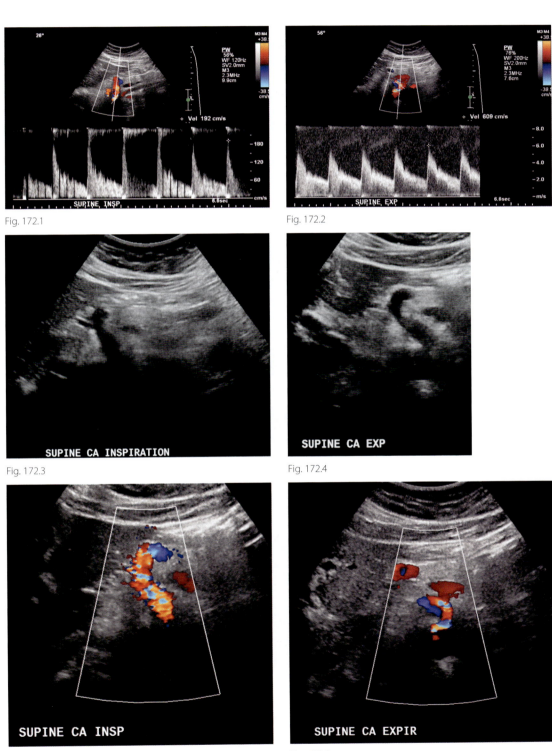

Fig. 172.1

Fig. 172.2

Fig. 172.3

Fig. 172.4

Fig. 172.5

Fig. 172.6

Case 172 Median Arcuate Ligament Syndrome (Celiac Artery Compression Syndrome)

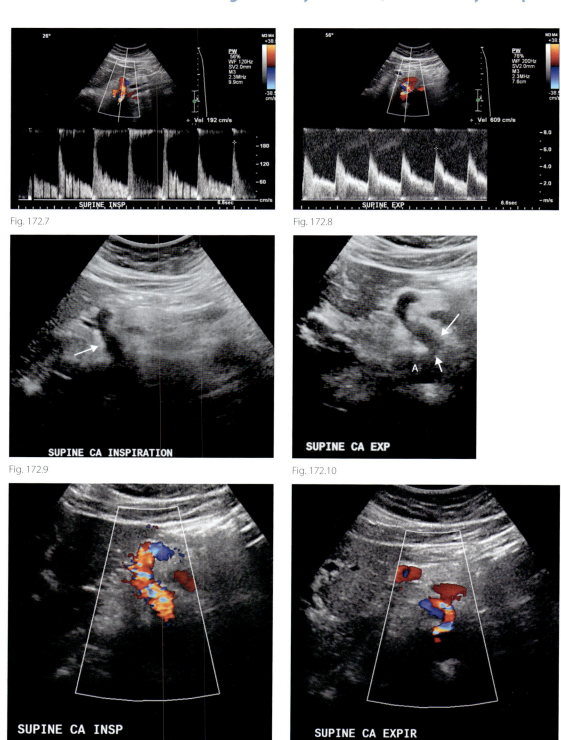

Fig. 172.7

Fig. 172.8

Fig. 172.9

Fig. 172.10

Fig. 172.11

Fig. 172.12

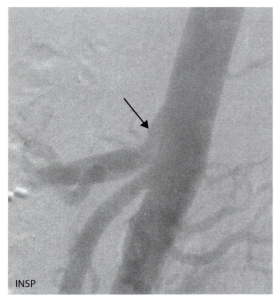

Fig. 172.13

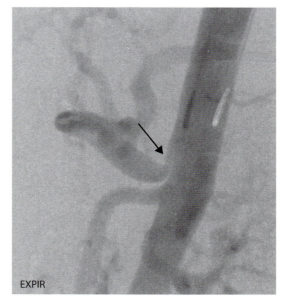

Fig. 172.14

Imaging Findings

▶ Increased peak systolic velocity (PSV) in the celiac artery (CA) in expiration (609 cm/s) (Fig. 172.8) compared to inspiration (192 cm/s) (Fig. 172.7)

▶ Straight course of CA on grayscale (arrow in Fig. 172.9) and on color Doppler (Fig. 172.11) during inspiration, with a "fishhook" appearance on expiration seen on both grayscale (long arrow in Fig. 172.10) and on color Doppler (Fig. 172.12). The origin of the CA is narrowed on expiration (short arrow in Fig. 172.10) with post-stenotic dilatation. Aorta (A)

▶ Narrowing and "fishhook" or angled appearance of CA (arrow in Fig. 172.14) on angiogram obtained in expiration compared to CA (arrow in Fig. 172.13) on inspiratory angiogram confirms US findings

Differential Diagnosis

▶ Celiac artery stenosis
▶ Postprandial changes
▶ Compensatory flow

Teaching Points

▶ The median arcuate ligament (MAL) is a fibrous band that connects the diaphragmatic crura and usually crosses over the aorta above the CA. If the MAL crosses the aorta more inferiorly and anterior to the CA, it can cause compression of the CA in expiration due to upward movement of the diaphragm resulting in recurrent abdominal pain
▶ Clinical presentation
  ▪ Abdominal pain (± postprandial)
  ▪ Nausea
  ▪ Weight loss
  ▪ Midepigastric bruit—worse during expiration, standing, or exercise
  ▪ Symptoms most common in 20- to 40-year-old females
▶ However, compression of the CA by the MAL can be an incidental finding, and some patients are completely asymptomatic
▶ US findings
  ▪ Normal PSV in CA during inspiration
  ▪ Elevated PSV in CA during expiration
  ▪ Straight or more vertical orientation of CA during inspiration
  ▪ "Fishhook" or angled appearance of CA with narrowing of origin during expiration
  ▪ PSV will return to normal if the patient is scanned in the erect position, even in expiration. Hence, scanning in the upright position will increase the specificity of the US findings

- Celiac artery stenosis
  - Commonly accepted Doppler criteria: PSV > 200 cm/s or PSV three times aortic PSV
  - Focal narrowing of the vessel lumen and color Doppler aliasing
  - PSV and configuration of CA will not change during respiration or in the erect position
- Diagnosis of chronic mesenteric ischemia requires > 60% narrowing in at least two of the three mesenteric vessels
- In the postprandial state or in patients with stenosis of the superior mesenteric artery or inferior mesenteric artery, elevated PSV in the CA due to increased or compensatory flow may be noted throughout the respiratory cycle without evidence of vessel narrowing

Management

- Dynamic US is the first-line imaging modality
  - CT angiography or angiography can also be used for diagnosis
- Laparoscopic surgical decompression with division/resection of the MAL
- Percutaneous intervention with angioplasty and/or stenting of the CA is indicated only for the treatment of residual or recurrent stenosis following laparoscopic surgical decompression
- Demonstration of the anatomic anomaly and respiratory changes is not necessarily predictive of symptoms or response to intervention
  - Imaging findings may be incidental, and the narrowing of the CA during expiration may not be the cause of the patient's pain
- Hence, not all patients respond to surgery
- Pain relief may not be durable in all patients
- Response tends to be better in older patients

Further Reading

1. Wolfman D, Bluth EI, Sossaman J. Median arcuate ligament syndrome. *J Ultrasound Med*. 2003; 22: 1377–1380.
2. Jimenez JC, Harlander-Locke M, Dutson EP. Open and laparoscopic treatment of median arcuate ligament syndrome. *J Vasc Surg*. 2012; 56: 869–873.

History

▶ 69-Year-old female with acute-onset, severe hypertension (Figs. 173.1–173.4)

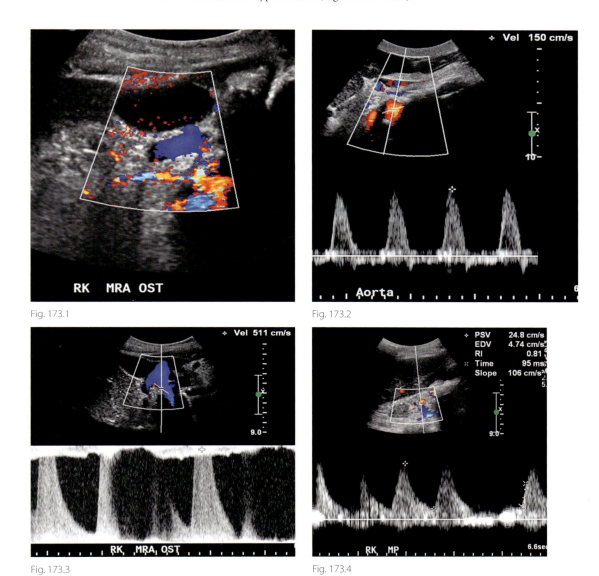

Fig. 173.1

Fig. 173.2

Fig. 173.3

Fig. 173.4

Case 173 Renal Artery Stenosis

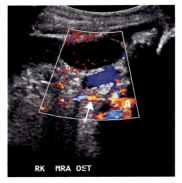

Fig. 173.5

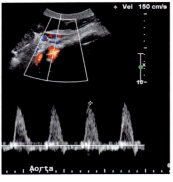

Fig. 173.6

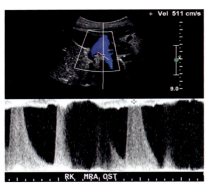

Fig. 173.7

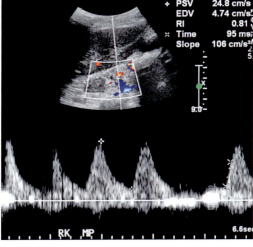

Fig. 173.8

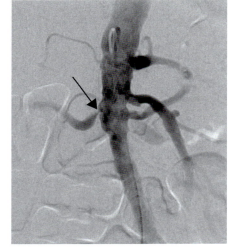

Fig. 173.9

Imaging Findings

► Transverse color Doppler image demonstrating color aliasing and narrowing of the origin of the right renal artery (RA) (arrow in Fig. 173.5). Aorta (A)
► Peak systolic velocity (PSV) is 511 cm/s at the origin of the right RA (Fig. 173.7) and is 150 cm/s in the aorta proximal to the origin of the right RA (Fig. 173.6), yielding an RA to aortic PSV ratio of 3.41
► Note delayed systolic upstroke in the spectral Doppler waveform (Fig. 173.8) of an interlobar RA with a prolonged acceleration time (AT) of 95 ms
► Angiogram demonstrating high-grade stenosis at the origin of the right RA (arrow in Fig. 173.9)

Differential Diagnosis

► Renal artery stenosis (RAS) due to fibromuscular dysplasia
► Takayasu arteritis
► Dissection of renal artery

Teaching Points

► RAS leads to renovascular hypertension (RVHT) through activation of the renin–angiotensin cascade
  ▪ Accounts for < 1% of all hypertensive patients in the United States
► In the United States, RVHT is caused primarily by atherosclerosis (90%) and fibromuscular dysplasia (FMD) (10%)
  ▪ Atherosclerotic RAS occurs predominately in men > 50 years of age; narrowing found at the origin of the RAs; may be bilateral in older patients
  ▪ FMD most commonly affects the middle or distal third of the RA; occurs predominantly in young to middle-aged women; 50% bilateral

- Takayasu arteritis is the most common cause of RVHT in India
- Other causes include dissection, radiation therapy, and neurofibromatosis
▶ Presentation
  - Rapid onset of severe, accelerated hypertension (HTN)
    • Diastolic blood pressure > 110 mm Hg
  - Lack of response to triple-drug therapy
  - Early or late age onset of HTN
  - Absence of family history of essential HTN
  - HTN in the setting of renal failure, abdominal or flank bruit, asymmetric renal size
  - Recurrent or flash pulmonary edema
▶ Diagnosis requires documentation of RAS plus physiologic abnormality
  - Angiogram with measurement of renal vein renin levels is the gold standard
  - Structural narrowing can be documented on MR angiography or CT angiography
  - US potentially can provide both structural and physiologic information
▶ Direct US findings
  - Increased PSV > 200–250 cm/s at site of stenosis in main RA
    • CORAL Trial used > 300 cm/s
  - PSV ratio between RA and aorta > 2–3.5
  - May be difficult to see entire length of renal artery, especially the origin, in as many as 20–30% of patients depending on body habitus
  - Intravenous US contrast agents (currently not approved for this use by the U.S. Food and Drug Administration) can be used to salvage nondiagnostic examinations
▶ Indirect US findings
  - Delayed systolic acceleration in the intraparenchymal RAs
    • Acceleration index (AI) < 300 cm/s^2
    • AT > 70 ms
    • Tardus parvus waveform
  - Can get a spectral Doppler waveform from the intraparenchymal renal arteries in nearly all patients
  - Not a sensitive finding: older age, long-standing HTN, calcified vessels, diabetes, and atherosclerosis reduce the incidence of tardus parvus waveforms distal to a stenosis
  - Not a specific finding: a tardus parvus waveform indicates that there is a proximal stenosis, but does not identify where
    • Unilateral: origin of RA
    • Bilateral: aortic stenosis, aortic coarctation, bilateral RAS
▶ RVHT due to FMD
  - Arteritis of unknown etiology
  - Occurs most commonly in women between the ages of 25 and 50 years
  - Beaded appearance with narrowing and increased PSV of middle third of main RA
  - Distal tardus parvus waveforms in the intraparenchymal renal arteries usually present when there is significant luminal narrowing of the main RA in young patients
  - Assess for intracranial aneurysms
  - HTN responds well to percutaneous or surgical revascularization

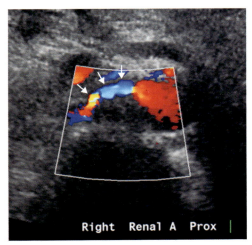

Fig. 173.10

Note "string of pearls" or beaded appearance (arrows in Fig. 173.10) of the right renal artery in this 36-year-old female with RVHT due to FMD.

► Takayasu arteritis
  ▪ Inflammatory disease of unknown etiology causing thickening of the arterial wall and luminal narrowing at the origins of major branch vessels from the aorta
  ▪ Often involves innominate, carotid, and subclavian arteries; patients present with cold hands and decreased pulses, sometimes called "pulseless disease"
  ▪ Ages 15–30 years, eight times more common in females
  ▪ Smooth hypoechoic thickening of the arterial walls with long-segment narrowing of lumen beginning at origin from aorta, increased PSV, often bilateral
  ▪ Treated with steroids and chemotherapy
► Renal artery dissection
  ▪ Rare cause of RVHT
  ▪ Usually associated with aortic dissection

Management

► Traditionally, arterial bypass graft or stenting was believed to cure RVHT with either elimination of or significant reduction in anti-hypertensive medications and salvage or stabilization of renal function
  ▪ However, intervention may not improve HTN or renal function if the kidney is small; has a thin, echogenic renal cortex; or resistive index > 0.8
► Data from the CORAL Trial indicate that current medical therapy has better outcome than either surgical or percutaneous intervention for RVHT due to atherosclerosis
► Intervention is now only definitively recommended, usually with angioplasty, for patients with RVHT secondary to FMD
  ▪ Angioplasty with stenting may be performed for acute RA dissection
  ▪ If medical therapy fails, some clinicians recommend intervention for patients with severe HTN or flash pulmonary edema, but there is little evidence-based data

Further Reading
1. Wang SY, Scoutt LM. US evaluation of renovascular hypertension. *US Clinics* 2011: 6: 491–511.
2. Cooper CJ, Murphy TP, Cutlip DE, et al. Stenting and medical therapy for atherosclerotic renal–artery stenosis. *N Engl J Med*. 2014; 370: 13–22.

History

▶ 8-Year-old male presenting with hypertension (Figs. 174.1–174.3)

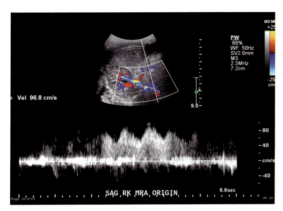

Fig. 174.1

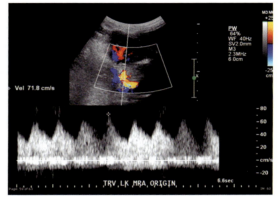

Fig. 174.2

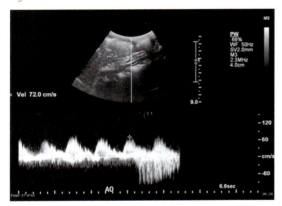

Fig. 174.3

Case 174 Aortic Coarctation With Tardus Parvus Waveforms in the Bilateral Main Renal Arteries and the Abdominal Aorta

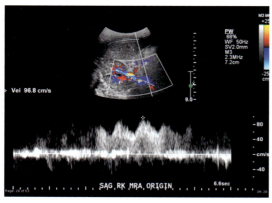

Fig. 174.4

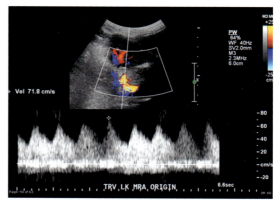

Fig. 174.5

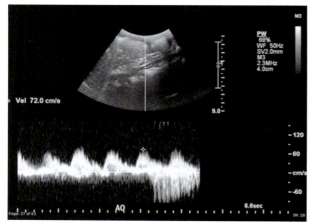

Fig. 174.6

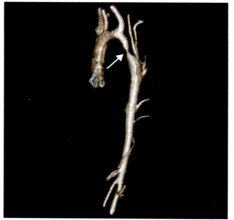

Fig. 174.7

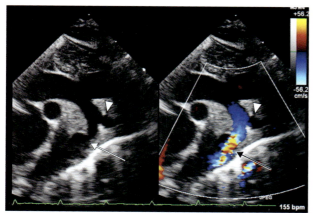

Fig. 174.8

Imaging Findings

▶ Tardus parvus waveforms are present in the right and left main renal arteries as well as the aorta (Figs. 174.4–174.6). There is no evidence of narrowing or focal color aliasing in the main renal arteries to suggest renal artery stenosis

▶ Volume-rendered magnetic resonance angiography (MRA) image (Fig. 174.7) demonstrates narrowing of the thoracic aorta (arrow) distal to the origin of the left subclavian artery diagnostic of aortic coarctation

► Split-screen image from a cardiac echo (Fig. 174.8) confirms narrowing of the descending aorta (arrow in left grayscale image) distal to the origin of the left subclavian artery (arrowheads) with focal color aliasing (arrow in right color Doppler image) indicating high-velocity flow at the stenosis

Differential Diagnosis

► Congenital aortic valvular stenosis
► Midaortic syndrome
► Williams syndrome
► Takayasu arteritis
► Renal artery stenosis

Teaching Points

► Tardus parvus (TP) arterial spectral Doppler waveforms are characterized by a slow, horizontal systolic upstroke and rounding or blunting of the systolic peak (tardus) with decreased peak systolic velocity (parvus)
  ▪ Indicate a relatively severe more proximal or upstream stenosis
  ▪ More pronounced the more distal one samples to the stenosis
  ▪ Assessed by "gestalt" (visual inspection), prolonged acceleration time, or decreased systolic acceleration index
  ▪ Distribution of the TP waveform will help localize the stenosis
► In this case, a TP spectral Doppler waveform is present in the abdominal aorta as well as in both main renal arteries, indicating that the stenosis is upstream or proximal to the abdominal aorta
  ▪ In a child, aortic coarctation is the most common cause
  ▪ Other causes include congenital aortic valve stenosis, aortic stenosis, subvalvular aortic stenosis, and aortic webs
  ▪ In adults, aortic valvular stenosis is the most common cause of this constellation of findings
► Aortic coarctation: congenital anomaly, associated with bicuspid aortic valve (30%), circle of Willis aneurysms (10%), ventricular septal defect, atrial septal defect, patent ductus arteriosus, and Turner syndrome
  ▪ 5–8% of all congenital heart defects
  ▪ More common in males
► Two types of aortic coarctation
  ▪ Preductal (infantile)
    • Descending aorta receives flow from the ductus arteriosus
    • Presents in infancy with congestive heart failure when the ductus closes
    • If severe, can be life-threatening
  ▪ Postductal (adult)
    • Presents later in childhood or as young adult with hypertension, shortness of breath, dizziness, diminished lower extremity pulses, and/or intermittent claudication
    • Rib notching and aortic silhouette figure of 3 contour on chest X-ray
► Midaortic syndrome
  ▪ Unknown etiology
  ▪ Presents in children with narrowing of the abdominal aorta and visceral (including renal) branch vessels
► Williams syndrome
  ▪ Genetic deletion from chromosome 7 resulting in decreased elastin production
  ▪ Can result in segmental narrowing of the aorta with resultant downstream TP waveforms including renal arteries
► Takayasu arteritis
  ▪ Granulomatous vasculitis causing marked intimal fibrosis and narrowing of the origins of the large branches off the aorta, sometimes narrowing of the aorta as well
  ▪ Could cause TP waveforms in the main renal arteries and would be a consideration in a young to middle-aged woman of Asian descent with hypertension
  ▪ Would expect to see stenosis at the origins of the main renal arteries
  ▪ Rare in children and males
  ▪ Less likely to demonstrate a TP waveform in the abdominal aorta
► Renal artery stenosis (RAS)
  ▪ Bilateral RAS could cause bilateral TP waveforms in the intraparenchymal renal arteries
  ▪ Increased PSV at the origins of the main renal arteries
  ▪ Normal aortic waveform
  ▪ Children unlikely to have bilateral RAS (slight association with neurofibromatosis)

Management

► Corrected surgically with either resection or placement of a graft or patch

► Angioplasty for restenosis following surgery

► 10% recurrence rate post surgical repair and 20% following angioplasty

Further Reading

1. Chaubal N, Dighe M, Shah M. Sonographic and color Doppler findings in aortoarteritis (Takayasu arteritis). *J Ultrasound Med.* 2004; 23: 937–944.

2. Kimura-Hayama ET, Meléndez G, Mendizábal AL, et al. Uncommon congenital and acquired aortic diseases: Role of multidetector CT angiography. *RadioGraphics.* 2010; 30(1): 79–98.

History

▶ 65-Year-old female with hematuria (Figs. 175.1–175.6)

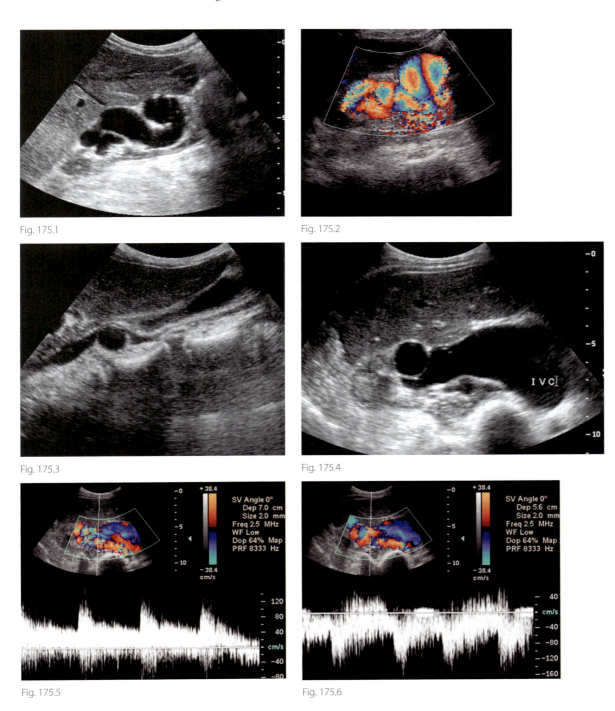

Fig. 175.1

Fig. 175.2

Fig. 175.3

Fig. 175.4

Fig. 175.5

Fig. 175.6

Case 175 Congenital Renal Arteriovenous Malformation

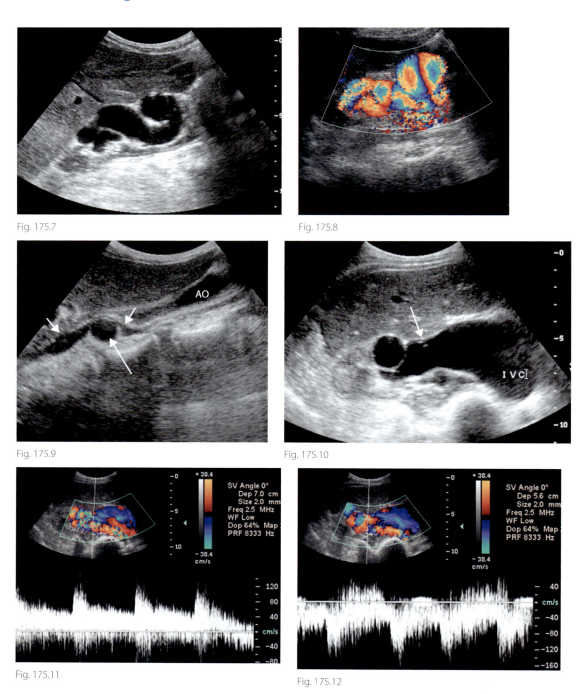

Fig. 175.7

Fig. 175.8

Fig. 175.9

Fig. 175.10

Fig. 175.11

Fig. 175.12

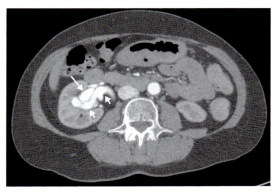

Fig. 175.13

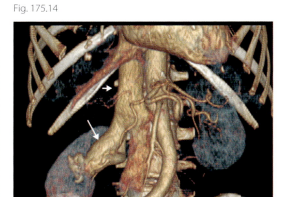

Fig. 175.14

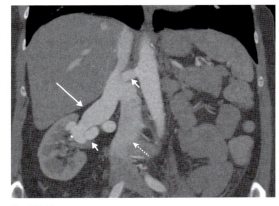

Fig. 175.15

Fig. 175.16

Imaging Findings

▶ Grayscale (Fig. 175.7) and color Doppler (Fig. 175.8) images reveal markedly dilated vessels in the right renal hilum, with color aliasing and soft tissue color bruit (color pixels located outside the lumen of the dilated, tortuous vessels) in Fig. 175.8 indicating high-velocity, turbulent flow

▶ Sagittal grayscale image (Fig. 175.9) demonstrates marked dilatation of the right main renal artery (long arrow) as it courses posterior to the inferior vena cava (short arrows). Aorta (AO)

▶ Transverse grayscale image (Fig. 175.10) demonstrates massive dilatation of the right renal vein (arrow) and inferior vena cava (IVC)

▶ Note increased end diastolic velocity (EDV) in the right renal artery (Fig. 175.11) with pulsatile high-velocity flow in the right renal vein (Fig. 175.12)

▶ Arterial phase images from a CT angiogram (Fig. 175.13–175.15) confirm enlarged right renal artery (short arrows) with early filling of the enlarged right renal vein (long arrows in Fig. 175.13 and 175.15) but no enhancement of the left renal vein (long arrow in Fig. 175.14). Note decreased density of contrast enhancement in the infrarenal IVC (dashed arrow in Fig. 175.15) due to reflux of contrast from the right renal vein

▶ Three-dimensional volume-rendered coronal CT (Fig. 175.16) showing enlarged right renal vein (long arrow) and IVC (short arrow)

Differential Diagnosis

▶ Varices

Teaching Points

▶ Abnormal communication between renal artery and vein, termed malformation (AVM) if congenital and fistula (AVF) if acquired
  ▪ Congenital AVM < 25%
    • Cirsoid AVM: most common, multiple arterial feeders, dilated "corkscrew" appearance
    • Cavernous: single arterial feeder
  ▪ Acquired approximately 75%
    • Most have a single dominant feeding artery and draining vein

- ▶ Etiology of acquired AVFs
  - ▪ Renal biopsy (most common)
  - ▪ Surgery
  - ▪ Trauma
  - ▪ Erosion from malignancy—especially renal cell carcinoma
- ▶ Presentation
  - ▪ Gross hematuria (75%)
  - ▪ Microscopic hematuria
  - ▪ Flank pain often secondary to blood clot obstructing the collecting system
  - ▪ Hypertension
  - ▪ High-output congestive heart failure
  - ▪ Flank bruit
  - ▪ May be asymptomatic and incidentally detected on imaging
- ▶ US findings
  - ▪ Dilated feeding artery—single or multiple
  - ▪ Dilated draining vein ± IVC (dependent on volume of shunted blood)
    - • Focal dilatation of draining vein may mimic pseudoaneurysm
  - ▪ Soft tissue color bruit
  - ▪ Turbulent flow with spectral broadening and increased PSV and EDV in feeding artery
  - ▪ Pulsatile high-velocity flow in draining vein (i.e., "arterialization" of venous spectral Doppler waveform)
- ▶ Varices
  - ▪ Dilated serpiginous retroperitoneal veins surrounding kidney with minimally phasic low-velocity waveform; would not have pulsatile high-velocity flow
  - ▪ Normal flow pattern in renal artery

Management

- ▶ Embolization with coils
- ▶ Partial or total nephrectomy for symptomatic patients if embolization unsuccessful

Further Reading

1. Chimpiri AR, Natarajan B. Renal vascular lesions: Diagnosis and endovascular management. *Semin Intervent Radiol.* 2009; 26(3): 253–261.
2. Cura M, Elmerhi F, Suri R, et al. Vascular malformations and arteriovenous fistulas of the kidney. *Acta Radiol.* 2010; 51(2): 144–149.

History

▶ 48-Year-old female with hepatitis C presents with worsening liver function tests (Figs. 176.1 and 176.2)

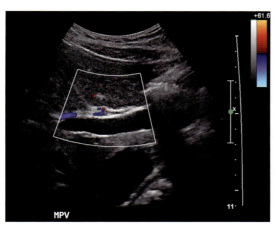

Fig. 176.1

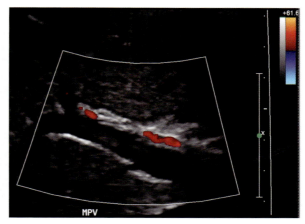

Fig. 176.2

Case 176 False-Positive Diagnosis of Portal Vein Thrombosis Due to Poor Technique

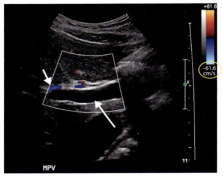

Fig. 176.3

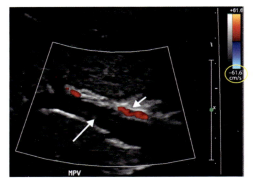

Fig. 176.4

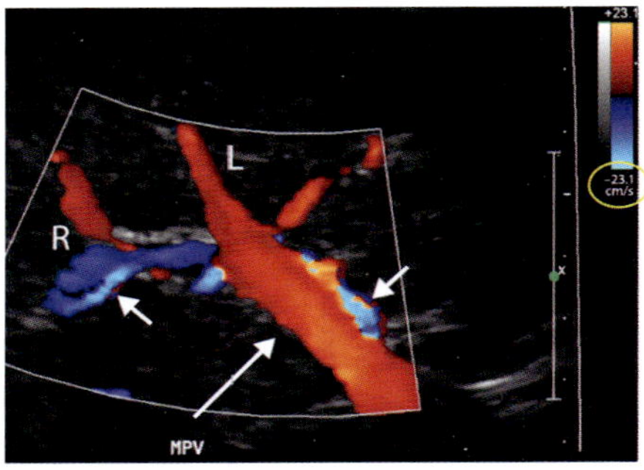

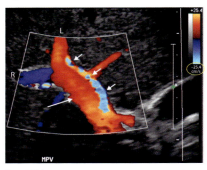

Fig. 176.5

Fig. 176.6

Imaging Findings

► No color flow is detected in the main portal vein (PV) (long arrows in Figs. 176.3 and 176.4). Note low-level internal echoes seen best near long arrow in Fig 176.4 that could be misconstrued as acute portal vein thrombosis (PVT). Color flow is noted in the main hepatic artery (HA) (short arrows in Figs. 176.3 and 176.4)

► However, the scale is extremely high (61 cm/s; yellow circles in Figs. 176.3 and 176.4), which decreases the sensitivity of color Doppler for detection of low-velocity flow. In addition, the PV in image A is nearly perpendicular to the insonating US beam, which also decreases the sensitivity of color Doppler for the detection of flow

► When the color Doppler scale is decreased (23.1 cm/s in Fig. 176.5 and 25.4 cm/s in Fig. 176.6, yellow circles), blood flow is readily detected in the main (long arrows), right (R), and left (L) PVs, and color aliasing is noted in the HA (short arrows), indicative of relatively higher velocity flow

Differential Diagnosis

► Portal vein thrombosis
► Slow flow in the portal vein

Teaching Points

► Risk factors for PVT: slow PV flow (often secondary to portal hypertension and/or cirrhosis), hypercoagulable states, intestinal inflammation/infection, sepsis, malignancy, volume depletion (especially acute), and trauma
► US findings of PVT
  ▪ Echogenic material within the PV (acute PVT is typically hypoechoic to anechoic, whereas chronic thrombus tends to be more echogenic)
  ▪ Intraluminal echoes due to PVT may be difficult to distinguish from artifactual low-level echoes, which are commonly observed in the PV due to slow flow, reverberation artifact, partial volume averaging, or poor penetration
  ▪ Acute PVT typically will cause expansion of the PV
  ▪ Absence of detectable blood flow on Doppler interrogation; color void if non-occlusive
  ▪ Periportal collaterals (cavernous transformation) in chronic PVT

- Slow PV flow is common in patients with portal hypertension before complete reversal of flow occurs
- US findings of slow PV flow
  - Swirling or slow-moving intraluminal echoes without shadowing or comet tail artifact on grayscale imaging, best seen in main PV
  - Color Doppler US may not be adequately sensitive to detect very slow flow, and it is least sensitive for the detection of flow if the vessel is oriented 90° to the insonating US beam or parallel to the transducer surface
  - Hence, if no flow is noted in the PV on color Doppler and no thrombus is seen on grayscale images, the possibility of slow flow should be considered
- Techniques for optimization of color Doppler machine settings for the detection of low-velocity, low-volume flow include the following
  - Decreasing the pulse repetition frequency or scale
  - Increasing the gain until limited by noise or motion artifact (i.e., when color pixels are detected outside the vessel walls)
  - Decreasing the size of the color box
  - Using a straight rather than steered (angled) color box
  - Decreasing the wall filter
  - Increasing color write priority
  - Decreasing transducer frequency may improve penetration and aid in detection of blood flow in deeper structures such as the PV. However, note that increasing transducer frequency improves detection of blood flow in superficial vessels
  - Increasing ensemble length (number of color Doppler pulses per line of color Doppler information)
- Spectral and power Doppler modes are more sensitive than color Doppler for the detection of blood flow
- Patient maneuvers to improve detection of PV flow
  - Position: ensure that the PV is not perpendicular to the US beam. Because the Doppler frequency shift is directly proportional to the cosine of the Doppler angle, color Doppler is least sensitive for the detection of blood flow when the vessel is perpendicular to the US beam because the cosine of 90° is zero
  - Imaging post breath hold and release: "holding" a deep breath will increase intra-abdominal pressure and reduce flow in the PV. When the breath is released, flow will increase in the PV and be easier to detect
  - Postprandial imaging: eating will increase portal flow
- Aliasing (wrap around of the spectral waveform or the color spectrum from light yellow to light turquoise) occurs when the frequency shift exceeds the Doppler scale
  - In this case, aliasing occurred in the higher velocity HA when the scale was decreased (short arrows in Fig. 176.6)

Management

- If no flow is detected in the PV on color Doppler and no internal echoes are seen on grayscale, the sonographer must ensure that all Doppler machine settings have been adjusted to maximize the detection of low-velocity flow to avoid mistaking slow flow in a patent PV for anechoic PVT
- If portal venous flow is still not identified, contrast-enhanced MR or CT are more sensitive for the detection of PV flow than Doppler US and should be performed to confirm the diagnosis
- Contrast-enhanced US, although not approved for this use by the U.S. Food and Drug Administration, can also be used to increase the sensitivity of US for the detection of flow in the portal vein and exclude PVT

Further Reading
1. Desser TS, Jedrzejewicz T, Haller MI. Color and power Doppler sonography: Techniques, clinical applications, and trade-offs for image optimization. *Ultrasound Q.* 1998; 14: 128–149.
2. Middleton WD. Color Doppler: Image interpretation and optimization. *Ultrasound Q.* 1998; 14: 194–209.

Case 177

History

▶ 82-Year-old female with severe abdominal pain (Figs. 177.1–177.3)

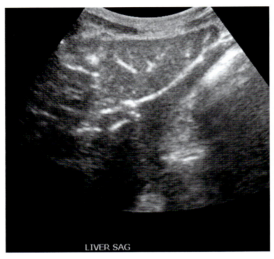

Fig. 177.1

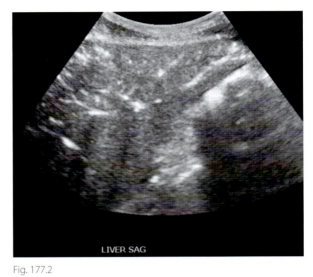

Fig. 177.2

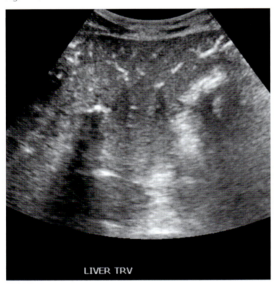

Fig. 177.3

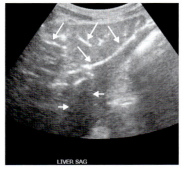

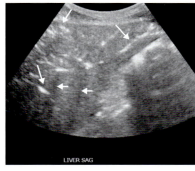

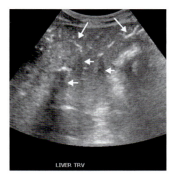

Fig. 177.4   Fig. 177.5   Fig. 177.6

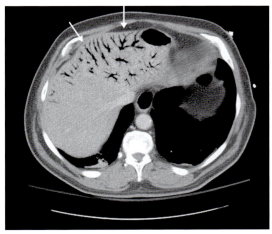

Fig. 177.7

Imaging Findings

▶ Peripheral echogenic branching linear structures predominantly in the left lobe of the liver (long arrows in Figs. 177.4–177.6)
▶ Several demonstrate "dirty" shadowing (short arrows in Figs. 177.4–177.6)
▶ Contrast-enhanced CT scan demonstrating extensive portal venous gas (arrows in Fig. 177.7) in the left lobe of the liver in this patient with mesenteric ischemia

Differential Diagnosis

▶ Pneumobilia
▶ Hepatic artery calcification

Teaching Points

▶ Gas in the portal vein (PV) is most commonly associated with mesenteric ischemia; other etiologies include the following
  ▪ Intra-abdominal infection/inflammation (diverticulitis, perforated peptic ulcer, emphysematous cholecystitis, inflammatory bowel disease, sepsis)
  ▪ Bowel distention due to obstruction, ileus, or iatrogenic procedures such as endoscopy
  ▪ Blunt trauma or barotrauma
  ▪ Idiopathic (15%)
▶ Prognosis depends on etiology
  ▪ Mortality rate is 75–90% if bowel ischemia is the cause
  ▪ Less ominous finding in the setting of trauma, bowel distention, or post procedures
▶ US more sensitive than CT for diagnosis of PV gas

► US findings
  ▪ Branching, echogenic linear areas extending peripherally in the hepatic parenchyma with "dirty" shadowing or reverberation artifact

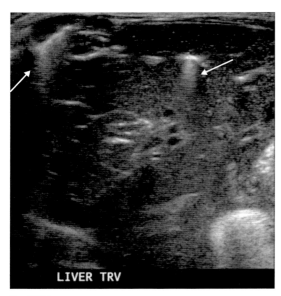

Fig. 177.8

Echogenic linear peripheral foci with dirty reverberation artifact (arrows in Fig. 177.8) in a premature infant with PV gas due to necrotizing enterocolitis
  ▪ Echogenic areas may become "patchy" or poorly defined as gas diffuses through the hepatic capillaries

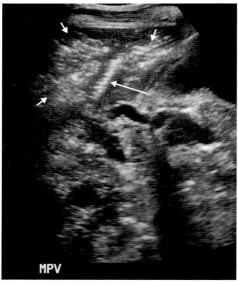

Fig. 177.9

In this 74-year-old female with infarcted bowel, the echogenic foci of PV gas have become "patchy" and confluent (short arrows in Fig. 177.9), although gas in the left PV appears linear (long arrow in Fig. 177.9)
  ▪ Tiny, mobile, round echogenic intraluminal foci within PV
    • Represent the actual gas bubbles
    • Will flow peripherally
    • Easiest to visualize in main, right, or left PVs

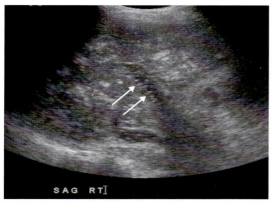

Fig. 177.10

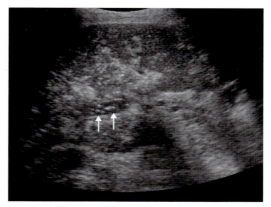

Fig. 177.11

Note multiple tiny echogenic "dots" or bubbles of gas in the main PV (arrows in Fig. 177.10) and right PV (arrows in Fig. 177.11). Although some of the peripheral hyperechoic foci are linear, much of the echogenic gas has a more infiltrative or diffuse pattern as it permeates into the liver parenchyma.

- Pencil-thin vertical "spikes" on spectral Doppler PV waveform
  - Considered a pathognomonic finding for bubbles of gas in the PV

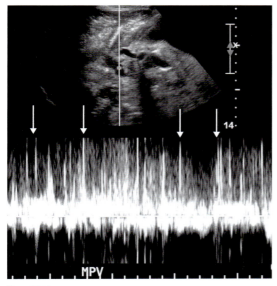

Fig. 177.12

This 58-year-old female presented with severe abdominal pain. Note numerous thin vertical spikes (arrows in Fig. 177.12) on spectral Doppler waveform in the main portal vein (MPV), an artifact due to the high reflectivity of the gas bubbles in the MPV.

► Pneumobilia
- Branching echogenic linear structures in liver
- Adjacent to PV
- Will not fill in with color
- Typically more central rather than peripheral within the hepatic parenchyma
- Normal PV spectral Doppler waveform
- Patients less severely ill, often s/p interventions such as common bile duct (CBD) exploration, endoscopic retrograde cholangiopancreatography, or CBD stent placement

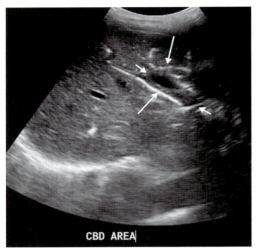

Fig. 177.13

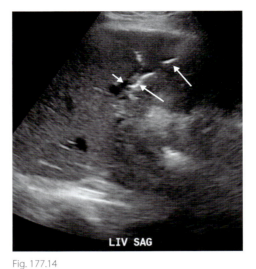

Fig. 177.14

In this patient status post cholecystectomy and common bile duct exploration, linear echogenic streaks of air are seen in the intrahepatic bile ducts (long arrows in Figs. 177.13 and 177.14), adjacent to the anechoic portal veins (short arrows in Figs. 177.13 and 177.14).

▶ Heavily calcified hepatic arteries
- Branching linear echogenic structures within hepatic parenchyma
- May be quite focal and "dot-like"
- Central or peripheral
- Two parallel echogenic lines
- Posterior shadowing sharper and denser than "dirty" shadowing from air
- Normal PV spectral Doppler waveform
- Asymptomatic
- Evidence of severe peripheral vascular disease elsewhere

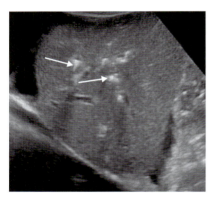

Fig. 177.15

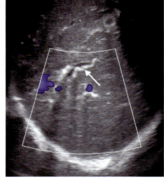

Fig. 177.16

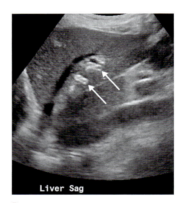

Fig. 177.17

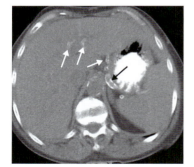

Fig. 177.18

Note numerous echogenic foci with ring-down or comet tail artifact associated with the portal triads in a 68-year-old female presenting with abdominal pain (arrows in Fig. 177.15). On a more longitudinal plane, these elongate and roughly parallel the PVs but are more irregular and tortuous (arrow in Fig. 177.16) than pneumobilia, which would also give rise to linear echogenicity in the portal triads adjacent to the PVs. Further imaging demonstrates two parallel echogenic lines (arrows in Fig. 177.17) separated by a hypoechoic layer consistent with calcification in the hepatic arterial walls, as confirmed on non-contrast-enhanced CT scan (Fig. 177.18) demonstrating mural calcification in the left intrahepatic and extrahepatic main hepatic arteries (white arrows). The splenic artery is also heavily calcified (black arrow in Fig. 177.18).

Management

▶ Dependent on etiology and clinical presentation

▶ Contrast-enhanced CT and/or CT angiography to confirm findings and assess the bowel, followed by surgery in acutely ill patients with possible bowel ischemia

Acknowledgment

Figure 177.12 reprinted with permission from Scoutt LM. Ultrasound: Vascular in Approach to Diagnosis: A Case-Based Imaging Review. In: Baumgarten DA, Bhalla S, Salkowski LR, et al., eds. ARRS, Reston VA; 11–27, Image D.

Further Reading

1. Sebastia C, Quiroga S, Espin E, et al. Portomesenteric vein gas: Pathologic mechanisms, CT findings, and prognosis. *RadioGraphics*. 2000; 20: 1213–1224.
2. Oktar SO, Karaosmanoğlu D, Yücel C, et al. Portomesenteric venous gas: Imaging findings with an emphasis on sonography. *J Ultrasound Med*. 2006; 23: 1051–1058.

Case 178

History

▶ 57-Year-old male with liver cirrhosis and prior placement of a transjugular intrahepatic portosystemic (TIPS) shunt presents with newly appearing ascites (Figs. 178.1–178.4)

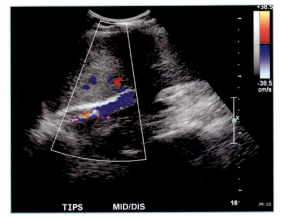

Fig. 178.1

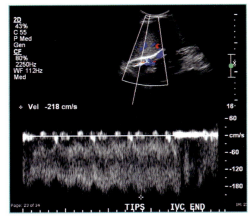

Fig. 178.2

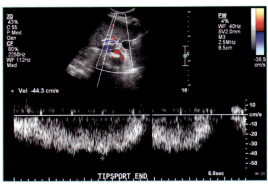

Fig. 178.3

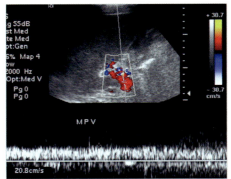

Fig. 178.4

Case 178 Transjugular Intrahepatic Portosystemic Shunt (TIPS) Stenosis

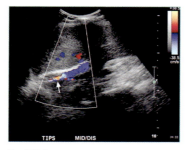

Fig. 178.5

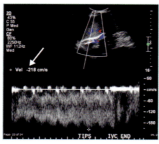

Fig. 178.6

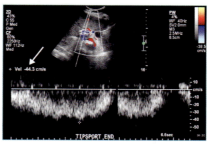

Fig. 178.7

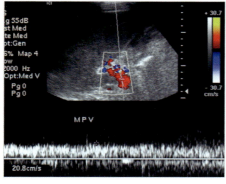

Fig. 178.8

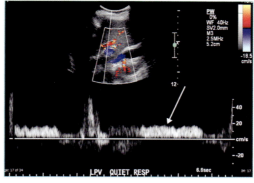

Fig. 178.9

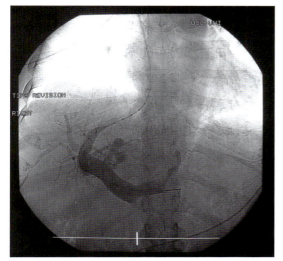

Fig. 178.10

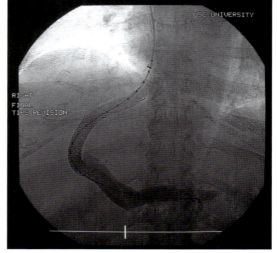

Fig. 178.11

Imaging Findings

▶ Narrowed lumen, color aliasing, and elevated peak systolic velocities (218 cm/s) in the distal TIPS shunt near the hepatic venous end (arrows in Figs. 178.5 and 178.6)

▶ Markedly decreased velocity in the proximal shunt (44 cm/s) with velocity gradient of 147 cm/s across the shunt (arrow in Fig. 178.7)

▶ Slow-velocity flow (21 cm/s) in the main portal vein (MPV) (Fig. 178.8)

▶ Hepatopetal flow in the left portal vein (LPV) (arrow in Fig.178.9)

▶ Newly appearing ascites

▶ Angiographic revision with angioplasty and additional stent graft placement (Figs. 178.10 and 178.11)

Differential Diagnosis

► Normal study
► TIPS thrombosis

Teaching Points

► TIPS shunts: preferred alternative to surgical portosystemic shunts for complications of portal hypertension (variceal bleeding, intractable ascites)
► Placement of metallic stent between hepatic and portal vein to divert blood flow from high-pressure portal venous into system circulation
  ▪ Avoids major surgery
  ▪ No alteration in extrahepatic vascular anatomy
► Indications
  ▪ Variceal bleeding
  ▪ Intractable ascites
  ▪ Intractable pleural effusion
  ▪ Budd–Chiari syndrome
  ▪ Hepatorenal syndrome
  ▪ Bridge to transplantation
► Contraindications
  ▪ Severe hepatic encephalopathy
  ▪ Right-sided heart failure
► TIPS stenosis: thought to be primarily secondary to neointimal or pseudointimal hyperplasia; much more common on the hepatic venous side of the shunt
► Doppler US criteria suggesting TIPS stenosis
  ▪ Reappearance of gastroesophageal varices, reaccumulation of ascites, pleural effusion
  ▪ Failure to fill the entire lumen with flow on color flow imaging
  ▪ Elevated velocities within the TIPS > 200 cm/s with a gradient between proximal, mid, and distal portions (> 50 cm/s)
  ▪ Decreased velocity in the main portal vein (< 30 cm/s)
  ▪ Velocity in TIPS < 50–60 cm/s
  ▪ Either increase or decrease in TIPS velocity by 50–60 cm/s since prior exam
  ▪ Hepatopetal flow within the right and left portal veins
► Early experience involved placement of bare stents with patency rate of only 40–60% one year after placement
► Expanded polytetrafluoroethylene (PTFE)-covered stents are now used exclusively with a patency rate of 80–90% one year after placement
► Normal US findings after placement of a TIPS shunt or stent
  ▪ Color or power Doppler flow identified within the entirety of the shunt
  ▪ Normal velocities within the shunt: from 90 to 190 cm/s or from 100 to 200 cm/s
  ▪ No gradient within the shunt (< 50 cm/s variation in velocity)
  ▪ Hepatopetal flow within the MPV (i.e., toward the shunt) with elevated velocities within the MPV (> 40 cm/s)
  ▪ Hepatofugal flow in the right and left portal veins (i.e., toward the shunt)
► TIPS occlusion: no flow in the shunt on color, power, or spectral Doppler US
  ▪ Decreased and/or reversed flow in MPV
  ▪ Hepatopetal flow in LPV

Management

► Selected cases of TIPS stenosis can be treated with balloon angioplasty or thrombolysis as well as additional stent graft placement
► If interrogating PTFE-covered stents immediately post placement, be aware of an artifact with shadowing caused by air bubbles embedded within the wall of the stent that may mimic thrombosis
  ▪ Delay baseline study until 48–72 h

Further Reading

1. Benito A, Bilbao J, Martinez-Cuesta A, et al. Doppler ultrasound for TIPS: Does it work? *Abdominal Imaging*. 2003; 29: 45–52.
2. Sajja KC, Dolmatch BL, Rockey DC. Long term follow-up of TIPS created with expanded poly-tetrafluoroethylene covered stents. *Dig Dis Sci*. 2013; 58(7): 2100–2106.

History

▶ 82-Year-old female presenting with sepsis and abnormal liver function tests (Figs. 179.1–179.4)

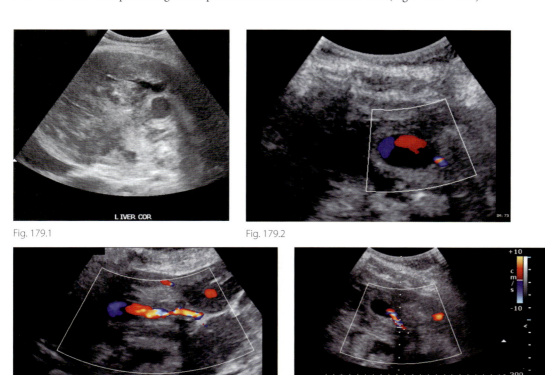

Fig. 179.1

Fig. 179.2

Fig. 179.3

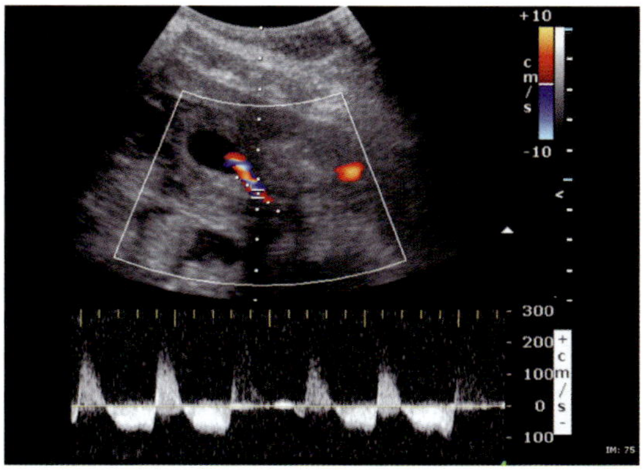

Fig. 179.4

Case 179 Mycotic Pseudoaneurysm Arising From the Main Hepatic Artery

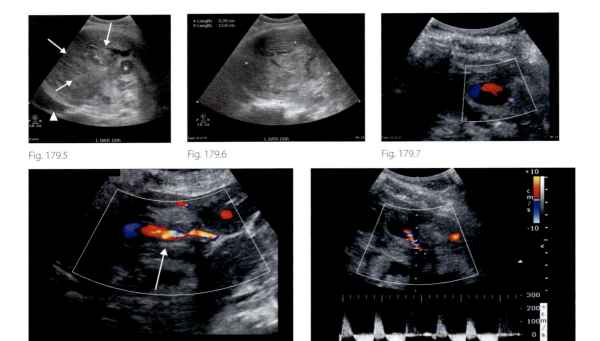

Fig. 179.5

Fig. 179.6

Fig. 179.7

Fig. 179.8

Fig. 179.9

Imaging Findings

▶ Large heterogeneous echogenic ill-defined area in the right lobe of the liver consistent with parenchymal hemorrhage (arrows in Fig. 179.5; calipers in Fig. 179.6)
▶ Small right pleural effusion (arrowhead in Fig. 179.5)
▶ Note adjacent round, anechoic cystic structure (asterisk in Fig. 179.5) that fills in on color Doppler imaging (Fig. 179.7) with a swirling, "yin-yang" pattern consistent with a pseudoaneurysm (PSA)
▶ There is a long neck (arrow in Fig. 179.8) to the PSA with a pulsatile bidirectional "to-and-fro" spectral Doppler waveform (Fig. 179.9)
▶ The neck could be traced back to the main hepatic artery (HA) (not shown)
▶ The patient subsequently died secondary to rupture of the PSA

Differential Diagnosis

▶ Hepatic artery aneurysm
▶ Hepatic hematoma secondary to trauma or rupture/bleeding from a liver mass such as an adenoma, hepatocellular carcinoma, or metastasis

Teaching Points

▶ PSAs of the HAs can occur following trauma, iatrogenic injury from endovascular interventions, liver transplantation, infection, pancreatitis, and connective tissue disease (e.g., polyarteritis nodosa)
▶ The wall of a PSA is composed of either compacted surrounding soft tissues or only one or two of the three arterial layers: intima, media, and adventitia
▶ US findings
  ▪ Anechoic, round cystic structure
  ▪ Internal echoes if partially or completely thrombosed
  ▪ Swirling blood flow pattern on color Doppler, termed "yin-yang" appearance
  ▪ Vascular channel or neck connecting PSA to artery of origin
    • Neck may be thick or thin

- Spectral Doppler waveform from a thin neck will demonstrate a "to-and-fro" pattern, with flow heading toward the PSA during systole and away from the PSA during diastole
- Highly variable waveform pattern in a thick neck
- Rupture may result in surrounding parenchymal hemorrhage
  - Heterogeneous, often echogenic, although echogenicity will depend on time course
- HA aneurysm
  - Fourth most common site of intra-abdominal aneurysms
  - 80% present with catastrophic rupture
  - A true aneurysm has a full-thickness arterial wall composed of all three arterial layers
  - Arise directly from the HA
    - Focal or fusiform
    - No "yin-yang" flow pattern
    - No neck or "to-and-fro" spectral Doppler waveform pattern
- Spontaneous hepatic hemorrhage
  - Echogenicity variable depending on time course:
  - Most common causes: trauma (including iatrogenic) or underlying hepatic mass (adenoma, hepatocellular carcinoma, and metastasis)
    - Linear anechoic laceration variably present in setting of trauma
    - Underlying hepatic mass may be masked by hemorrhage

Management

- Treatment of mycotic PSAs consists of long-term antibiotic therapy and coil embolization
- Emergent surgery or percutaneous intervention in the setting of rupture and massive hemorrhage

Further Reading

1. Casillas VJ, Amendola MA, Gascue A, et al. Imaging of nontraumatic hemorrhagic hepatic lesions. *RadioGraphics*. 2000; 20: 367–378.
2. O'Driscoll D, Olliff SP, Olliff JF. Hepatic artery aneurysm. *Br J Radiol*. 1999; 72: 1018–1025.

Case 180

► 36-Year-old male, day 4 status post renal transplantation, who presents with pain over transplant and oliguria (Figs. 180.1–180.6)

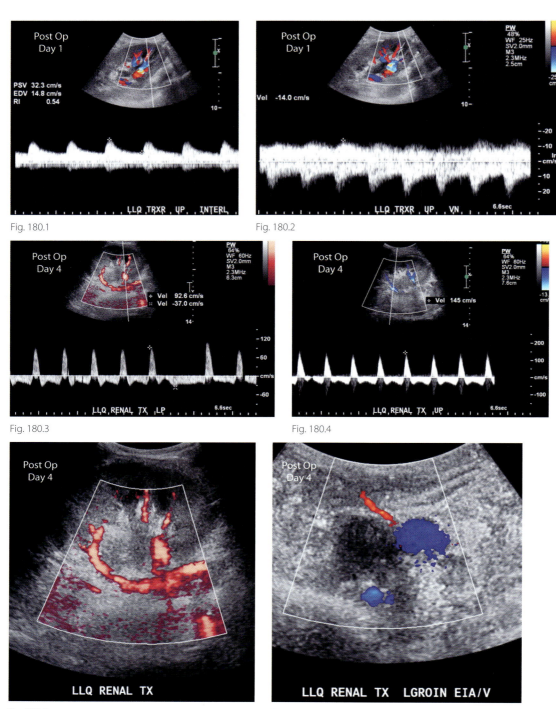

Fig. 180.1

Fig. 180.2

Fig. 180.3

Fig. 180.4

Fig. 180.5

Fig. 180.6

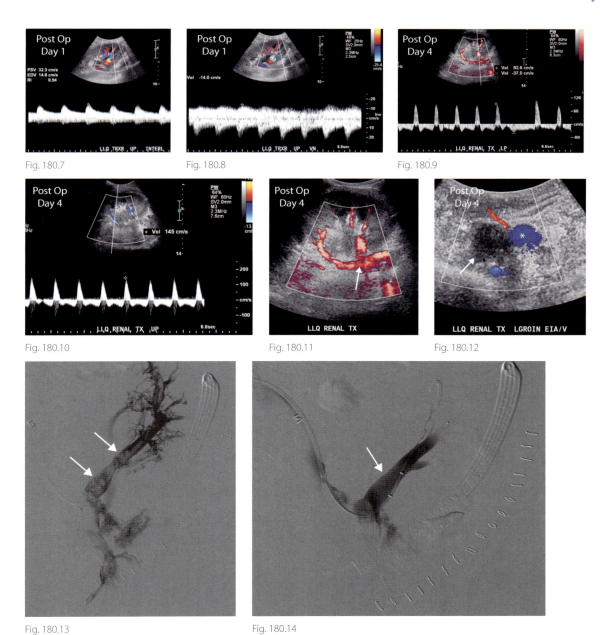

Fig. 180.7

Fig. 180.8

Fig. 180.9

Fig. 180.10

Fig. 180.11

Fig. 180.12

Fig. 180.13

Fig. 180.14

Imaging Findings

▶ Spectral Doppler waveforms in the intraparenchymal renal arteries (Fig. 180.7 and below baseline on Fig. 180.8) are normal on postoperative day 1 with continuous forward diastolic flow and a resistive index (RI) of 0.54. Normal intraparenchymal venous flow is also present (caliper in Fig. 180.8, above baseline)

▶ On postoperative day 4, the arterial waveforms are markedly abnormal with reversed diastolic flow (Figs. 180.9 and 180.10). No intraparenchymal venous flow was detectable. In the absence of venous flow, this arterial waveform pattern is highly suggestive of renal vein thrombosis

▶ Power Doppler image (Fig. 180.11) reveals a single vessel (arrow) in the renal hilum, confirmed to be the renal artery on spectral Doppler (not shown). The main renal vein could not be identified

▶ Transverse color Doppler image (Fig. 180.12) demonstrating flow in the recipient external iliac artery (asterisk). No flow is seen in the external iliac vein (arrow), which is distended with hypoechoic thrombus

- After several hours of thrombolysis, venogram (Fig. 180.13) demonstrates non-occlusive filling defects in the main renal vein (arrows), consistent with renal vein thrombosis
- Following several more hours of catheter-directed thrombolysis, there was complete resolution of the thrombus in the main renal vein (arrow in Fig. 180.14)

Differential Diagnosis

- Compression of renal parenchyma by subcapsular fluid collection (Page kidney phenomenon)
- Hyperacute rejection
- Acute tubular necrosis (ATN)
- Renal artery thrombosis

Teaching Points

- Renal vein thrombosis (RVT) occurs in 1–4% of renal transplants
  - Most often within the first postoperative week
  - If not treated, will result in graft loss
- Presentation
  - Acute pain over allograft
  - Hematuria
  - Abrupt cessation of urine output
- Risk factors
  - Hypercoagulable states
  - Hypovolemia, hypotension
  - Kinking of vascular pedicle
  - Compression of renal vein by mass/fluid collection such as hematoma or lymphocele
  - Technical difficulties at surgery
  - Propagation of common femoral or external iliac vein thrombosis
- US findings
  - Enlarged allograft
  - Effacement of the renal sinus and pelvis, loss of corticomedullary differentiation, and decreased parenchymal echogenicity
  - Absence of flow in the parenchymal and main renal veins on color, power, and spectral Doppler US
  - Main renal vein distended with echogenic, hypoechoic, or even anechoic thrombus, depending on time course
  - Reversal of diastolic flow in the intraparenchymal and main renal arteries

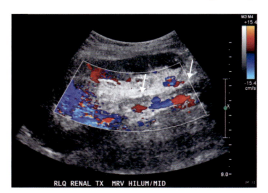

Fig. 180.15

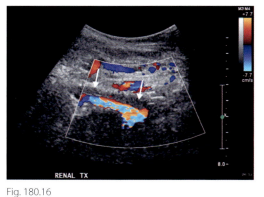

Fig. 180.16

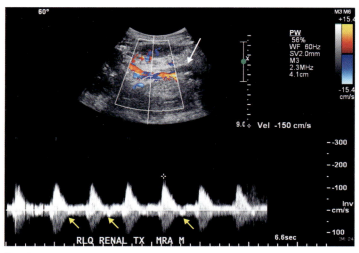
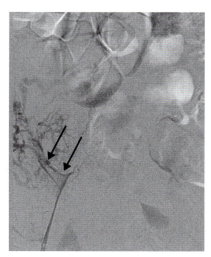

Fig. 180.17   Fig. 180.18

Color Doppler US images of the transplanted kidney in the right lower quadrant demonstrating absence of flow in the main renal vein (white arrows in Figs. 180.15–180.17), which is filled with hypoechoic thrombus. Spectral Doppler waveform of the main renal artery (Fig. 180.17) has a high resistance pattern with a short period of flow reversal in early diastole (yellow arrows). Venogram demonstrates filling defects in the main renal vein (arrows in Fig. 180.18), confirming the diagnosis of RVT.

▶ Reversed diastolic flow in the renal arteries is a nonspecific finding indicating increased peripheral vascular resistance
  ▪ If venous flow is preserved, consider hyperacute rejection, severe ATN, and peritransplant fluid collection (usually subcapsular hematoma) compressing the renal parenchyma or hilar vessels (Page kidney phenomenon)
    • Hyperacute rejection extraordinarily rare due to HLA matching
    • Severe ATN uncommon in living related donor transplants without major intraoperative complications
    • Surgical decompression warranted for subcapsular fluid collections that compress or deform the renal parenchyma resulting in reversal of diastolic flow
▶ Renal artery thrombosis
  ▪ Occurs in < 1% of renal transplants
  ▪ Presents with pain and anuria
  ▪ Risk factors: vessel size mismatch, small vessels (more common in pediatric transplants), hypercoagulable states, hypotension, hypovolemia, and kinking of vessel
  ▪ US findings: no arterial or venous flow in the main renal artery, main renal vein, or in the parenchymal vessels
  ▪ Surgical emergency

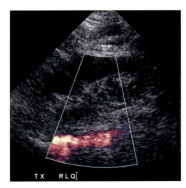
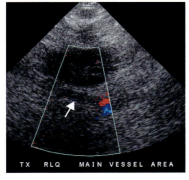
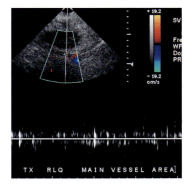

Fig. 180.19   Fig. 180.20   Fig. 180.21

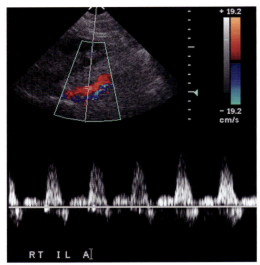

Fig. 180.22

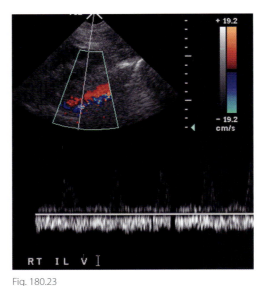

Fig. 180.23

This 54-year-old female presented with acute onset of anuria 10 hours post renal transplantation. No vascularity is noted in the renal hilum or parenchyma on power Doppler (Fig. 180.19). There is a hypoechoic tubular structure in the region of the vascular pedicle (arrow in Fig. 180.20) without evidence of blood flow on color (Fig. 180.20) or spectral Doppler (Fig. 180.21), consistent with thrombosis of the main renal artery. Note normal waveforms in the recipient external iliac artery (Fig. 180.22) and vein (Fig. 180.23).

Management

► Non-occlusive RVT: systemic anticoagulation
► Occlusive RVT: surgical exploration with thrombectomy or percutaneous thrombolysis
► If diagnosis is delayed, nephrectomy of a nonviable graft is necessary to prevent superinfection

Further Reading

1. Sutherland T, Temple F, Chang S, et al. Sonographic evaluation of renal transplant complications. *J Med Imaging Radiat Oncol.* 2010; 54: 211–218.
2. Hedegard W, Saad WEA, Davies MG. Management of vascular and nonvascular complications after renal transplantation. *Tech Vasc Interventional Rad.* 2009; 12: 240–262.
3. Rodgers SK, Sereni CP, Horrow MM. Ultrasonographic evaluation of the renal transplant. *Radiol Clin North Am.* 2014; 52: 1307–1324.
4. Zarzour JG, Lockhart ME. Ultrasonography of the renal transplant. *US Clinics.* 2014; 9(4): 683–695.

History

▶ 44-Year-old male presents with delayed graft function postoperative day 2 following deceased donor renal transplantation with approximately 18 hours of cold ischemic time for the renal allograft (Figs. 181.1–181.3)

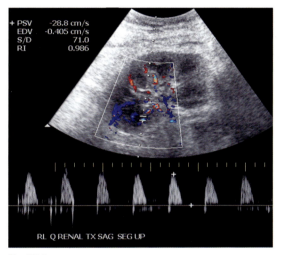

Fig. 181.1

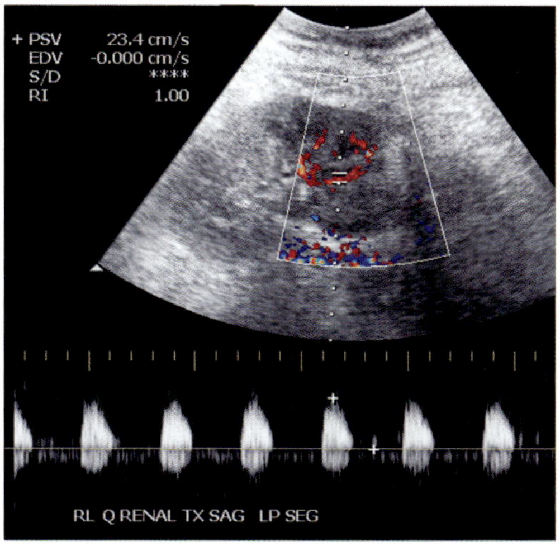

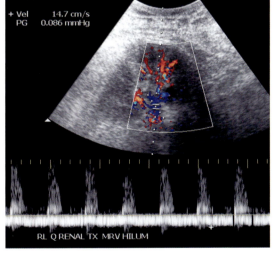

Fig. 181.2

Fig. 181.3

Case 181 Acute Tubular Necrosis in a Renal Transplant

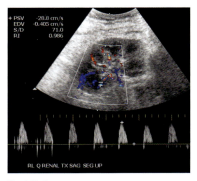

Fig. 181.4

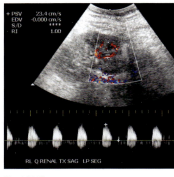

Fig. 181.5

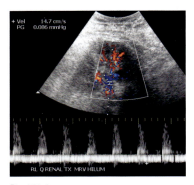

Fig. 181.6

Imaging Findings

▶ Spectral Doppler US images show elevated resistive indices (RI) (1.0) with complete absence of diastolic flow in the parenchymal arteries in the upper and lower poles of the transplanted kidney (Figs. 181.4 and 181.5)

▶ The main renal vein is patent (Fig. 181.6)

Differential Diagnosis

▶ Renal vein thrombosis
▶ Hyperacute or acute rejection
▶ Perinephric fluid collection resulting in Page kidney physiology

Teaching Points

▶ Acute tubular necrosis (ATN) is a major cause of delayed graft function in renal transplants
  ▪ Most commonly presents within the first 3 days postoperatively
  ▪ More common post deceased donor rather than living related donor transplantation
  ▪ Incidence increasing as donor criteria have been expanded due to organ shortage to allow transplantation of kidneys from sicker patients
    • "Stressed" kidneys will develop ATN earlier and more severely
▶ Risk factors
  ▪ Prolonged cold ischemic time
  ▪ Transplantation of stressed kidney from older donor, especially with prolonged, debilitating illness
  ▪ Excessive blood loss or hypotension during surgery
▶ US findings
  ▪ Elevated RIs, > 0.70–0.80 in parenchymal arteries (± main renal artery depending on severity)
  ▪ Diastolic flow can be completely absent and even reversed in severe cases
  ▪ Normal venous flow
  ▪ Swelling of allograft
  ▪ Cortical echogenicity may be increased or decreased, ± loss of renal sinus echoes
▶ Other causes of absent or reversed diastolic flow in the early postoperative state include the following
  ▪ Renal vein thrombosis (RVT)
  ▪ Large perinephric or subcapsular fluid collections (Page kidney physiology)
  ▪ Hyperacute rejection
  ▪ Severe hydronephrosis
  ▪ Acute rejection and drug toxicity
    • Usually occur after 10–14 days
▶ The main role of US in evaluating a patient with delayed graft function in the early postoperative period is to exclude the previously mentioned causes of graft dysfunction and elevated RI
  ▪ Identification of venous flow in the main and parenchymal renal veins excludes RVT
    • Diastolic flow usually reversed with RVT
    • Distinction is critical because RVT requires immediate thrombectomy or anticoagulation

- A perinephric or subcapsular fluid collection that compresses or distorts the renal cortex will be observed in patients with Page kidney physiology
  - Increased peripheral vascular resistance accounts for the decreased diastolic flow: decreased, absent, or reversed depending on severity
  - IR drainage or surgical decompression may be required if renal function is impaired
- Dilatation of the intrarenal collecting system is diagnostic of hydronephrosis
  - Rx: nephrostomy or ureteral stent
- Hyperacute rejection is extremely uncommon but usually occurs intraoperatively or immediately postoperatively and is a diagnosis of exclusion
  - Arterial and venous flow may be difficult to detect, likely due to a combination of thrombosis of the vessels and severe vasospasm, mimicking renal artery thrombosis
- Acute rejection and drug toxicity are rare before days 10–14 post-transplantation
  - Decreased diastolic flow much more common than absent or reversed flow
- Imaging features of ATN, drug toxicity, and hyperacute or acute rejection are almost identical on grayscale and on color and spectral Doppler US

Management

- Biopsy is indicated in differentiating ATN, acute rejection, and drug toxicity
- Supportive therapy
- Dialysis

Further Reading

1. Akbar SA, Jafri SZ, Amendola MA, et al. Complications of renal transplantation. *RadioGraphics*. 2005; 25: 1335–1356.
2. Sutherland T, Temple F, Chang S, et al. Sonographic evaluation of renal transplant complications. *J Med Imaging Radiat Oncol*. 2010; 54: 211–218.

Case 182

► 47-Year-old male with right lower quadrant renal transplant 1 month ago presents with worsening renal function (Figs. 182.1–182.4)

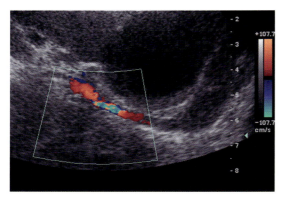

Fig. 182.1

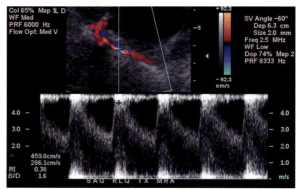

Fig. 182.2

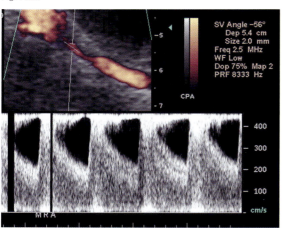

Fig. 182.3

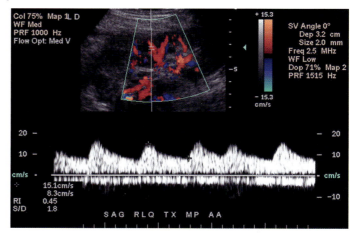

Fig. 182.4

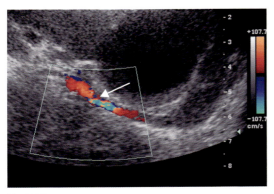

Fig. 182.5

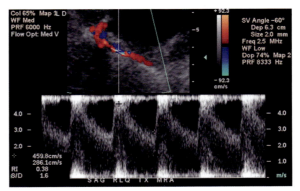

Fig. 182.6

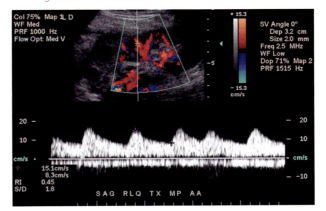

Fig. 182.7

Fig. 182.8

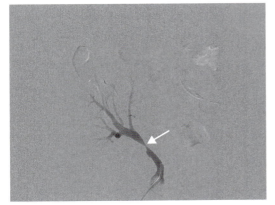

Fig. 182.9

Fig. 182.10

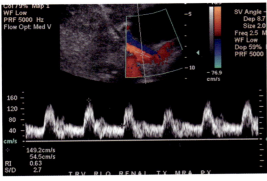

Fig. 182.11

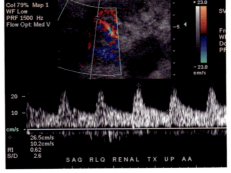

Fig. 182.12

Imaging Findings

▶ Narrowing of the main renal artery to the transplant on color and power Doppler US (arrows in Figs. 182.5 and 182.7) with aliasing and elevated peak systolic velocities (PSV) of 459.8 cm/s (Fig. 182.6)
▶ Tardus parvus waveform in the intraparenchymal renal artery (Fig. 182.8)
▶ Narrowing of the main renal transplant artery on pre-angioplasty angiogram (arrow in Fig. 182.9). The patient underwent successful dilatation of the transplant renal artery (arrow in Fig. 182.10)
▶ Normal spectral Doppler waveform of the main renal transplant artery post angioplasty with PSV of 149 cm/s (Fig. 182.11) and normalized waveforms with normal sharp systolic upstroke in the intrarenal parenchymal vessels (Fig. 182.12)

Differential Diagnosis

▶ Arteriovenous fistula
▶ Torqueing
▶ Compartment syndrome
▶ Iliac artery stenosis

Teaching Points

▶ Most common vascular complication following renal transplantation, occurring in up to 10% of cases
  ▪ More common following living related donor transplantation rather than deceased donor
▶ Typically at the surgical anastomosis of the vessel
▶ Can result in persistent hypertension and graft dysfunction, but often discovered during surveillance when patient is asymptomatic
▶ US findings
  ▪ Narrowing of the vessel on grayscale or color Doppler US
  ▪ Focal aliasing on color or spectral Doppler within the transplant main renal artery with elevated PSV (typically > 250 cm/s)
  ▪ Increased ratio of the PSV of the transplant main renal artery relative to the iliac artery (typically > 2:1)
  ▪ Delayed systolic upstrokes in intrarenal spectral Doppler waveforms causing a "tardus parvus" (TP) waveform
▶ Increase in PSV of the transplant artery is sensitive for renal artery stenosis (RAS); however, not specific. Specificity increased when TP waveform is present in intraparenchymal vessels
▶ Arteriovenous fistula: occurs usually after a renal biopsy, demonstrating a US "color bruit" (disorganized color flow vascularity adjacent to the site of the fistula) with arterialization of the vein and increased velocities and diastolic flow within the artery. Would not show TP waveform
▶ Other causes of increased PSV post renal transplantation
  ▪ Normal due to increased flow, angle of origin, edema around anastomosis (transient); would not see TP waveform in parenchymal vessels
  ▪ Torqueing, compression, compartment syndrome, rare, immediate post-op, can cause graft dysfunction. Usually associated with increased velocity and narrowing of main renal vein; might see TP waveform in intraparenchymal vessels
  ▪ Iliac artery stenosis might cause TP waveform but not narrowing or increased velocity in MRA, although if close to the anastomosis could be confused with renal artery stenosis at the anastomosis

Management

▶ In most cases, transplant RAS can be treated with angiography with balloon angioplasty
▶ Refractory cases following unsuccessful angioplasty may require surgical revision

Further Reading

1. Jimenez C, Lopez MO, Gonzalez E, et al. Ultrasonography in kidney transplantation: Values and new developments. *Transplant Rev.* 2009; 23(4): 209–213.
2. Krishnamoorthy S, Gopalakrishnan G, Kekre NS, et al. Detection and treatment of transplant renal artery stenosis. *Indian J Urol.* 2009; 24(1): 56–61.

History

▶ 35-Year-old female with a left lower quadrant renal transplant and status post percutaneous biopsy for renal failure (Figs. 183.1–183.3)

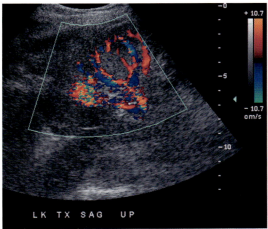

Fig. 183.1

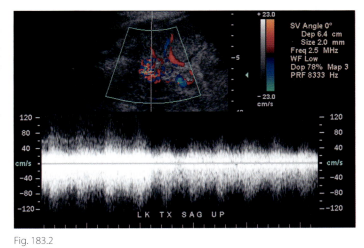

Fig. 183.2

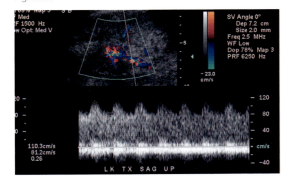

Fig. 183.3

Case 183 Post-Biopsy Arteriovenous Fistula in a Renal Transplant

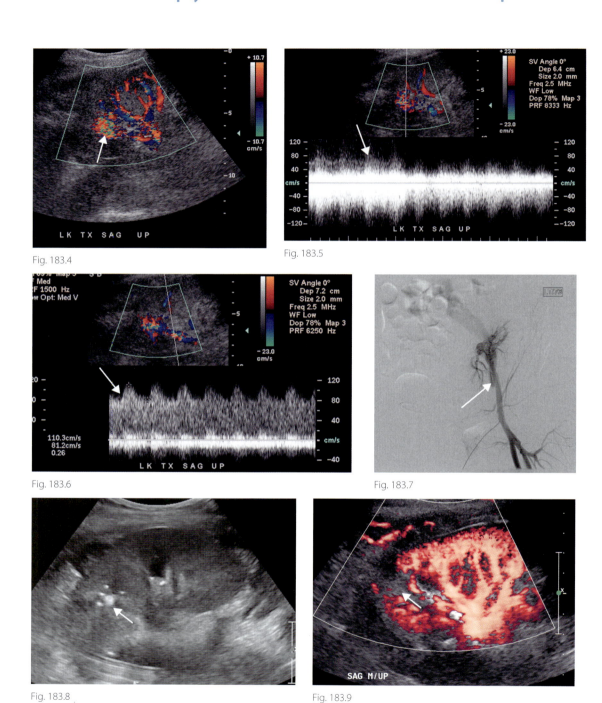

Fig. 183.4

Fig. 183.5

Fig. 183.6

Fig. 183.7

Fig. 183.8

Fig. 183.9

Imaging Findings

▶ Focal area of increased color flow on color Doppler US (CDUS) with color mosaic/aliasing in the upper pole of the left lower quadrant transplanted kidney indicative of a sonographic soft tissue bruit due to soft tissue vibration and pressure changes (arrow in Fig. 183.4)

▶ Note pulsatile increased velocity flow in draining vein (arrow in Fig. 183.5) and low-resistance waveform in the feeding artery with increased systolic and diastolic flow (arrow in Fig. 183.6)

- Note early draining vein on angiogram (arrow in Fig. 183.7)
- Post-embolization US demonstrates echogenic foci from coils (arrow in Fig. 183.8) and successful embolization with absence of flow in the previous upper pole arteriovenous fistula (AVF), resulting in focal area of infarction (arrow in Fig. 183.9)

Differential Diagnosis

- Transplant post-biopsy pseudoaneurysm (PSA)
- Transplant renal artery stenosis (RAS)

Teaching Points

- Most common intrarenal complication and following renal biopsies, typically when the biopsy needle traverses both a small artery and a vein
  - Incidence relates to the size of the needle and location of the biopsy; higher if needle tip is in renal sinus, and lower if in renal cortex
  - Association with the development of a pseudoaneurysm
- US findings
  - Grayscale: may see dilated venous outflow, mimicking small renal cyst or PSA
  - Color Doppler: aliasing at the site of the AVF, including in the adjacent soft tissues (sonographic soft tissue "bruit"), color mosaic
  - Spectral Doppler: low resistive indices near the site of the AVF
  - Elevated velocities and spectral broadening in the involved artery
  - "Arterialization" of the venous waveform of the draining vein
  - Waveforms at other parenchymal locations may be normal
- Post-biopsy PSA: cystic structure at the site of biopsy with "yin-yang" appearance on CDUS and "to-and-fro" flow within the neck of the PSA. Waveforms in adjacent/feeding arteries or draining veins will be normal. Could see soft tissue bruit due to high-velocity flow, although less common than with AVF
- RAS: suspected when the peak systolic velocity in the renal artery (RA) is
  - 250 cm/s with a velocity gradient between RA and iliac artery > 2:1
  - Tardus parvus waveform seen downstream
  - Uncommon to see color soft tissue bruit due to high-velocity flow at the site of stenosis

Management

- 70% of renal AVFs are relatively small and spontaneously resolve, making conservative management the appropriate primary choice in the majority of patients
- Large AVFs can result in hypertension, congestive heart failure, hematuria, and loss of graft function, thus requiring treatment via the following
  - Endovascular embolization
  - Surgery reserved for cases unsuccessfully treated by endovascular embolization

Further Reading

1. Lorenzen J, Schneider A, Regier M, et al. Post-biopsy arteriovenous fistula in transplant kidney: Treatment with superselective transcatheter embolization. *Eur J Radiol*. 2012; 81(5): e721–e726.
2. Deane C, Cowan N, Giles J, et al. Arteriovenous fistulas in renal transplants: Color Doppler ultrasound observations. *Urol Radiol*. 1992; 13: 211–217.

Case 184

History

▶ 46-Year-old male with renal transplant presents with hematuria 1 week following renal biopsy for worsening renal function (Figs. 184.1–184.4)

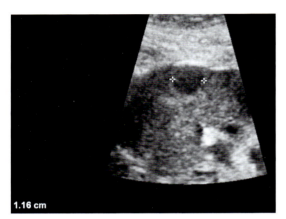

Fig. 184.1

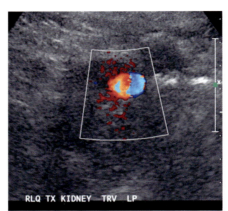

Fig. 184.2

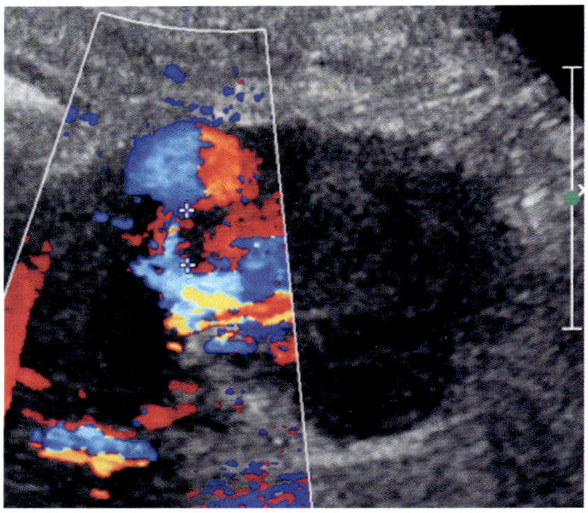

Fig. 184.3

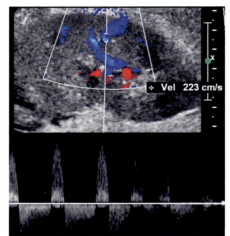

Fig. 184.4

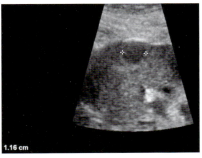

Fig. 184.5

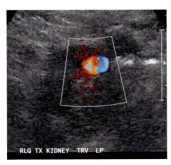

Fig. 184.6

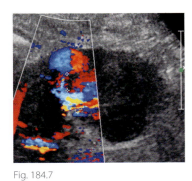

Fig. 184.7

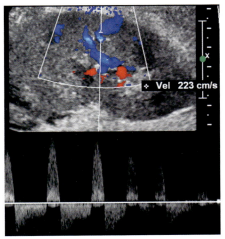

Fig. 184.8

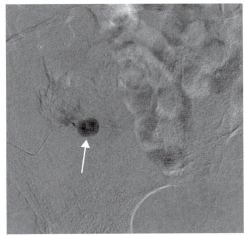

Fig. 184.9

Imaging Findings

▶ Anechoic, round 1.2-cm structure (calipers in Fig. 184.5) in the renal parenchyma with slight increased through-transmission fills in with color in a classic pseudoaneurysm (PSA) "yin-yang" color Doppler pattern (blue on one side and red on the other; Fig. 184.6)
▶ The neck (calipers in Fig. 184.7) demonstrates a "to-and-fro" spectral Doppler waveform pattern (Fig. 184.8) with flow going toward the PSA in systole and below the baseline or away from the PSA during diastole
▶ Digital subtraction angiogram (Fig. 184.9) demonstrating the PSA (arrow) prior to embolization

Differential Diagnosis

▶ Arteriovenous fistula
▶ Extrarenal pseudoaneurysm

Teaching Points

▶ Pseudoaneurysms (PSAs) and arteriovenous fistulas (AVFs) are well-recognized complications of percutaneous biopsy of renal transplant allografts
  ▪ AVFs more common than PSAs
  ▪ PSAs occur when there is laceration of the arterial wall
  ▪ AVFs result from simultaneous injury to an intrarenal artery and vein
▶ Clinical presentation
  ▪ Asymptomatic, particularly if small
  ▪ Pain
  ▪ Gross hematuria occurs in up to 5–7% of patients
    • Usually resolves spontaneously
    • Massive or persistent hematuria should alert the clinician to the possibility of a PSA or AVF

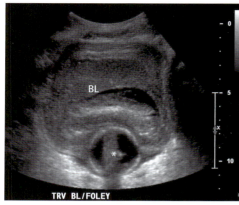

Fig. 184.10

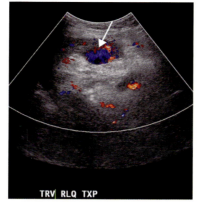

Fig. 184.11

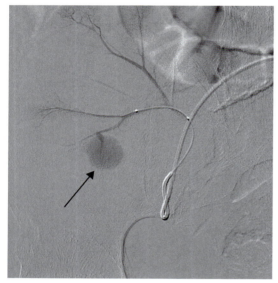

Fig. 184.12

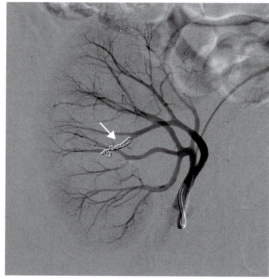

Fig. 184.13

This 66-year-old male presented with gross hematuria several weeks following biopsy of his renal transplant. The urinary bladder (BL) is almost completely filled with echogenic material, consistent with blood clot (Fig. 184.10). Foley catheter (asterisk). Color Doppler image of the transplanted kidney reveals a round vascular structure in the renal parenchyma (arrow in Fig. 184.11). Although the classic "yin-yang" color Doppler pattern of a PSA is not observed, there is no color aliasing or adjacent soft tissue color bruit to suggest high-velocity, turbulent flow as would be seen with an AVF. Selective digital subtraction angiogram (Fig. 184.12) demonstrates a contrast-filled outpouching (arrow) arising from an intrarenal artery, with no evidence of an early draining vein, consistent with a PSA. The feeding artery of the PSA was embolized using microcoils (arrow in Fig. 184.13) with no residual filling of the PSA.

▶ US findings of PSA
  ▪ Simple or complex, round anechoic to hypoechoic cystic structure on grayscale
  ▪ "Yin-yang" pattern on color Doppler, representing a flow vortex of swirling blood within a patent PSA sac
  ▪ Color void indicates thrombus within a partially thrombosed PSA
  ▪ "To-and-fro" spectral Doppler waveform pattern if the neck to the PSA is narrow, with flow heading toward the PSA during systole and away from the PSA during diastole
  ▪ A turbulent low-resistance spectral Doppler waveform pattern may be observed if the neck of the PSA is wide
  ▪ Exam should attempt to demonstrate the vessel of origin as well as the length and width of the neck. The neck of the PSA is most accurately evaluated on grayscale US because color blooming artifact will exaggerate size
▶ Diagnosis
  ▪ US is sufficient in most cases to diagnose a PSA and to differentiate a PSA from an AVF, although they may occur together
  ▪ Contrast-enhanced CT and MR usually not required
    • However, if performed, CT or MR will demonstrate a contrast-filled saccular arterial outpouching from an intrarenal artery
    • May help delineate exact location (main trunk or side branch), dimension of neck, and evaluate distal circulation (single end artery, multiple collateral vessels, or coexistent AVF)

- ► Arteriovenous fistulas
  - ■ Soft tissue color Doppler bruit due to perivascular tissue vibrations from high-velocity, turbulent flow
  - ■ Dilatation of draining vein may create a focal anechoic cystic area that fills in with color mimicking a PSA except that there will be no "yin-yang" color Doppler pattern of swirling blood flow and color aliasing is more likely to be observed
  - ■ Dilated "feeding" artery with high peak systolic and end diastolic velocity, a low-resistance spectral Doppler waveform pattern due to distal shunt/pressure gradient
  - ■ "Arterialization" of the spectral Doppler waveform in the draining vein with high-velocity pulsatile flow
- ► An extrarenal arterial PSA is a distinct entity
  - ■ Prevalence: < 1% of renal transplant patients
  - ■ Primarily occur at the arterial anastomosis
  - ■ Usually develop secondary to poor surgical technique and/or perivascular infection

Management

- ► Routine use of US to guide renal transplant biopsy to ensure biopsy of the lower pole parenchyma and thus avoid the larger hilar or extrarenal vessels has dramatically reduced the incidence of post biopsy complications such as AVFs and PSAs
  - ■ Currently, when AVFs and PSAs develop post biopsy, they arise from the intraparenchymal vessels and therefore tend to be small, posing less risk
- ► Many post biopsy PSAs will thrombose and resolve spontaneously
- ► Treatment recommended if the PSA is enlarging, persistent, arises from the main renal artery or hilar arteries (i.e., not surrounded by renal parenchyma), or is > 2 cm in diameter due to increased risk of rupture and hemorrhage
- ► Treatment options
  - ■ Selective embolization to minimize loss of functioning allograft tissue
  - ■ The arterial branch is embolized proximal and distal to the PSA neck
  - ■ Surgery, either partial or total nephrectomy, as a last resort

Acknowledgment

Figures 184.4 and 184.8 reprinted with permission from Mathur M, Ginat DT, Rubens D, Scoutt LM. Evaluation of organ transplants. In: Pellerito JS, Polak JF, eds. *Introduction to Vascular Ultrasonography*, 6th ed. New York: Elsevier; 2012: p. 592, Figure 34-14B.

Further Reading

1. Kobayashi K, Censullo ML, Rossman LL, et al. Interventional radiologic management of renal transplant dysfunction: Indications, limitations, and technical considerations. *RadioGraphics*. 2007; 27(4): 1109–1130.
2. Onur MR, Dogra V. Vascular complications of renal transplant. *Ultrasound Clin*. 2013; 8: 593–604.
3. Rodgers SK, Sereni CP, Horrow MM. Ultrasonographic evaluation of the renal transplant. *Radiol Clin North Am*. 2014; 52: 1307–1324.
4. Zarzour JG, Lockhart ME. Ultrasonography of the renal transplant. *US Clinics* 2014; 9(4): 683–695.

Case 185

History

▶ 18-Year-old male with liver failure 9 days post liver transplantation (Figs. 185.1–185.3)

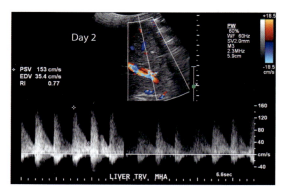

Fig. 185.1

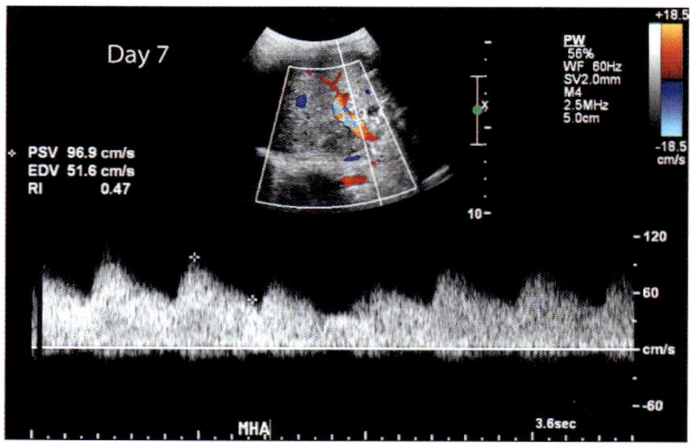

Fig. 185.2

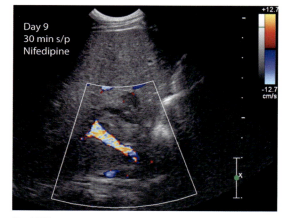

Fig. 185.3

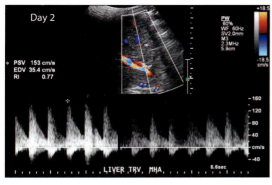

Fig. 185.4

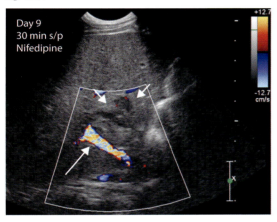

Fig. 185.6

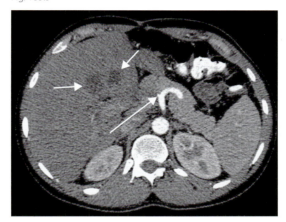

Fig. 185.7

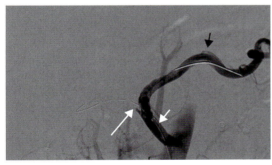

Fig. 185.8

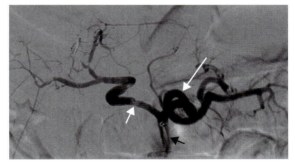

Fig. 185.9

Imaging Findings

▶ Postoperative day 2 (Fig. 185.4): main hepatic artery (MHA) waveform is essentially normal, with normal peak systolic velocity (PSV) and sharp systolic upstroke. Resistive index (RI) is slightly elevated at 0.77. The patient is tachycardic

▶ Postoperative day 7 (Fig. 185.5): interval development of a tardus parvus waveform with delayed systolic upstroke and diminished PSV in the MHA with increased diastolic flow and significantly decreased RI of 0.47

▶ Postoperative day 9 (Fig. 185.6): nonvisualization of MHA even following administration of nifedipine, a vasodilating agent; complex fluid collection (short arrows) in left hepatic lobe consistent with infarct/hematoma/abscess/biloma; patent main portal vein (long arrow)

▶ Thrombosis of common hepatic artery (HA) (long arrow in Fig. 185.7) at its origin from the celiac axis and complex fluid collection (short arrows) in the left lobe of the liver confirmed on CT angiogram

▶ Digital subtraction angiogram (Fig. 185.8) demonstrates complete occlusion of the HA (long white arrow) at its origin from the celiac axis (short white arrow); the splenic artery (black arrow) is patent.

► Angiogram (Fig. 185.9) demonstrating revascularization of the hepatic arterial tree following 4 days of transcatheter intra-arterial tissue plasminogen activator infusion. The main HA is now patent: note minor vessel diameter mismatch at the hepatic artery anastomosis (short white arrow); celiac axis (black arrow); splenic artery (long white arrow)

Differential Diagnosis

► Vasospasm
► High-grade hepatic artery stenosis (HAS)
► Hypotension
► Suboptimal study (obesity, ascites)

Teaching Points

► Occurs in up to 10% of liver transplant patients
  ▪ More common in children
  ▪ Second leading cause of graft failure in early postoperative period
  ▪ Significant mortality and graft loss if not treated
► Risk factors
  ▪ Increased cold ischemic time of donor liver
  ▪ Blood type incompatibility
  ▪ Small donor or recipient vessels, complex arterial reconstructions
  ▪ Hypotension
  ▪ Hypercoagulable states
  ▪ Acute rejection
  ▪ Hepatic artery stenosis
► Complications
  ▪ Because the hepatic artery provides the sole blood supply to the bile ducts in the transplanted liver, often complicated by bile duct ischemia/necrosis resulting in bile duct strictures, bilomas, abscesses
  ▪ Hepatic infarcts
  ▪ Liver failure
► Normal HA spectral Doppler waveform
  ▪ Rapid systolic upstroke with continuous forward diastolic flow and RI 0.5–0.7
  ▪ RIs < 0.4 are almost always due to proximal arterial stenosis or collateral flow from occlusion
► US findings
  ▪ No flow in MHA on color, spectral, or power Doppler
  ▪ Optimize technique: small color box, low wall filter, increase gain, low pulse repetition frequency (PRF), and low scale
  ▪ Evaluate main, right, and left HAs
  ▪ Children may develop arterial collaterals, typically having a tardus parvus pattern (acceleration time > 80 ms and a RI < 0.5)
  ▪ ± Biliary ductal dilatation, strictures
  ▪ ± Complex cystic liver lesions (bilomas, infarcts, abscesses)
► Tardus parvus HA waveforms or RI < 0.5 concerning for impending hepatic artery thrombosis (HAT) or HAS
  ▪ Most specific after 48 hours because reperfusion injury can cause similar waveforms
  ▪ Tardus parvus waveforms should prompt careful search for proximal HA stenosis
► Vasospasm, hypotension, poor acoustic windows, or severe HAS may result in false-positive diagnosis of HAT because Doppler US may not be able to detect extremely low-velocity, low-volume flow
  ▪ Reimaging following administration of nifedipine, a potent vasodilator, or intravenous US contrast agents (currently not approved by the U.S. Food and Drug Administration for this use) reduces false-positive Doppler examinations

Management

► Angiography (CT, magnetic resonance, or conventional) to confirm US findings or if US study suboptimal
► Thrombolytic therapy, thrombectomy, retransplantation

Further Reading

1. Shin DS, Padia SA, Kwan SW, et al. Catheter-directed thrombolysis for hepatic artery thrombosis following liver transplantation. *J Vasc Intervent Radiol.* 2014; 25(3, Supplement): S124.
2. Crossin JD, Muradali D, Wilson SR. US of liver transplants: Normal and abnormal. *RadioGraphics.* 2003: 23; 1093–1114.

History

▶ 22-Year-old female 1 year status post liver transplant with elevated liver function tests (Figs. 186.1–186.3)

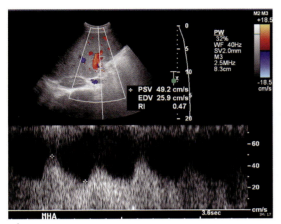

Fig. 186.1

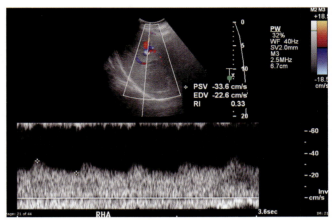

Fig. 186.2

Fig. 186.3

Case 186 Hepatic Artery Stenosis in a Liver Transplant

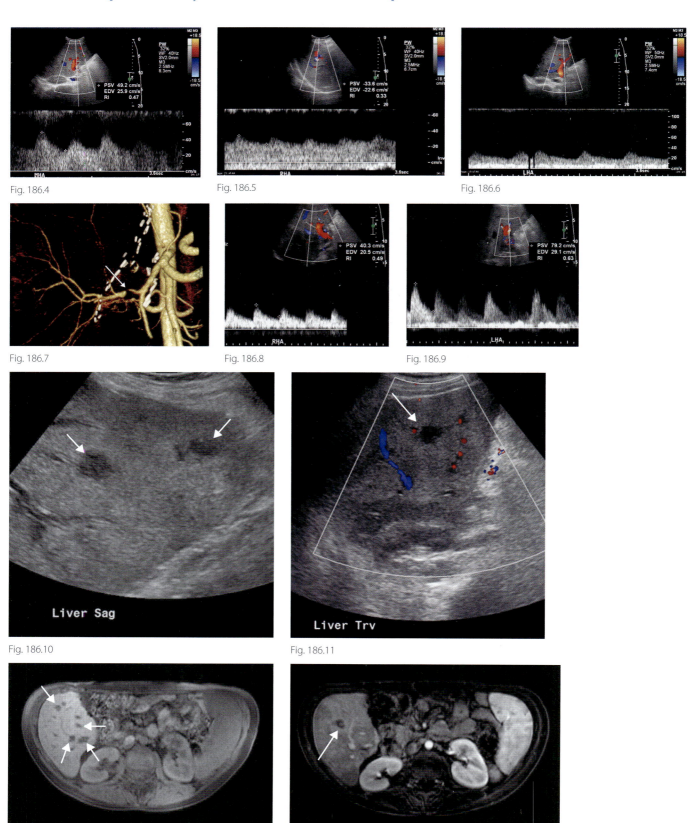

Fig. 186.4

Fig. 186.5

Fig. 186.6

Fig. 186.7

Fig. 186.8

Fig. 186.9

Fig. 186.10

Fig. 186.11

Fig. 186.12

Fig. 186.13

Imaging Findings

▶ Note tardus parvus spectral Doppler waveforms (delayed systolic acceleration with rounding of systolic peak) in the main (Fig. 186.4), right (Fig. 186.5), and left (Fig. 186.6) hepatic arteries suggestive of a proximal hepatic artery stenosis (HAS)

▶ Peak systolic velocity (PSV) in the main hepatic artery (HA) is 49.2 cm/s (Fig. 186.4). No focal area of increased PSV was found in the visualized main HA to confirm the diagnosis of HAS, likely because the anastomosis was more central and obscured by overlying bowel gas

▶ Three-dimensional volume-rendered image from a CT angiogram of the abdomen demonstrates a very high-grade focal stenosis of the proper HA at the surgical anastomosis (arrow in Fig. 186.7)

▶ Spectral Doppler waveforms obtained from the right (Fig. 186.8) and left (Fig. 186.9) hepatic arteries following balloon angioplasty of the main HA demonstrate resolution of the tardus parvus appearance with return of the normal sharp systolic upstroke and normal PSV

▶ Several days later, the patient presented with fever. Grayscale (Fig. 186.10) and color Doppler (Fig. 186.11) images demonstrated several new hypoechoic, avascular liver lesions (arrows) consistent with hepatic abscesses

▶ T1 fat-sat pre- and post-contrast-enhanced MR images (Figs. 186.12 and 186.13) confirm the presence of numerous low-signal ring-enhancing focal liver lesions (arrows), primarily in segment 5, most consistent with abscesses. These lesions resolved after several weeks of antibiotic therapy

Differential Diagnosis

▶ Celiac artery stenosis
▶ Aortic stenosis
▶ Hepatic artery thrombosis (HAT) with collateral flow
▶ Reperfusion injury

Teaching Points

▶ HAS is the second most common vascular complication post hepatic transplantation
  ▪ Estimated incidence of 5–11%
  ▪ More common in children
  ▪ Often occurs within 3 months of transplantation
▶ Etiology
  ▪ Scarring/fibrosis
  ▪ Acute rejection
  ▪ Injury to HA from surgical clamps or intra-arterial catheters
▶ Risk factors
  ▪ Difference in caliber of recipient and donor HA
  ▪ Small HA
  ▪ Prolonged cold ischemic time of donor liver
  ▪ ABO incompatibility
  ▪ Cytomegalovirus infection
▶ The biliary system in hepatic transplant recipients is perfused solely by the HA
▶ Consequently, patients with HAS may present with biliary ischemia and/or necrosis
▶ Clinical presentation
  ▪ Bile duct strictures, bile leaks, and bilomas
  ▪ Superinfection may lead to liver abscess and/or sepsis
  ▪ Hepatic infarcts
  ▪ May result in HAT with hepatic dysfunction and graft loss
▶ Doppler US is the first-line imaging study, and diagnostic criteria for HAS include the following
  ▪ PSV > 200–300 cm/s at the stenosis (anastomosis)
  ▪ Tardus parvus spectral Doppler waveforms distal to the stenosis (acceleration time ≥ 80 ms)
  ▪ Resistive index (RI) < 0.5
▶ Celiac artery stenosis or aortic stenosis
  ▪ Tardus parvus spectral Doppler arterial waveforms are indicative of a more proximal stenosis
  ▪ Hence, TP waveforms in the HAs may be observed in patients with celiac artery stenosis or aortic stenosis
  ▪ However, increased PSV in the main HA will not be noted
▶ Hepatic artery thrombosis
  ▪ Absence of arterial flow in the main and intraparenchymal HAs
  ▪ Although usually a surgical emergency, collateral arterial flow to the liver parenchyma will develop in some patients, most commonly in children
  ▪ TP waveforms are typically seen in the intraparenchymal HAs when reconstituted by collateral flow
  ▪ However, no flow will be noted in the main HA in the porta hepatis

- ▶ Reperfusion injury following hepatic transplantation
  - ▪ Increased diastolic flow (RI < 0.5–0.6) may be seen when vasodilatation occurs with reperfusion injury
  - ▪ ± Delay in systolic upstroke, simulating TP waveform
  - ▪ No increased PSV in main HA
  - ▪ Reperfusion injury typically resolves within 48 hours
  - ▪ Hence, TP waveforms in the HAs are much more specific for HAS or even impending HAT when observed > 48 hours post-transplantation

Management

- ▶ TP waveforms in the HAs > 48 hours post-transplantation should prompt further evaluation with contrast-enhanced US or CT/MR/ conventional angiography to exclude HAS, even if a focal increase in PSV in the main HA is not documented because visualization of a more central arterial anastomosis may be obscured by shadowing from overlying bowel gas
- ▶ Treatment of HAS: balloon angioplasty, surgical revision, and/or retransplantation

Acknowledgment

Figures 186.1, 186.2, 186.4, and 186.5 are reprinted with permission from Scoutt LM, Revzin MV, Thorisson H, Hamper UM. Ultrasound evaluation of the portal and hepatic veins. In: Zierler RE, Dawson DL, eds. *Strandness's Duplex Scanning in Vascular Disorders*, 5th ed. Philadelphia: Lippincott, Williams & Wilkins; 2015: Figures 22.43B and 22.43C.

Further Reading

1. Crossin JD, Muradali D, Wilson SR. US of liver transplants: Normal and abnormal. *RadioGraphics*. 2003; 23: 1093–1114.
2. McNaughton DA, Abu-Yousef MM. Doppler US of the liver made simple. *RadioGraphics*. 2011; 31: 161–188.
3. Bhargava P, Vaidya S, Dick AAS, et al. Imaging of orthotopic liver transplantation. *Am J Roentgenol*. 2011; 196: WS15–WS25.

History

▶ 46-Year-old liver transplant recipient presenting with abnormal liver function tests (Figs. 187.1–187.4)

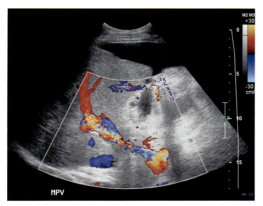

Fig. 187.1

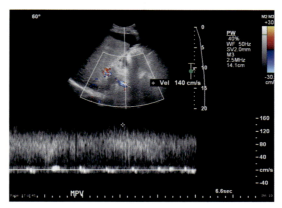

Fig. 187.2

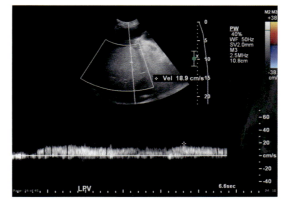

Fig. 187.3

Fig. 187.4

Case 187 Portal Vein Stenosis Status Post Liver Transplantation

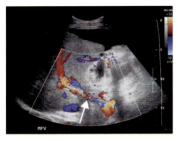

Fig. 187.5

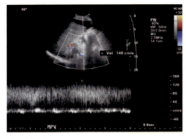

Fig. 187.6

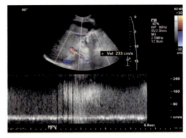

Fig. 187.7

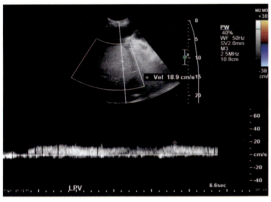

Fig. 187.8

Imaging Findings

▶ Narrowing of the main portal vein (MPV) (arrow in Fig. 187.5) at the anastomosis with focal color aliasing and post stenotic dilatation
▶ The velocity in the MPV is 233 cm/s in the narrowed segment (Fig. 187.7), significantly higher than in the proximal segment (140 cm/s in Fig. 187.6)
▶ Velocity in the left portal vein is normal (18.9 cm/s in Fig. 187.8) with normal respiratory variation

Differential Diagnosis

▶ Donor–recipient vessel size mismatch
▶ Portal venous fistula

Teaching Points

▶ Incidence of portal vein stenosis is approximately 1% after liver transplantation
  ▪ More common following pediatric and living donor liver transplants
▶ Risk factors
  ▪ Small vessel size
  ▪ Intraoperative portal vein (PV) reconstruction
  ▪ Prior PV surgery or PV thrombosis
  ▪ Misalignment of vessels
  ▪ Faulty surgical technique
  ▪ Excessive vessel length
▶ Clinical presentation
  ▪ Asymptomatic
  ▪ Abnormal liver function tests
  ▪ Portal hypertension with gastrointestinal bleeding, splenomegaly, and/or PV thrombosis/occlusion
▶ US findings
  ▪ Diagnostic US criteria somewhat controversial
  ▪ Narrowing of PV lumen, especially over a long segment

- Diameter of PV at stenosis < 50% of diameter of prestenotic segment
  - Lumen < 2.5 mm
  - Post-stenotic dilatation
  - Focal color aliasing
  - PV velocity > 125–155 cm/s
  - 2.5- to 3-fold increased PV velocity compared to prestenotic segment
  - Increase in velocity > 60 cm/s at the site of stenosis
- Donor and recipient MPV size mismatch
  - Abrupt change in caliber of MPV over a short segment
  - If donor MPV is smaller than recipient MPV, may be associated with increased velocity and color aliasing
  - Best seen on grayscale imaging
  - Long segment of narrowing and post-stenotic dilatation favors portal vein stenosis
  - Correlate with operative findings
  - Present on immediate postoperative baseline examination
- Hepatic artery (HA) to PV fistula
  - Increased PV velocity with color aliasing, likely pulsatile
  - No narrowing
  - Increased systolic and diastolic flow in the HA

Management

- CT or MR angiography with three-dimensional reconstruction can confirm focal narrowing of the PV
- Treatment: percutaneous transhepatic balloon angioplasty or surgical revision if symptomatic

Further Reading

1. Huang TL, Cheng YF, Chen TY, et al. Doppler ultrasound of postoperative portal vein stenosis in adult living donor transplantation. *Transplant Proc.* 2010; 42: 879–881.
2. Caiado A, Blasbalg R, Marcelino AS, et al. Complications of liver transplantation: Multimodality imaging approach. *RadioGraphics.* 2007; 27: 1401–1417.

Index

Figures are indicted by *f* and tables by *t*.

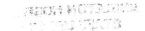

Pelvic inflammatory disease
    appendicitis and, 249
    endometritis with RPOC and, 49
    peritoneal inclusion cyst and, 40
    tubal ectopic pregnancy and, 100
    tubo-ovarian abscesses and, 7
Pelvic kidney, crossed fused renal ectopia and, 261, 262
Pelvic lymphadenopathy, Krukenberg tumors and, 18
Pena-Shokeir syndrome (pseudo-trisomy 18), trisomy 18 and, 213, 214
Penile implant, Peyronie disease and, 427
Pentalogy of Cantrell, omphalocele and, 176
Pentoxifyline, for Peyronie disease, 427
Perforated appendix
    pelvic abscess from, tubo-ovarian abscesses and, 8
    tubo-ovarian abscesses and, 7
Pericardial cyst, congenital diaphragmatic hernia and, 181, 182
Pericardial tamponade, for aortic dissection, 550
Perigestational hemorrhage (PGH), 82f, 83–84, 83f
Perinephric abscess
    diffuse large B-cell lymphoma and, 373, 375
    perinephric hematoma after renal biopsy and, 266
Peripheral artery disease (PAD), 562, 563–65, 563f
    portal venous gas and, 614
Peripheral vascular disease, emphysematous cholecystitis and, 300
Periportal lymphadenopathy, cholangiocarcinoma and, 313
Peritoneal carcinomatosis, from malignant melanoma, 332f, 333f, 334–36, 334f, 335f
Peritoneal inclusion cyst, 39f, 40–41, 40f, 41f
    hydrosalpinx and, 4, 5
Peritoneal tuberculosis, peritoneal carcinomatosis from malignant melanoma and, 334, 336
Peritonitis
    chemical, dermoid cyst and, 38
    chronic bacterial, peritoneal carcinomatosis from malignant melanoma and, 334
    meconium, 222
PET. See Positron emission tomography
Peyronie disease, 426f, 427, 427f
PGH. See Perigestational hemorrhage
Pheochromocytoma, 343
    adrenal myelolipoma and, 347, 348
Physiologic gut herniation, 95f, 96–97, 96f
Physiologic hydronephrosis of pregnancy, UVJ calculus and, 382
Physiologic implantation hemorrhage in uterus, incomplete pregnancy and, 114
Placenta accreta, 131
Placenta increta, 131
Placental abruption, 134f, 135–37, 135f, 136f
    hydranencephaly and, 139
    TTS and, 220
Placental tumors, 135
Placenta percreta, 130f, 131–33, 131f, 132f
Placenta previa, 131, 132, 133
Plantaris tendon rupture, 485f, 486–87, 486f
    gastrocnemius muscle tear and, 489, 490

Pleural effusions
    OHSS with heterotopic pregnancies and, 108
    pedunculated subserosal leiomyoma and, 64
    TIPS stenosis and, 618
PMB. See Postmenopausal bleeding
Pneumaturia, emphysematous cystitis and, 395
Pneumobilia, portal venous gas and, 611, 613
Polycystic kidneys. See also Autosomal dominant polycystic kidney disease; Autosomal recessive polycystic kidney disease
    trisomy 13 and, 216
Polycystic ovarian disease (PCOS)
    EH and, 60
    endometrial cancer and, 25
    OHSS with heterotopic pregnancies and, 107, 108
    ovarian torsion and, 46, 47
Polycythemia, RCC and, 369
Polydactyly, ARPKD and, 198
Polyhydramnios
    Beckwith-Wiedemann syndrome and, 206
    esophageal atresia and, 184, 185
    hydranencephaly and, 140
    meconium pseudocyst and, 222, 223
    TTS and, 219, 220
Polyorchidism, adenomatoid tumor of epididymis and, 424
Polyps
    cervical, 75
    endocervical, 74
    endometrial, 56f, 57–58, 57f, 58f
        EH and, 60
        endometrial cancer and, 25, 26
    gallbladder
        adenomyomatosis and, 241
        tumefactive sludge in gallbladder and, 291, 292
Polytetrafluorethylene (PTFE), 618
Polyvinyl chloride, cholangiocarcinoma and, 313
Popliteal artery (PA)
    insufficiency, 554f, 555–56, 555f
    TP waveforms and, 558, 558f
Popliteal artery aneurysm (PAA)
    Baker cyst and, 429, 430
    soft tissue mass and, 492, 493
    thrombosis of, 551f, 552–53, 552f
Popliteal cyst. See Baker cyst
Porcelain gallbladder, 302f, 303–4, 303f, 304f
    adenomyomatosis and, 241, 242
    emphysematous cholecystitis and, 300
    gallbladder adenocarcinoma and, 307
Portal hypertension
    Caroli disease and, 244
    gallbladder wall thickening and, 238
    portal vein stenosis and liver transplantation and, 648
    PVT and, 608
Portal vein, 617
    fistula, 648
    stenosis, liver transplantation and, 647f, 648–49, 648f

Urinary tract infection
emphysematous cystitis and, 393*f*
staghorn calculus and, 356
urothelial carcinoma of ureter and, 390
Urothelial carcinoma
pyonephrosis and, 378
UPJ calculus and, 384
of ureter, 389*f*, 390–91, 390*f*
of urinary bladder, 386*f*, 387–88, 387*f*, 388*f*
Uterine artery angiogram, for myometrial arteriovenous fistula, 28
Uterine artery embolization, for lipoleiomyoma, 23
Uterine fibroid embolization (UFE), for pedunculated subserosal leiomyoma, 66
Uterine leiomyomas, placental abruption and, 136
Uterine serositis, tubo-ovarian abscesses and, 7
Uterine/visceral perforation, misplaced IUD and, 52
Uterovesical junction (UVJ)
calculus, 381*f*, 382–85, 382*f*, 383*f*, 384*f*
urothelial carcinoma of urinary bladder and, 388
Uterus
adenomyosis of, 19*f*–20*f*
physiologic implantation hemorrhage in, incomplete pregnancy and, 114
septate, 67*f*, 68–71, 68*f*, 69*f*, 70*f*
interstitial ectopic pregnancy and, 104
UVJ. *See* Uterovesical junction

VA. *See* Vertebral artery
VACTERL. *See* Vertebral, anal atresia, cardiac, tracheoesophageal fistula, renal, limb
Vaginal bleeding
with cervical cancer, 72*f*, 74
with cervical incompetence with hourglass membranes, 123*f*
with EH, 59*f*
with endometrial cancer, 24*t*, 25
with endometrial polyp, 56*f*
with endometritis with RPOC, 48*f*, 49
with incomplete pregnancy, 112*f*
with molar gestation with IUP, 116
with myometrial arteriovenous fistula, 27*f*, 28
with PGH, 82*f*
placental abruption and, 136
with pregnancy in C-section scar, 109*f*, 111
with tubal ectopic pregnancy, 98*f*, 100
Vaginal spotting
with anembryonic gestation, 85*f*
EH and, 60
with misplaced IUD, 51*f*
Varices, congenital AVM and, 605, 606
Vasculitis
chronic mesenteric ischemia and, 589, 590
SMA dissection and, 586, 587
Vasospasm, HAT and liver transplantation and, 642

VCUG. *See* Voiding cystourethrogram
Vein of Galen malformation, 145*f*, 146–47, 146*f*, 147*f*
Venogram
for DVT, 505*f*, 506
for hemodialysis fistula failure, 578, 578*f*
Veno-occlusive disease, gallbladder wall thickening and, 238
Ventricular septal defect
aortic coarctation and, 601
TGA and, 171
Ventriculomegaly
DWM and, 149
TR and, 503
trisomy 13 and, 217
Verapamil, for Peyronie disease, 427
Vertebral, anal atresia, cardiac, tracheoesophageal fistula, renal, limb (VACTERL), esophageal atresia and, 185, 186
Vertebral artery (VA)
pre-steal waveform in, 530*f*, 531–33, 531*f*, 532, 533*f*
TP waveforms in, 520*f*, 521–22, 521*f*
Vesicoureteral reflex, MCDK and, 191
Visceromegaly, Beckwith-Wiedemann syndrome and, 207
Voiding cystourethrogram (VCUG), for PUVs, 201
Von Hippel-Lindau syndrome
RCC and, 369
renal angiomyolipoma and, 255
Von Meyenburg complexes. *See* Biliary hamartomas

WES sign, emphysematous cholecystitis and, 300
Whirlpool sign, with ovarian torsion, 46
Williams syndrome, aortic coarctation with TP waveforms and, 600
Wilms tumor
Beckwith-Wiedemann syndrome and, 207
horseshoe kidney and, 258
Wilson disease, medullary nephrocalcinosis and, 269

Xanthogranulomatous pyelonephritis (XGP)
for staghorn calculus, 359
staghorn calculus and, 356, 357

Yin-yang appearance
AAA and, 537
AVF and, 576
in kidney transplantation, 635
CFA PSA and, 570, 572
myometrial arteriovenous fistula and, 28
PSA in kidney transplantation and, 637, 638, 639
Yolk sac
interstitial ectopic pregnancy and, 103
IUP and, 80, 81
OHSS with heterotopic pregnancies and, 107
PGH and, 83, 84
tubal ectopic pregnancy and, 99